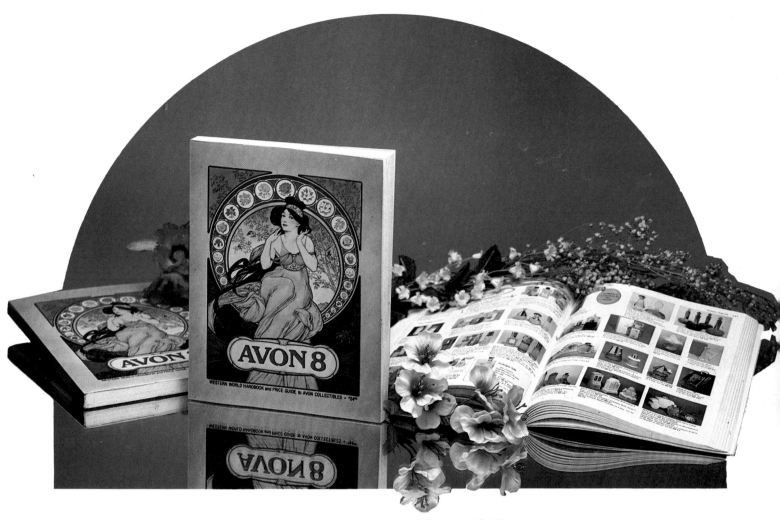

Western World
Handbook and Price Guide
to Avon Collectibles

Produced by Western World Publishing
and the
Western World Avon Collectors Club

Printed in the United States of America
by Western World Publishing
Pleasant Hill, California U.S.A.

ISSN 0192-4060   •   ISBN 0-931864-08-9
©1985 Western World Publishing

from the
PUBLISHER'S DESK

In 1968 an article on Avon collecting appeared in the Western Collector, a magazine then published by Western World. From that article, penned from his Den of Antiquity in Clayton, New Jersey, Jack Wiseburn made the hobby of collecting Avon known to the world.

Nearly 17 years have passed. During that time seven Western World Avon collecting books have been published, each increasing in size, content and usability to the collecting community. Now, the latest and largest of that famed series, Avon-8, presents more than 13,000 items pictured in full color, described and priced to reflect today's economy.

Our Senior Editors, *Doyle Darch* and *Dorothy Bernard* have teamed with Art Director *Sylvia McCann* and Final Layout Artist *Floyd Busby*, to produce this extraordinary book on Avon collecting.

As with all of the Western World Handbooks and Price Guides to Avon Collectibles, the Market Price **(MP)** represents the median price from all sections of the country. The Original Price is the Avon Company's first issued price, and later prices may vary.

As the new publisher of the Western World books, I would especially like to thank *Joe Weiss*, the originator and former publisher of this splendid series of Avon books, for his help and guidance.

Special gratitude is due my wife, *Ellen*, for her dedication and hard work in making Avon-8 a reality.

Our sincere gratitude is expressed to the many contributors, many of whom allowed us to photograph portions of their prized collections to grace the pages of Avon-8. There are too many to list, but special mention and thanks to (in alphabetical order):

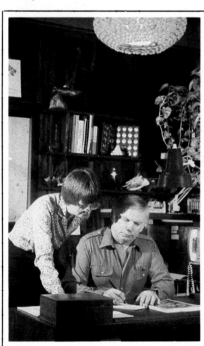

Don & Netta Bryant	Dick & Beverly Pardini
Doyle & Jeanne Darch	Ray Potter
Shirley Fairbanks	Betty Roddy
Ron & Pat Federico	Bob & Dorothy Rudolph
George Gaspar	Clyde & Darlene Sisson
Jerry Graham	Jenny Stanley
Garnet & Bud Harter	Mike & Linda Stone
Bud & Roz Hoover	Leonard Talys
Joe Kunch	Maynard Watson
Nick & Marci LaToof	Jean Williams
Ray & Ralphie Lintz	Lilliebelle Willsey
Ozie & Cynthia Nicholas	

In addition, we must also thank Carolyn Schlaefer, Sherry Sheppard, Dede Smith, Gloria Johnson, Keri Martinez and Angela Gregory for their contributions..
... And a very special thanks to Margit Bernhus, to whom this book is dedicated with love.

Floyd P. Busby
Western World Avon Collectors Club

Table of CONTENTS

the AVON Story

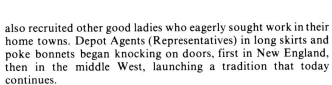

By Dorothy Bernard

The concept that built a company from a tiny one-man operation to a cosmetic giant can be credited to its founder, David Hall McConnell. That company was the California Perfume Company, later to be known as the Avon Company.

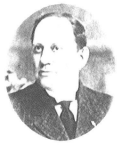

Mr. David H. McConnell

The Avon story begins in the 1880's when a New York book salesman, Mr. D.H. McConnell, developed a sales aid his woman customers liked very much — that was to present each of them an inexpensive little bottle of perfume. When Mr. McConnell determined that the perfumes he offered were often more in demand than his books, he decided to manufacture and sell perfumes direct to consumers in their homes. A Perfume Set, he decided, would be the perfect product to start with.

Mr. McConnell had great courage, but almost no capital when he started his perfume business in June of 1886. A small 20 x 26 foot room at 126 Chambers Street in New York City had to suffice for the manufacturing, shipping and office work necessary to market the "Little Dot" Perfume Set. He had one stenographer in his employ and he himself filled the position of bookkeeper, cashier, correspondent, shipping clerk, office boy and manufacturing chemist.

The name on the door read "California Perfume Company" — a name suggesting the perfume-filled air of a far-away state with its sunshine and its flowers.

At first, only five fragrances were manufactured — *Violet, White Rose, Heliotrope, Lily of the Valley* and *Hyacinth.* These were the natural perfume of the flower, made the natural way with the process used by the large French perfumers.

When the quality level of his perfumes was realized, David McConnell found that he needed help in distributing them.

In his book-selling days, Mr. McConnell had gone into homes in all parts of the country and had been touched by the struggle so many women were having to "make ends meet." In those days, women with homes and children to care for had little or no chance to earn the extra money so many of them needed for the comfort of their families.

He believed with all his heart in the direct-selling method of offering needed products to customers in their own homes. He had proved by his own experience that this was a satisfying and stimulating way of earning money. Convinced that it would be a dignified and pleasant way for women to earn, he resolved to employ women to sell his perfumes door-to-door. This was a truly radical concept in 1886. In those days everyone knew a woman's place was in the home answering doors, not knocking on them.

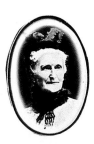

Mrs. P.F.E. Albee

At about the time that noted Lady from France first raised her torch over New York Harbor, another lady carried the first sample case of CPC perfumes. Her name was Mrs. Persus Foster Eames Albee (pronounced All-bee), a 50 year old widow from Winchester, New Hampshire, who needed money to support her children.

Mrs. Albee, the only General Agent (now called District Manager), traveled a large territory by train and by horse drawn wagon selling the perfumes to the women of several northeastern states. During this period she also recruited other good ladies who eagerly sought work in their home towns. Depot Agents (Representatives) in long skirts and poke bonnets began knocking on doors, first in New England, then in the middle West, launching a tradition that today continues.

This method of direct selling has been of great advantage to generations of Avon women and their families. Since this system was put into practical operation by Mrs. Albee, she has been given the title of "Mother of the California Perfume Company."

If you'd told Mrs. Albee that she was a "business pioneer" and that women the world over would follow in her footsteps for scores of years to come, she'd probably never have believed you.

But that's just what happened.

Mr. McConnell soon found it necessary to increase his perfume fragrances and, as business grew, additional items were added to the line. Among the first were *Shampoo Cream, Witch Hazel Cream, Hair Tonic, Bay Rum, Lait Virginal (a milky bath), Bandoline (to keep waves in a woman's hair), Face Powder, Shaving Soap* and *Baby Powder.* Soon after, Extracts and many other household products were manufactured and sold.

From the very beginning the quality products were sold with a *"money back guarantee."* This was a most unusual policy in those days.

Here is a chronological review of some of the highlights in the *Avon Company's* growth and progress.

1886 The *California Perfume Company* was started in one small room in a six floor building below Union Square in New York City.

1888 Business had grown to occupy an entire floor. *Violet Water* and *Violet Almond Meal,* a powdered toilet soap, were added to the line.

1894 The entire six floors of the building were used for manufacturing. Construction of a new laboratory was started in Suffern, 30 miles north of New York City.

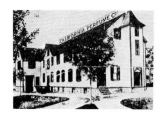

1895 A *Branch* distribution office was opened in Luzerne, Pennsylvania. It was phased out in 1934.

1896 As his efforts and hard work won their way to the front, the manufacturing end of the company grew out of David McConnell's hands. He secured the services of Adolph Goetting, a man who had been in the perfume business for 25 years and had the reputation for making the finest perfumes in the American market. In order to secure his services he was obliged to buy out his business and close up his laboratory. The Suffern Laboratory was enlarged and additional *Branch* offices were opened in Davenport, Iowa and Dallas, Texas. The first catalog, consisting of text only, was issued on November 2, 1896.

1898 A fourth *Branch* office was opened at 504 Mission Street in San Francisco, California. It was destroyed by the 1906 earthquake and fire, but immediately reopened at 16th and Landers Streets in San Francisco.

1899 A second addition to the Suffern Laboratory was a brick building, doubling the size of the existing one.

1903 A Kansas City, Missouri Branch was opened, eliminating the need for the outgrown Branches in Iowa and Texas. There were 48 General Agents and over 10,000 Depot Agents. *The Great Oak,* a brief history of the California Perfume Company by David McConnell, was printed and in 1945 it was reprinted and distributed to Avon employees and Representatives.

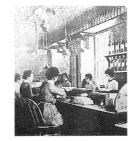

From a 1902 Catalog.....

1905 Representatives were introduced to their own magazine, the *Outlook.* It was published continuously until 1974 when the *Avon Calling* publication took its place. The *Catalogs,* at that time, dscribed 117 different products — among them two types of rouge, liquid and cake. In those days women used rouge, but in secret.

1906 The first CPC advertisement was seen in *Good Housekeeping* Magazine and featured Roses Perfume.

1909 The Home Office moved from Chambers Street to larger quarters at 31 Park Place in New York City.

1913 The *CPC Depot Agent,* an independent business woman, could earn bonus awards. One of the first prizes was a *Fireless Cookstove* that cooked by the heat of stone slabs and boasted a thick aluminum lining.

1914 The first International Branch and Laboratory opened in Montreal, Canada.

1915 The California Perfume Company had a large line of products and, according to the standards of beauty at that time, it was very handsome. Flowers, cupids, bows and lace were litho-graphed on package wrappers and perfume bottles were tied with ribbons. When plans for the 1914-1915 Panama Pacific Exposition in San Francisco were formulated, the Company was invited to exhibit. This was a world's fair and prizes were given for the best articles exhibited in various classifications. The entire line of CPC perfumes, toilet articles and household products was entered in competition with similar products from every corner of the globe. To David McConnell's delight, his company was awarded the Gold Medal, both for *Quality of Products* and *Beauty of Packaging.* A facsimile of the Gold Medal was proudly shown on packages for several years afterward.

1916 On January 27th the California Perfume Company incorporated in the State of New York.

1921 Representatives had a wonderful new selling tool, the color-plate catalog, showing actual size photos of the products offered. It was a great step forward from the first method of "show and tell" when a Representative carried a suitcase full of products from home to home.

1922 The San Francisco Branch closed and joined Kansas City.

1925 The Suffern Laboratory had grown twenty times its original size and was servicing 25,000 Representatives.

1926 The Home Office moved from Park Place to larger quarters at 114 Fifth Avenue located near Union Square in Greenwich Village.

1928 As distribution spread into almost all of the 48 States, the name California Perfume Company seemed too regional for such a far-reaching Company. A line of new products called *Avon* was introduced and included a toothbrush, a cleaner and a talc.

1929 It was decided that a complete new line of *Beauty* and *Household* products be introduced. Because an entirely new line should look the part, artists and designers were called in. A new trademark *"Avon"* with the *Ann Hathaway*

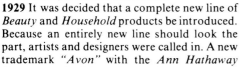

Cottage worked into the word was accepted. Blue, white and silver, olive and black were the colors chosen for the *Avon Line.* The *Household Line* was named *"Perfection"* and given its own trademark. The packages were dressed in orange, white and brown. By Christmastime everything was ready and the new line

was introduced to delighted Representatives and their customers.

1931 The first group of Avon Cosmetics was tested and approved by *Good Housekeeping.* As the Good Housekeeping Seals appeared on packaging, the Gold Medal facsimilies were dropped. By 1936 Good Housekeeping completed their tests and approved *all* Avon and Perfection products that came within their scope.

1932 Three week campaigns replaced 4-week campaigns and less-than-regular price *Specials* were introduced.

1936 Management felt that something more could be done to make the Avon Products even more desirable. Because their quality could not be improved, it was decided to modernize the packages by redesigning them. The word *"Avon"* for the trade-mark was retained, but the design was changed to the "A" with the flower underneath. The color scheme of the packages and labels were changed entirely. Avon cosmetics were dressed in turquoise, gold and white. Toiletries were dressed in green and white. The men's line was changed to maroon and cream. In October 1936 Representatives received news of the impending changes in the form of a fold-out Broadside, illustrating Avon Gift Sets in their "new dress." In November 1936 shipping of products in their newly designed jars, bottles, tubes and boxes started and the changeover was entirely completed at the end of Summer 1937. *Avon Products, Inc.* became a wholly owned subsidiary and Distributor of the CPC.

1937 The name *California Perfume Company* no longer appeared. Labels read *Avon Products, Distributor.* The Home Office moved to 30 Rockefeller Plaza in New York. David McConnell dies at age 79 and David McConnell, Jr. becomes Avon's second president.

1939 A third distribution center opened in Los Angeles.

1941 After 9 additions to the original building, the Suffern Laboratory is torn down to make way for larger, more up-to-date buildings.

1942 During World War II much of Suffern's assembly line work was devoted to the Armed Forces. Because of the many restrictions on packaging, it is sometimes difficult to accurately date some of the items issued during the war years. Many substitutions in packaging were made without prior notice. Plastic bottle closures replaced metal ones and many products were temporarily discontinued. Lipsticks were stripped of their pretty metal cases and were enclosed in heavy cardboard or plastic cases. Representatives were required to obtain an empty tube for every full Shaving Cream or Toothpaste tube sold.

1944 Space became so crowded at the Suffern Laboratory that the Lipstick and Rouge Division was moved to nearby Middletown, N.Y. and assumed the name of *Allied Products.*

1946 Gone were World War II restrictions on packaging. Once again lipsticks were available in metal containers and new products and packaging began to appear. On March 21st the CPC name was legally changed to *Avon Allied Products, Inc.* and *Allied Products, Inc. Avon Products, Inc.* remained a wholly-owned subsidiary and continued to use the word *Distributor* on labels.

1947 The opening of a new laboratory in Pasadena, California marked the last year *Montreal* appeared on labels. Labels were changed to read *New York-Pasadena.* Branch offices opened at the Merchandise Mart in Chicago.

1950 On December 31st Allied Products and Avon Allied Products, Inc. merged and assumed the name *Avon Products, Inc.* The word *Distributor* was dropped from the label and in 1951 labels read *Avon Products, Inc., New York-Pasadena.* Today, the word *Distributor* only appears on labels when the product is made by an outside vendor. A few are *Candles, Room Fresheners* and *Decrative Gifts.*

1954 Avon took its first step off the North American continent by establishing operations in Pureto Rico and Venezuela.

1955 *Sales Brochures* were introduced to support the campaign selling effort.

1968 A new marketing concept took place. Representatives in the west and some mid-western states began calling on customers every two weeks. After the new two-week program proved successful, other Divisions joined the plan. The eastern states completed the conversion in March 1969.

6

The AVON Story

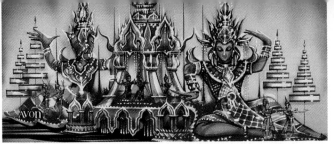

1971 Jewelry was introduced in the U.S. Avon is now the *largest distributor of costume jewelry in the world!*

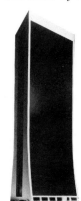

1972 Avon moved into new World Headquarters at 9 West 57th Street in New York.
1973 Avon welcomed a wholly-owned subsidiary — *Family Fashions by Avon,* a company selling wearing apparel by mail from Newport News, Virginia.
1979 In April *Tiffany & Co.,* noted jewelers, was joined to the Avon company. Sales topped *two billion dollars* for the year. *Roses to the Winners,* created as a tribute to women in sports, was the theme of Avon's first Pasadena Tournament of Roses Parade entry in 1979. The 1980 Parade entry was a tribute to *The World of Music* and featured Frank Sinatra. In 1981 the Avon entry, *Autumn Splendor,* was a Grand Prize winner. The 1982 Avon entry in the Rose Parade was titled *Beauty of the Orient.* Leslie Kin Kawai, the 1981 Rose Queen, appeared on the float — which was dedicated by Avon to the Representatives and Managers in Avon's Japanese market. The 1983 Avon New Year's Day entry was a floral presentation of Egyptian antiquity titled the *Dawn of Beauty.* For the third time in their five years of entry to the Rose Parade, Avon won a major prize for their float. They were awarded the Isabella Coleman Award, given for the Most Effective Presentation of Total Decoration. *Firebird* was the title of Avon's sixth entry into the world famous Pasadena Rose Parade. As a salute to the Arts, the 1984 *Firebird* float was named for the well known Stravinsky ballet score.

The **1985** Avon entry in the Rose Parade (shown above-right) was titled *"International Beauty",* saluting the rich diversity of American culture. A tribute to the contribution of Eastern countries to the American melting pot, the majestic float featured 14-foot-high replicas of graceful Thai dancers and Thai-American women. The striking float was awarded the *Directors Trophy* for Excellence of Craftsmanship, Overall Design and Floral Construction.

1982 Avon launched another corporate venture; the creation of *Great American Magazines, Inc.,* a direct mail magazine subscription business. Further diversification took place with the merger of **Mallinckrodt, Inc.,** manufacturers of health care products, specialty chemicals and flavors and fragrances.
1983 More expansion at Avon with the addition of *James River Traders,* a direct-mail line of men's fashionable clothing.
1984 *Ultra Fit Hosiery* was introduced in Campaign 1 and was the most successful new product introduction in the history of Avon, with sales of 7 million units. In Campaign 22 the hosiery name was changed to *Avon Style and Fit.*

From that humble beginning in 1886, the McConnell idea has grown into a multi-billion dollar business, affecting the lives of millions of people around the world. The company now offers about 700 different products and the number of Avon Representatives the world over totals one and a half million.

Like a story from the Arabian Nights — a tiny perfume business has grown into a giant corporation — a story that began with a single Perfume Set.......

That's the story of AVON

AVON COLLECTING

with Dorothy Bernard

Since 1969, when the first *Western World Handbook* was published, one of our great assets in determining prices has been readers who will quote specific prices for collectibles. It is, of course, the buyer and seller of Avon collectibles who determine the price. What a buyer is willing to pay for a collectible — and what a seller is willing to sell his collectible for — are the determining factors. With information gathered from all corners of the nation, our *Handbook and Price Guide* represents the national median in pricing.

Regular Price (shown preceding the **MP**) reflects Avon's price at original issue date. Later Avon prices may increase or decrease from the original issue price.

MP *(Market Price)* reflects empty containers, except for tubes, and where the product is an integral part of the container

— for example, soap dishes and Sunshine Rose Candle. **MP** does not include the box unless it is necessary to the collectible, such as in sets and boxed soaps.

MP followed by an asterisk (*) tells you that the item was still available from Avon at time of publication and the **MP** is the same as you would pay for the full, mint product at Avon's special pricing. Because of generally increasing prices, you will often find the **MP*** is the same amount, or more, than the original issue price.

If you are a new collector, you may find that *Western World Handbook* prices vary in relationship to current Market Prices. Even an expert cannot keep up with the changing values brought on by the discontinuance or re-introduction of Avon containers or just the effects of inflation. And we must all contend with the variations in value dependant on the condition of the item. Even though Market Prices at times seem puzzling, they give us a good overview of what's happening to the general price picture.

Mint, full and boxed items continue to be most in demand and draw the highest price. The *mint condition bottle* is empty, without flaked paint, cracks, or chips, has all labels, correct lid and all accessory parts.

Bottles with cracks, chips or missing labels are affected in value. A slight chip on a common bottle would reduce its value about 50%, on a rare bottle about 25%. Badly chipped, or bottles without labels, on the other hand, are very severely penalized — generally, about 75% for the rare bottle and 90% for the common one.

There's always a reason for occasional changes in Market Prices. For example, increased interest in collecting Perfection, paper items, older samples and demonstration aids have caused these items to increase greatly in value, as has appreciation of different packaging issued during wartime or a glass strike, containers issued for only a short time or special Christmas or Anniversary packaging.

Clubs and Chapters are an ideal place to make your Avon wants and needs known. And one of the primary functions of Western World has been to provide Club Members with a Market Place where buyers and sellers of collectibles can meet to Buy, Sell or Trade. The WWAC Newsletter offers you Free Ads and the opportunity to do your own Market Survey. Whether at your Club or in the Newsletter, Avon-8 and the Free Ads are a hard combination to beat!

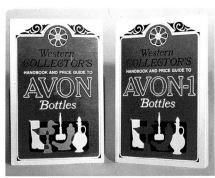

1969 Avon Handbook and **Avon-1**, *the reprinted edition. 96 pages, in black & white and color, with 84 items shown. Only 5,000 of the original edition were produced. Avon-1 was so popular, it was reprinted nine times! Original price $3.95.*

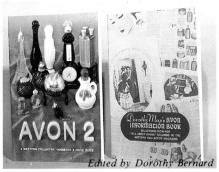

Edited by Dorothy Bernard

1971 Avon-2, *First of the all-color Western World Avon Collectors Books. 96 pages with hundreds more items. Original price $4.95* **1971 Dorothy May Bernard Information Book,** *a premium featuring our Senior Editor's columns from Western World's original magazine, the Western Collector.*

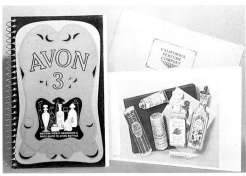

1973 Avon-3, *176 pages with some 2,000 Avon items was the first spiral bound book. Edited by Shirley Mae Onstot, famed Avon collector. Original price $9.95. The* **1917 CPC Catalog** *reproduction, never sold, a premium with purchase of Avon-3.*

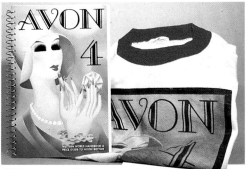

1975 Avon-4, *224 pages, all in full color, with over 3,000 Avon collectibles. Original price $12.95. The full-color* **Avon-4 T-Shirt** *was a premium with a purchase of Avon-4 at a 1975 National Avon Show and Sale. Original price $5.95 Edited by Dorothy Bernard.*

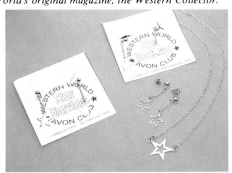

1976 Earrings and **Open Star Necklace** *in both gold and silver were created and distributed by Western World as a premium for the W'World Newsletter. Sold at $3.95 for the Earrings, and $9.95 for the Necklace. One year only, 1976.*

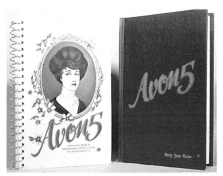

1977 Avon-5, *320 pages, all color, over 6,000 Avon collectibles shown. Spiral bound. Original price $14.95.* **Avon-5 Deluxe Edition,** *red cloth binding with owner's name imprinted in gold. Original price $21.95. Edited by Dorothy Bernard*

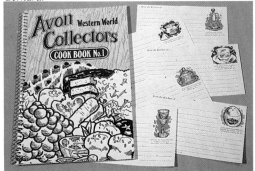

1978 Western World Cook Book No. 1. *96 pages with recipes from W'World Avon Club Members. Original price $4.95.* **1977 Recipe Cards,** *24 to the set featuring Avon collectibles on each card. Given as a premium or a gift. Original price $1.50 per set.*

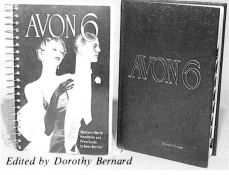

Edited by Dorothy Bernard

1979 Avon-6, *448 pages, all in full-color, with more than 9,000 Avon items cataloged. Original price $19.95. The* **Avon-6 Deluxe Edition,** *brown leather grain cover, tabbed index and satin marker. Original price $27.95. Sold by mail only.*

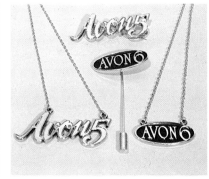

1977-1979 Avon-5 & Avon-6 Jewelry Premiums. *Given to bulk purchasers of Avon-4 and Avon-5 books in recognition of outstanding sales effort. Avon-5 jewelry available as Brooch or Necklace, Avon-6 jewelry as Stickpin or Necklace. Never sold.*

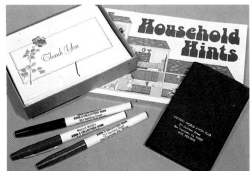

1975-77-79 Western World Merchandise Gifts *Felt pens with Avon-4 and Avon-5. Purse or pocket notebooks with Avon-4, -5 and -6. Thank You Notes and Household Hints book given with Avon-6 bulk purchases. Never sold.*

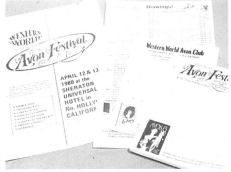

1979 and 1980 Western World Avon Collectors Festival *held at the Sheraton Universal Hotel in Universal City, California. Programs and Souvenir Scratch Pads shown. An Avon Plant Tour, Show & Sale, Dinner Banquet and Displays were featured.*

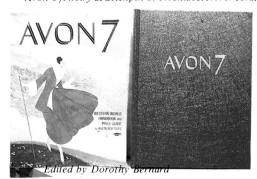

Edited by Dorothy Bernard

1981 Avon-7, *all color, in new, larger size. Sewn binding, over 12,000 Avon collectibles, 288 pages. Original price $22.95.* **Avon-7 Deluxe Edition** *with burgundy leather grain, padded cover, gilt edges, satin marker, gold stamped. Original price $29.95*

CPC DEPOT AGENT

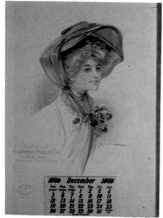

1909 *CPC Calendar, customer gift with purchase* **MP $200.**

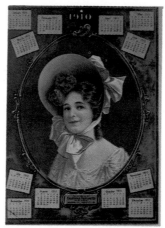

1910 *CPC Calendar, customer gift with purchase* **MP $200.**

In the 1800's Avon ladies were called Depot Agents. Managers were called Traveling Agents, and then General Agents. If a Depot Agent sold $250.00 worth of products she was offered the opportunity to become a General Agent. No easy task in those days when the most expensive item in the line was 40 cents.

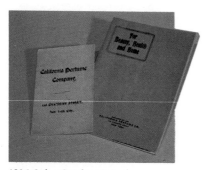

1896 *Sales Catalog, issued November 2nd, 30 pages, text only* **MP $400 to $500.**
1906 *Sales Catalog* **MP $400 to $500.**

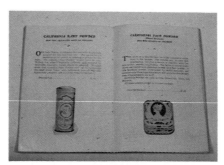

1906 *Sales Catalog (left) shown open*

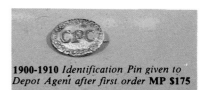

1900-1910 *Identification Pin given to Depot Agent after first order* **MP $175**

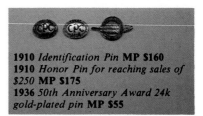

1910 *Identification Pin* **MP $160**
1910 *Honor Pin for reaching sales of $250* **MP $175**
1936 *50th Anniversary Award 24k gold-plated pin* **MP $55**

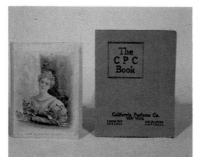

1898 *Second Sales Catalog, issued in November, 60 pages* **MP $400 to $500**
1917 *Smaller size of large Sales Catalog, text only, to leave with customers, 40 pages* **MP $300**

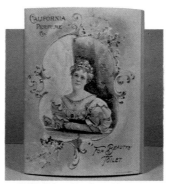

1900 *Sales Catalog, 64 pages* **MP $400 to $500**

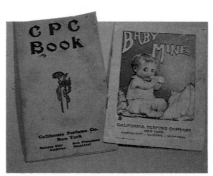

1914 *Sales Catalog* **MP $350**
1923 *Baby Booklet to record baby's development, given with baby product purchase* **MP $150**

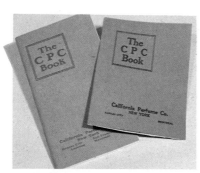

1915 *Sales Catalog* **MP $300**
1923 *Smaller size of large Sales Catalog, 32 pages* **MP $250**

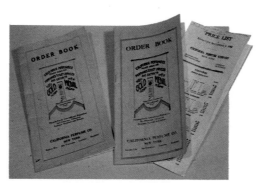

1916 *Order Book* **MP $55**
1922 *Order Book* **MP $60**

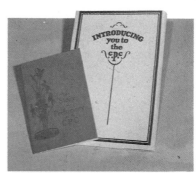

1916 *The Story of Perfumery and the CPC booklet* **MP $50**
1928 *Introducing You to the CPC booklet, 30 pages, given to new Representatives* **MP $30**

In the late 1800's Goetting & Co. Perfumes were distributed by CPC and only sold in stores. Hinze Ambrosia, Inc. was a wholly-owned subsidiary from 1902-1954.

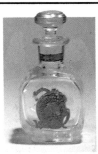

1898 *Goetting & Co. Perfume (sold only in stores)* **MP $200**

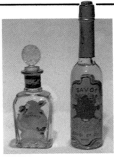

1898 *Goetting's Perfume* **MP $200**
1898 *Savoi Et Cie & Co. Florida Water 3½oz* **MP $225**

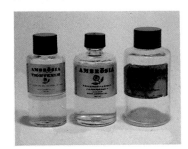

1900's *Ambrosia Skin Care bottles (Sold only in stores)* **MP $150 each**

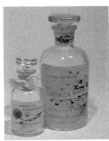

1961 *Reproductions of 1890 bottles for display in Branch Museums. Extract of Carnation* **MP $200,** *Florida Water* **MP $250**

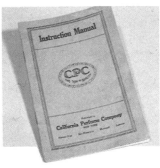

1921 *Representative's Instruction Manual 8"x5¼"* **MP $40**

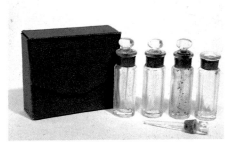

1920 *Perfume Demonstrator. American Ideal, Daphne, Roses, Trailing Arbutus* **MP $350 complete**

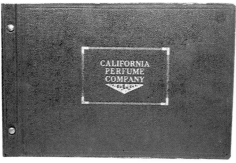

1915-20 *Sales Catalog* **MP $230 each complete catalog.**

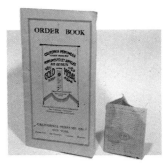

1923-25 *Order Book* **MP $30**
1926 *"One Minute Please" folder* **MP $10**

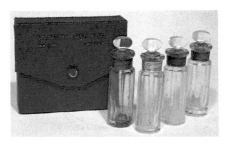

1924 *Perfume Demonstrator. Mission Garden, Vernafleur, Trailing Arbutus & Daphne shown* **MP $350 complete**

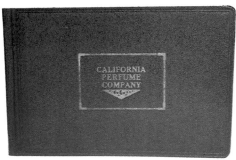

1920-22 *Sales Catalog (no screws in binding)* **MP $225 each**

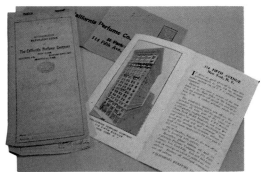

1926 *Order Book* **MP $30**
1926 *CPC envelope, Fifth Ave. replacing Park Pl. address* **MP $12 as shown**
1926 *Pamphlet regarding new Home Office address at 114 Fifth Ave.* **MP $32**

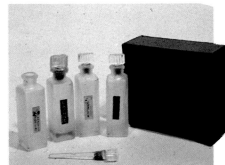

1928 *Perfume Demonstrator. Vernafleur, Trailing Arbutus, Daphne & Mission Garden shown* **MP $350 complete**
(See also pgs. 280-81 for Avon Fragrance Demonstrators)

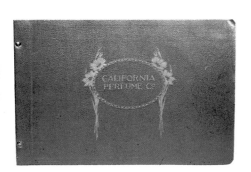

1922-29 *Sales Catalog* **MP $200 each complete catalog**

(See also pg. 285 for Avon catalogs)

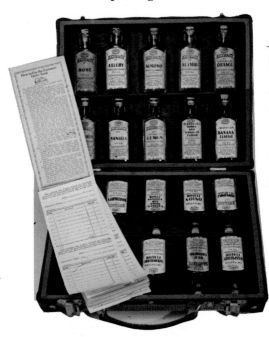

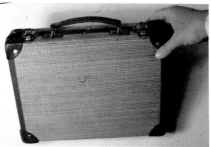

1912 Sales Manager's Demonstration Case. 20 food extracts & colorings **MP $2,000, $90 each bottle** *(shown closed above)*
1930 Order Book **MP $25**

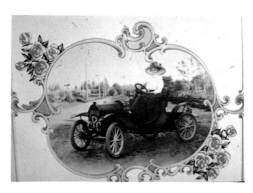

1911 Brush Runabout motor car, won by Effie Miller, Oregon Depot Agent for her fine sales record.

1913 Sales Manager's Demonstration Case, 14"x10"x4" **MP $200,** *Sales Manager's Contract* **MP $25** ⬇

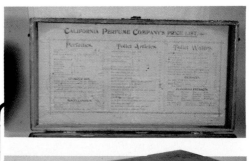

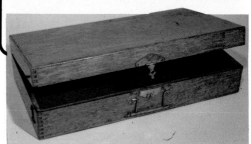

1897 Depot Agent's Demonstration Case holds variety of products **MP $250**

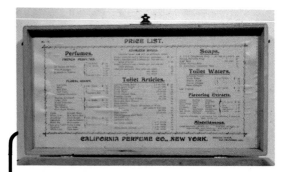

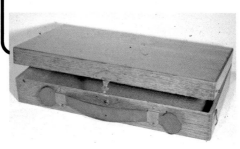

1900 Depot Agent's Demonstration Case **MP $225** *(price list on inner lid shown above)*

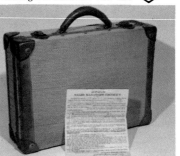

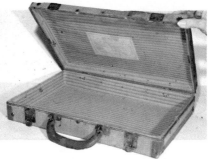

1915 Sales Manager's Demonstration Case, 17"x11"x4" **MP $200**

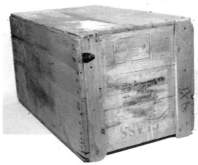

1919 CPC wooden Shipping Case, 27"x14½"x14" **MP $75**

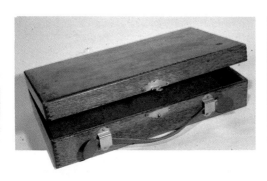

1900's Depot Agent's Demonstration Case **MP $200**

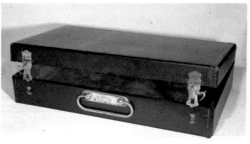

1920's Sales Manager's Demonstration Case **MP $175**

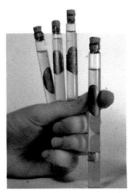

1890 *Perfumes, Oriental, Orange Blossom and two called Parfum, each 15¢* **MP $200 each**

CPC PERFUMERY

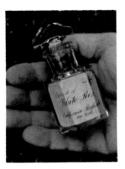

1893 *Extract of White Rose 1 oz 40¢* **MP $180**

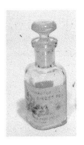

1902 *Extract of Sweet Pea Perfume 1 oz 40¢* **MP $175**

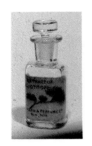

1908 *Extract of Heliotrope Perfume 1oz 50¢* **MP $160**

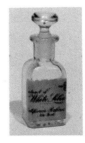

1900 *Extract of White Lilac Perfume 1 oz 40¢* **MP $175**

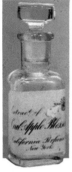

1900-1908 *Extract of Crab Apple Blossom Perfume 1 oz 50¢* **MP $175**

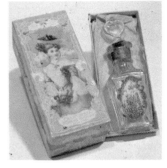

1908 *Perfume, in choice of fragrances 1oz 50¢* **MP $180, $230 boxed**

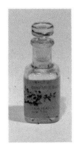

1908 *Extract of Crab Apple Blossom 1 oz 60¢* **MP $160**

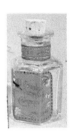

1909 *White Rose Perfume 50¢* **MP $155**

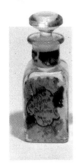

1910 *Perfume 1 oz 50¢* **MP $175**

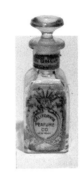

1915 *Rose Geranium Perfume 1 oz 50¢* **MP $155**

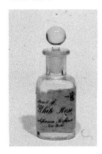

1905 *Extract of White Rose Perfume 1 oz 50¢* **MP $170**

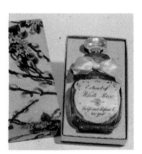

1908-1910 *Extract of White Rose Perfume 2oz 90¢* **MP $180, $230 boxed**

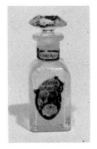

1915 *White Rose Perfume 1oz 50¢* **MP $155**

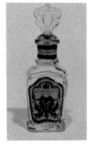

1912 *White Rose Perfume ½ oz. Sold in Gift Set* **MP $135**

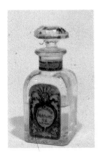

1916 *White Rose Perfume 2 oz 90¢* **MP $165**

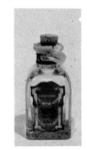

1918 *White Rose Perfume 2oz $1* **MP $160**

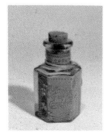

1908-1909 *New Mown Hay Perfume. Sold only in Atomizer Set.* **MP $160**

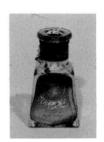

1910 *Lou Lillie Perfume 1 oz. Sold only in Atomizer Set.* **MP $160**

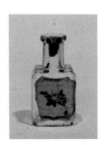

1906 *Rose Perfume. Sold only in Little Folks Set.* **MP $100**

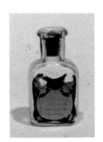

1914 *White Rose Perfume. Sold only in Little Folks Set.* **MP $80**

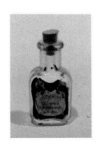

1914 *Heliotrope Perfume. Sold only in Little Folks Set.* **MP $80**

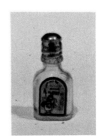

1923 *Heliotrope Perfume. Sold only in Little Folks Set.* **MP $75**

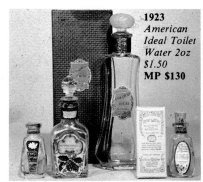

1923
*American
Ideal Toilet
Water 2oz
$1.50*
MP $130

1915 *Lotus Cream Sample* **MP $85**
1919 *Lily of The Valley Perfume 1 oz 50¢*
MP $130
1924 *Rose Water, Glycerine & Benzoin
Sample* **MP $75, $95 boxed**

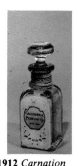

1912 *Carnation
Perfume 1 oz 50¢*
MP $150

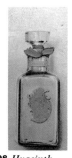

1908 *Hyacinth
Perfume 1 oz 50¢*
MP $175

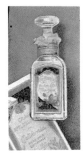

1917 *Crab Apple
Blossom Quadruple
Extract Perfume
½ oz 90¢* **MP $150,
$175 boxed**

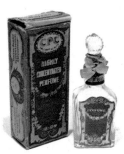

1918 *Concentrated Perfume
½ oz. Choice of 21
fragrances 50-75¢*
MP $140, $165 boxed

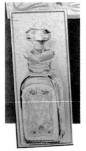

1916 *Carnation Triple
Extract Perfume 1 oz
50¢* **MP $150,
$175 boxed**

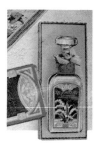

1915 *Lily of The Valley
Triple Extract Perfume
1 oz 90¢* **MP $155,
$175 boxed**

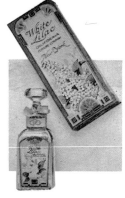

1915 *White Lilac Triple
Extract Perfume 1 oz 90¢*
MP $150, $175 boxed

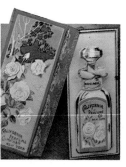

1915 *White Rose
Quadruple Extract
Perfume 1 oz $1.10*
MP $150, $175 boxed

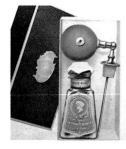

1910 *Perfume, in choice of
27 fragrances & Perfect
Atomizer 90¢ to $2.40*
MP $185, $215 boxed
*Perfect Atomizer, separate
40¢* **MP $30**

CPC PERFUMERY

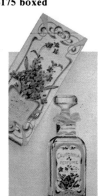

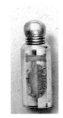

1909 *Musk
Perfume Atomizer
Bottle 1 oz*
MP $175

1914 *Heliotrope
Triple Extract
Perfume 1 oz 50¢*
**MP $145, $175
boxed**

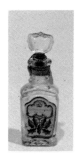

1914 *Carnation
Perfume ½ oz.
Sold only in
Box No. 2 Gift
Set* **MP $80**

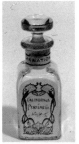

1910 *Carnation
Perfume 1 oz
50¢* **MP $160**

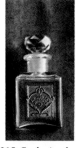

1915 *Crab Apple
Blossom or
Trailing Arbutus
Perfume 2 oz
embossed label
$2.25* **MP $180**

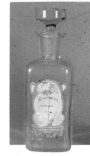

1915 *California
Bouquet Perfume 8 oz
$3.25* **MP $180**

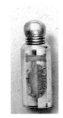

1908 *Traveler's
Bottle, 8 frag.
60¢* **MP $140**

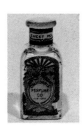

1916 *Sweet Pea
Perfume 1 oz 90¢*
MP $150

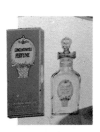

1923 *Concentrated
Perfume in 9 frag. ½ oz
Roses shown 59¢*
MP $115, $135 boxed

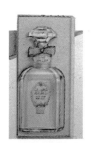

1923 *1 oz Perfume in 9
frag. Lily of The Valley
shown $1.17* **MP $125,
$150 boxed**

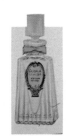

1925 *1 oz Perfume in
6 frag. Crab Apple
Blossom shown $1.17*
MP $120

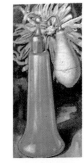

1928 *Perfume &
Atomizer $2.25*
MP $150

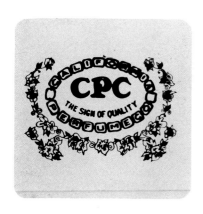

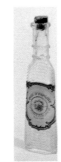

1902 Peau D'Espagne French Perfume, trial size 25¢ **MP $190**

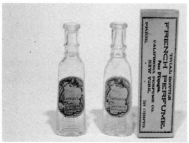

1917 Peau D'Espagne, trial size 50¢ **MP $145**
1915 Peau D'Espagne, trial size 25¢ **MP $155, $180 boxed**

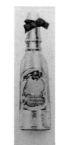

1917 Le Parfum des Roses, trial size 50¢ **MP $145**

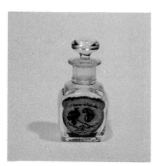

1905-1910 L'Odeur De Violette 2 oz $1.90 **MP $190**

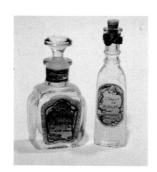

1910 L'Odeur De Violette 2 oz $1.90 **MP $170**
1915 L'Odeur De Violette, trial size 25¢ **MP $155**

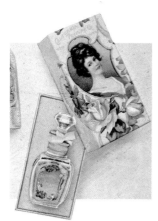

1917-1920 Le Parfum des Roses ½ oz $1 **MP $155, $180 boxed**

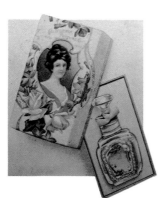

1917-1920 L'Odeur De Violette 1 oz $1.90 **MP $155, $180 boxed**

T O I L E T W A T E R

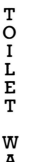

1902 California Eau de Cologne 2 oz 35¢ **MP $200**

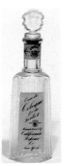

1906 White Rose Toilet Water 4 oz 65¢ **MP $180**

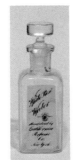

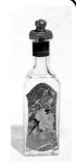

1910 White Rose Toilet Water 2 oz 35¢ **MP $160**

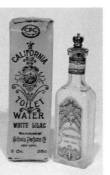

1915 White Lilac Toilet Water 2 oz 35¢ **MP $150, $175 boxed**

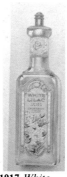

1917 White Lilac Toilet Water 2 oz 75¢ **MP $140**

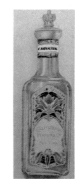

1917 Carnation Toilet Water 2 oz 75¢ **MP $140**

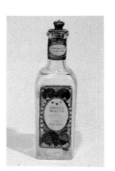

1914 Carnation Toilet Water 4 oz 65¢ **MP $150**

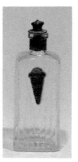

1926-1929 Crab Apple Blossom Toilet Water 4 oz $1.08 **MP $95**

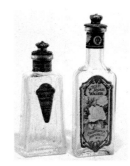

1926 White Rose Toilet Water 2 oz 59¢ **MP $95**
1917 White Rose Toilet Water 2 oz 75¢ **MP $140**

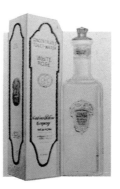

1923 White Rose Toilet Water 2 oz 59¢ **MP $105, $125 boxed**

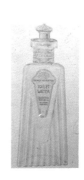

1926 Lily of the Valley Toilet Water 2 oz 59¢ **MP $95**

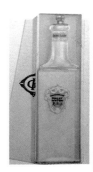

1923 Crab Apple Blossom Toilet Water 2 oz 59¢ **MP $105, $125 boxed**

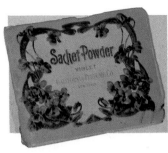
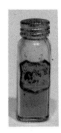
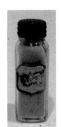

1908 *Sachet Powder Envelope. Violet (shown) White Rose, Heliotrope 25¢* **MP $50**

1902 *White Rose Sachet Powder 25¢* **MP $130**

1902 *Heliotrope Sachet Powder 25¢* **MP $130**

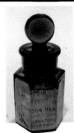

Lavender Salts

Lavender Salts was used for the relief of sick and nervous headaches, faintness, nausea, shortness of breath, dizziness, seasickness and many other every-day ills. The combination glass and rubber stopper prevented evaporation.

1888 *Lavender Salts 35¢* **MP $275**

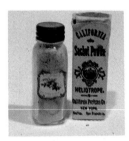
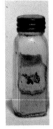
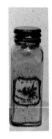
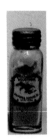

1908 *Heliotrope Sachet Powder 25¢* **MP $125, $150 boxed**

1908 *Rose Sachet Powder 25¢* **MP $125**

1910 *Rose Sachet Powder 25¢* **MP $125**

1910 *Heliotrope Sachet Powder 25¢* **MP $125**

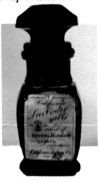
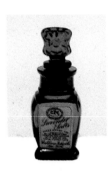

1893 *Lavender Salts 35¢* **MP $250**

1911 *Lavender Salts 35¢* **MP $225**

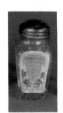
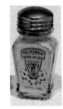
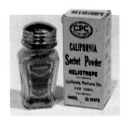

1915 *Carnation Sachet 25¢* **MP $95**

1915 *White Lilac Sachet 25¢* **MP $95**

1922 *Heliotrope Sachet 25¢* **MP $90, $115 boxed**

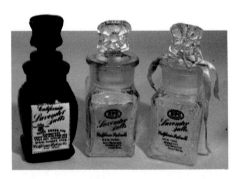

1906 *Lavender Salts, Label reads: "These Goods are guaranteed under the Pure Food & Drug Act June 30, 1906." 35¢* **MP $240**
1920 *Lavender Salts 50¢* **MP $130**
1917 *Lavender Salts 35¢* **MP $130**

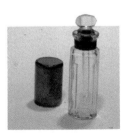
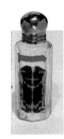
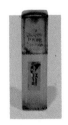

1923 *Perfume Flaconette ¼ oz 48¢* **MP $95**

1915 *Traveler's Bottle 1 oz 60¢* **MP $130** *(See 1908 Traveler's Bottle p. 12)*

1926 *Perfume Flaconette in 8 fragrances 1 oz 59¢* **MP $95**

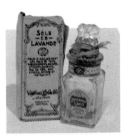
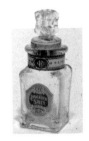

1923 *Lavender Salts 49¢* **MP $115, $140 boxed**

1925 *Lavender Salts 50¢* **MP $100**

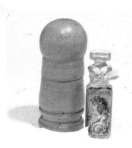

1912 *Perfume with wooden holder 60¢* **MP $225 complete, $135 Bottle only**

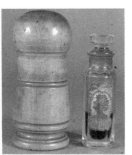

1910 *Perfume with wooden holder 60¢* **MP $225 complete, $135 Bottle only**

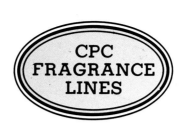

CPC FRAGRANCE LINES

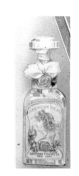

1914 *Perfume, intro size 60¢* **MP $140, $165 boxed**

1914 *Perfume 1 oz $2, 2 oz $3.75* **MP $140 each**

AMERICAN IDEAL

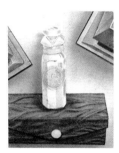

1917 *Perfume, intro size 75¢* **MP $135, $160 boxed**

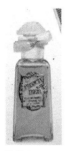

1917 *Perfume 1 oz $2.50* **MP $135**

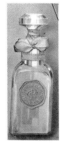

1923 *Perfume 2 oz $4.75* **MP $135**

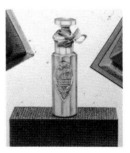

1923 *Perfume, intro size 75¢* **MP $125, $150 boxed**

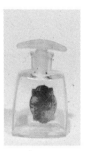

1925 *Perfume 1 oz $2.40* **MP $125**

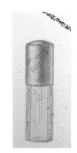

1928 *Perfume Flaconette $1.10* **MP $95**

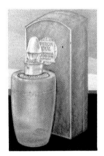

1928 *Perfume 1 oz $2.40* **MP $125, $150 boxed**

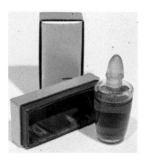

1930 *Perfume 1 oz $2.40* **MP $110, $135 boxed**

(See 1941 Perfume p. 46)

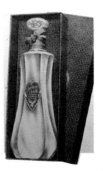

1923 *Toilet Water 2 oz $1.50* **MP $135, $160 boxed**

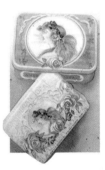

1914 *Toilet Soap 50¢* **MP $95, $60 Soap only**

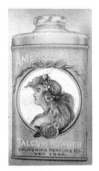

1914 *Talcum Powder 4 oz 35¢* **MP $85**

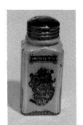

1907-08 *Powder Sachet 50¢* **MP $125**

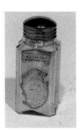

1908 *Powder Sachet 50¢* **MP $125**

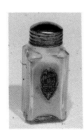

1918 *Powder Sachet 50¢* **MP $95**

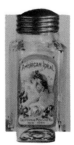

1914 *Powder Sachet 50¢* **MP $100**

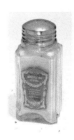

1920 *Powder Sachet $1.25* **MP $95**

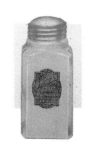

1923 *Sachet Powder $1.25* **MP $90**

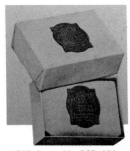

1919 *Soap 50¢* **MP $70**

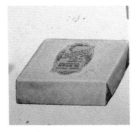

1923 *Soap 48¢* **MP $65**

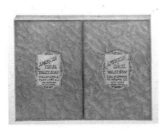

1926 *Boxed Toilet Soaps 96¢*
MP $80

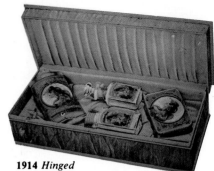

1914 *Hinged*
Box holds Talcum, 1 oz
Perfume, Sachet Powder and Soap $4
MP $500

.....AMERICAN IDEAL

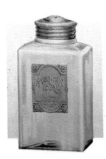

1918 *Talcum*
Powder 3½oz 75¢
MP $100

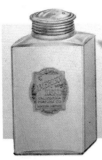

1923 *Talcum*
Powder 3½ oz 72¢
MP $95

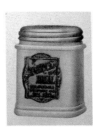

1918 *Cream Deluxe*
$1 **MP $60**

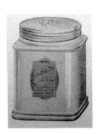

1923 *Cream Deluxe*
96¢ **MP $50**

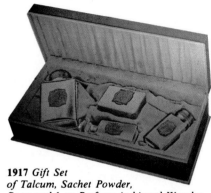

1917 *Gift Set*
of Talcum, Sachet Powder,
Soap and 1 oz Perfume in hinged Wooden
Box $5.50 **MP $400**

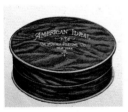

1915 *Face Powder,*
white or flesh colored
75¢ **MP $65**

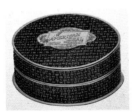

1923 *Face Powder 96¢*
MP $55

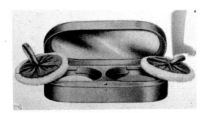

1920 *Double Compact, Face*
Powder or Rouge $1.50 **MP $60**

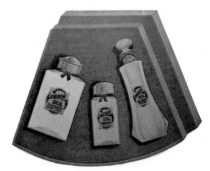

1923 *Threesome Set. Talcum, Sachet*
Powder and 2 oz Toilet Water $3.95
MP $335

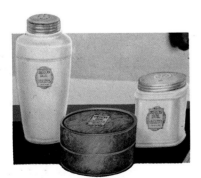

1928 *Talcum 76¢* **MP $75**
1928 *Face Powder $1* **MP $40**
1928 *Cream Deluxe $1* **MP $40**

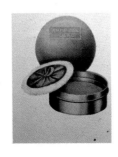

1920 *Compact,*
Compressed Face
Powder or Rouge
75¢ **MP $40**

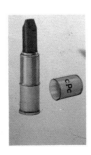

1928 *Lipstick*
$1 **MP $20**

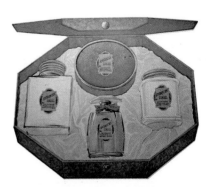

1926 *Foursome Set. Talcum, Face*
Powder, Cream Deluxe and 1 oz Perfume
$6.50 **MP $360**

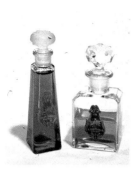 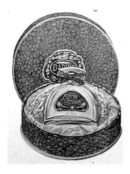 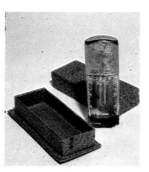 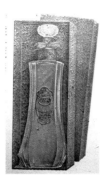 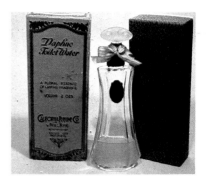

1916 *Perfume 1 oz $1.90*
2 oz $3.45 **MP $160**
1919 *Perfume 4 oz $6.50*
MP $215

1926 *Perfume 1 oz $1.85*
MP $135, $160 boxed

1928 *Perfume Flaconette $1*
MP $95

1920 *Toilet Water*
2 oz $1.50 **MP $135,**
$155 boxed

1926 *Toilet Water 2 oz (shown with*
outer box, left) $1.20 **MP $180**
as shown

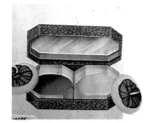 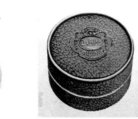 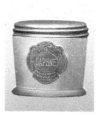 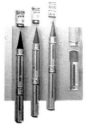 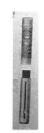

1917 *Double Vanity Box. Face Powder and*
Rouge Compacts $1 **MP $60**
1917 *Vanity Rouge Compact (also available*
with powder) 50¢ **MP $45**

1917 *Face Powder*
75¢ **MP $65**

1917 *Cerate*
75¢ **MP $60**

1917 *Eyebrow Pencils,*
Br, Blk, Blonde 30¢
Lipstick 50¢
MP $25 each

1923 *Lipstick*
39¢ **MP $20**

DAPHNE

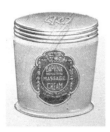 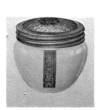 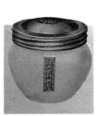 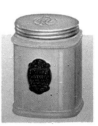 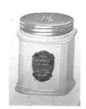

1923 *Cerate*
72¢ **MP $55**

1923 *Rolling Massage*
Cream 69¢ **MP $55**

1926 *Cerate (shown)*
or Derma Cream 75¢
MP $50

1926 *Massage*
Cream 75¢ **MP $50**

1928 *Massage*
Cream 70¢
MP $45

1928 *Cerate*
(shown) or Derma
Cream 75¢
MP $45

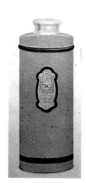 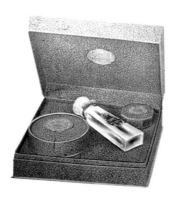 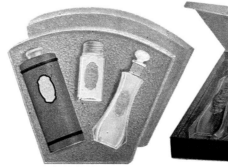 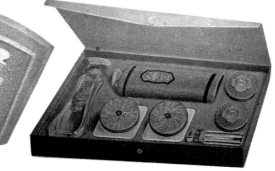

1920 *Talcum Powder*
4 oz 48¢ **MP $65**

1917 *Daphne Set. Face*
Powder, Perfume 1 oz &
Rouge $3.50 **MP $325**

1923 *Daphne Threesome.*
Talcum & Sachet Powders, Toilet
Water 2 oz $3.20 **MP $325**

1926-28 *Septette Gift. Cerate & Derma Creams,*
Face Powder & Rouge Compacts, Talcum, Toilet
Water & Perfume Extract $2.95 **MP $450**

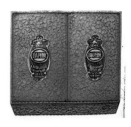

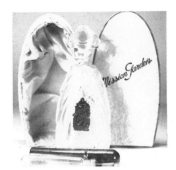

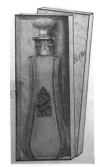

MISSION GARDEN

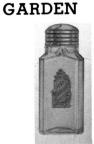

1926 Bath Salts 98¢
MP $75

1926 Boxed Soaps 72¢
MP $70

1922 Perfume 1½ oz $4.95
MP $210, $300 boxed

*1922 Toilet Water
2 oz $2.25 MP $130,
$160 boxed*

*1922 Sachet
Powder $1.75*
MP $90

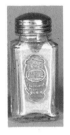

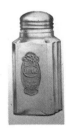

JARDIN D' AMOUR

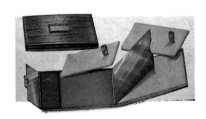

*1922 Sachet
96¢ MP $85*

*1920 Sachet
96¢ MP $90*

*1926 Sachet
$1 MP $75*

*1926 Vanity Compact, Rouge & Powder
$2.25 MP $45*

DAPHNE

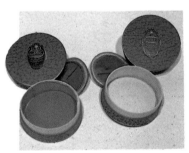

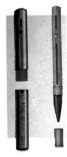

*1926 Ensemble Set. Brow Pencil, Rouge,
Face Powder, Lipstick $2.25 MP $200*

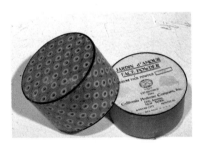

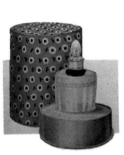

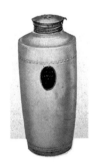

1923 Single Rouge Compact 39¢
MP $40
1923 Face Powder 72¢ **MP $40**

*1926 Lipstick 39¢
Eyebrow Pencil
29¢ MP $20 each*

*1926 Adherent Face
Powder $1.25 MP $75*

*1926 Perfume 1 oz $3.50,
2 oz $6.50 MP $115,
$150 boxed*

1926 Talcum $1.00
MP $60

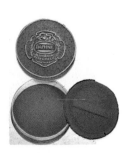

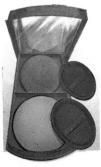

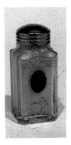

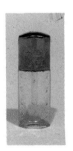

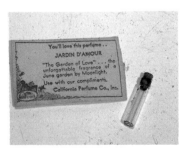

*1926 Single Compact,
Rouge or Face
Powder 39¢ MP $35*

*1926 Duplex
Compact, Rouge
& Face Powder
98¢ MP $45*

*1929 Powder
Sachet $1.25*
MP $75

*1929 Perfume
Flaconette $1.10*
MP $110

1932 Perfume Sample **MP $25**

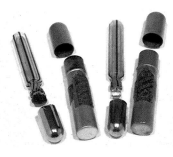

1925-26 *Perfume Flaconettes and Holders* $1.20 each **MP $90 each**

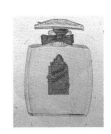

1925 *Perfume 1 oz* $2.85 **MP $140**

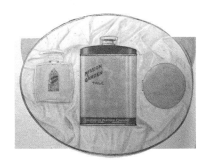

1925 *Threesome Set. Perfume 1 oz, Talc & Twin Compact* $7 **MP $310**

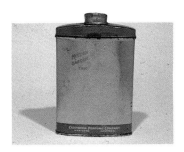

1925 *Talc 4 oz* 75¢ **MP $95**

MISSION GARDEN

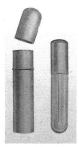

1922 *Flaconette Perfume & Brass Holder* 98¢ **MP $100**

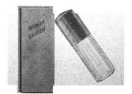

1927 *Perfume Flaconette* $1.20 **MP $95, $125 boxed**

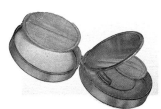

1923 *Twin Compact* $1.48 **MP $55**

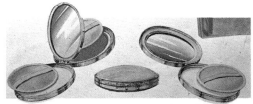

1925 *Twin Compact* $1.48 **MP $50**

1925 *Single Compact* 98¢ **MP $45**

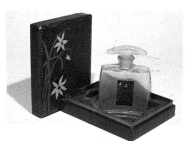

1925 *Perfume 1 oz* $2.10 **MP $140**

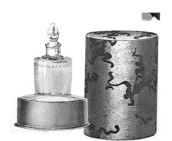

1926 *Perfume 1 oz* $2.19 **MP $115, $160 boxed**

NARCISSUS

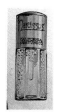

1926 *Perfume Flaconette* 84¢ **MP $95**

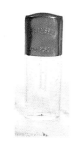

1927 *Perfume Flaconette* $1 **MP $95**

NATOMA ROSE

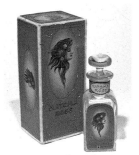

1914 *Perfume 1 oz* 75¢ **MP $145, $175 boxed**

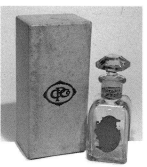

1914 *Perfume 2 oz* $1.40 **MP $150, $180 boxed**

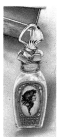

1915 *Box N, Perfume ½ oz* 75¢ **MP $140, $170 boxed**

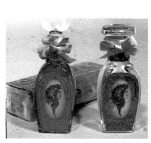

1915 *Perfume 1 oz* $1.40 **MP $135, $160 boxed**
1916 *Perfume 1 oz* $1.40 **MP $120, $145 boxed**

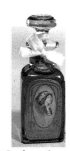

1918 *Perfume 1 oz* $1.40 **MP $135**

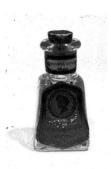
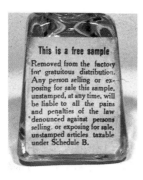

1915 *Perfume Sample* **MP $160** *(Back of bottle also shown with "Free Sample" label)*

....NATOMA ROSE

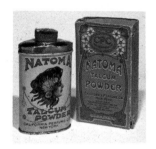
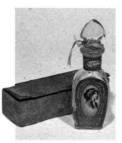

1914 *Talcum Powder 25¢*
MP $100, $130 boxed

1920 *Perfume ½ oz 75¢*
MP $135, $165 boxed

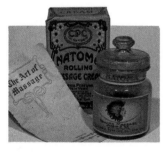
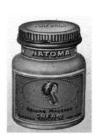

1914-20 *Rolling Massage Cream
5 oz 50¢* **MP $160, $185 boxed,**
Art of Massage Booklet **MP $20**

1920 *Rolling Massage
Cream 5 oz 75¢*
MP $120

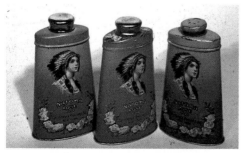

1915 *Talcum 4 oz 35¢* **MP $80**
1918 *Talcum 4 oz 35¢* **MP $90**
1921 *Talcum 4 oz 35¢* **MP $80**

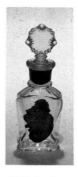
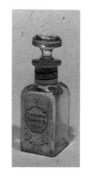
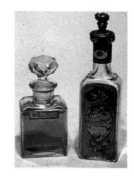
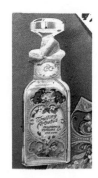

1913 *Perfume
1 oz 60¢*
MP $200

1912 *Perfume
1 oz 50¢*
MP $150

1915 *Perfume 2 oz $3.75*
MP $200
1915 *Toilet Water 2 oz 75¢
4 oz $1.50* **MP $135**

1914 *Perfume 1 oz
$1.10* **MP $140,
$185 boxed**

TRAILING ARBUTUS

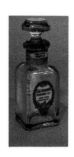
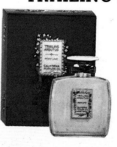
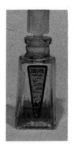
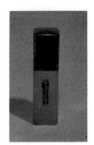

1923 *Perfume 1 oz
$1.17* **MP $120**

1925 *Perfume 1 oz &
2 oz $1.17 & $2.10*
MP $140, $165 boxed

1926 *Perfume
2 oz $2.10*
MP $125

1926 *Perfume
Flaconette 59¢*
MP $95

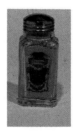
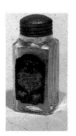
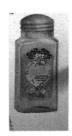
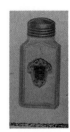

1918 *Sachet
Powder 75¢*
MP $100

1917 *Sachet
Powder 60¢*
MP $100

1914 *Sachet
Powder 60¢*
MP $110

1923 *Sachet
Powder 72¢*
MP $90

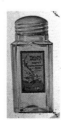
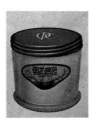

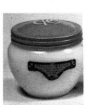

1925 *Sachet
Powder 72¢*
MP $90

1925 *Vanishing
Cream, 2 & 4 oz
size 33¢ & 59¢*
MP $50 each

1925 *Cold Cream,
Reg. & Dbl. size
33¢ & 59¢* **MP $50
each**

1928 *Cold Cream
69¢* **MP $45**

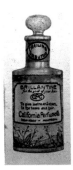
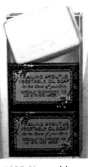
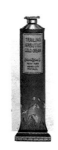
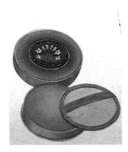
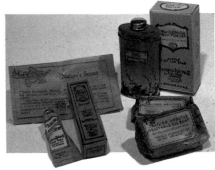

*1923 Brilliantine
2 oz 39¢* **MP $120**

*1925 Vegetable
Oil Soap, 3 cakes
39¢* **MP $100**

*1925 Cold Cream,
tube 23¢* **MP $30**

*1928 Rouge, cardboard
40¢* **MP $30**

1925 Cold Cream Sample **MP $60., $85
boxed, $15 Folder**
*1915 Talcum Powder Sample, Eng. & French
Label* **MP $100, $125 boxed**
1925 Vegetable Oil Soap Sample **MP $75**

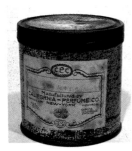
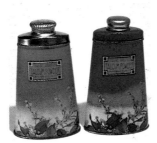
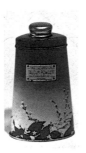
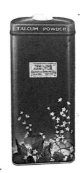
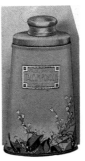
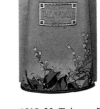

*1917 Talcum Powder
1 lb. to refill powder
containers 89¢* **MP $130**

*1914 only, Talcum Powder 4 oz
25¢* **MP $120**
*1923 Talcum Powder dark
blue label, 4 oz 35¢*
MP $75

*1923 Talcum Powder
4 oz, light blue
label 35¢* **MP $75**

*1925 Talcum
Powder 1 lb. 89¢*
MP $80

*1915-20 Talcum Powder
4 oz 25¢* **MP $100, $125 boxed**

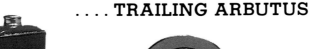

. . . . TRAILING ARBUTUS

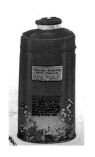
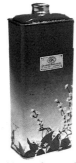
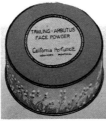
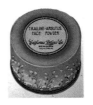
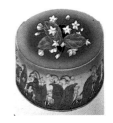

*1925 Bath Powder
4¾ oz 35¢* **MP $75**

*1925 Bath Powder
1 lb. 89¢* **MP $80**

1923 Face Powder 33¢
MP $45

1925 Face Powder 33¢
MP $40

1928 Face Powder 35¢
MP $40

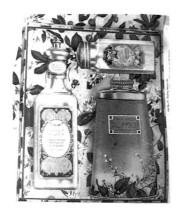
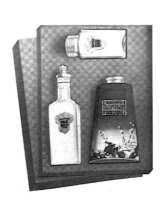
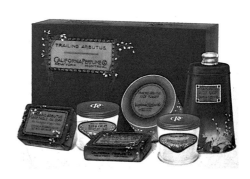

*1914 Set 'T' 4 oz Sprinkle-top Toilet
Water, Sachet Powder, 4 oz Talcum
Powder $2.50* **MP $390**

*1923 Threesome Set. 2 oz Toilet
Water, 4 oz Talc & Sachet Powder
$1.85* **MP $300**

*1925 Sextette Set. 2 Vegetable Oil Soaps,
Cold Cream, Face Powder, Vanishing
Cream and Talcum Powder $1.59* **MP $280**

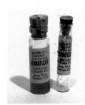
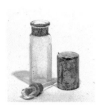
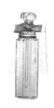
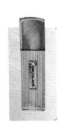
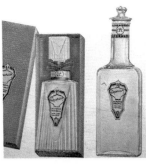
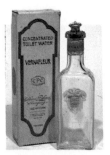
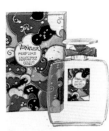

1920 *Fragrance Sample* **MP $85**
1923 *Fragrance Sample* **MP $85**

1925 *Perfume Flaconette 1/4 oz 48¢* **MP $100**

1923 *Perfume Flaconette 1/4 oz 48¢* **MP $90**

1928 *Perfume Flaconette 69¢* **MP $95**

1926 *Perfume 1 oz $1.44* **MP $125, $150 boxed**
1926 *Toilet Water 2 oz 74¢* **MP $95**

1923 *Toilet Water 2 oz 59¢* **MP $105, $125 boxed**

1925 *Perfume 1 oz $1.45* **MP $140, $165 boxed**

VERNAFLEUR

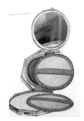
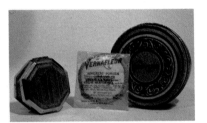
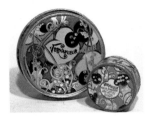
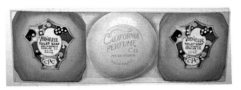

1928 *Double Compact $1.50* **MP $45**

1928 *Single Compact $1* **MP $35**
1923 *Face Powder Sample* **MP $20**
1923 *Adherent Face Powder 48¢* **MP $40**

1925 *Adherent Face Powder 48¢* **MP $40**
1925 *Face Powder Sample* **MP $45**

1928 *Toilet Soap, 3 cakes 70¢* **MP $100**

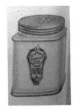
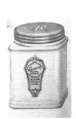
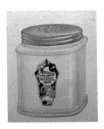
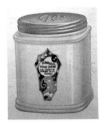
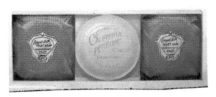

1923 *Tissue Creme, small 48¢, large 89¢* **MP $50**

1923 *Nutri-Creme, small 48¢, large 89¢* **MP $50**

1928 *Nutri-Creme, regular 50¢ double 90¢* **MP $45 each**

1928 *Tissue Creme, regular 50¢ double 90¢* **MP $45 each**

1925 *Toilet Soap, 3 cakes 69¢* **MP $100**

1928 *Bath Set. Dusting Powder, Bath Salts 10 oz, 2 Toilet Soaps $3.50* **MP $250**

VERNAFLEUR

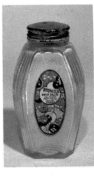
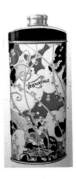
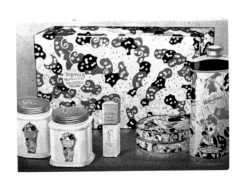
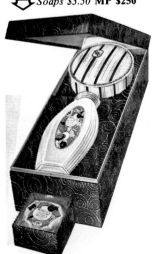

1923 *Vernatalc 4 oz 39¢* **MP $75**

1925 *Bath Salts 10 oz 75¢* **MP $85**

1926 *Vernatalc 4 oz 39¢* **MP $65**

1928 *Quintette Set. Tissue Creme, Nutri-Creme, Perfume, Face Powder & Vernatalc $2.25* **MP $330**

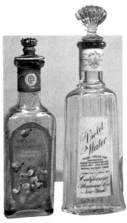

1918 *Toilet Water 2 oz 75¢*
MP $125
1906 *Violet Water 2 oz 75¢*
MP $180

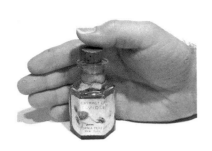

1900 *Extract of Violet Perfume 1 oz 40¢, 2 oz 75¢* **MP $185**

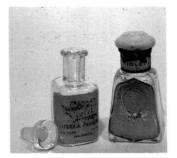

1908 *Perfume Extract 2 oz 90¢* **MP $175**
1910 *Atomizer Set Perfume Bottle* **MP $150**

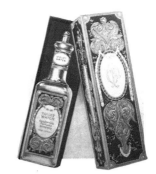

1914 *Violet Toilet Water 2 oz 65¢* **MP $150, $175 boxed**

VIOLET

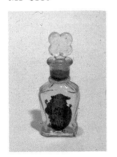

1908 *Perfume ½ oz (Gift Set bottle)* **MP $150**

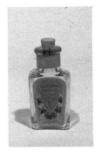

1914 *Perfume (Set H bottle)* **MP $145**

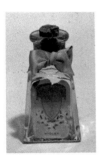

1916 *Perfume 1 oz $1* **MP $140**

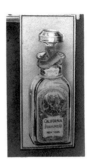

1915 *Perfume 1 oz 90¢* **MP $150, $175 boxed**

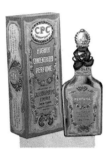

1917 *Perfume ½ oz 50¢* **$140, $170 boxed**

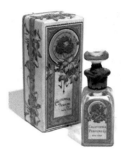

1918 *Perfume 1 oz 90¢* **MP $140, $175 boxed**

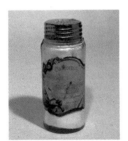

1906 *Talcum 3½ oz 25¢* **MP $125**

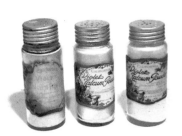

1908 *Talcum Powder 3½ oz 25¢* **MP $110**
1920 *Talcum Powder 3½ oz 25¢* **MP $95**
1920 *As above, with Food & Drug Act lable* **MP $95**

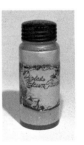

1923 *Talcum Powder 3½ oz 25¢* **MP $90**

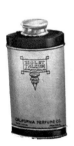

1923 *Talcum 3½ oz 23¢* **MP $80**

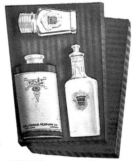

1923 *Threesome Set. Talcum, Toilet Water 2 oz and Sachet Powder $1.40* **MP $300**

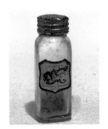

1910 *Sachet Powder 25¢* **MP $125**

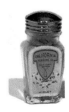

1914 *Sachet Powder 25¢* **MP $90**

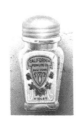

1915 *Sachet Powder 25¢* **MP $90**

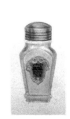

1923 *Sachet Powder 49¢* **MP $85**

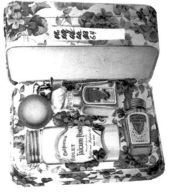

1914 *Gift Set H. Talcum, Perfume 1 oz, Atomizer, Sachet Powder $1.35* **MP $375**

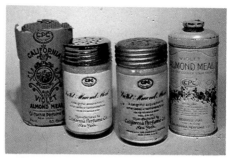

1914 *Almond Meal 3½ oz 50¢* **MP $100, $130 boxed**
1920 *Almond Meal 3¾ oz 50¢* **MP $90**
1923 *Almond Meal 4 oz 48¢* **MP $80**

.....VIOLET

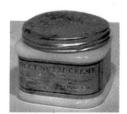   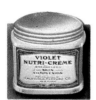

1910 *Nutri-Creme 50¢*
MP $60

1915
*Nutri-Creme
small 50¢*
MP $55

1914
*Nutri-Creme
double size 90¢*
MP $55

In the early 1900's Violet
Nutri-Creme was intro-
duced as a true skin
food. It was called
"The Queen of
Complexion Creams".

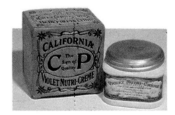

1920 *Nutri-Creme 50¢* **MP $50,
$65 boxed**

  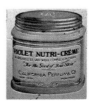 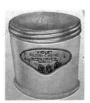

1923
*Nutri-Creme
small 49¢*
MP $45

1923
*Nutri-Creme
double size 89¢*
MP $45

1925
*Nutri-Creme
89¢* **MP $45**

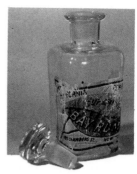

Bay Rum

Bay Rum was in the CPC-
Avon line for more than sixty
years. Whether used for its
curative powers, as a hair
tonic or simply as an after
shave lotion, Avon collectors
have labeled Bay Rum as a
highly prized collectible.

1898 *Bay Rum 1 pint $1.25*
MP $240

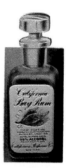 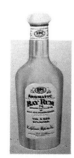 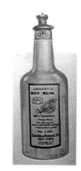

1915 *Bay Rum
4 oz 40¢*
MP $130

1918 *Bay Rum 4 oz
75¢ 8 oz $1.50, pint
$3.00* **MP $110 each**

1923 *Bay Rum 4 oz
47¢, 8 oz 84¢, pint
$1.44* **MP $105**

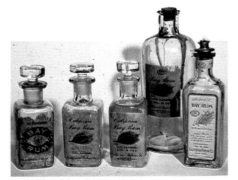 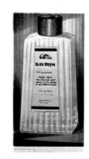

1896 *Bay Rum 4 oz 40¢* **MP $200**
1908 *Bay Rum 4 oz 40¢* **MP $170**
1912 *Bay Rum 4 oz 40¢* **MP $150**
1915 *Bay Rum 16 oz $1.44* **MP $160**
1927 *Bay Rum 4 oz 50¢* **MP $100**

1930 *Bay Rum 4 oz
52¢* **MP $75**

(See also pg. 228)

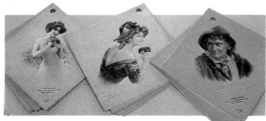

1914 *Shaving Leaves, Pad of 50 sheets 15¢* **MP $75**
1915 **MP $70**
1923 **MP $55**

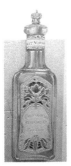 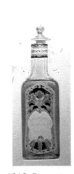 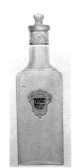 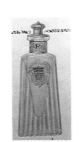 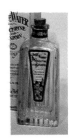 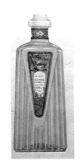 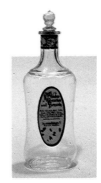

1914 *Lait Virginal Milk Bath 2 oz 65¢, 4 oz $1.25, 8 oz $2.00* **MP $135 each**

1918 *Benzoin Lotion 2 oz 90¢ and 4 oz $1.75* **MP $105 each**

1923 *Benzoin Lotion 2 oz 59¢* **MP $100**

1926 *Benzoin Lotion 2 oz 59¢* **MP $90**

1928 *Rosewater Glycerin and Benzoin Lotion 4 oz 48¢* **MP $80**

1925 *Rosewater Glycerin and Benzoin Lotion 48¢* **MP $90**

1924 *Rosewater Glycerin and Benzoin Lotion 4 oz $1.14* **MP $100**

CPC TOILETRIES

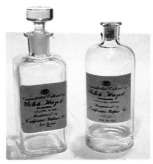 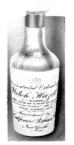 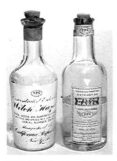 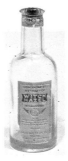 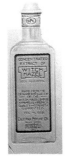 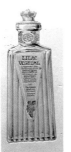 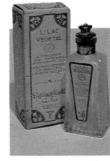

1909 *Witch Hazel Extract 16 oz 75¢* **MP $160**
1915 *Witch Hazel Extract 16 oz 95¢* **MP $125**

1915 *Witch Hazel Extract 4 oz 25¢* **MP $110**

1912 *Witch Hazel Extract 4 oz 25¢* **MP $125**
1920 *Witch Hazel Extract 4 oz 39¢* **MP $90**

1923-27 *Witch Hazel 4 oz 39¢* **MP $85**
8 oz 69¢ **MP $85**
32 oz $3.25 **MP $100**

1926 *Witch Hazel 4 oz 39¢* **MP $80**
8 oz 69¢ **MP $80**
Pint $1.20 **MP $85**

1927 *Lilac Vegetal 2 oz 59¢* **MP $90**, *4 oz $1.08* **MP $90**

1928 *Lilac Vegetal 2 oz 59¢, 4 oz $1.08* **MP $80, $100 boxed**

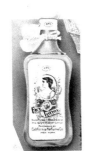 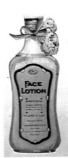 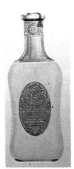 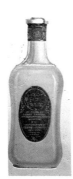 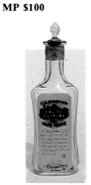 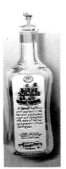 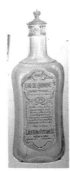 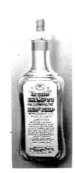

1912 *Face Lotion, white or pink 6oz $1* **MP $110**

1917 *Face Lotion, white or pink 6oz $1* **MP $95**

1923 *Face Lotion, white or pink, 6oz 97¢* **MP $80**

1926 *Liquid Face Powder 97¢* **MP $75**

1902 *Eau de Quinine Hair Tonic 65¢* **MP $135**

1915 *Eau de Quinine Hair Tonic 65¢* **MP $110**

1923 *Eau de Quinine Hair Tonic 6 oz 69¢* **MP $95**

1915 *Liquid Shampoo 35¢* **MP $100**

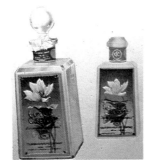 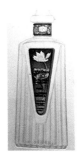 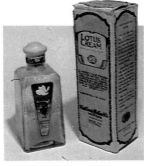 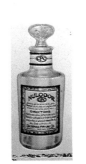 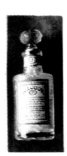 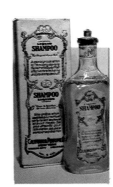

1917 *Lotus Cream 12 oz $1.25* **MP $150**
1917 *Lotus Cream 4 oz 50¢* **MP $125**

1925 *Lotus Cream 50¢* **MP $80**

1927 *Lotus Cream 4 oz 48¢* **MP $80, $100 boxed**

1926 *Nulodor 33¢* **MP $110**

1928 *Nulodor 35¢* **MP $100**

1923 *Liquid Shampoo 6 oz 48¢* **MP $90, $115 boxed**

CPC ELITE POWDERS

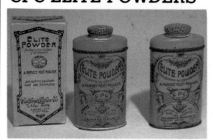
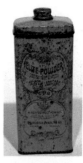

1920 *Elite Powder 25¢* MP $70, $90 boxed
1923 *Elite Powder 24¢* MP $65, $85 boxed

1923 *Elite Powder
1 lb. 89¢* MP $65

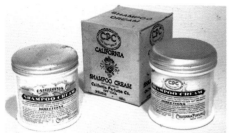
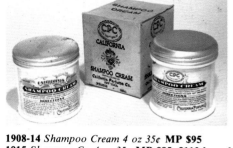

1900 *Shampoo Cream 35¢*
MP $115

1908-14 *Shampoo Cream 4 oz 35¢* MP $95
1915 *Shampoo Cr. 4 oz 35¢* MP $85, $110 boxed

CPC CREAMS

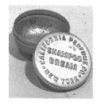

1908 *Shampoo Cream
Sample* MP $60

1915
*Bandoline Hair
Dressing 35¢*
MP $85

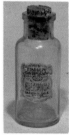
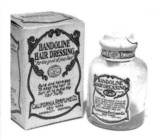

1922 *Bandoline
Hair Dressing
4 oz 45¢*
MP $85

1923 *Bandoline Hair Dressing
2 oz 24¢, 4 oz 45¢* MP $80,
$100 boxed

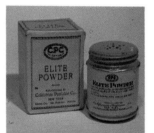
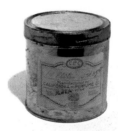

1914 *Elite Powder 25¢*
MP $80, $100 boxed

1917 *Elite Powder 1 lb. to
refill powder containers
89¢* MP $125

(See also Elite Powders pg. 157)

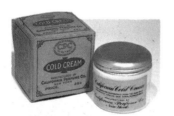
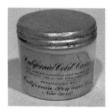
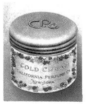
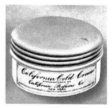
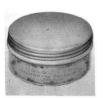
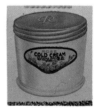

1906 *Cold Cream 2 oz 25¢*
MP $90, $115 boxed

1908 *Cold Cream
2oz 25¢* MP $90

1915 *Cold
Cream, small
25¢* MP $80

1906-08 *California
Cold Cream
double size 45¢*
MP $90

1917 *Cold
Cream, triple
size 65¢*
MP $80

1926 *Rose
Cold Cream
63¢* MP $60

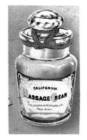
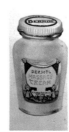
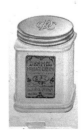
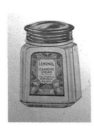
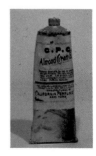
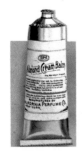
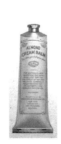
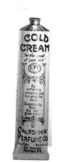

1908-15 *Massage
Cream 75¢*
MP $110

1920 *Dermol
Massage Cream
$1.00* MP $85

1923 *Dermol
Massage Cream
96¢* MP $75

1926-30 *Lemonol
Cleansing Cream
50¢* MP $60

1910 *Almond
Cream 2 oz
25¢, 6 oz 50¢*
MP $100

1915 *Almond
Cream Balm 2 oz
25¢, 6 oz 50¢*
MP $55. each

1918 *Almond
Cream Balm
30¢* MP $55

1923 *Cold
Cream, small
23¢, large 45¢*
MP $55 each

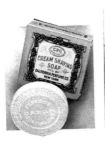 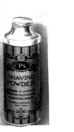 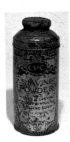 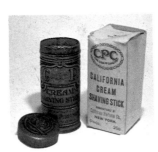 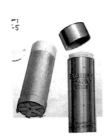 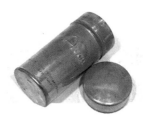

1915 *Cream Shaving Soap 25¢* **MP $75**

1915 *Shaving Powder 2 oz 35¢* **MP $55**

1927 *Shaving Powder 2 oz 33¢* **MP $35**

1915 *Cream Shaving Stick in metal container 35¢* **MP $60, $75 boxed**

1918 *Bayberry Shaving Stick 33¢* **MP $55**

1934-36 *Shaving Stick 36¢* **MP $40**

CPC MEN'S TOILETRIES

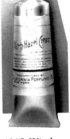 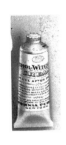 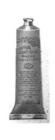 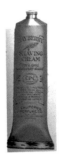 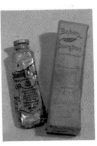 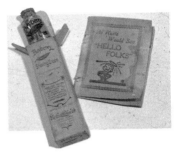

1915 *Witch Hazel Cream small 25¢* **MP $55**

1917 *Menthol Witch Hazel Cream (small) 25¢* **MP $55**

1918 *Menthol Witch Hazel Cream 35¢* **MP $55**

1918 *Bayberry Shaving Cream 35¢* **MP $55**

1918 *Bayberry Shaving Cream Sample* **MP $70, $100 boxed**

1923 *Bayberry Shaving Cream Sample* **MP $65, $95 boxed**

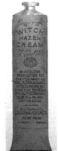 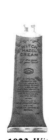 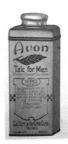 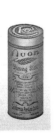 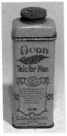 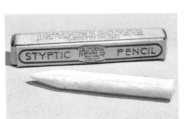 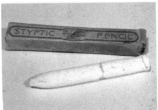

1923 *Witch Hazel Cream, triple size 59¢* **MP$55**

1923 *Witch Hazel Cream, small size 30¢* **MP $55**

1928 *Avon Talc for Men 25¢* **MP $40**

1928 *Avon Shaving Stick 35¢* **MP $45**

1929 *Avon Talc for Men 25¢* **MP $40**

1923 *Styptic pencil 10¢* **MP $20 boxed**

1925 *Styptic Pencil 10¢* **MP $18 boxed**

Shaving Cabinet No. 9 came out for Christmas selling in 1931 and was available for only about one year. The Shaving Cabinet, pictured in black and white, appears on a special insert page that was added to the 1930 Sales Catalog. The white metal cabinet was cleverly constructed to comfortably hold 3 regular size Avon Shaving requisites:

A bottle of Toilet Water for the ladies, a Gold Plated Gem Safety Razor and two extra blades. In addition, there was a slot for a shaving brush. Three holes in the top of the cabinet provided ventilation. A mirror was positioned on the outside of the cabinet door. Product copy on the catalog page states, "The Cabinet, complete with fittings is offered at a special price — which is less than the container alone would cost if it could be bought in the stores."

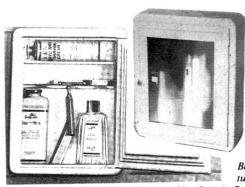

1930 *Shaving Cabinet No. 9 (white enamel 8x6½x2⅜" deep) sold with contents: Bayberry Shaving Cream, tube 35¢, Talc for Men 35¢, Styptic Pencil 10¢, 2 oz White Rose Toilet Water for the ladies 75¢, gold plated Gem Safety Razor and 2 extra blades. $2.50* **MP $270, $100 cabinet only**

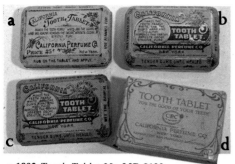

a-1892 *Tooth Tablet* 25¢ **MP $120**
b-1906 *Tooth Tablet* 25¢ **MP $110**
c-1900-06 *Tooth Tablet* 25¢ **MP $115**
d-1915 *Tooth Tablet* 25¢ **MP $90**

CPC
TOOTH PRODUCTS

In the 1890's the Tooth Tablet was the only dental product offered by the California Perfume Company.

In the early 1900's Tooth Wash was introduced as an antiseptic cleanser of the mouth and teeth. A few drops in a glass of water provided a pleasant tasting mouthwash.

The CPC dentifrice line rapidly expanded to include regular Tooth Powder, Dental Cream and Sen Den Tal Cream. The Sen Den Tal Cream contained a breath fragrance similar to Sen-Sen and was advertised as a mildly abrasive dentifrice and breath purifier. Toothbrushes were added to the line in 1928 and were the first items to carry the 'Avon' name.

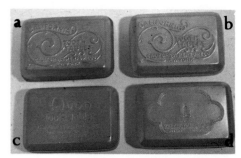

a-1921 *Tooth Tablet* 24¢ **MP $75**
b-1923 *Tooth Tablet* 24¢ **MP $75**
c-1934 *Tooth Tablet* 35¢ **MP $60**
d-1936 *Tooth Tablet* 36¢ **MP $60**

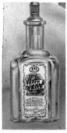

1915 *Tooth Wash* 25¢ **MP $105**

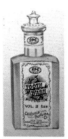

1920 *Tooth Wash* 35¢ **MP $100**

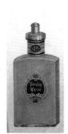

1923 *Tooth Wash* 33¢ **MP $90**

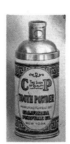

1910-1923 *Tooth Powder* 25¢ **MP $70**

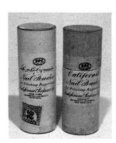

1920-22 *Nail Powder* 25¢, then 24¢ **MP $60** (2 different labels shown)

CPC
NAIL
CARE

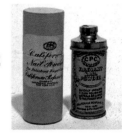

1916 *Nail Powder* 25¢ **MP $60**
1923 *Radiant Nail Powder* 24¢ **MP $50**

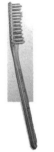

1928 *Avon Toothbrush ass't colors.* 50¢ **MP $20**

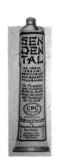

1918 *Sen Den Tal Cream* 50¢ **MP $60**

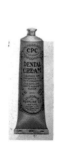

1915 *Dental Cream* 25¢ **MP $60**

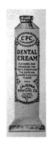

1923 *Dental Cream* 35¢ **MP $55**

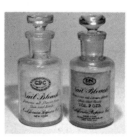

1912 *Nail Bleach* 25¢ **MP $115**
1915 *Nail Bleach* 2 oz 25¢ **MP $115**

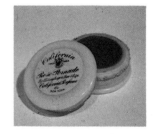

1904 *Rose Pomade* 25¢ **MP $125**

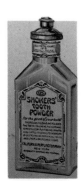

1915 *Smoker's Tooth Powder* 50¢ **MP $125**

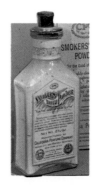

1923 *Smoker's Tooth Powder* 2¾ oz 25¢ **Mp $110, $135 boxed**

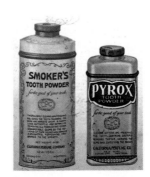

1925 *Smoker's Tooth Powder* 48¢ **MP $55**

1925 *Pyrox Tooth Powder* 24¢ **MP $45**

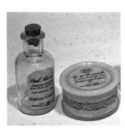

1920 *Nail Bleach* 25¢ **MP $100**
1920 *Rose Pomade* 25¢ **MP $85**

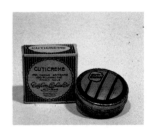

1924 *Cuti-Creme* 30¢ **MP $40, $50 boxed**

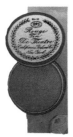 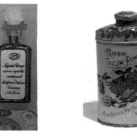 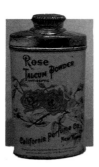 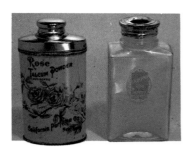 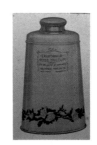

1915 *Rouge Tin De Theatre 25¢* **MP $50**

1915 *Liquid Rouge 25¢* **MP $95**

1908-10 *Rose Talcum Antiseptic Powder 3½ oz 25¢* **MP $110**

1912-14 *Rose Talcum Antiseptic Powder 3½ oz 25¢* **MP $105**

1910-1912 *Rose Talcum Antiseptic Powder 3½ oz 25¢* **MP $100**
1920 *California Rose Talcum 3½ oz 72¢* **MP $95**

1923 *California Rose Talcum 4 oz 33¢* **MP $75**

CPC FACE & BODY POWDERS

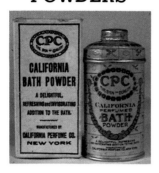 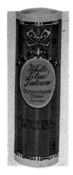 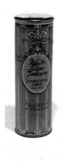 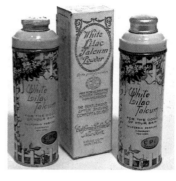 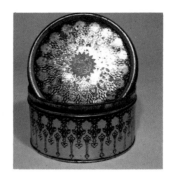

1914 *Bath Powder 4½ oz 25¢* **MP $70, $85 boxed**

1917 *White Lilac Talcum 4 oz 25¢* **MP $60**

1918 *White Lilac Talcum 4 oz 25¢* **MP $60**

1912 *White Lilac Talcum 4 oz 25¢* **MP $80, $95 boxed**
1920 *White Lilac Talcum 4 oz 24¢* **MP $70, $85 boxed**

1926 *Body Powder $1.19* **MP $80**

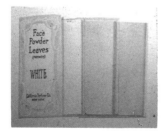 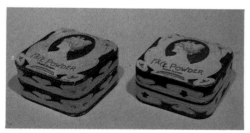 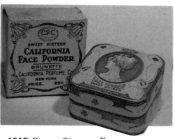 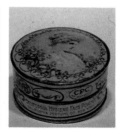

1911 *Face Powder Leaves. Scented paper with Face Powder on one side in 3 shades. Rose, white or rachel, 72 leaves per book. 20¢* **MP $40**

1914 *Sweet Sixteen Face Powder 25¢* **MP $60**
1906 *Sweet Sixteen Face Powder 25¢* **MP $70**

1918 *Sweet Sixteen Face Powder 35¢* **MP $50, $70 boxed**

1914 *Hygiene Face Powder white, pink or brunette 50¢* **MP $85**

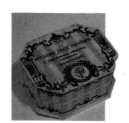 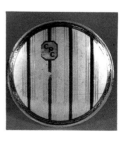 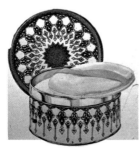 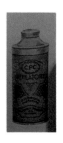 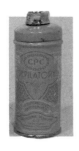 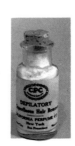

1915 *Hygiene Face Powder 3 tints 50¢* **MP $65**

1925 *Dusting Powder $1* **MP $80**

1926 *Body Powder $1.19* **MP $80**

1917 *Depilatory 50¢* **MP $65**

1920 *Depilatory 50¢* **MP $65**

1915 *Depilatory 50¢* **MP $100**

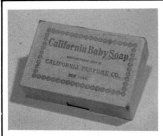

1896 *California Baby Soap 15¢*
MP $95

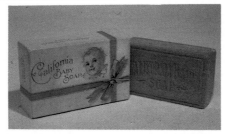

1905 *California Baby Soap 15¢* **MP $85**

BABY SOAP

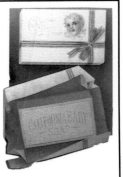

1914 *California Baby Soap 4 oz 15¢*
MP $50

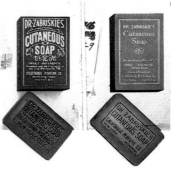

Dr. Zabriskie's Cutaneous Soap
1915 *25¢* **MP $50**
1923 *24¢* **MP $45**

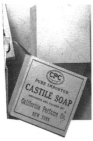

1915 *Castile Soap 25¢* **MP $60**

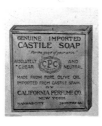

1925 *Castile Soap 33¢* **MP $50**

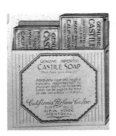

1928 *Castile Soap, 2 cakes 50¢* **MP $50**

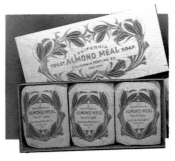

1906 *Toilet Almond Meal Soap, 3 cakes 25¢* **MP $100**

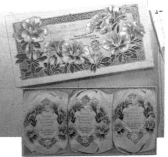

1906 *Almond, Buttermilk & Cucumber Soap, 3 cakes 40¢* **MP $125**

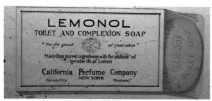

1920 *Lemonol Toilet & Complexion Soap, 3 cakes 45¢* **MP $110**

1923 *Lemonol Toilet Soap, 12 per carton $1.65* **MP $125**

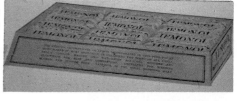

CPC SOAPS

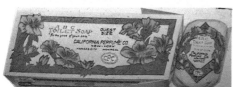

1923 *ABC Toilet Soap 6 guest size cakes 48¢* **MP $110**

1926 *Almond Bouquet Toilet Soap, 3 cakes 30¢* **MP $100**

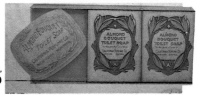

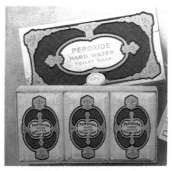

1915 *Peroxide Hard Water Toilet Soap, 3 cakes 50¢* **MP $100**

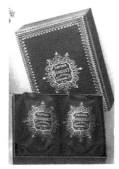

1906 *Savona Bouquet Soap, 2 cakes 50¢* **MP $100**

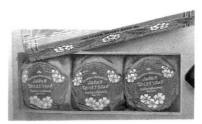

1906 *Japan Toilet Soap, 3 cakes 25¢* **MP $125**

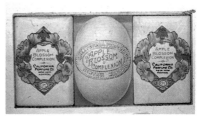

1926 *Apple Blossom Complexion, 3 cakes 69¢* **MP $100**

(See also pg. 167)

CPC GIFT SETS

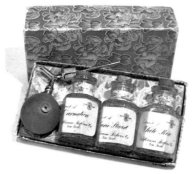

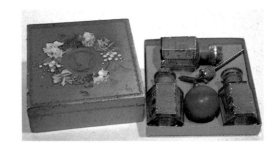

1900 *Atomizer Box. Three 1 oz Perfumes & Atomizer. Choice of 27 fragrances $1.35* **MP $600**

1908-10 *CP Atomizer set. Three 1 oz Perfumes & Atomizer. $1.50-$6 depending on choice of 34 fragrances* **MP $525**

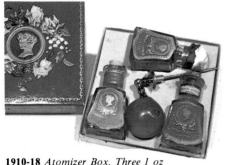

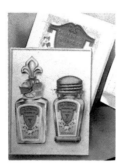

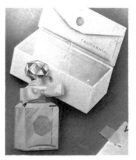

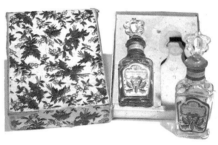

1910-18 *Atomizer Box. Three 1 oz Perfumes & Perfect Atomizer. $1.50-$6 depending on choice of 31 fragrances* **MP $500**

1915-16 *Gift Box No. 2. Perfume 1/2 oz & Sachet Powder in White Lilac, Violet, Heliotrope or White Rose. $50¢* **MP $270**

1914 *Gift Box F. Crab Apple Blossom or Trailing Arbutus Perfume 2 oz $2.25* **MP $225, $250 boxed**

1912 *Gift Box A. Two 1/2 oz Perfumes, choice of 6 fragrances 50¢* **MP $325**

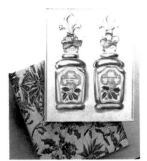

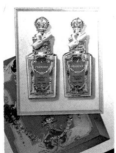

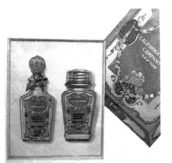

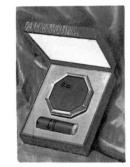

1915 *Gift Box A. Two 1/2 oz Perfumes in a choice of Violet, White Rose, Carnation, White Lilac, Heliotrope and Lily of the Valley. 50¢* **MP $310**

1917 *Gift Box No. 3. Two 1/2 oz Perfumes, choice of fragrances. 95¢* **MP $320**

1923 *Gift Box No. 2. Perfume 1/2 oz & Sachet Powder in Violet, Heliotrope or Carnation. 97¢* **MP $245**

1928 *Vanity Set. Lipstick & Compact $2.40* **MP $75**

SETS FOR BABY

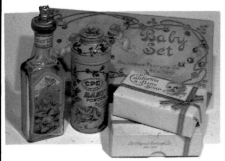

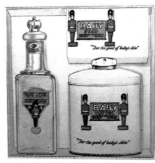

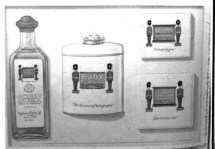

1914 *Baby Set, Powder, Soap & Violet Water 2 oz 75¢* **MP $300**
Baby Powder 25¢ **MP $70**
Baby Soap 15¢ **MP $55**
Violet Water 35¢ **MP $125**

1922 *Baby Set. Soap, Powder & Violet Toilet Water 2 oz 99¢* **MP $250**
Soap 23¢ **MP $55**
Powder 29¢ **MP $70**
Toilet Water 2 oz 48¢ **MP $100**

1925 *Baby Set. Supreme Olive Oil 4 oz, Baby Powder 4 oz, Boric Acid & Castile Soap 5 oz $1.78* **MP $350**
Supreme Olive Oil **MP $115**
Baby Powder 29¢ **MP $70**
Baby Soap 23¢ **MP $55** *Boric Acid 23¢* **MP $75**

CPC CHILDREN'S SETS

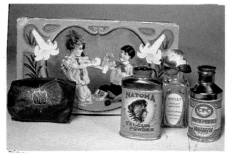

1914 *Juvenile Set. Minatures, Savona Bouquet Soap, Natoma Talcum, Violet Water & Tooth Powder. 50¢* **MP $500**

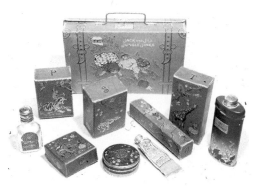

1926 *Jack & Jill Jungle Jinks. Trailing Arbutus Talcum & Daphne Perfume. Apple Blossom Soap, Cold Cream, Sen Den Tal Cream & Toothbrush. $1.50* **MP $400, $75 box only**

LITTLE FOLKS SETS

Combination sets of 4 gem bottles of perfume, packaged especially as a set for children. The same 4 odors are used in each set. Each bottle is kidded and ribboned, the box is artistically lithographed in 7 colors and each is gold embossed. The perfumes are regular CPC Triple Extracts.

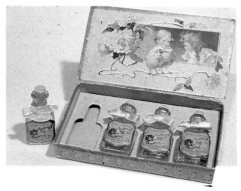

1912 *Little Folks Set. Violet, White Rose, Carnation & Heliotrope Perfume 40¢* **MP $550, $100 each bottle**

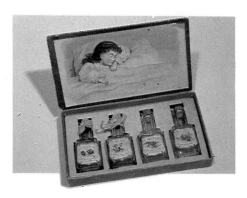

1906 *Little Folks Set. Violet, White Rose, Carnation & Heliotrope Perfume 40¢* **MP $550, $100 each bottle**

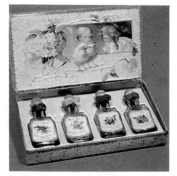

1911 *Little Folks Set. Violet, White Rose, Carnation & Heliotrope Perfume 50¢* **MP $550, $100 each bottle**

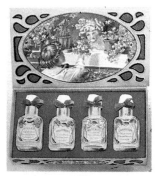

1914 *Little Folks Box. Violet, White Rose, Carnation & Heliotrope Perfume 50¢* **MP $400, $80 each bottle**

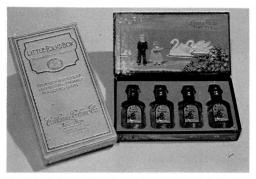

1923 *Little Folks Gift Box. Violet, Carnation, White Lilac & Heliotrope Perfumes 69¢* **MP $375,** *as shown,* **$75 each bottle**

(See also Little Folks p. 101)

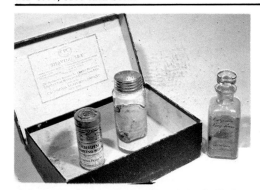

1912-14 *Shaving Set. Cream Shaving Stick, Violet Talcum. Bay Rum 4 oz (shown). Not shown are Tube Menthol Witch Hazel Cream, White Lilac Water 2 oz, Styptic Pencil and Shaving Pad $1.50* **MP $550**

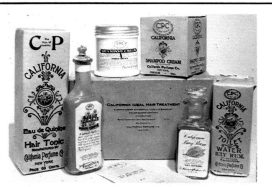

CPC MEN'S SETS

1915 *Ideal Hair Treatment Set. Eau de Quinine Hair Tonic, Shampoo Cream, Bay Rum 4 oz $1.35* **MP $450**

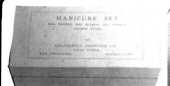
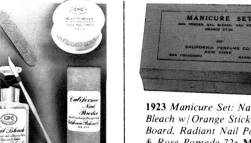
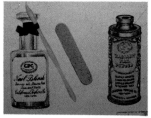

1915 Manicure Set: Nail Bleach w/Cuticle Stick, Rose Pomade, Nail Powder and Emery Board 65¢ **MP $260 boxed**

1915 Nail Bleach with Cuticle Stick 25¢ **MP $110**
1915 Rose Pomade 25¢ **MP $85**
1915 Nail Powder, paper box 25¢ **MP $45** ⇦

1923 Manicure Set: Nail Bleach w/Orange Stick, Emery Board, Radiant Nail Powder & Rose Pomade 72¢ **MP $260**

Nail Bleach 2oz with Orange Wood Stick 24¢ **MP $110**
4 oz 72¢ **MP $130**   *8 oz $1.23* **MP $150**   *16 oz $1.95* **MP $200**
Radiant Nail Powder 24¢ **MP $50**
Rose Pomade 24¢ **MP $85**

CPC MANICURE SETS

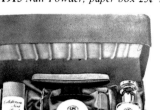
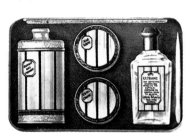
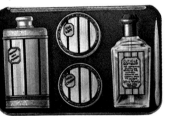

Radiant Nail Powder 24¢ **MP $45**
Nail White 30¢ **MP $40**
Cuti-Creme 30¢ **MP $40**
Cutrane 30¢ **MP $90**

1914 Complete Manicure Set: Buffer, Scissors, File, Nail Bleach, Nail Powder & Rose Pomade, Orange Wood Stick & 6 Emery Boards $3.00 **MP $400 as shown**

1924-26 Manicure Set: Radiant Nail Powder, Nail White, Cuti-Creme & Cutrane ⇦ *$1.20* **MP $240**

1928 Boudoir Manicure Set. Radiant Nail Powder, Nail White, Nail Cream & Cuticle Softener ⇦ *$1.20* **MP $225**

Radiant Nail Powder 30¢ **MP $45**
Nail White 30¢ **MP $40**
Nail Cream 30¢ **MP $40**
Cuticle Softener or Cuticle Remover 30¢ **MP $75**

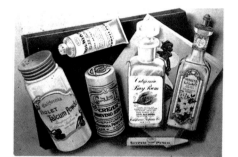
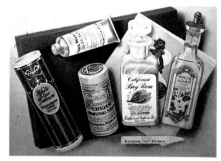
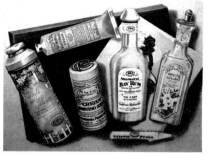

1915 Gentlemen's Shaving Set: Menthol Witch Hazel Cream, Violet Talcum Powder, Cream Shaving Stick, Bay Rum, White Lilac Toilet Water, Styptic Pencil & Shaving Pad, 50 sheets $1.50 **MP $525**

1918 Gentlemen's Shaving Set: White Lilac Talcum, other items identical to those seen in 1915 set $2.35 **MP $480 complete**

GENTLEMEN'S SETS

1919 Gentlemen's Shaving Set: Menthol Witch Hazel Cream, White Lilac Talcum, Cream Shaving Stick, Bay Rum 4 oz, White Lilac Toilet Water, Styptic Pencil & Shaving Pad. 50 sheets $2.25 **MP $480 complete**

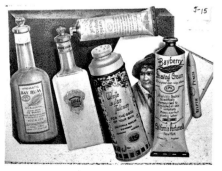
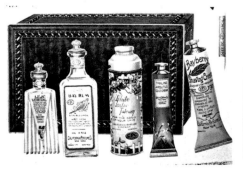
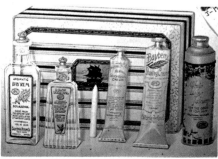

1923 Gentlemen's Shaving Set: White Lilac Toilet Water, Bay Rum 4 oz, White Lilac Talcum, Menthol Witch Hazel Cream, Bayberry Shaving Cream, Styptic Pencil and Shaving Pad $1.95 **MP $425 complete**

1927 Humidor Shaving Set: Lilac Vegetal, Bay Rum 4 oz, White Lilac Talcum, Menthol Witch Hazel Cream or Trailing Arbutus Cold Cream, Bayberry Shaving Cream & Styptic Pencil $1.95 **MP $400 complete**

1928 Humidor Shaving Set: Bay Rum 4 oz, Lilac Vegetal, Styptic Pencil, Witch Hazel Cream, Bayberry Shaving Cream, White Lilac Talcum or CPC Talc for Men $2.25 **MP $400 complete**

PERFECTION

COLORINGS

Throughout the early years, Sales Catalogs encouraged the use of CPC baking products for guaranteed "perfect results" and "perfection in baking." It is not surprising, then, that in 1920 the Company chose the name **Perfection** for the CPC baking line. **Concentrated Colorings** and **Coloring Set** introduced the newly designed Perfection packaging, followed by **Flavoring Extracts** and **Baking Powder** in 1923.

Between 1928 and 1929 two household products, **Avon Maid Powdered Cleanser** and **Auto Lustre**, were introduced in new Avon packaging. During this transition, it was decided that the household product line have its own name.

In 1930 the entire baking and household lines were introduced in orange, brown and white Perfection packaging. For ten years the basic packaging remained the same, but each item was issued under **five** different labels.

Exceptions were **Powdered Cleaner**, issued with **four** different labels, and **Auto Polish**, (formerly Auto Lustre) discontinued in 1936, issued with only two. These two products did not join the Perfection line until 1933 when their original Avon containers were depleted.

Sales Catalogs are useless in determining when label changes took place.

During the entire ten year period, the company continued to utilize the 1930 catalog picture of products.

The following guide will tell you when your 1930-1940 Perfection product was issued.

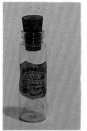

1902 *Vegetable Coloring (chocolate shown) from Set* **MP $50 ea. bottle, $500 boxed set of 8**

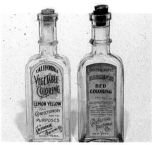

1900-08 *Vegetable Coloring, 8 colors, shown in Lemon Yellow 2oz 25¢, 4oz 45¢* **MP $120**
1908-14 *Harmless Coloring, 8 colors, shown in Red 2oz 25¢ 4oz 45¢* **MP $95**

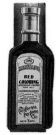

1915-17 *Harmless Coloring, 8 colors, shown in Red 1oz 20¢, 2oz 35¢* **MP $60**

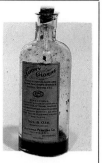

1918-20 *Savory Coloring 8oz (rare) 69¢* **MP $125**

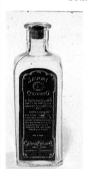

1923 *Savory Coloring 3oz 33¢* **MP $50**

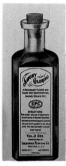

1918-20 *Savory Coloring 3oz (rare) 33¢* **MP $80**

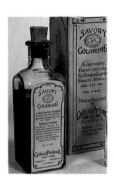

1920 *Savory Coloring 3oz (rare) 35¢* **MP $55, $75 boxed**

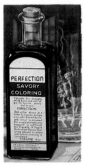

1930 *Savory Coloring 4oz 50¢* **MP $40**

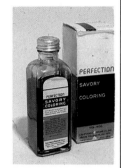

1934 *Savory Coloring 4oz 35¢* **MP $20, $28 boxed**

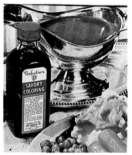

1941-47 *Savory Coloring 4oz 35¢* **MP $18**

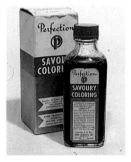

1945-46 *Savoury Coloring 4 oz (rare spelling) 39¢* **MP $22, $27 boxed**

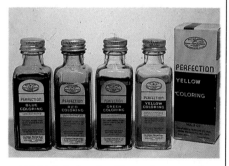

1934-36 *Colorings 2oz blue, red, green, yellow 25¢ each* **MP $20 each, $25 boxed**

COLORINGS — In May 1900, Avon for the first time offered the nation's cooks vegetable colorings in red, green, yellow, lilac, violet, orange and two shades of brown.

Dorothy Bernard's
1930's PERFECTION LABEL DATING GUIDE

1930-33	An Avon Product Made by California Perfume Co., Inc. New York-Montreal
1933-34	An Avon Product California Perfume Co., Inc. New York-Montreal
1934-36	California Perfume Co., Inc. Avon Products, Inc., Div. New York-Montreal
1936-39	Avon Products, Inc., Div. California Perfume Co., Inc. New York-Montreal
1939-40	Avon Products, Inc. Distributor New-York-Montreal-Kansas City Los Angeles

In 1941 Perfection household items were introduced in newly designed brown, green and white packaging and baking products in brown, red and white. Labels read: **Avon Products, Inc., Distributor, New York-Montreal**. This packaging remained in the line for **only one** year and is extremely difficult to find.

By late 1942 all Perfection items were issued in wartime cardboard or glass containers. Following the war, products continued in wartime packaging until most were discontinued between 1947-48. The 8 remaining products were re-issued in packaging identical to introductory packaging of 1941, except that **Pasadena** replaced **Montreal** on the label. **Baking Powder, Savory Coloring, Mending Cement** and **Furniture Polish** were discontinued by 1953 and **Liquid Shoe White, Spots-Out, Powdered Cleaner** and **Mothicide** were discontinued in 1957.

1941

1920

PERFECTION

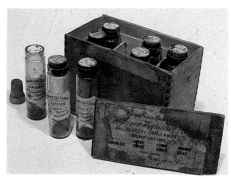

1908-10 *Combination Box of 8 harmless Food Colorings 50¢* **MP $415 complete, $45 box only, $45 each bottle**

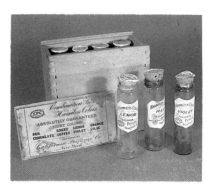

1910-15 *Combination Box of 8 harmless Food Colorings 50¢* **MP $375 complete, $40 box only, $40 each bottle**

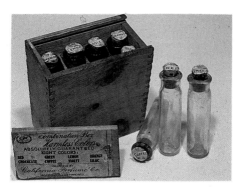

1915-20 *Combination Box of 8 harmless Colors (N.Y.-Montreal label) 60¢* **MP $340 complete, $36 box only, $36 each bottle**

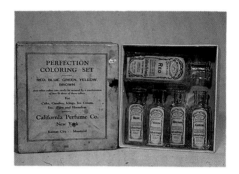

1920-30 *Perfection Coloring Set. Cardboard box holds 2oz red, ½oz each green, yellow, blue & brown 74¢* **MP $280, $50 each bottle**

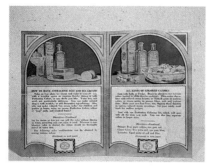

1920-30 *Perfection Coloring Set. Folder* **MP $35**

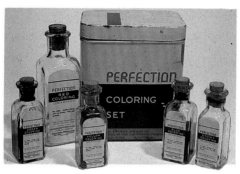

1930-33 *Coloring Set. 2oz red, ½oz each green, yellow, brown & blue. Metal container 85¢* **MP $160 set. Bottles each MP $25, box MP $20**

COLORING SETS

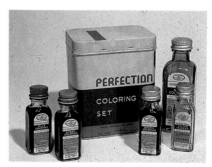

1934 only *Coloring Set. (An Avon Product CPC label) 2oz red, ½oz each brown, green, blue & yellow 85¢* **MP $160 set. Bottles each MP $25, box MP $25**

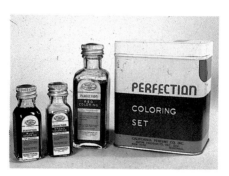

1934-37 *Coloring Set. (CPC/Avon Div. label) 2oz red, ½oz each blue, brown, green & yellow 85¢* **MP $145 set. Bottles each MP $20, box MP $20**

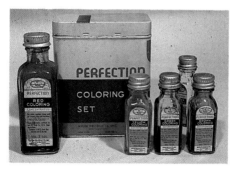

1939-40 *Coloring Set. (Avon Prod. Inc., Dist. label) 2oz red, ½oz each yellow, green, brown & blue 85¢* **MP $120 set. Bottles each MP $18, Box MP $18**

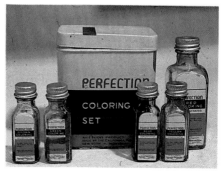

1941 only *Coloring Set. 2oz red, ½oz each brown, yellow and green & blue with matching lids 85¢* **MP $150 set. Bottles each MP $18, $25 with colored lids. Box MP $18**

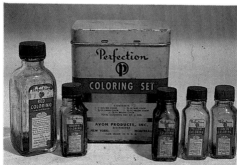

1941-47 *Coloring Set. 2oz red, ½oz each brown, blue, yellow, green 85¢* **MP $100. Bottles each MP $12, box $20**

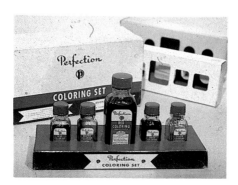

1943-45 *Coloring Set. Same bottles as 1941 (left) but issued in cardboard "Victory Packaging" 98¢* **MP $160**

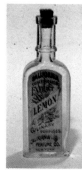
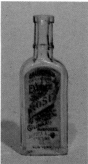
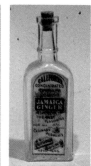
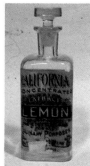
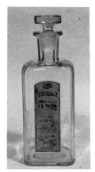
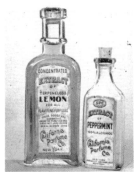
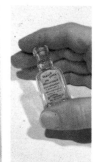

1898-1902 *California Extract 2oz 25¢, 16oz $1.75, 32oz $3.25* **MP $110, $150 Qt.**

1898-1902 *California Extract, 22 flavors (Rose shown) see size & prices (left)* **MP $110, $150 Qt.**

1902-08 *California Extract (Jamaica Ginger shown) 4oz 45¢* **MP $125**

1902-08 *California Extract (Lemon shown) 16oz $1.75* **MP $175**

1912 *Extract of Terpeneless Lemon 16oz $1.75* **MP $150**

1908 *Concentrated Extract of Terpeneless Lemon Extract 4oz 45¢* **MP $90**
1917 *Extract of Peppermint 2oz 55¢* **MP $60**(N.Y.-Kansas City-San Francisco-Montreal)

1910 *Vanilla, Tonka & Vanillin Sample 1 tsp.* **MP $175**

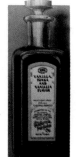
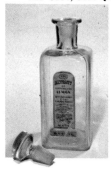
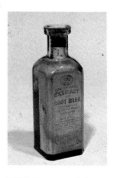
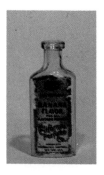
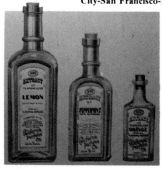
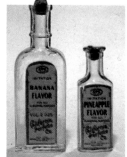

1915-17 *Flavoring Extracts. Vanilla, Tonka & Vanillin (shown) 16oz $3.25* **MP $100** w/glass stopper

1915 *Extract of Terpeneless Lemon 16oz $3.25* **MP $100**

1915 *Extract of Root Beer (rare) 2oz 45¢* **MP $150**

1915-18 *Imitation Banana Flavoring 2oz 25¢* **MP $75**

1915-17 *Flavoring Extracts (Lemon & Peppermint shown) 4oz 45¢, 2oz 25¢* **MP $70 each**
1917 *Extract of Terpeneless Orange 1oz 30¢ (new label address)* **MP $60**

1918 *Imitation Banana Flavoring 2oz 45¢* **MP $60** (N.Y.-Kansas City-S'Francisco-Montreal)
1918 *Imitation Pineapple Flavor 1oz 25¢* **MP $60**

- FLAVORINGS -

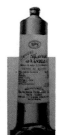
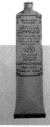
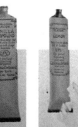
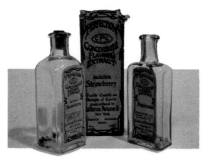
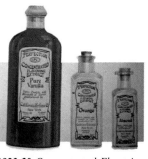
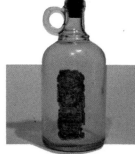

1918 *No-Alcohol Flavoring Compound of Vanilla. Sm. 30¢ Lg. 55¢* **MP $50 each**

1923 *No-Alcohol Flavor, Vanilla Compound large 45¢* **MP $30**

1923 *No-Alcohol Flavor, Lemon shown, small 24¢* **MP $30**

1922 *Imitation Strawberry Flavoring (rare) 4oz 90¢* **MP $125, $150 boxed**
1923 *Flavoring Extract (Peppermint shown) 4oz 90¢* **MP $55**

1923-30 *Concentrated Flavoring Extracts: Qt. $6.25, Pt. $3.25 (shown), 8oz $1.75, 4oz 90¢ (shown), 2oz 45¢ (shown), 1oz 25¢* **MP $55 each, $100 Qt.**

1923 *Flavoring Extract (Orange shown) 1 Qt. $6.25* **MP $125 with mint label**

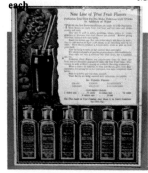
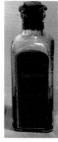
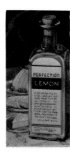
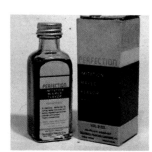
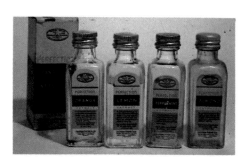

1923 *True Fruit Flavors in Lemon, Loganberry, Orange, Grape, Cherry and Raspberry 2oz 39¢, 4oz 74¢, 8oz $1.44* **MP $55 each, $25 Paper Flyer**

1923 *True Fruit Raspberry Flavor 2oz 39¢, 4oz 74¢, 8oz $1.44* **MP $55**

1930 *Flavoring Extract, shown in Lemon, 2oz 50¢, 4oz 75¢, 8oz $1.45* **MP 25¢ ea.**

1933-34 *Imitation Maple Flavor (An Avon Product/CPC label) 2oz 40¢* **MP $25, $30 boxed**

1934-36 *Flavoring Extract (CPC/Avon, Div.) Orange, Lemon, Peppermint, Almond 2oz 40¢* **MP $20, $25 boxed**

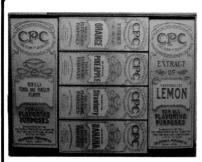 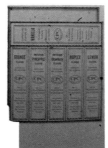 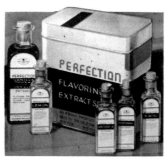 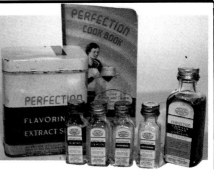

1915 *Box X, Flavoring Extract Set: two 2oz bottles and four 1oz bottles in choice of 18 flavors $1* **MP $460, $70 each bottle**

1918 *Box N.A. No-Alcohol Flavoring Set: 1 lg. tube Vanilla & 5 sm. tubes Orange, Strawberry, Maplex, Pineapple & Lemon flavors $2* **MP $400 boxed sets/Tubes $50 ea**

1930-33 *Flavoring Set. 2oz Vanilla, Tonka & Vanillin, ½oz each Lemon, Wintergreen, Peppermint & Almond Extracts (shown) $1* **MP $175 set. Bottles each $25, metal can $25**

1933-34 *Flavoring Set. Metal can, Recipe Book, 2oz Vanilla, Tonka & Vanillin, ½oz each, Lemon, Wintergreen, Peppermint & Almond Extracts (shown) $1* **MP $170 set. Bottles each $25, metal can MP $25, Cook book MP $20**

FLAVORING SETS

A 1908 catalog states: "CP Flavoring Extracts are not only guaranteed to be the most natural, and the most concentrated flavoring extracts on the market today, but also to be truthfully labelled and put up in full measure bottles.

In the making of the CP Vanilla Extract, only the very highest grade of Mexican Vanilla beans are used.

In the making of the CP Lemon and Orange Extracts, all of the 'terpene' is removed from the oils of lemon and orange before bottling. This 'terpene' is a fatty substance which has absolutely no flavoring properties, and is consequently valueless. The extraction of the terpene also removes a certain bitterness which is sometimes mistaken for strength.

CP Extract of Jamaica Ginger is not only the best possible Ginger for flavoring cakes, etc.; but Jamaica Ginger is also one of the old standby family remedies for stomach-ache, cholic and indigestion."

The first Flavoring Extract Set was introduced in 1915. It consisted of six bottles of flavorings in a choice of 18 different flavors. Some of the unusual flavorings were Celery, Cinnamon, Nutmeg, Onion, Pistachio and Rose.

Flavoring Extract Sets were in the CPC-Avon line until 1947 when they were discontinued.

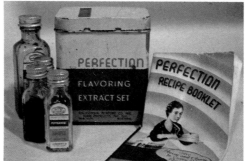 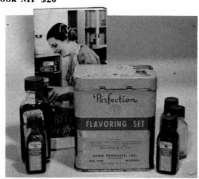

1934-36 *Flavoring Set. (CPC/Avon, Div.) Recipe Booklet, 2oz Vanilla, choice of four ½oz flavorings $1* **MP $150 set. $20 ea. bottle, $20 Recipe Booklet, $20 Metal Can**

1941-47 *Flavoring Set. Recipe Book, 2oz Vanilla, choice of four ½oz flavorings $1* **MP $100 set. $12 ea. bottle, $20 Recipe Book, $15 Metal Can**

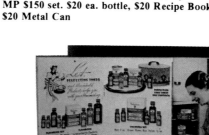 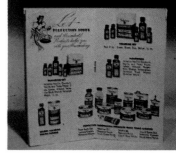

1941-42 *Perfection Recipe Booklet* **MP $20**

1943-47 *Perfection Recipe Booklet, wartime issue (eliminates Olive Oil, Cake Chest & 8oz Vanilla)* **MP $20**

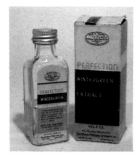 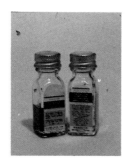 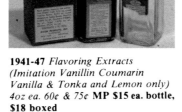 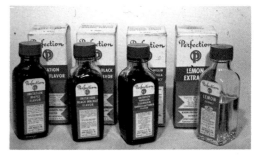

1934 only *Flavoring Extract (An Avon Product/CPC label) Peppermint shown 2oz 40¢* **MP $25, $30 boxed**

1934-36 *Vanilla, Tonka & Vanillin Extract Sample ¼oz* **MP $35**
1939-40 *Imitation Vanillin Coumarin Vanilla & Tonka Extract Sample ¼oz* **MP $35**

1941-47 *Flavoring Extracts (Imitation Vanillin Coumarin Vanilla & Tonka and Lemon only) 4oz ea. 60¢ & 75¢* **MP $15 ea. bottle, $18 boxed**

1941-47 *Food Flavorings: Maple, Black Walnut, Vanilla and Lemon 2oz each (Orange, Wintergreen, Peppermint & Almond not shown) 40¢* **MP $12, $15 boxed**

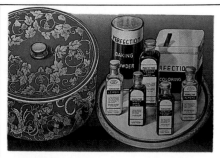

1933-38 *Cake Chest contains 1lb Baking Powder, Coloring Set, 4oz Vanilla Extract & 2oz ea. Lemon, Almond, Maple & Black Walnut Extracts & Cookbook $3.50* **MP $385** *complete and full,* **$50** *Cake Chest only*

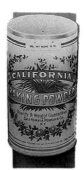

1915-20 *Baking Powder 16oz 55¢* **MP $60**

BAKING POWDER

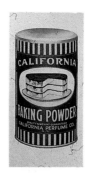

1920-23 *California Baking Powder 16oz 55¢* **MP $70**

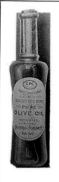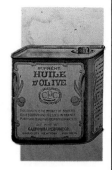

1915 *Olive Oil, table size $1* **MP $125**

1923 *Huile D'Olive pint $1.35* **MP $60**

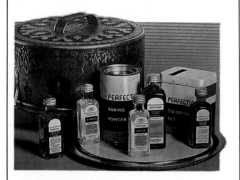

1938-41 *Cake Chest. Same contents as 1933 Set, but newly designed Cake Chest & labeling $3.50* **MP $325** *complete and full,* **$40** *Cake Chest only*

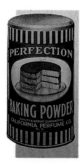

1923-25 *Baking Powder 16oz 45¢* **MP $55**

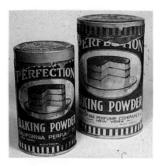

1925-28 *Baking Powder 8oz 24¢* **MP $55**
1928-29 *Baking Powder 16oz 45¢* **MP $60**

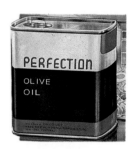

1930-33 *Olive Oil, pint $1.35* **MP $45**

OLIVE OIL

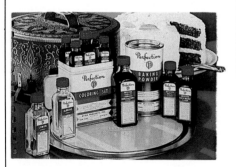

1941-42 *Cake Chest. Same contents as 1938 above but new package design $3.95* **MP $265** *complete,* **$40** *Cake Chest only*

CAKE CHESTS

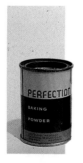

1930-34 *Baking Powder Sample (An Avon Product Label)* **MP $50**

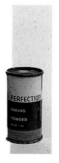

1936-39 *Baking Powder Sample* **MP $50**

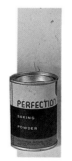

1934-36 *Baking Powder Sample* **MP $50**

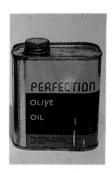

1934-36 *Olive Oil 16oz $1.35* **MP $40** *(Avon Products, Inc., Div. added to label)*

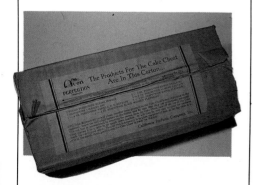

1930's *Avon/Perfection Carton contained all Cake Chest Set contents* **MP $40**

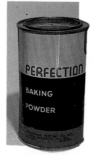

1934-36 *Baking Powder 16oz 45¢* **MP $35** *(1930-34 as above with an Avon Product label)*

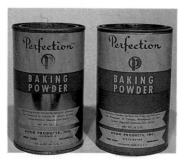

1941-43 *Baking Powder 16oz 45¢* **MP $40**
1943-47 *Baking Powder (wartime issue) 16oz 45¢* **MP $45** *(1947-50 Same as above with Pasadena label)*

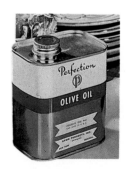

1941 only *Olive Oil, pint $1.35* **MP $50** *(rare)*

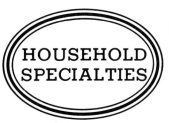

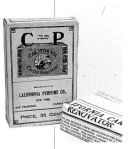

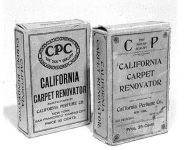

1906-08
Carpet
Renovator
35¢ **MP $85**

1915-20 *Carpet Renovator, 1 cake 35¢*
MP $75
1908-14 *Carpet Renovator, 1 cake 35¢*
MP $80

MACHINE OIL

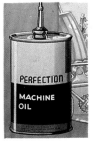

MACHINE OIL-A general purpose lubricant for vacuum cleaners, sewing machines, lawn mowers, typewriters, squeaky doors, automobile springs — wherever metal needs lubrication or protection.

1930-34 *Machine Oil 3oz 25¢* **MP $32 (An Avon Product Label)**

CPC/PERFECTION CLEANERS

In the CPC/Avon line for more than 60 years, this cleaner was the first CPC household product introduced and one of the last Perfection products to be discontinued.

1893 *It was manufactured under the name of* **California Carpet Renovator,** *because that was its original purpose.*

1898 *The catalog relates that* **California Carpet Renovator** *is also an excellent cleaner for curtains, blankets, fine dresses, woodwork, furniture, window shades and patent leather shoes. One cake provides two gallons cleaning solution.*

1908 *The Catalog refers to the product now as* **CP Renovator,** *a preparation for cleaning and brightening many articles. Put up like a cake of soap with directions on the wrapper of each cake.*

1920 *Because of WWI,* **C P Renovator** *is discontinued, then re-introduced in* **1925** *under the name of* **Easy Cleaner.** *Newly designed packaging, featuring the* **E-Z Maid** *girl, contains two cakes of soap.*

1928 *Both the original product form and name is changed to* **Avon Powdered Cleaner.** *New blue packaging features* **Avon Maid,** *but continues to carry the oval CPC logo.*

1930 *Product is issued in a canister-designed package and the cottage* **Avon** *logo replaced the CPC oval.*

1933 **Avon Powdered Cleaner** *joins the* **Perfection** *line in brown, white and orange packaging.*

1941 *Packaging is again updated as a circled* **P** *logo replaces Avon on the label.* **Perfection Powdered Cleaner** *remained in the line until* **1957** *when it was discontinued.*

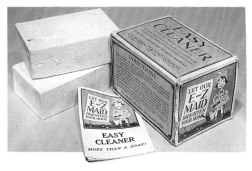

1924-28 *Easy Cleaner Naptha Bar Soaps, two ½lb cakes 33¢* **MP $100 boxed,** *Easy Cleaner Folder* **MP $25**

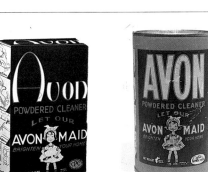
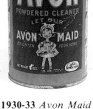

1928-30 *Avon Maid Powdered Cleaner (with CPC oval) 12oz 25¢* **MP $80**

1930-33 *Avon Maid Powdered Cleaner 16oz 35¢* **MP $75**

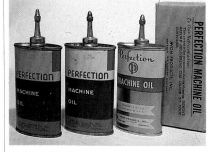

1934-36 *Machine Oil 3oz 26¢* **MP $28, $35 boxed**
1936-39 *Machine Oil 3oz 26¢* **MP $25, $32 boxed** *(Avon Prod. Div. label)*
1941-42 only *Machine Oil 3oz 26¢* **MP $35, $42 boxed**

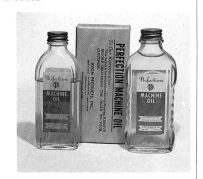

1943-44 *Machine Oil 3oz 29¢* **MP $35, $40 boxed**
1944-48 *Machine Oil 3oz 29¢* **MP $30, $35 boxed**

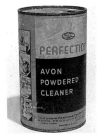

1936 only *Powdered Cleaner 16oz 35¢* **MP $65**

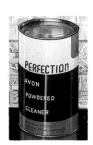

1933-34 *Powdered Cleaner 16oz 35¢* **MP $45** *(An Avon Product Label)*

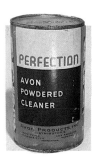

1939-41 *Powdered Cleaner (Los Angeles added to label) 16oz 35¢* **MP $50**

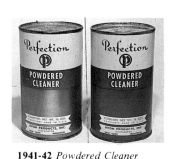

1941-42 *Powdered Cleaner (Montreal label) 16oz 35¢* **MP $40**
1947-57 *Powdered Cleaner 16oz 39¢* **MP $20** *(Pasadena label)*

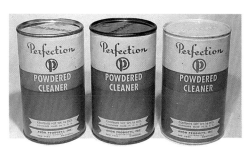

1942-47 *Powder Cleaners 16oz, issued with silver, bronze or white lid 35¢* **MP $25 each**

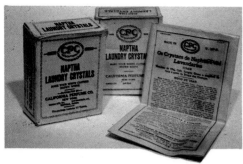

1914-18 *Naptha Laundry Crystals, 13 per box 25¢*
MP $60
1920 *Naptha Laundry Crystals, 13 per box (Gold Medal Award on box & folder in German, English, Spanish, French, Italian & Portuguese) 25¢*
MP $50, $25 Folder

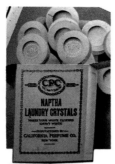

1918-20 *Naptha Laundry Crystals, 13 per box 25¢* **MP $50**

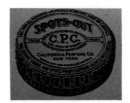

1918-21 *Spots-Out ½lb 35¢, 1lb 65¢* **MP $75**

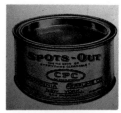

1921-29 *Spots-Out ½lb 33¢, 1lb 59¢* **MP $50**

SPOTS OUT
Spots Out was a cleansing paste used to remove dirt, grease and other spots from anything that was washable — especially recommended for cleaning the upholstery of automobiles. It was not harmful to hands because it was free from acids, grit, sand or caustic materials.

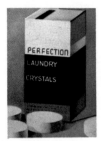
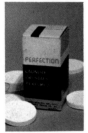

1930-33 *Laundry Crystals 13 per box 25¢* **MP $45**

1936-39 *Laundry Crystals Perfumed 25¢* **MP $30 (Avon Products, Inc. Div.)**

LAUNDRY CRYSTALS

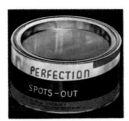

1930-33 *Spots-Out ½lb 40¢* **MP $25 (An Avon Product)**

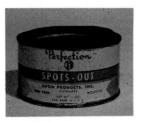

1941-42 *Spots-Out (Montreal label) ½lb 40¢* **MP $40**
1947-50 *Spots-Out, as above (Pasadena label)* **MP $20**

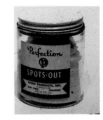

1943-47 *Spots-Out 9½oz 45¢* **MP $32**

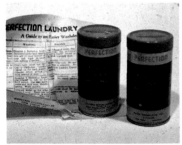

1934-36 *Laundry Crystals Perfumed, 13 per box 25¢* **MP $35 (CPC/Avon Div.)**
1939-40 *Laundry Crystals Perfumed 13 per box 25¢* **MP $25 (Avon Products, Inc., Dist.)**
1930's-40's *Laundry Guide Folder* **MP $20**

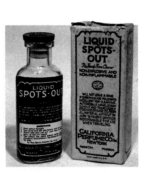

1925-29 *Liquid Spots-Out 4oz 37¢* **MP $45, $55 boxed**

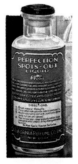

1929 only *Spots-Out Liquid 4oz 50¢* **MP $45**

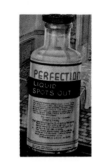

1930-33 *Liquid Spots-Out 4oz 50¢* **MP $40 (CPC on lid)**

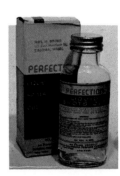

1933-34 *Liquid Spots-Out 4oz 40¢* **MP $40, $50 boxed**

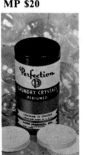
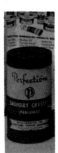

1941-42 *Laundry Crystals (perfumed) 13 per box 25¢* **MP $30**

1943-47 *Laundry Crystals (perfumed) 13 per box 29¢* **MP $30**

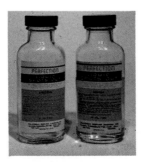

1934-35 *Liquid Spots-Out 4oz 40¢* **MP $35**
1936 *Liquid Spots-Out 4oz 40¢* **MP $40**

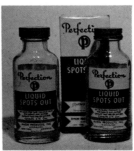

1941-42 *Liquid Spots-Out (smooth lid) 4oz 40¢* **MP $40**
1943-47 *Liquid Spots-Out (Montreal label) 4oz 50¢* **MP $25, $30 boxed**
1947-57 *Liquid Spots-Out (Pasadena label) 4oz 50¢* **MP $20, $25 boxed**

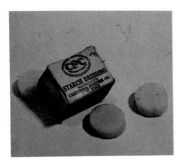

1911 *Starch Dressing Sample.*
MP $50

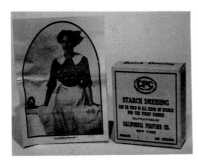

1911-15 *Starch Dressing, 25 tablets 25¢*
MP $70, Folder MP $15

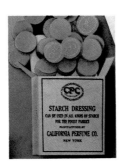

1915-20 *Starch Dressing, 25 tablets 25¢* **MP $50**

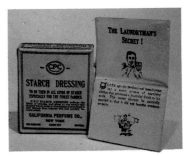

1920-23 *Starch Dressing (with S 'Francisco on label) 25 tablets 33¢* **MP $45, $15 Folder**

STARCH

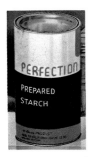

1930-33 *Prepared Starch 6oz 35¢* **MP $40 (An Avon Product)**

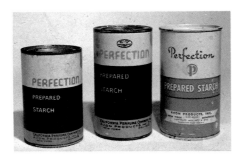

1934-36 *Prepared Starch 6oz 35¢* **MP $35**
1936 only *Prepared Starch 8oz 35¢* **MP $35** (Avon Products, Inc., Div.)
1943-45 *Prepared Starch 8oz cardboard 39¢* **MP $25**

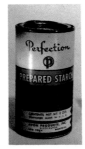

1941-43, then 1946-47 *Prepared Starch 8oz 35¢* **MP $20**

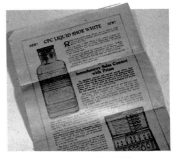

1926 *Representative's Flyer introducing new Liquid Shoe White* **MP $25**

SHOE WHITE

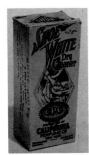

1918-20 *Shoe-White Dry Cleaner 25¢* **MP $100 boxed**

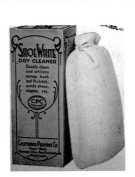

1920 *Shoe White Dry CLeaner 5oz 25¢* **MP $75 boxed**

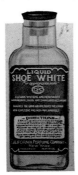

1926 *Liquid Shoe White 4oz 35¢* **MP $55**

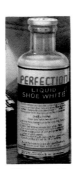

1930 *Liquid Shoe White 4oz 50¢* **MP $50**

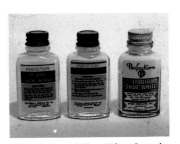

1934-35 *Liquid Shoe White Sample 4/5oz* **MP $40**
1935-36 *Liquid Shoe White Sample 4/5oz* **MP $40**
1941-42 *Liquid Shoe White Sample 4/5oz* **MP $50**

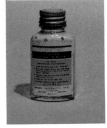

1939-40 *Liquid Shoe White Sample 4/5oz* **MP $40**

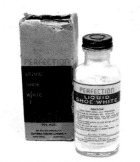

1932-33 *Liquid Shoe White 4oz 50¢* **MP $45, $50 boxed (An Avon Product)**

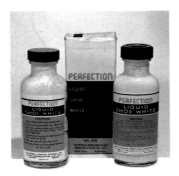

1934-36 *Liquid Shoe White (different labels & lids) 4oz 50¢* **MP $40, $45 boxed (CPC/Avon Products, Inc., Div.)**

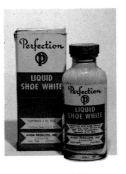

1941-42 *Liquid Shoe White (smooth lid) 4oz 37¢* **MP $20, $23 boxed**

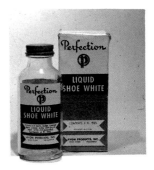

1947-57 *Liquid Shoe White 4oz 39¢* **MP $20, $23 boxed (Pasadena label)**

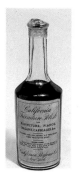 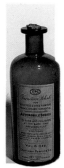 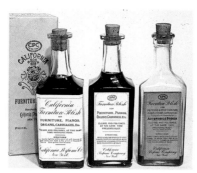 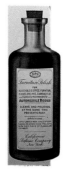 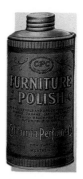 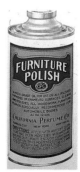 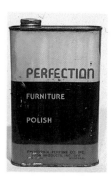

1908-10 *Furniture Polish 8oz 50¢* **MP $160**

1919 *Furniture Polish, rare amber bottle 8oz 60¢* **MP $160. $125 clear glass**

1910 *Furniture Polish 8oz 50¢* **MP $160 $180 boxed**
1915 *Furniture Polish 8oz 50¢* **MP $150**
1918 *Furniture Polish 8oz 50¢* **MP $135**

1918-20 *Furniture Polish 8oz 60¢* **MP $125**

1916-17 & 1921-24 *Furniture Polish, lg. 48¢, qt. $1.20* **MP $60**, *½ gal $2.25* **MP $75**

1927 *Furniture Polish 12oz 48¢, qt. $1.20* **MP $50 each**

1934-36 *Furniture Polish 1 qt. $1.15* **MP $65** *(CPC/Avon label)*

FURNITURE POLISH

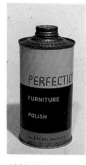 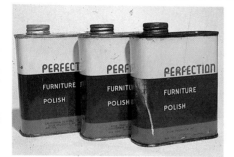 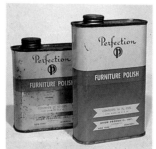 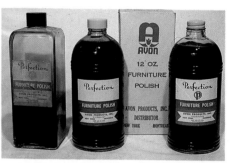

1930-33 *Furniture Polish 12oz 75¢, qt. $1.25* **MP $35** *(An Avon Product)*

1934-36 *Furniture Polish 12oz 75¢* **MP $35** *(CPC/Avon label)*
1936-39 *Furniture Polish 12oz 75¢* **MP $30** *(Avon/CPC label)*
1939-40 *Furniture Polish 12oz 75¢* **MP $30** *(Avon, Dist. label)*

1941-42 *Furniture Polish 12oz 60¢ (rare)* **MP $45** *(Montreal label)*
1942 only *Furniture Polish 16oz $1.29* **MP $45**

1943-44 *Furniture Polish 12oz 69¢* **MP $45**
1944-45 *Furniture Polish (plastic cap) 12oz 69¢* **MP $45, $50 boxed**
1946-47 *Furniture Polish (metal cap) 12oz 69¢* **MP $45, $50 boxed**

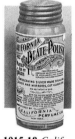 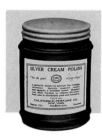 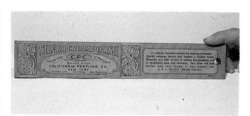 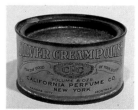 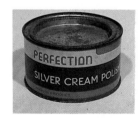

1915-18 *California Plate Polish 4oz 35¢* **MP $90**
1902-15 *(not shown) Same container, no oz. on front 25¢* **MP $150**

1919 *Silver Cream, 6oz Polish 30¢* **MP $65**

1920-22 *Silver Cream Polish, Manufacturer's sample label* **MP $35**

1922-29 *Silver Cream Polish 8oz 30¢, 16oz 54¢* **MP $50**

1930-33 *Silver Cream Polish 8oz 35¢* **MP $30** *(An Avon Product)*

SILVER POLISH

MENDING CEMENT

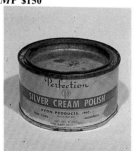 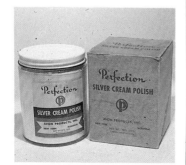 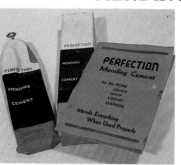 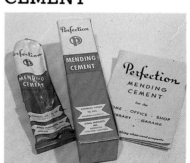

1941-42 *Silver Cream Polish ½lb 35¢* **MP $25**
1947-51 *As above, (Pasadena label)* **MP $20**
1951-53 *In glass (not shown) 8oz 49¢* **MP $25**

1943-47 *Silver Cream Polish (wartime pkg.) 10½oz 49¢* **MP $30, $38 boxed**

1933-41 *Mending Cement, large tube 25¢* **MP $20, $25 boxed, Flyer MP $10**

1941-47 *Mending Cement 25¢* **MP $12, $15 boxed, Flyer MP $5**
1947-50 *As above (Pasadena label) 29¢* **MP $12**

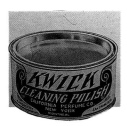 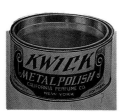

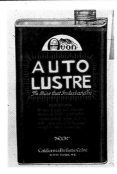 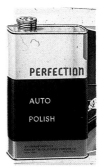 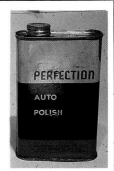

1922 *Kwick Cleaning Polish ½lb 24¢, 1lb 45¢* **MP $50**

1928-30 *Kwick Metal Polish ½lb 24¢* **MP $40**

1929 *Auto Lustre Sample (rare)* **MP $100**

1929-33 *Auto Lustre 16oz 75¢* **MP $75**

1933 *Auto Polish 8oz 75¢* **MP $55 with short issue label**

1934-36 *Auto Polish 16oz 75¢* **MP $40**

KWICK METAL

AUTO POLISH

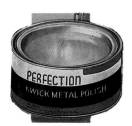 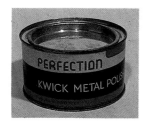 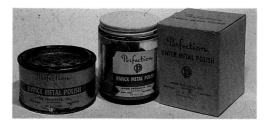 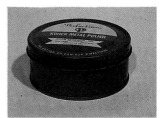

1930-33 *Kwick Metal Polish ½lb 35¢* **MP $35 (An Avon Product)**

1933-34 *Kwick Metal Polish ½lb 35¢* **MP $35**

1941-42 *Kwick Metal Polish ½lb 35¢* **MP $25**
1943-46 *Kwick Metal Polish (wartime pkg.) 8oz 39¢* **MP $35, $40 boxed**

1946-47 *Kwick Metal Polish 13oz (rare)* **MP $75 (Montreal label)**

MOTHICIDE

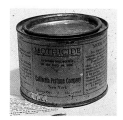 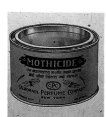 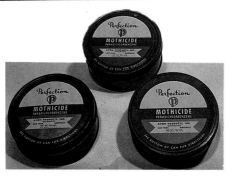 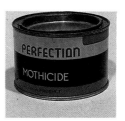 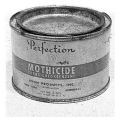

1923-26 *Mothicide ½lb 48¢* **MP $40**

1926-30 *Mothicide ½lb 48¢* **MP $40**

1946-47 *Mothicide, shown with 3 different lids, 8½oz 55¢* **MP $30 each**

1933-34 *Mothicide ½lb 50¢* **MP $35**

1941-42 *Mothicide ½lb 50¢* **MP $40**

MOTH PROOFER

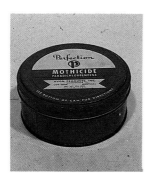 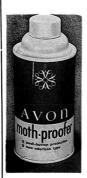 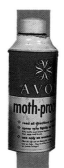 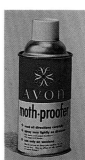 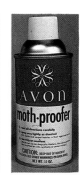

1942-46 *Mothicide (wartime pkg.) 8oz 55¢* **MP $30, $45 boxed with folder. $7 folder only**

1947-48 *Mothicide 8½oz 55¢* **MP $28**
1948-58 *Mothicide, as above (Pasadena label)* **MP $22**

1956 *Avon moth-proofer 12oz $1.89* **MP $10**
1960 *(same can 11oz) $1.89* **MP $12**
1961 *Avon moth-proofer 11oz $1.89* **MP $5**
1963 *Avon moth-proofer 11oz $1.89* **MP $5**
1967 *Avon moth-proofer 11oz $1.89* **MP $4**

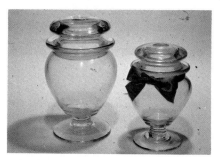

1914-21 *Lavender Fragrance Jar 6¾" high*
$4.25 complete **MP $155**
1921-34 *American Beauty Fragrance Jar*
$2.95 **MP $130**

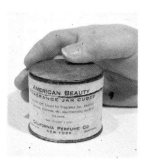

1923 *American Beauty*
Fragrance Jar Cubes 48¢
MP $50

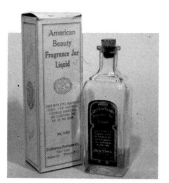

1923 *American Beauty*
Fragrance Jar, Liquid 4oz 96¢
MP $115, $140 boxed

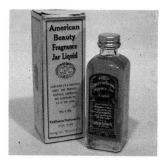

1925 *American Beauty*
Fragrance Jar Liquid 4oz 96¢
MP $100, $125 boxed

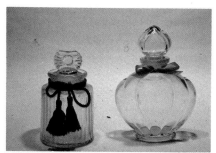

1934-42 *American Beauty Fragrance Jar,*
complete $2.75 **MP $100**
1948 *Fragrance Jar, Clear stopper $3.50*
MP $75 (short issue)

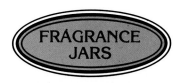

FRAGRANCE JARS

CPC/Avon Fragrance Jars are among Avon's finest designs. A combination of scented liquid and ammoniated cubes created a pleasing fragrance — they were also used for faintness and dizziness.

In 1943, because of Suffern's heavy war production, the 1934 Fragrance Jar was discontinued. No sales catalogs were issued from 1943 to 1946, instead revised price lists were provided and were added by the Representative to her 1942 catalog.

The 1945 pottery Jar insert page shows the lid with white roses and green leaves. Porosity caused the discontinuance of the Jar in May 1945. It was reissued in 1946 with white roses and white leaves on the lid and was discontinued a short time later. Since few of the 1943-1946 insert pages were kept, pictures of the pink ceramic jars are now quite rare

A heart-shaped Jar was introduced for Christmas 1948. Because moisture collected in the clear glass stopper — in 1949 a frosted stopper appeared to improve the appearance. The beautiful Rose Fragrance Jar remained in the line until the late 1950's. Although the Fragrance Jar was not pictured in Avon's 1957 catalog, it was sold until 1958 when stock was depleted.

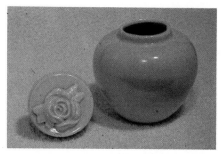

1946 *Rose Fragrance Jar, all white lid $2.95*
MP $90

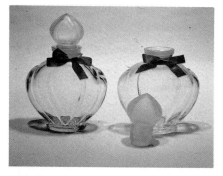

1949 *Rose Fragrance Jar, translucent frosted*
lid $3.50 **MP $50**
1951 *Rose Fragrance Jar, frosted lid $3.50*
MP $35

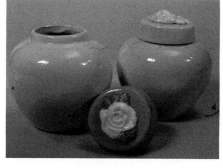

1945 *Rose Fragrance Jar, rose top, green*
leaves $2.95 **MP $85**
1946 *Rose Fragrance Jar, pink top, white*
leaves $2.95 **MP $75**

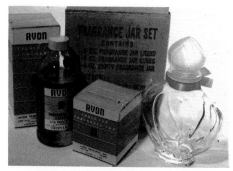

1949 *Fragrance Jar Set $3.50* **MP $95**
1949 *Refill Liquid 6oz $1.39* **MP $20**
1949 *Refill Cubes 3oz 85¢* **MP $20**

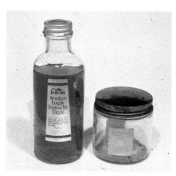

1934-36 *American Beauty Fragrance*
Jar Liquid 6oz $1.25 **MP $45**
1939-41 *American Beauty Fragrance*
Jar Cubes 3oz 75¢ **MP $35**

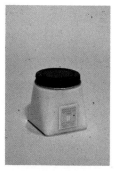

1937-39 *American*
Beauty Fragrance Jar
Cubes 3oz 75¢ **MP $25**

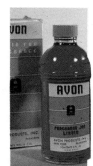

1937-53
Fragrance Jar
Liquid 6oz $1.25
MP $20, $25
boxed

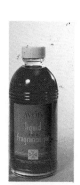

1954-58
Rose
Fragrance
Liquid 6oz
$1.39 **MP $18**

Dorothy Bernard's

CPC/AVON LABEL DATING GUIDE:

Until an established CPC/Avon product was re-issued in newly designed packaging, its original catalog picture (called a pick-up) was shown in succeeding catalogs for a period of sometimes several years. This is notably apparent, for example, in the Perfection Line. Because of this, the CPC and Avon Catalogs through the 1950's fail to reveal the many different label changes that took place over the years. Labels serve an important function in helping to date CPC/Avon bottles within a particular time period.

1886-88 CALIFORNIA PERFUME COMPANY
New York

1888-98 As Above
(with Eureka Trademark)

1898-04 CALIFORNIA PERFUME COMPANY
New York-San Francisco-Dallas

1904-11 CALIFORNIA PERFUME COMPANY
New York-San Francisco-Kansas City
(with CP logo circled within Eureka TM)

1911-15 CALIFORNIA PERFUME COMPANY
New York-San Francisco-Kansas City
(with oval CPC logo)

1915-23 CALIFORNIA PERFUME COMPANY
New York-San Francisco-Kansas City-Montreal

1923-27 CALIFORNIA PERFUME COMPANY
New York-Kansas City-Montreal

1927-30 CALIFORNIA PERFUME COMPANY, INC.
New York-Montreal

1930-34 CALIFORNIA PERFUME COMPANY, INC.
New York-Montreal
(with Cottage "A" logo)

1934-36 CALIFORNIA PERFUME COMPANY, INC.
AVON PRODUCTS, INC., DIV.
New York-Montreal

1936-39 AVON PRODUCTS, INC., DIV.
CALIFORNIA PERFUME CO., INC.
New York-Montreal
(with Tulip "A" logo)

1939-47 AVON PRODUCTS, INC., DIST. OR DISTRIBUTOR
New York-Montreal

1947-51 AVON PRODUCTS, INC., DIST.
New York-Pasadena

1951-57 AVON PRODUCTS, INC.
New York-Pasadena

1957-67 AVON PRODUCTS, INC.
New York, N.Y.

1967-72 AVON PRODUCTS, INC.
New York, N.Y. 10020

1972... AVON PRODUCTS, INC.
New York, N.Y. 10019

Note: The Home Office location appears on all packaging, either New York, or N.Y., depending upon label space. Very early labels may also carry the 126 Chambers Street address. Occasionally, when space was adequate, a few bottle labels and Perfection containers listed an added Branch office. Luzerne may be seen on 1915-1934 labels and Los Angeles 1939-47. Boxes most always listed all Branch offices.
(See Perfection Guide pg. 34)

1888-1904

1904-1911

1911-1930

1929

1930-1936

1936-53

1940's

1953

1976

1978...

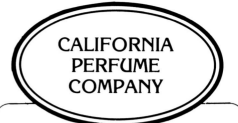

Dorothy Bernard's
CPC FRAGRANCE DATING GUIDE

1886 *Heliotrope (discontinued 1928)*
Hyacinth (1922)(re-intro 1974)
Lily of the Valley (1954)(re-intro 1963)
Violet (1928)(re-intro 1972)
White Rose (1940)

1890 *Orange Blossom (1895)*
Oriental (1895)

1890-96 *Bay Rum (1950)(re-intro 1962)*
Carnation (1930)
Crab Apple Blossom (1930)
Eau de Cologne (1925)
Florida Water (1922)
Lavender (1925)(re-intro 1939)
Lou Lillie (1910)
Sweet Cologne (1916)
Sweet Pea (1925)
White Heliotrope (1920)

1896-98 *L'Odeur de Violette (1920)*
Le Parfum des Roses (1920)
Musk (1925)
Peau d' Espagne (1920)
White Lilac (1925)

1900 *Bouquet Marie (1910)*
Frangipani (1910)
Golf Club (1910)
Golf Violet (1922)
Jack Rose (1922)
Jockey Club (1925)
Marie Stuart (1910)(also spelled Stewart)
May Blossom (1910)
New Mown Hay (1922)
Rose Geranium (1925)(re-intro 1942)
Stephanotis (1910)
Trailing Arbutus (1948)
Tube Rose (1912)
Venetian Carnation (1925)
Ylang, Ylang (1910)

1905 *California Bouquet (1922)*
Treffle (1920)

1906 *Roses (1925)*

1907 *American Ideal (1935)(re-intro 1941)*

1910 *Honeysuckle (1925)(re-intro 1966)*

1914 *Natoma Rose (1925)*

1916 *Daphne (1928)*

1922 *Mission Garden (1928)*

1923 *Vernafleur (1940)*

1925 *Lilac Vegetal (1936)(renamed Lilac 1936)*
Narcissus (1940)

1926 *Jardin d' Amour (1939)*
(renamed Garden of Love 1939)

(For Avon Fragrance Line, dating see: Women's and Girl's pg. 46, Men's pg. 214)

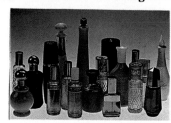

Dorothy Bernard's
FRAGRANCE DATING GUIDE FOR WOMEN and GIRLS

1929 *Ariel*

1930 *391 Perfume (renamed Bolero 1934)*

1934 *Bolero*
Cotillion
Gardenia (re-intro 1972)
Jasmine

1935 *Pine*
Rose (formerly Roses)
Topaze (re-intro 1959)

1936 *Lucy Hays (Mrs. McConnell's maiden name)*
Lilac (re-intro 1963 — formerly Lilac Vegetal)

1937 *Courtship*

1938 *Marionette*

1939 *Ballad*
Garden of Love (formerly Jardin d'Amour)

1940 *Sonnet (re-intro 1972)*

1941 *American Ideal, changed to Apple Blossom same year (re-intro 1974)*

1942 *Attention*
Orchard Blossom
Rose Geranium

1945 *White Moire*

1946 *Crimson Carnation*
Here's My Heart (re-intro 1957)

1947 *Golden Promise*
Swan Lake
Wishing (re-intro 1963)

1948 *Happy Hours*
Quaintance

1949 *Flowertime*

1950 *Luscious*
To A Wild Rose

1951 *Forever Spring*

1952 *Young Hearts (for Girls)*

1954 *Bright Night*

1955 *Nearness*
Merriment (for Girls)

1956 *Elegante*
Persian Wood (first Avon Aerosol Cologne)
Daisies Won't Tell (for Girls)

1957 *Here's My Heart*
Floral

1959 *Topaze*

1960 *Buttons 'n Bows (for Girls)*

1961 *Somewhere*
Skin-So-Soft (Bath line)

1962 *Occur!*

1963 *Wishing*
Lilac
Lily of the Valley

All products of the same fragrance and package design are found under the proper name unique to that particular line.

1964 *Pretty Peach (for Girls)*
Rapture

1965 *Hawaiian White Ginger*
Unforgettable

1966 *Honeysuckle*
Regence

1967 *Blue Lotus*
Brocade
Miss Lollypop (for Girls)

1968 *Charisma*
Silk & Honey (Bath Line)

1969 *Bird of Paradise*
Elusive
Her Prettiness (for Girls)
Lemon Velvet
Lights and Shadows
Patterns
Strawberry (Bath line)

1970 *Hana Gasa*
Sea Garden (Bath line)
Small World (for Girls)

1971 *Field Flowers*
Moonwind

1972 *Carnation*
Flower Talk (for Girls)
Gardenia
Mineral Springs (Bath line)
Roses, Roses
Sonnet
Violet

1973 *Imperial Garden*
Patchwork
Raining Violets
Sweet Honesty

1974 *Apple Blossom*
Hyacinth
Magnolia
Pink & Pretty (for Girls)
Timeless

1975 *Come Summer*
Queen's Gold
Unspoken

1976 *Emprise*

1977 *Ariane*
Candid
Delicate Daisies (for Girls)

1978 *Blue Tranquility (Bath line)*
Frivolie (Bath line)
Sun Blossoms
Tempo

1979 *Hello Sunshine (for Girls)*
Tasha
Zany

1980 *Country Breeze*
Foxfire
Shower 'Scape (Bath line)
Sportif
Wild Jasmine

1981 *Little Blossom (for Girls)*
Odyssey
Toccaro

1982 *Soft Musk*
Fantasque

1983 *Light Accents*
(Willow, Tea Garden, Amber Mist)
Pavi Elle

1984 *Pearls & Lace*
Vivage

(See Page 45 for CPC Fragrance Guide......
Page 214 for Men's Fragrance Guide)

AVON FRAGRANCE LINES

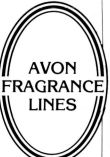
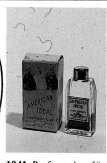

1941 *Perfume 1oz 20¢ introductory, then 75¢ (sold only 4 months)* **MP $100, $140 boxed**

AMERICAN IDEAL

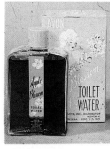
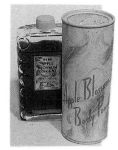

1941 *Toilet Water 2 oz $1.04* **MP $40, $50 boxed**

1941 *Cologne 6oz $1* **MP $80**
1941 *Body Powder 5oz 65¢ MP $26*

APPLE BLOSSOM

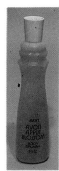
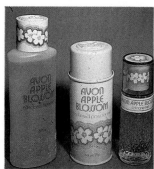

1977 *Body Splash 8oz $5* **MP 50¢**

1974 *After Bath Freshener 8oz $4* **MP 75¢**
1974 *Powder Mist 7oz $4* **MP $1**
1974 *Cologne Mist 2oz $4.25* **MP $1.25**

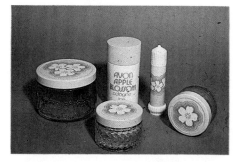

1974 *Cologne Gelee 3 oz $4* **MP $1**
1978 *Cologne Ice 1 oz $3.75* **MP $1**
1974 *DemiStik .19 oz $1.75* **MP 50¢**
1975 *Cream Sachet .66 oz $3* **MP 50¢**
1974 *Cream Sachet .66oz $2.50* **MP $1.25**

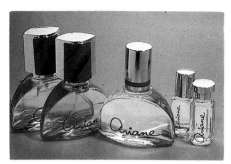

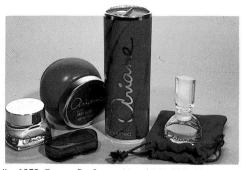

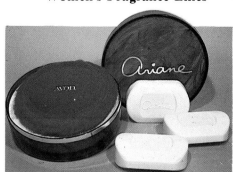

1977 *Cologne Spray 1.8oz marked "First Edition."*
Sold only at sales meetings. *$7.50* **MP $8**
1977 *Cologne Spray 1.8oz $7.50* **MP $9***
1978 *Cologne 2oz $6.50* **MP $1**
1978 *Purse Concentre .33oz $4* **MP $1**
1977 *Cologne .33oz $3* **MP $1**

1978 *Creme Perfume .66oz $4.50* **MP 50¢**
1978 *Skin Softener 5oz $6* **MP $3***
1978 *Talc 3.5oz* **MP $3***
1977 *Perfume 1/4oz $15* **MP $10**
1977 *Solid Perfume Compact .2oz $3.75* **MP $1**

1977 *Beauty Dust 6oz $8.50* **MP $3**
1978 *Boxed Soaps, three 3oz cakes $7* **MP $5**

Ariane

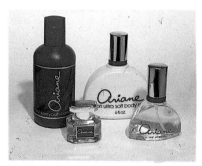

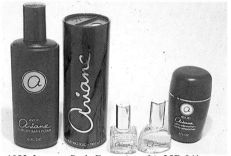

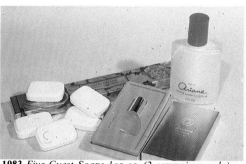

1979 *Bath Foam 6 oz $5.50* **MP 50¢**
1979 *Light Perfume .5 oz $7* **MP $1**
1979 *Soft Body Satin 6oz $5* **MP 50¢**
1979 *Cologne Spray 1oz $7* **MP $6***

1982 *Luxury Bath Foam 6 oz $6,* **MP $4***
1982 *Bonus Size Talc 5 1/4 oz (1 campaign only)*
$3.50 **MP $1**
1981 *Cologne .33 oz $4* **MP $1**
1982 *Cologne .33oz $4.50* **MP $2.50***
1982 *Ultra Sensation Body Smoother 3oz $6*
MP $5*

1983 *Five Guest Soaps 1oz ea. (2 campaigns only)*
$6 **MP $4**
1983 *Light & Lavish Cologne 6oz $7.50*
MP $6*
1983 *Perfume .33oz $13* **MP $11***
(See also Awards pg. 295)

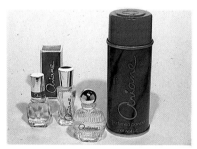

1978 *Cologne .33oz $3* **MP $1.50**
1979 *Cologne .33oz $3* **MP $1**
1980 *Cologne .33oz $3.50* **MP $1**
1979 *Powder Mist 4oz $5* **MP $3***

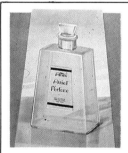

1929 *Perfume 1oz*
$2.50 **MP $125,**
$150 boxed

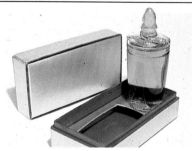

1929 *Toilet Water 2oz $1.75*
MP $115, $145 boxed

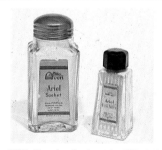

1929 *Powder Sachet 78¢* **MP $60**
1933 *Bath Salts Sample* **MP $75**

ARIEL

Attention

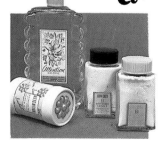

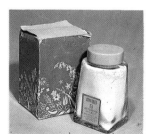

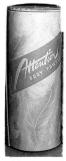

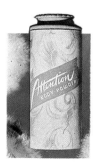

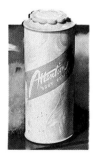

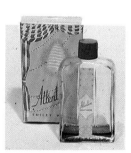

1943 *Cologne 6oz $1* **MP $80**
1944-45 *Sachet, cardboard*
1 1/4oz $1.15 **MP $20**
1943 *only Sachet 1 1/4oz $1.15* **MP $28**
1942-47 *Sachet 1 1/4oz $1.15* **MP $20**

1943 only *Sachet 1 1/4oz*
57¢ **MP $35 in 57th**
Anniversary box

1944-46 *Body*
Powder 5oz
65¢ **MP $25**

1943 only *Body*
Powder 5oz
65¢ **MP $30**

1947 only *Body*
Powder 5oz
65¢ **MP $30**

1942 only *Toilet Water*
2 oz $1.04 **MP $45**
$60 in Xmas Box

*Available from Avon at time of publication

Bird of Paradise

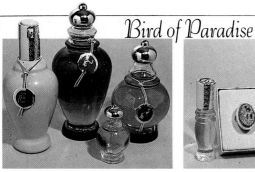

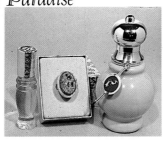

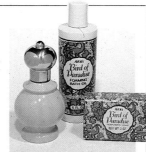

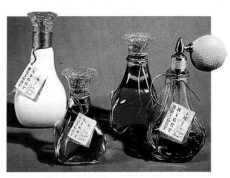

1969 Cologne Fluff 3oz $5 MP $3
1969 Emollient Oils 6 oz $5 MP $4
1969 Cologne 4 oz $5 MP $3
1970 Half-ounce Cologne $1.75
MP $2

1970 Rollette .33 oz $3 MP $1.50
1970 Perfume Glace Ring $10
MP $10
1970 Cologne Mist 3 oz $6 MP $1

1976 Cologne Spray 2.7 oz
$7 MP $2
1974 Foaming Bath Oil 6 oz
$5 MP $1
1975 Soap 3 oz $1.25 MP $1

1958 Cologne Mist 3 oz $2.75 MP $24
1955 Toilet Water 2 oz $2 MP $22
1955 Cologne 4 oz $2.50 MP $22
1955 Cologne w/Atomizer 4 oz $3.50 MP $36

(See also Awards pg. 308)

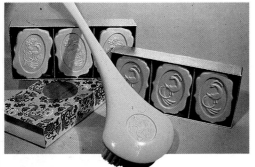

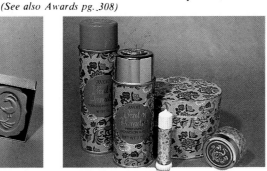

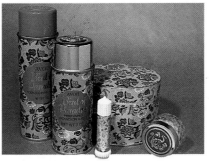

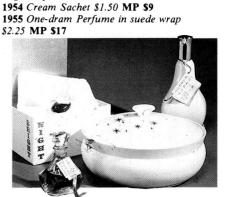

1972 Boxed Soap, three 3 oz cakes with embossed
flowers $4 MP $6
1970 Boxed Soap, three 3 oz cakes, no flowers
$4 MP $7
1970 Bath Brush and 5 oz Soap $6 MP $9

1971 Hair Spray 7 oz $1.50 MP $4
1971 Powder Mist 7 oz $4 MP $2
1974 DemiStik .19 oz $2 MP 50¢
1969 Beauty Dust 6 oz $5 MP $5
1975 Cream Sachet .66 oz $3 MP $1

1955 Powder Sachet .9 oz $1.50 MP $13
Also 1¼ and 1½oz (rare) MP $25
1955 Rare issue of Powder Sachet with
ridged cap $1.50 MP $22
1954 Cream Sachet $1.50 MP $9
1955 One-dram Perfume in suede wrap
$2.25 MP $17

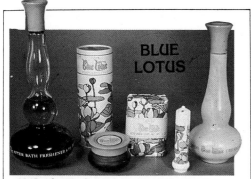

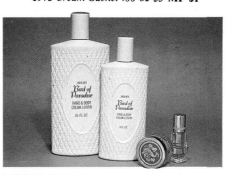

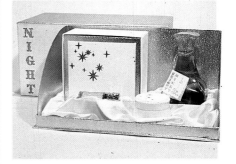

1971 Perfumed Talc 3½ oz $1.35 MP 50¢
1970 Cream Sachet .66 oz $3 MP $1
1972 Emollient Mist 4 oz $3 MP $2
1971 Foaming Bath Oil 6 oz $4 MP $2
1971 Perfumed Skin Softener 5 oz $4 MP $4

1974 Hand & Body Cream Lotion 16oz $5
MP $1
1972 Hand & Body Cream Lotion 8oz $3 MP $1
1979 Creme Perfume .66oz $3.50 MP $1
1979 Purse Concentre .33oz $3 MP $1

1956 Beauty Dust 8 oz in hinged box with
bow-tied ⅝ dram fragrance $2.50 MP $40
1954 Gift Perfume with crystal stopper and
neck tag ½ oz $7.50 MP $90
1959 Beauty Dust 6 oz $2.95 MP $14
1958 Cologne Mist 3 oz $2.75 MP $21

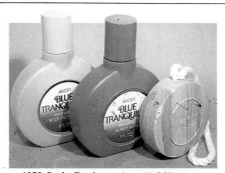

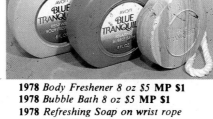

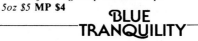

BLUE LOTUS

1967 After Bath Freshener 6 oz $3 MP $5
1970 Talc 3½ oz $1.10 MP $3
1969 Cream Sachet .66oz $2.50 MP $2
1969 Soap 3oz 49¢ MP $4
1969 DemiStik $1.50 MP $2
1969 Cream Lotion 5oz $2 MP $2

1978 Body Freshener 8 oz $5 MP $1
1978 Bubble Bath 8 oz $5 MP $1
1978 Refreshing Soap on wrist rope
5oz $5 MP $4

BLUE TRANQUILITY

1955 Melody Set. Beauty Dust 8oz,
Cologne 4oz, Cream Sachet & 1 dram
Perfume $8.75 MP $100

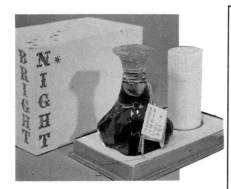

1956 Magic Hours Set. 2oz Toilet Water and Cologne Stick $3.50 MP $50

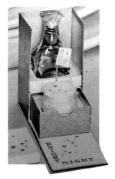

1957 Bright Night Gem Set. Toilet Water 2 oz and Cream Sachet $3.50 MP $45

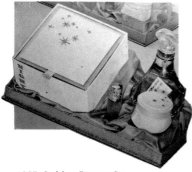

1957 Golden Beauty Set. Contains same items as Melody Set (p. 48) $8.95 MP $90

B R I G H T   N I G H T

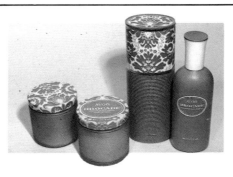

1968 *Skin Softener 5 oz $4 MP* **$4**
1968 *Skin Softener 5 oz $4 MP* **$10**
1968 *Cologne Mist 3 oz refillable $6 MP* **$4**
1967 *Cologne Mist Refill 3 oz $4 MP* **$3**

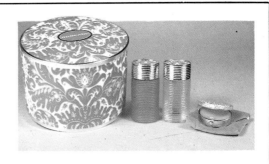

1971 *Beauty Dust 6 oz $5 MP* **$5**
1968 *Perfume Oil ½ oz $6 .MP* **$9**
1969 *Cologne ½ oz $1.75 MP* **$4**
1968 *Perfume Glace with Purse $5.50 MP* **$10**

BROCADE

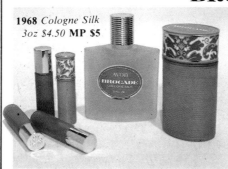

1968 *Cologne Silk 3oz $4.50 MP* **$5**

1971 *Rollette .33oz, 4-A design on lid, $3 MP* **$6**
1967 *Rollette .33oz $3 MP* **$3** • 1968 *Rollette .33oz, glass strike issue, vertical ribbing, $3* MP **$10** • 1968-69 *Rollette .33oz, patterned lid, issued in various Sets MP* **$7** • 1967 *Cologne 4oz $6 MP* **$7**

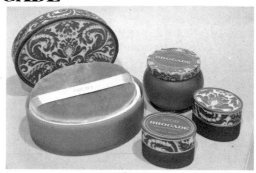

1967 *Beauty Dust, plastic 6oz $6 MP* **$11**
1968 *Perfumed Skin Softener, glass strike issue 5oz $4 MP* **$17**
1968 *Cream Sachet .66oz, label on bottom $3 MP* **$6**
1967 *Cream Sachet .66oz, label on lid $3 MP* **$7**

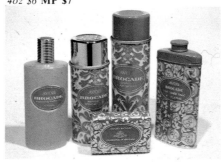

1968 *Foaming Bath Oil 6 oz $4.50 MP* **$2**
1970 *Powder Mist 7 oz, different labeling than 1968 issue, $4 MP* **$2**
1971 *Hair Spray 7 oz $1.50 MP* **$4**
1968 only *Talc 2¾ oz, Perfumed Pair Set, MP* **$5**
1968 only *Soap 3 oz, Perfumed Pair Set, MP* **$5**

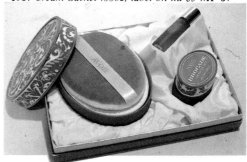

1967 *Deluxe Gift Set. Beauty Dust 6oz, Perfume Rollette .33oz & Cream Sachet .66oz $12.95 MP* **$43**

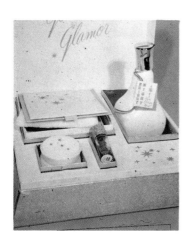

1958 Golden Glamor Set. 8 oz Beauty Dust, 3 oz Cologne Mist, Cream Sachet and 1 dram Perfume $8.95 MP $95

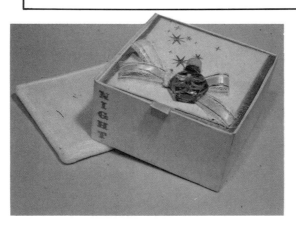

1957-58 Beauty Dust 8 oz in hinged box with bow-tied ⅝ dram fragrance $2.50 MP $35, $20 Beauty Dust only

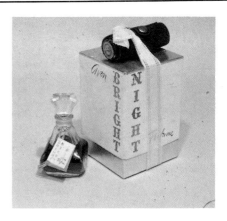

1954 Perfume Set. Perfume ½ oz and 1 dram Perfume in suede wrap $7.50 MP $140

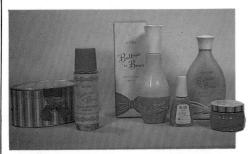

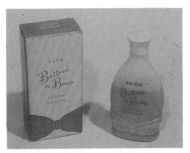

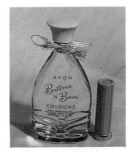

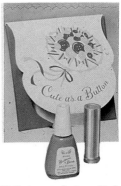

1960 *Beauty Dust, cdbd. 4 oz $2.25* **MP $20**
1962 *Roll-On Deodor, gl. 1¾ oz 89¢* **MP $10**
1960 *Cologne Mist 2½ oz 89¢* **MP $12, $15 boxed**
1961 *Nail Polish 69¢* **MP $7**
1962 *Bubble Bath plastic 4 oz $1.35* **MP $9**
1960 *Cream Sachet .66 oz $1.35* **MP $11**

1962 *Cream Lotion 4 oz*
$1.35 **MP $9, $13 boxed**

1960 *Cologne 2 oz*
$1.35 **MP $16**
1961 *Lipstick 89¢* **MP $6**

1962 *Cute as a Button, Pink Nail Polish & Lipstick $1.58* **MP $20**

Buttons 'n Bows

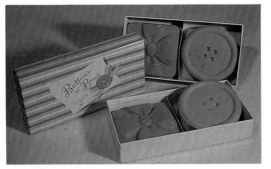

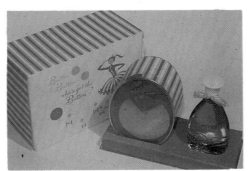

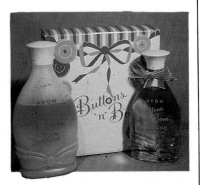

1961 *Boxed Soaps $1.35* **MP $27, $30** *with emb. thread on button*

1961 *Button, Button. Beauty Dust 4 oz and Cologne 2 oz $3.60* **MP $45**

1962 *Pretty Choice. 2 oz Cologne and choice of Cream Lotion or Bubble Bath, 4 oz each $2.70* **MP $33**

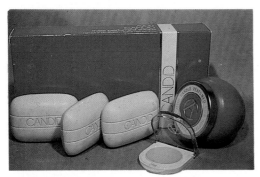

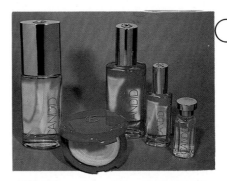

CANDID

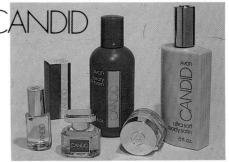

1977 *Boxed Soaps three 3 oz $7* **MP $6**
1977 *Skin Softener 5 oz $6* **MP $3***
1977 *Solid Perfume Compact .2 oz $3.75* **MP $1**

(See also Awards pg. 309)

1977 *Cologne Spray 1.8 oz $7.50* **MP $9***
1977 *Cologne 2 oz $6.50* **MP 50¢**
1977 *Purse Cologne .5 oz $3* **MP $2**
1977 *Cologne .33 oz $3* **MP $1**
1978 *Pressed Powder Compact $4* **MP $J**

1979 *Purse Concentre .33 oz $4* **MP $1**
1979 *Light Perfume .5 oz $7* **MP 50¢**
1979 *Bath Foam $5.50* **MP $3**
1979 *Creme Perfume .66 oz $4.50* **MP 50¢**
1979 *Soft Body Satin 6 oz $5* **MP 50¢**

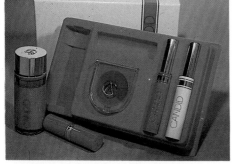

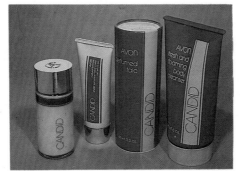

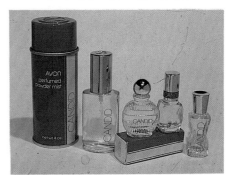

1976 *Color Collection $15.25* **MP $7**
  Makeup 1.5 oz $3.50 **MP $1**
  Cheek Color .15 oz $3.50 **MP 75¢**
  Lip Color $2.25 **MP 75¢**
  Eye Color .25oz $3 **MP 75¢**
  Mascara .25 oz $3 **MP 75¢**

1977 *Under-Makeup Moisturizer 2 oz. $3.50* **MP $1**
1978 *Face Color 1.5 oz $3.50* **MP 50¢**
1977 *Talc 3½ oz $3* **MP $2***
1977 *Foaming Body Clnsr. 6 oz $4.50* **MP 50¢**

*Available from Avon at time of publication

1979 *Powder Mist 4 oz $5* **MP $3***
1979 *Cologne Spray 1 oz $7* **MP $6***
1980 *Cologne .33 oz $3.50* **MP 50¢**
1978 *Cologne .33 oz $3* **MP $1**
1979 *Cologne .33 oz $3* **MP $1**

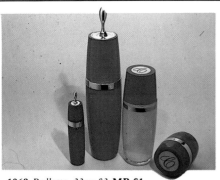

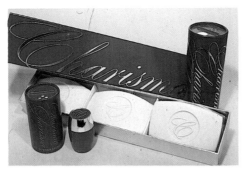

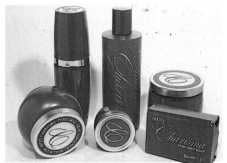

1968 *Rollette .33oz $3* **MP $1**
1968 *Cologne Mist 3oz $4.50* **MP $2**
1969 *Cologne Silk 3 oz, frosted $4.50*
MP $5, MP $3 clear glass
1968 *Cream Sachet .66 oz $3* **MP $1**

1975 *Powder Sachet 1¼ oz $3.50* **MP $1.50**
1969 *Half-ounce Cologne $1.75* **MP $2**
1970-74 *Boxed Soap, 3 3 oz cakes $3.50* **MP $7**
1970 *Talc 3½oz $1.35* **MP $2***

1974 *Skin Softener 5oz $4* **MP $3***
1976 *Cologne Spray 2.7oz $8* **MP $8.50**
1976 *Foaming Bath Oil 6oz $5.50* **MP $1**
1969 *Skin Softener, glass 5oz $4* **MP $4**
1975 *Cream Sachet .66oz $4.50* **MP $1**
1975 *Soap 3oz $1.25* **MP $1.25***

Charisma

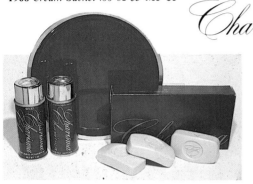

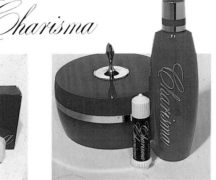

1972 *Powder Mist, all metal 7 oz $4* **MP $1**
1969 *Powder Mist, paper label 7 oz $4* **MP $5**
1970 *Tray 10" dia. $3* **MP $7**
1975-79 *Boxed Soap 3 3oz cakes $6* **MP $6**

1968 *Beauty Dust 6 oz $6* **MP $6**
1972 *DemiStik .19 oz* **MP $1**
1970 only *Foaming Bath Oil 6 oz $3.50* **MP $5**
1971 *As above but no red band on lid* **MP $2**

Cotillion

. . . one of Avon's most popular fragrances ever . . .

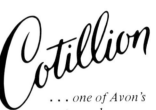

Mr. David H. McConnell

1934 *July 10th to 30th only, a customer gift Perfume, 2 drams, honoring David McConnell's 76th Birthday 20¢* **MP $85**
1935 *July 10th to 23rd only, a customer gift honoring David McConnell's 77th Birthday 20¢* **MP $85**
1936 *July only, a customer gift honoring David McConnell's 78th Birthday 20¢* **MP $85**
The 1936 Birthday Gift was the last of the series as Mr. McConnell died on January 20, 1937

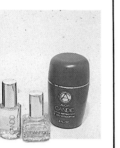

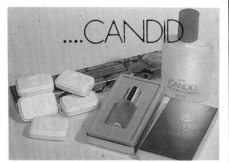

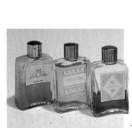

1982 *Luxury Bathfoam 6 oz $6* **MP $4***
1982 *Bonus Size Talc 5¼ oz $3.50* **MP $1**
1982 *Cologne .33 oz $4.50* **MP $2.50***
1981 *Cologne .33 oz $4* **MP $1**
1982 *Ultra Sensation Body Smoother 3 oz $6* **MP $5***

1975 *Powder Sachet 1¼oz $3.50* **MP $1**
1976 *Rollette .33oz $4.50* **MP $1**
1977 *Cologne Spray 1.8 oz $6.50* **MP $2**
1976 *Xmas-wrapped Soap 3 oz $2.25* **MP $2**

(See also Awards pg. 306)

1937 *Customer gift, with additional purchase 20¢* **MP $85**

1939 *Customer gift, with additional purchase 20¢* **MP $75**

Add $10 to all MP's if boxed

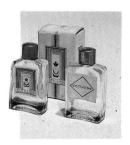

....CANDID

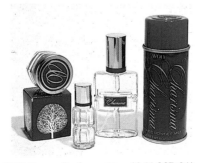

1983 *Five Guest Soaps 1 oz each (2 campaigns only) $6* **MP $4**
1983 *Light & Lavish Cologne 6 oz $7.50* **MP $6***
1983 *Perfume .33 oz $13* **MP $11***

1979 *Creme Perfume .66oz $3.50* **MP $4***
add $1 to MP for 1980 Christmas box
1979 *Purse Concentrate .33oz $3* **MP $1**
1979 *Cologne Spray 1.8oz $6* **MP $1**
1979 *Powder Mist 4oz $4.50* **MP 50¢**

(See more perfumes on p. 56)

***Available from Avon at time of publication*

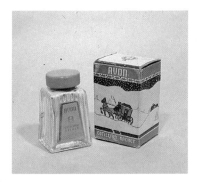

1937 Powder Sachet $1.04 **MP $26,**
$45 in Xmas Box

... Cotillion

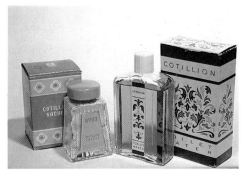

*1937 Powder Sachet 1½ oz $1.04. Sold in special
box as "Good Will Gesture" for 20¢* **MP $26,
$45 boxed**
*1939 Toilet Water 2 oz. Special packaging sold
from May 2 to May 22, 1939 only. 20¢ with
another purchase.* **MP $45, $60 boxed**

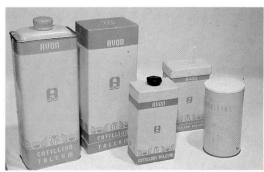

1939-43 Talc (metal) 14½ oz $1.04 **MP $25**
1943-44 Talc (cdbd.) 14½ oz $1.19 **MP $40**
1944-45 Talc (cdbd.) 2¾ oz 37¢ **MP $30**
1943-44 Talc (cdbd.) 2¾oz 37¢ **MP $30**
1947 Talc 2¾oz 39¢ **MP $30**

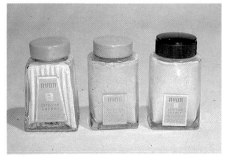

1937-38 Powder Sachet 1½oz $1.04 **MP $26**
1939 Powder Sachet 1¼oz $1.04 **MP $20**
1943 Powder Sachet 1¼oz $1.15 **MP $20**

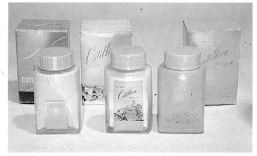

1943 Powder Sachet 1¼oz $1.15 **MP $20, $30 boxed**
1946 Powder Sachet 1¼oz $1.19 **MP $18, $28 boxed**
1946 Powder Sachet 1¼oz $1.19 **MP $25, $35 boxed**

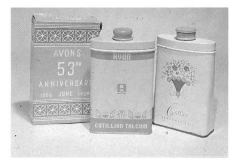

1939 Talc 2¾ oz, 53rd Anniversary Box **MP $33**
1938-42 Talc only 37¢, 1943-50 39¢ **MP $15**
1957 Talc 2¾ oz 69¢ **MP $6**

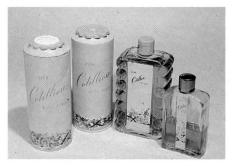

1946 Body Powder 5 oz 65¢ (rare) **MP $40**
1947 Body Powder 4½ oz 75¢ **MP $22**
1946 Cologne 6 oz $1.50 **MP $50**
1946 Toilet Water 2 oz $1.19 **MP $38**

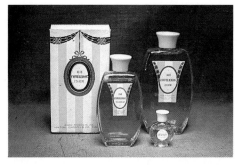

1950 Toilet Water 2 oz $1.75 **MP $25, $30 boxed**
1950 Perfume ⅛ oz (rare) $1.50 **MP $80, $100
boxed**
1950 Cologne 4 oz $1.75 **MP $25**

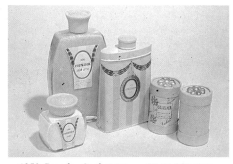

1950 Powder Sachet 1¼ oz $1.25 **MP $20**
1950 Cream Lotion 6 oz 89¢ **MP $30**
1950 Talc 2¾oz 43¢ **MP $12**
*1945 Powder Sachet, cardboard 1¼ oz
$1.15* **MP $22**
*1944 Powder Sachet, cardboard 1¼ oz
$1.15* **MP $22**

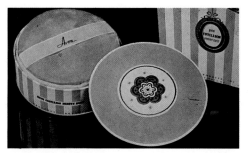

1951 Beauty Dust 6oz $1.75 **MP $23, boxed $30**

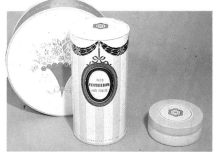

1953 Beauty Dust 6 oz $1.95 **MP $18**
1950 Body Powder 5 oz 75¢ **MP $22**
1951 Cream Sachet .66oz $1.25 **MP $18**

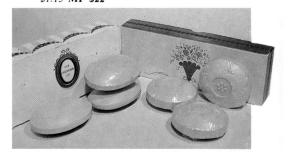

1950 Boxed Soaps, three 3 oz cakes 79¢ **MP $45**
1953 Boxed Soaps, three 3 oz cakes 89¢ **MP $40**

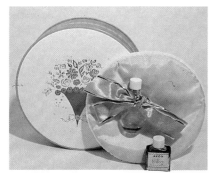

1956 *Beauty Dust with ⅝ dram bottle of matching fragrance* $1.95 **MP** **$40 complete,** **$12 bottle only**
1953 *Beauty Dust as above with ⅝ dram square bottle of fragrance* $1.75 **MP** **$45 complete, $17 bottle only**

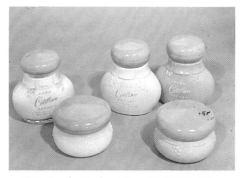

1953 *Powder Sachet 1¼ oz* $1.25 **MP $15**
1958 *Powder Sachet 1¼ oz* $1.50 **MP $12**
1957 *Powder Sachet 1¼ oz (white lettering)* $1.50 **MP $20**
1953 *Cream Sachet .66 oz* $1.25 **MP $15**
1958 *Cream Sachet .66 oz* $1.50 **MP $10**

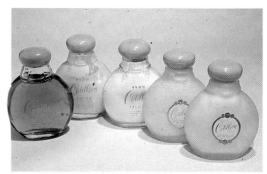

1954 *Bath Oil 4½ oz* $1.25 **MP $13**
1954 *Cream Lotion 4½ oz* 95¢ **MP $13**
1955 *Talc 3 oz* $1 **MP $15**
1958 *Body Powder 3 oz* $1 **MP $12**
1956 *Talc 3 oz* $1 **MP $14**

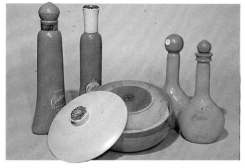

1959 *Perfumed Bath Oil 8 oz* $2.50 **MP $20**
1959 *Cologne Mist 3 oz* $2.95 **MP $23**
1959 *Beauty Dust 6 oz* $2.95 **MP $15**
1957 *Cologne Mist 3 oz* $2.50 **MP $25**
1958 only *Cologne Mist 3 oz (rare)* $2.50 **MP $55**

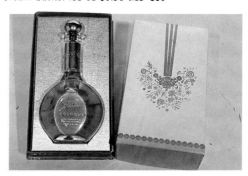

1959 only *Gift Cologne 4 oz (N.Y.-Pasadena label)* $2.50 **MP $75**

... Cotillion

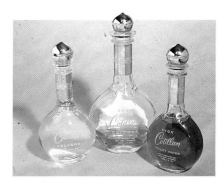

1961 *Cologne 2 oz* $1.50 **MP $23**
1953 *Cologne 4 oz* $2 **MP $20**
1953 *Toilet Water 2 oz* $1.50 **MP $18**

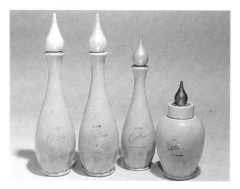

1961 *Perfumed Bath Oil 6 oz* $3 **MP $7**
1966 *Foaming Bath Oil 6 oz* $2.75 **MP $2**
1961 *Cream Lotion 4 oz* $1.50 **MP $5**
1961 *Body Powder 4 oz* $2.25 **MP $8**

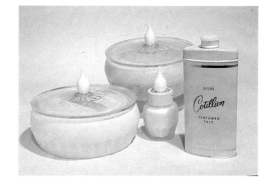

1961 *Beauty Dust 6 oz* $4 **MP $7, $10 with yellow container**
1961 *Powder Sachet .9 oz* $2 **MP $9**
1974 *Talc 3½ oz* $1.50 **MP 50¢**

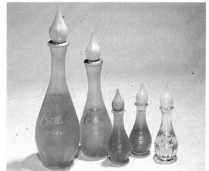

1961 *Cologne 4 oz* $3 **MP $12**
1961 *Cologne 2 oz* $2 **MP $3**
1963 *Perfume Oil for bath ½ oz* $4 **MP $12**
1964 *Perfume Oil ½ oz* $4 **MP $9**
1969 *Cologne ½ oz* $1.50 **MP $2**

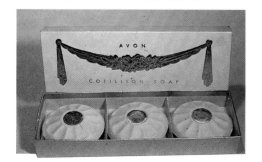

1961 *Boxed Soaps three 3 oz* $1.50 **MP $26**

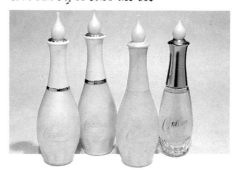

1971-75 *Cologne Mist 3 oz* $5 **MP $4**
1961 *Cologne Mist 3 oz* $4 **MP $7**
1975-76 *Cologne Mist 3 oz* $8 **MP $2**
1976-81 *Cologne Spray 2.7 oz* $7 **MP $1**

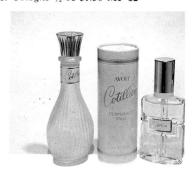

1967 *Cologne Silk 3 oz* $3.75 **MP $5**
1974 *Talc 3½ oz* $1.50 **MP 50¢**
1979 *Cologne Spray 1.8 oz* $6 **MP $1**

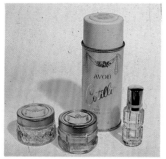

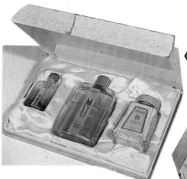

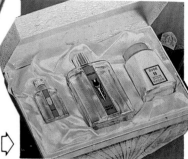

1938 *Cotillion Enchantment.*
1 dram Perfume, Toilet Water
2oz & Powder Sachet $2.95
MP $180

1964 *Skin Softener 5oz $3.25* **MP $1**
1966 *Hair Spray 7oz $1.50* **MP $1**
1977 *Foaming Bath Oil 6oz $4.50*
MP $1
1975 *DemiStik .19oz $2.50* **MP $1**

1975 *Cream Sachet .66oz $3* **MP $1**
1979 *Creme Perfume .66oz $3.50*
MP 50¢
1968 *Powder Mist 7oz $3.50* **MP $1**
1979 *Purse Concentre .33oz $3*
MP $1

1939 *Cotillion Enchantment.*
1 dram Perfume, Toilet Water 2oz
& Powder Sachet $2.95 **MP $180**

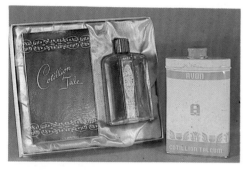

1940 *Cotillion Classic. Toilet Water 2 oz and Talc 2¾ oz $1.50* **MP $75**

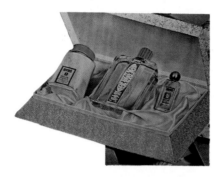

1940 *Cotillion Enchantment. Toilet Water 2 oz Powder Sachet and 1 dram Perfume $2.85* **MP $125**

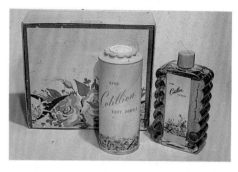

1946 *Cotillion Classic. Body Powder 5 oz and Cologne 6 oz $2.48* **MP $120**

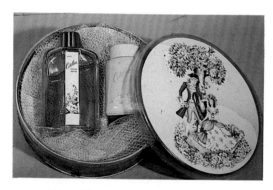

1946 *Cotillion Garland. Toilet Water 2 oz and Powder Sachet $2.84* **MP $85**

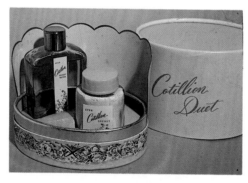

1947 *Cotillion Duet. Toilet Water 2 oz and Powder Sachet $2.39* **MP $75**

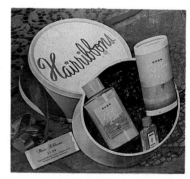

1948 *Hair Ribbons. Talc, Hand Lotion and ⅝ dram Perfume $1.59* **MP $80**

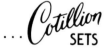

...*Cotillion* SETS

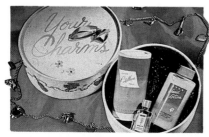

1949 *Your Charms. Talc, Hand Lotion and ⅝ dram Perfume $1.59* **MP $80**

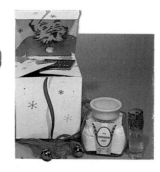

1951 *Jolly Surprise. Powder Sachet and 1 dram Perfume $1.99* **MP $50**

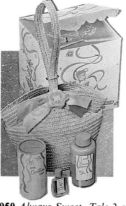

1950 *Always Sweet. Talc 2 oz, ⅝ dram Perfume, Cream Lotion 2 oz and Straw Handbag $2.39* **MP $100**

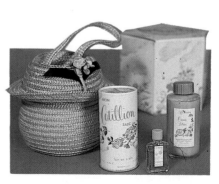

1951 *Always Sweet. Cotillion Talc 2 oz, Perfume ⅝ dram, Cream Lotion 2 oz and Straw Handbag $2.39* **MP $100**

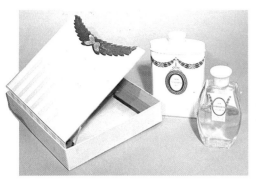

1950 *Cotillion Garland. Talc and Toilet Water 2 oz $1.85* **MP $60**

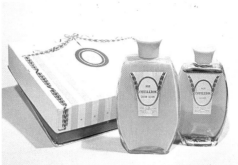

1950 *The Cotillion. Cream Lotion 6 oz and Cologne 4 oz $2.39* **MP $75**

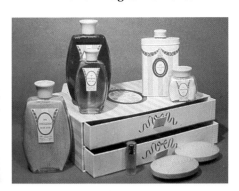

1950 *Bath Ensemble. Cream Lotion, Toilet Water, Bath Oil, Talc, Powder and Cream Sachets, 1 dram Perfume and 2 bars Soap $8.25* **MP $200**

... *Cotillion* SETS

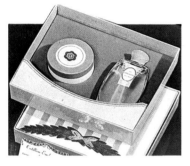

1951 *Cotillion Enchantment. Toilet Water 2 oz & Cream Sachet $2.50* **MP $60**

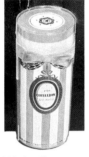

1952 *Cotillion Fantasy. Body Powder 5 oz and Cream Sachet $1.95* **MP $50**

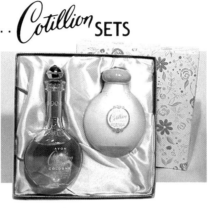

1953 *Cotillion Duet. Cologne 4 oz and Talc 3¼ oz $3* **MP $50**

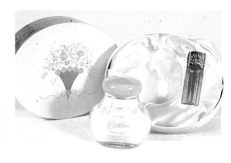

1953-56 *Cotillion Enchantment. 1¼ oz Powder Sachet and 1 dram Perfume $3* **MP $40**

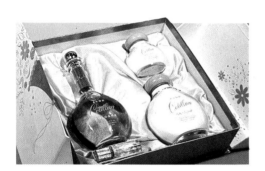

1953 *Cotillion Deluxe. Cologne 4 oz, 1 dram Perfume, Powder Sachet & Talcum $6* **MP $75**

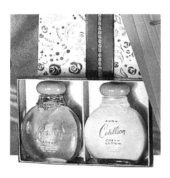

1954 *Cotillion Garland. Cream Lotion & Bath Oil 4½ oz each $2.15* **MP $38**

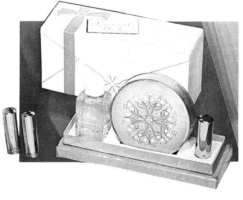

1954 *Special Date. Toilet Water ½ oz, Powder-Pak and Fashion Lipstick $1.95* **MP $41**

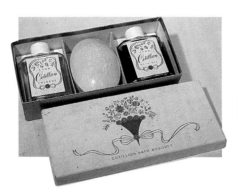

1956 *Bath Bouquet. Bath Oil, Cologne 2 oz each and 1 oz cake Soap $2.25* **MP $75**

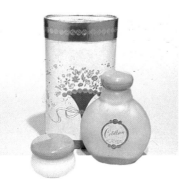

1956 *Cotillion Carol. Talc & Cream Sachet $2.25* **MP $36**

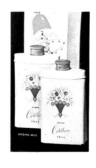

1956 *Singing Bells. 2 Talcs $1.10* **MP $20**

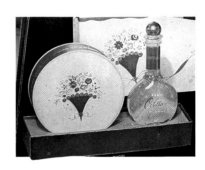

1956 *Princess. Cologne 4 oz and Beauty Dust 6 oz $3.95* **MP $68**

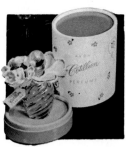

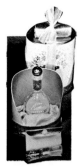

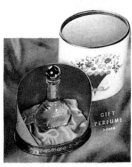

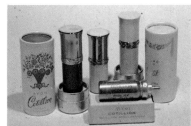

1948 *Gift Perfume 3 dr. $3 MP $110*

1951 *Gift Perfume 3 drams $3.50 MP $100, $125 boxed*

1957 only *Gift Perfume 3 drams and 1 dram Perfume in gold wrapper $6 MP $130, boxed with ribbon*

1953 *Gift Perfume 3 drams $4.50 MP $85, $105 boxed*

1960 *Spray Perfume 2 drams $2.95 MP $15, $20 boxed*
1960-61 *Spray Perfume 2 drams $2.95 MP $15*
1961-62 *Spray Perfume $3.50 MP $10, $14 boxed*
1960-63 *Spray Perfume Refills $1.75 & $2.25 MP $12 boxed*

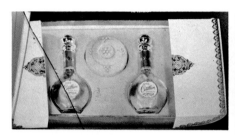

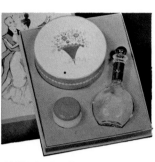

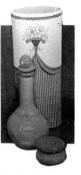

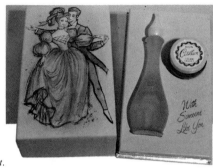

1957 *Cotillion Treasures. Bath Oil, Soap, Cologne $2.75* **MP $76**

1957 *The Cotillion. Beauty Dust, Cream Sachet & Cologne $4.95* **MP $70**

1958 *Cotillion Bouquet. Cologne Mist 3 oz & Cream Sachet $3.95* **MP $85**

1961 *With Someone Like You. Cologne 2 oz & Cream Sachet $4* **MP $22**

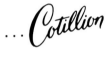

...*Cotillion*

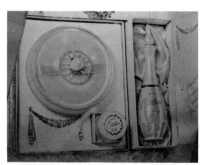

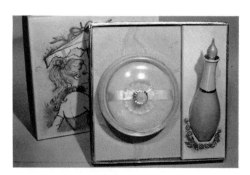

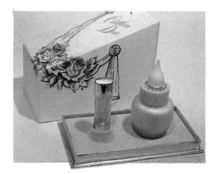

1961 *Cotillion Debut. Beauty Dust, Cream Sachet, Cologne Mist $10* **MP $35**

1963 *Debutante. Beauty Dust 6 oz, Cologne Mist 3 oz $8.50* **MP $25**

1964 *Cotillion Duo. Powder Sachet & 1 dram Perfume $3.98* **MP $22**

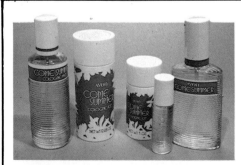

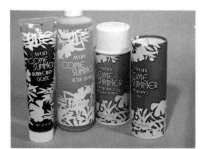

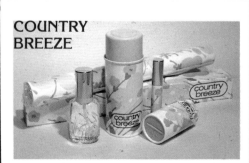

1975 *Cologne Mist 2 oz $5 MP $2*
1975 *Cologne Ice 2¼ oz $5 MP $5*
1976 *Cologne Ice (as above) 2 oz $5 MP $1*
1978 *Cologne Ice 1 oz $3.75 MP $2*
1977 *Touch of Cologne .33 oz $1.75 MP $1*
1977 *Cologne Spray 1.8 oz $5 MP $1*

1976 *Bubble Bath Gelee 4 oz $3.50 MP $2*
1975 *Body Splash 12 oz $5 MP $3*
1975 *Powder Mist 7 oz $4.50 MP $2*
1976 *Talc 3½ oz $2 MP $1*

COME SUMMER

COUNTRY BREEZE

1980 *Drawer Lining Paper & Powder Sachet 1¼oz $8.50 MP $4*
1980 *Cologne Spray 1oz $6 MP $1*
1980 *Powder Mist 4oz $4.50 MP 50¢*
1980 *Mini-Spray .33oz $4.50 MP $1*

(See also Awards pg. 310)

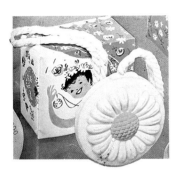

1959 *Daisy Soap $1.19*
MP $20, $25 boxed

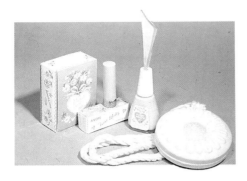

1960 *First Waltz Set. Pomade and Nail
Polish $1.25* **MP $22**
1960 *Nail Polish 69¢* **MP $8**
1962 *Soap $1.19* **MP $20, $24 boxed**

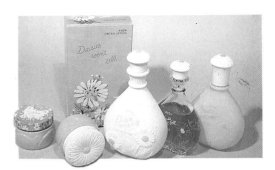

1959 *Cream Sachet .66 oz $1.19* **MP $15**
1963 *Cream Sachet .66 oz $1.10* **MP $11**
1962 *Cream Lotion 4 oz $1.19* **MP $7, $10 boxed**
1962 *Cologne 2 oz $1.19* **MP $7, $10 boxed**
1963 *Cologne Mist 2 oz $2.25* **MP $10, $13 boxed**

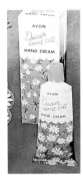

1958 *Hand Cream
1¾ oz 49¢*
MP $8, $10 boxed

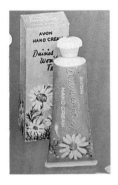

1962 *Hand Cream
1¾ oz 59¢*
MP $8, $10 boxed

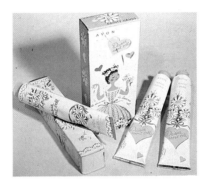

1956 *Hand Cream 1¾ oz. Sets only.*
MP $10, $15 boxed
1957 *Dainty Hands. 2 Hand Cream 1¾ oz
79¢* **MP $20, $8 each tube**

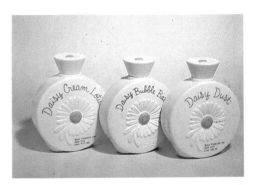

1958 *Cream Lotion 4 oz $1.19* **MP $10, $15 boxed**
1958 *Bubble Bath 4 oz $1.19* **MP $10, $15 boxed**
1958 *Daisy Dust 2 oz $1.19* **MP $10, $15 boxed**

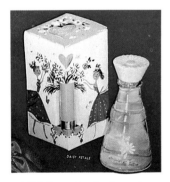

1957 *Daisy Petals. Pomade
Lipstick and Cologne 2 oz
$1.59* **MP $27**

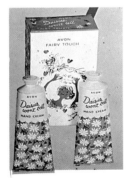

1958 *Fairy Touch. Two
Hand Cream 79¢*
MP $20, $8 each tube

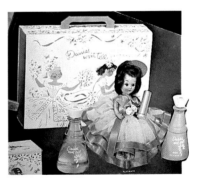

1956 *Playmate Cologne, Cream Lotion
2 oz each, Pomade Lipstick and Doll
$3.95* **MP $95 with case, Doll MP $40**

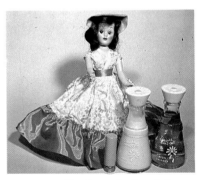

1957 *My Dolly. Cream Lotion, Cologne
2 oz each, Pomade Lipstick & Doll $3.95*
MP $95 boxed, $40 Doll only

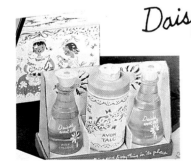

Daisies won't tell

1956 *Daisies Won't Tell Set. Cologne,
Bubble Bath 2 oz each, Talc 3¼ oz $2.25*
MP $70, Talc MP $25

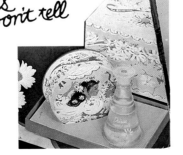

1956 *Miss Daisy. Cologne 2 oz
Beauty Dust $2.35* **MP $50**

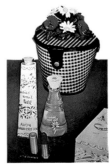

1956 *Little Charmer.
Plastic Handbag. Hand
Cream, Pomade
Lipstick and Cologne
2 oz $3.50* **MP $65**

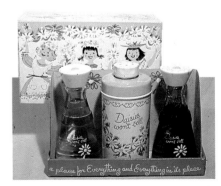

1957 *Daisies Won't Tell Set. Cologne and
Bubble Bath 2 oz each, Talc 3¼ oc $2.25*
MP $65, Talc MP $25

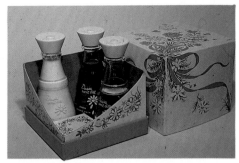

1957 One I Love. Cologne, Cream Lotion and Bubble Bath 2 oz each $2.49 **MP $57**

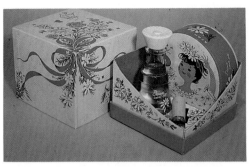

1957 Daisy Bouquet. Cologne 2 oz Beauty Dust and Pomade Lipstick $2.95 **MP $50**

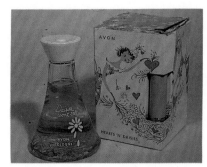

1958 Hearts 'N Daisies. Cologne 2 oz and Pomade Lipstick $1.59 **MP $25**

... Daisies won't tell

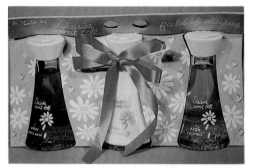

1958 Field of Daisies. Bubble Bath, Cream Lotion with red ribbon and Cologne 2 oz each $2.19 **MP $50**

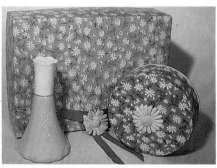

1958 Daisy Darling. Spray Cologne 1½ oz and Beauty Dust 4 oz $2.98 **MP $45**

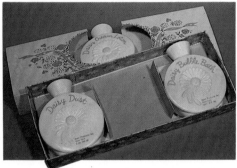

1959 Daisy Bouquet. Cream Lotion, Bubble Bath 4 oz each & Daisy Dust 2 oz $3.50 **MP $38**

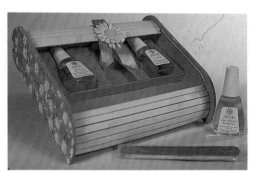

1959 Daisy Treasure Set. 5 Manicure items $2.75 **MP $60**

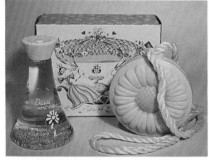

1961 Pretty Beginner. Cologne 2 oz and choice of Lotion, Bubble Bath, Shampoo, Daisy Dust or Soap $2.38 **MP $30, $40 with Soap**

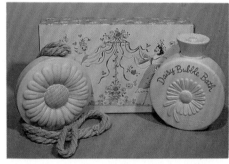

1960 Gay Daisies. Soap and choice of Bubble Bath, Cream Lotion or Shampoo 4 oz each or Daisy Dust 2 oz $2.35 **MP $37**

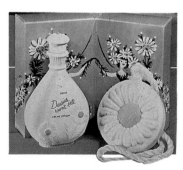

1962 First Recital. Soap and Choice of Cream Lotion, Bubble Bath 4 oz ea. or Daisy Dust 2 oz $2.38 **MP $35**

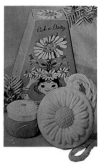

1963 Pick A Daisy. Soap & Cream Sachet $2.38 **MP $36**

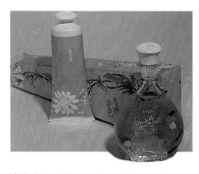

1963 Daisy Chain. Hand Cream 1¾ oz, Cologne 2 oz $1.78 **MP $24**

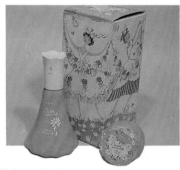

1959 Love Me Love Me Not. Spray Cologne 1½ oz and Cream Sachet $2.50 **MP $40**

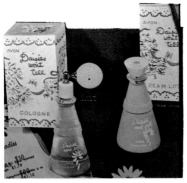

1956 *Cologne 2 oz with Atomizer*
$1.25 MP $20, $25 boxed
1956 *Cream Lotion 69¢* MP $15,
$18 boxed

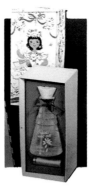

Daisies won't tell

1956 *Blossoms Set.*
Cologne 2 oz and
Pomade Lipstick
$1.59 MP $25

DELICATE DAISIES

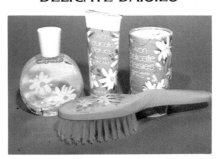

1977 *Cologne 2 oz $3.50* MP $1
1977 *Hand Cream 1.5 oz $2* MP 50¢
1977 *Talc 2 oz $2* MP 50¢
1977 *Hairbrush 7" long $5.50* MP $4

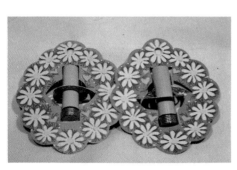

1956 *Beauty Dust with plain side 3.5 oz*
$1.19 MP $30

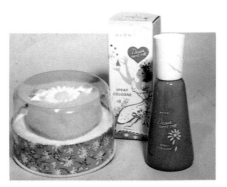

1956 *Beauty Dust 3.5 oz $1.19* MP $25
1958 *Beauty Dust 4 oz $1.49* MP $20

Elusive

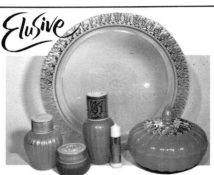

1970 *Tray $4* MP $10
1970 *Foaming Bath Oil 6oz $3.50* MP $2
1969 *Cream Sachet .66oz $3* MP $1
1969 *Cologne Mist 3 oz $6* MP $1
1970 *DemiStik .19 oz $1.75* MP $1
1969 *Beauty Dust 6 oz $6* MP $5

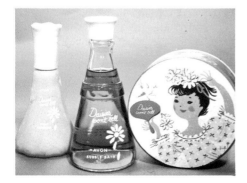

1957 *Gift Pomade (yellow) 59¢* MP $13,
Pomade only $4
1958 *Gift Pomade 59¢* MP $13,
Pomade only $4

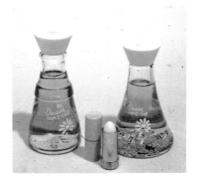

1959 *Fluff-On 4oz powder & puff $1.98*
MP $15
1957 *Spray Cologne 1.5oz $1.59* MP $14,
$16 boxed

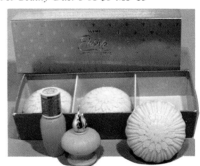

1970 *Boxed Soaps, three 3 oz cakes*
$3.50 MP $6
1969 *Rollette .33oz $3* MP $1
1969 *Half-ounce Cologne $1.75* MP $3

(See also Awards pg. 308)
(See also Stockholder's Gifts pg. 330)

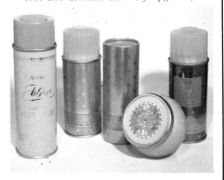

1958 *Spray Cologne 1½oz $1.59* MP $17
1956 *Bubble Bath 4oz $1.10* MP $12
1957 *Beauty Dust $1.29* MP $23

1956 *Cologne 2 oz (sets only)* MP $15
1962 *Pomade Lipstick 59¢* MP $4
1961 *Cologne 2 oz $1.19* MP $9

1970 *Hair Spray 7 oz $1.50* MP $3
1970 *Powder Mist 7 oz $4* MP $2
1971 *Talc 3½ oz $1.35* MP 50¢
1970 *Skin Softener 5 oz $4* MP $2
1972 *Powder Mist 7 oz $4* MP $1

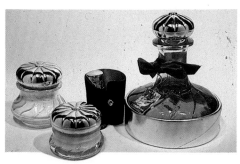

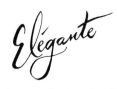

Elégante

An elegant collection of truly regal packaging and superb craftmanship in glass . . .

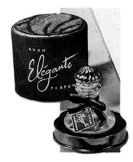

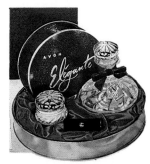

1957 Powder Sachet .9 oz $1.50 **MP $19**
1956 Cream Sachet .66 oz $1.50 **MP $13**
1956 Perfume 1 dram in suedene wrapper $2.25 **MP $18**
1956 Cologne 4oz $2.50 **MP $25, $40 boxed**

1956 Gift Perfume ½ oz $7.50 **MP $130,** **$85 bottle only**

1957 Sparkling Burgundy. Beauty Dust 6 oz, Cream Sachet, Cologne 4 oz & 1 dram Perfume $8.95 **MP $120**

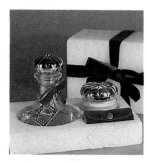

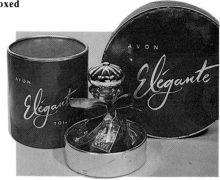

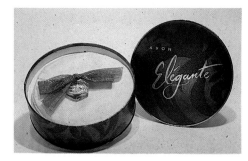

1957 Snow Dreams. Toilet Water 2 oz, Cream Sachet & 1 dram Perfume in suedene wrapper $5.50 **MP $80**

1957 Toilet Water 2oz $2 **MP $25, $40 boxed**
1956 Beauty Dust 6oz $2.25 **MP $22**

1957 Beauty Dust 6 oz & ⅝ dram Fragrance $2.25 **MP $35 complete**

emprise

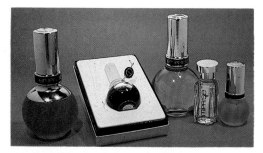

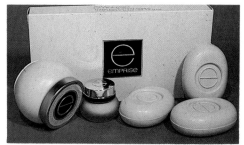

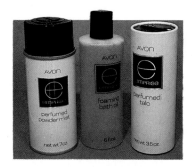

1976 Spray Cologne 1.8 oz $7.50 **MP $1**
1976 Perfume ¼ oz $15 **MP $8, $10 boxed**
1977 Cologne 2 oz $6.50 **MP $1**
1977 Cologne .33 oz $3 **MP $1.50**
1976 Purse Concentre .33 oz $5 **MP 75¢**

1976 Boxed Soaps, three 3 oz cakes $6 **MP $6**
1977 Skin Softener 5 oz $6 **MP 50¢**
1977 Creme Perfume, .66 oz $5 **MP 50¢**

1977 Powder Mist 7 oz $5 **MP $2**
1977 Foaming Bath Oil 6 oz $5.50 **MP $1**
1977 Talc 3½ oz $4 **MP 50¢**

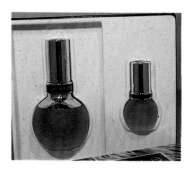

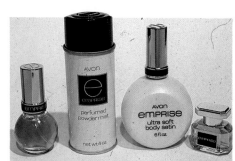

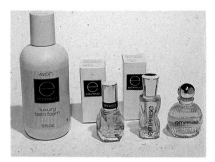

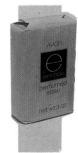

1977 Gift Set. Cologne Spray 1.8 oz and Purse Concentre .33 oz $11.50 **MP $4**

(See also Awards pg. 309)

1979 Cologne Spray 1 oz $7 **MP $1**
1979 Powder Mist 4 oz $5 **MP 50¢**
1979 Body Satin 6oz $5 **MP 50¢**
1979 Light Perfume .5oz $7 **MP $1**

1979 Bath Foam 6 oz $5.50 **MP 50¢**
1978 Cologne .33 oz $3 **MP $1**
1979 Cologne .33 oz $3 **MP $1**
1980 Cologne .33 oz $3.50 **MP $1**

1979 Perfumed Soap 3oz $1.50 **MP $1**

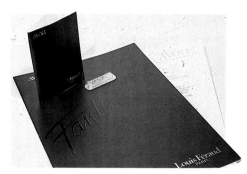

1982 Perfume Vial Sample MP 50¢
1982 Fantasque Brochure MP 50¢

Fantasque

Inspired by the French designer
Louis Feraud, a fragrance as
brilliant and beautiful as the
fashions that made Paris
famous.

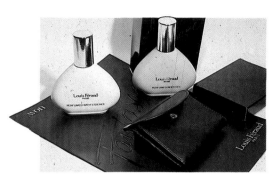

1983 Perfumed Bath Essence 4oz $14 MP $9.50*
1983 Perfumed Body Veil 4oz $14 MP $9.50*
1983 La Purse Fantasque, leather 3½"x4" $5 with
purchase MP $5

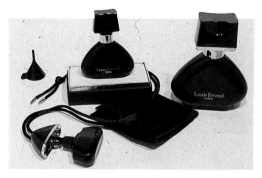

1982 Parfum Pendant with funnel in velvet pouch
.15oz $32 MP $25*
1982 Parfum .5oz $42 MP $35*
1982 Eau de Cologne Spray 1.7oz $22 MP $17*

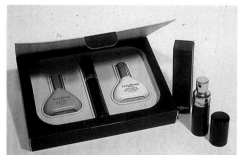

1983 Gift Collection. Perfumed Body Veil .5oz,
Eau de Cologne Flacon Spray .33oz & Perfumed
Bath Essence .5oz $6.50 with Fantasque purchase
MP $13 boxed
1983 Eau de Cologne Flacon Spray .5oz $13
MP $10*

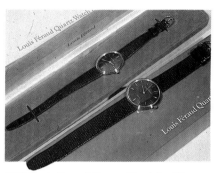

1983 Louis Feraud Quartz Watch for Women
$195 MP $195 boxed
1983 Louis Feraud Quartz Watch for Men
$195 MP $195 boxed

FLOWER TALK

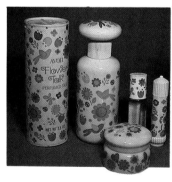

1972 Talc 3½oz $1.50
MP $3
1972 Cologne Mist 3oz
$5 MP $5
1973 Rollette .33oz
$1.75 MP $5
1972 DemiStik .19oz
$2 MP $3
1972 Cream Sachet
.66oz $2.50 MP $4

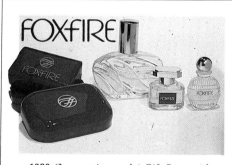

1980 (2 campaigns only) Gift Soap with
Case 3oz $6.50 MP $5
1980 Cologne 2oz $8 MP $1
1980 Light Perfume .5oz $7 MP 75¢
1981 Cologne .33oz $4 MP 50¢

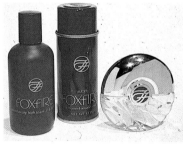

1980 Bath Foam 6oz $5 MP 50¢
1981 Powder Mist 4oz $5 MP $4*
1980 Cologne Spray 1.8oz $9.50 MP $8*

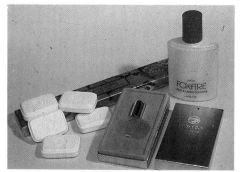

1983 Five Guest Soaps 1oz each (2 campaigns
only) $6 MP $4
1983 Light & Lavish Cologne 6oz $7.50 MP $6*
1983 Perfume .33oz $13 MP $11*

*Available from Avon at time of publication

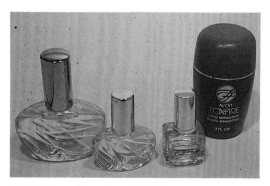

1982 Cologne Spray 1oz $9 MP $6*
1982 Fragrance Petite Cologne .33oz $4.50 MP $2.50*
1981 Classic Miniature Cologne .33oz $4 MP $1
1982 Ultra Sensation Body Smooter 3oz $6 MP $5*

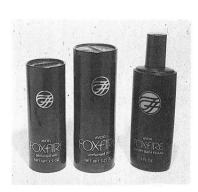

1981 Talc 3.5oz $3.50 MP $2*
1982 Talc, bonus size 5¼oz $3.50 MP $1
1982 Luxury Bath Foam 6oz $6 MP $4*

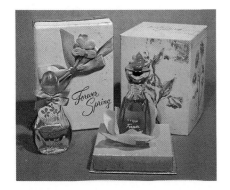

1951 *Perfume 3 dram $5* MP $95, $110 boxed
1956 *Perfume ½oz $5* MP $90, $105 boxed

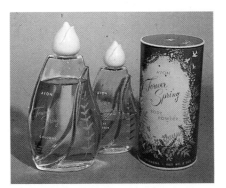

1951 *Cologne 4 oz $2* MP $21
1951 *Toilet Water 2 oz $1.50* MP $20
1951 *Body Powder 5 oz 85¢* MP $18

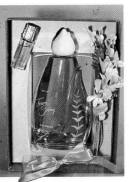

1951 *Spring Corsage. Cologne 4oz and 1 dram Perfume $4.50* MP $50

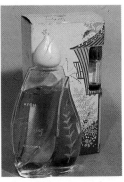

1951-53 *Spring Song. Cologne 4 oz and 1 dram Perfume $3.50* MP $50

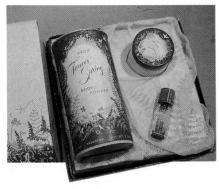

1952 *Forever Spring Set. Body Powder 5 oz, Cream Sachet and 1 dram Perfume $3.95* MP $65

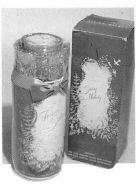

1952-53 *Spring Melody. Body Powder 5oz & Cream Sachet $1.95* MP $40

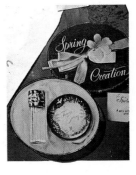

1953 *Spring Creation. Cream Sachet .66 oz & 1 dram Perfume $2.75* MP $42

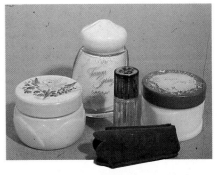

1956 *Cream Sachet .66 oz $1.25* MP $12
1951 *Powder Sachet 1¼ oz $1.25* MP $15
1951 *One dram Perfume in suedene wrapper $1.75* MP $20
1951 *Cream Sachet .66 oz $1.25* MP $14

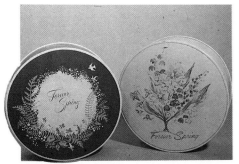

1951 *Beauty Dust 6 oz $1.75* MP $25
1956 *Beauty Dust 6 oz $1.95* MP $20

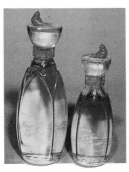

1956 *Cologne 4 oz $2* MP $19
1956 *Toilet Water 2 oz $1.50* MP $18

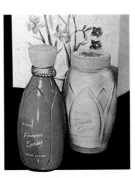

1956 *Spring Mood. Cream Lotion 4oz and Body Powder 4oz $1.95* MP $52

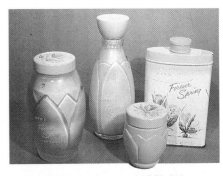

1956 *Body Powder 4 oz $1* MP $18
1956 *Cream Lotion 4 oz 95¢* MP $21
1958 *Talc 2¾ oz 69¢* MP $13
1956 *Powder Sachet .9 oz $1.25* MP $13

Forever Spring Springtime

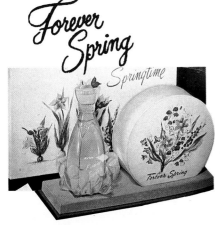

1956 *Springtime. Cologne 4 oz & Beauty Dust 6 oz $3.95* MP $52
(See also Awards pg. 306)

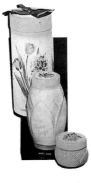

1956 *April Airs. Body Powder 4 oz & Cream Sachet $2.25* MP $42

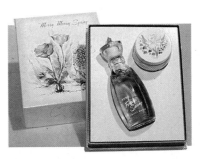

1956 *Merry, Merry Spring. Toilet Water 2 oz and Cream Sachet $2.75* MP $42

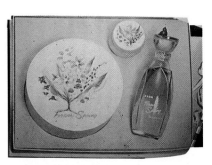

1957 *Spring Goddess. Beauty Dust 6 oz, Cream Sachet & Cologne 4 oz $4.95* MP $60

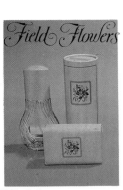

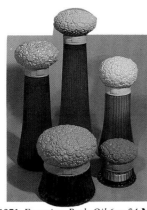

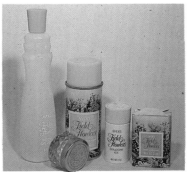

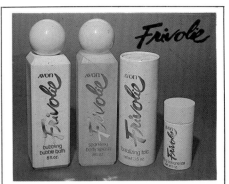

1980 *Cologne Spray 1.5 oz*
$6.50 **MP $1**
1980 *Talc 3.5 oz $2.50*
MP 50¢
1980 *Soap 3 oz $1.75*
MP $1

1971 *Foaming Bath Oil 6oz $4* **MP $2**
1972 *After Bath Freshener 8oz $4* **MP $2**
1971 *Cologne Mist 3oz $6* **MP $1**
1971 *Cologne Gelee 3oz $4* **MP $3**
1971 *Cream Sachet .66oz $3* **MP $2**

1976 *Body Splash 8 oz $5* **MP $1**
1975 *Cream Sachet .66 oz $3* **MP $1**
1971 *Powder Mist 7 oz $4* **MP $1**
1978 *Cologne Ice 1 oz $3.75* **MP $2**
1975 *Soap 3 oz $1.25* **MP $1**

1978 *Bubble Bath 8 oz $4.50* **MP $1**
1978 *Body Splash 8 oz $4.50* **MP $1**
1978 *Talc 3.5 oz $2* **MP 50¢**
1978 *Cologne Ice 1 oz $3.75* **MP $1**

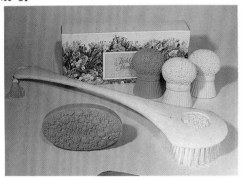

1971 *Bath Brush & 5 oz Soap $6* **MP $10**
1971 *Boxed Soaps, three 3 oz cakes*
$3.50 **MP $8**

(See also Awards pg. 308)

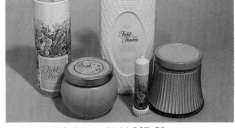

1971 *Talc 3½ oz $1.35* **MP 75¢**
1973 *Skin Softener 5 oz $4* **MP $1**
1972 *Cream Lotion 8 oz $3* **MP $1**
1973 *DemiStik .19 oz $2* **MP 50¢**
1971 *Skin Softener 5 oz $4* **MP $2.50**

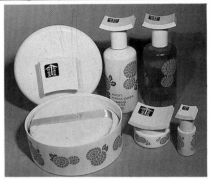

1970 *Beauty Dust 6oz $6* **MP $3**
1971 *Foaming Bath Oil 6oz $3.50* **MP $4**
1971 *Foaming Bath Oil 6oz (clear) $4* **MP $3**
1970 *Cream Sachet .66oz $3* **MP $2**
1970 *Rollette .33oz $3* **MP $2**

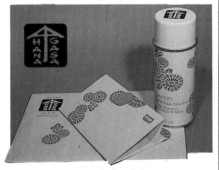

1970 *Gift Notes, 15 with 18 seals $2*
MP $7
1971 *Powder Mist 7 oz $4* **MP $2**

(See also Awards pgs. 307-308)

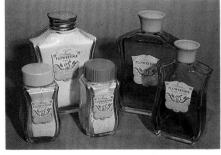

1949 *Powder Sachet, pink cap 1¼ oz $1.19* **MP $15**
1950 *Powder Sachet, blue cap 1¼ oz $1.19* **MP $20**
1949 *Talc 3¾ oz metal shaker 89¢* **MP $25**
1949 *Cologne 4oz $1.75* **MP $23**
1949 *Toilet Water 2 oz $1.25* **MP $30**

**F
L
O
W
E
R
T
I
M
E**

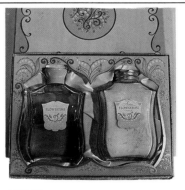

1949 *Flowertime Set. Cologne 4 oz,*
Talc 3¾ oz $2.75 **MP $62**

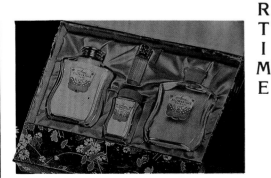

1950 *Flowers In the Wind. Talc, Powder*
Sachet, Cologne 1 dram Perfume $5.50 **MP $95**

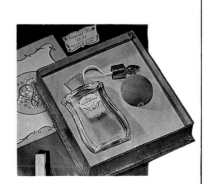

1951 *Fragrant Mist. Toilet Water 2 oz*
with Atomizer. **MP $60.**
Atomizer only $15

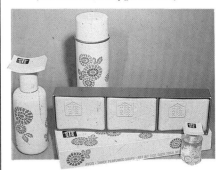

1970 *Cologne Mist 3 oz $6* **MP $2**
1971 *Hair Spray 7 oz $1.50* **MP $2**
1971 *Boxed Soaps, three 3 oz cakes*
$3.50 **MP $7**
1970 *Half-ounce Cologne $1.75* **MP $3**

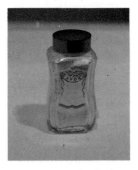

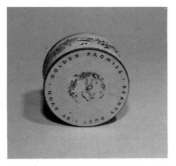

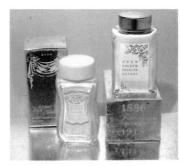

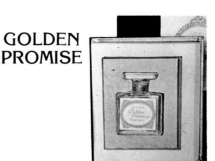

GOLDEN PROMISE

1952 only *Powder Sachet 1¼ oz $1.25* **MP $20**

1947-51 *Beauty Dust, all cardboard box (issued only in Sets)* **MP $25**

1952 *Powder Sachet 1¼ oz $1.25* **MP $16, $20 boxed**
1948 *Powder Sachet 1¼ oz $1.19 (sold to customers for 1 campaign in honor of 62nd Anniversary)* **MP $18, $35 boxed**

1954 *Perfume ½ oz $3.95* **MP $100, $130 boxed**

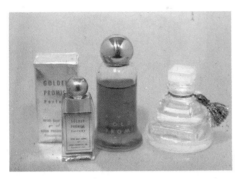

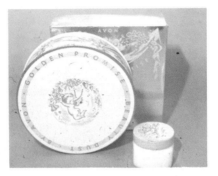

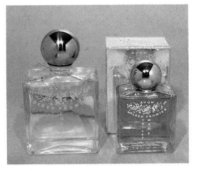

1947 *Perfume gift given to Pasadena Branch employees. Both bottle & box state "with best wishes of Avon Products, Inc., Pasadena, Cal."* **MP $100, $125 boxed**
1947 *Perfume ½ oz $5* **MP $100, $175 boxed**
1950 *Perfume 3 dram $4* **MP $125, $160 boxed**

1947 *Beauty Dust 6 oz $1.50* **MP $22, $27 boxed**
1953 *Cream Sachet, .66 oz $1* **MP $14**

1947 *Cologne 4 oz $2.25* **MP $23, $28 boxed**
1952 *Toilet Water 2 oz $1.50* **MP $23, $28 boxed**

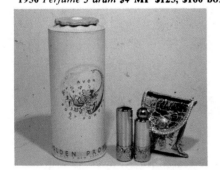

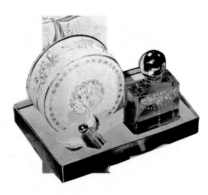

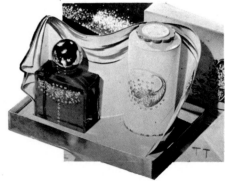

1947 *Body Powder 4½ oz 75¢* **MP $20**
1949 *Golden Duet. Lipstick & 1 dram Perfumette (glass) in gold metal case and gold pursette $2.50* **MP $50, Perfumette MP $25**

1947 *Golden Promise 3 piece Set. Beauty Dust, Cologne 4 oz and 1 dram Perfume $4.95* **MP $95**

1947 *Golden Promise 2 piece Set. Body Powder 4½oz & Cologne 4oz $2.95* **MP $60**

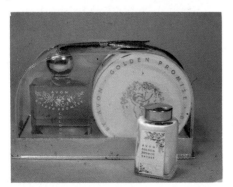

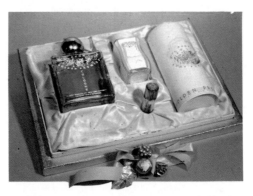

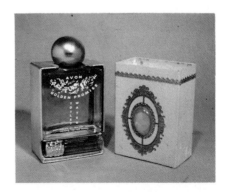

1950 *Golden Promise Set. Beauty Dust and Cologne 4oz $3.95* **MP $65**
1951 *Powder Sachet 1¼oz $1.25* **MP $20**

1952-53 *Deluxe Set. Cologne 4oz, Powder Sachet 1¼oz, Body Powder 4½oz and 1 dram Perfume $6.25* **MP $105**

1953 *Golden Jewel Set. Toilet Water 2oz and 1 dram Perfume $2.75* **MP $45**

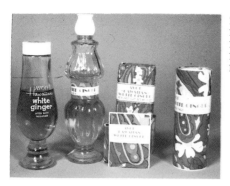

1965 After Bath Freshener 5 oz $2 **MP $9**
1967 After Bath Freshener 6 oz $2.50 **MP $4**
1969 Kwickettes, box of 14 $1.35 **MP $3**
1970 Soap 3 oz 60¢ **MP $1**
1970 Talc 3½ oz $1.10 **MP $1**

HAWAIIAN WHITE GINGER

1967 Beauty Dust 6oz $3 **MP $6**
1968 Cream Sachet .66oz $2 **MP $2**
1969 Cream Lotion 5oz $2 **MP $2**
1969 Cream Sachet .66oz $2.50 **MP $9**
1971 Cologne Mist 2oz $4.25 **MP $4**

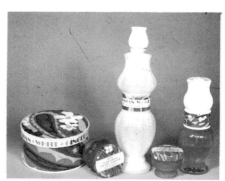

happy hours

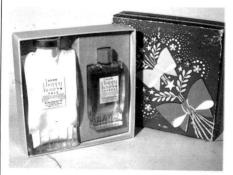

1948 Star Bouquet Set. Talc 2¾ oz and
Cologne 1 oz $1.25 **MP $80, $30 each
Talc or Cologne**

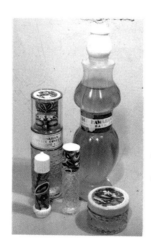

1973 Cologne Mist
2 oz $4.25 **MP $1**
1972 Bath Freshener
8 oz $3.50 **MP $1**
1970 DemiStik
.19 oz $1.75 **MP $1**
1972 Rollette
.33 oz $2.50 **MP $1**
1973 Cream Sachet
.66 oz $2.50 **MP $1**

(See also Awards pg. 307)

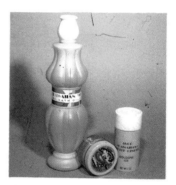

1968 Foaming Bath Oil 8 oz $3 **MP $1**
1975 Cream Sachet .66 oz $3 **MP $1**
1978 Cologne Ice 1 oz $3.75 **MP $1**

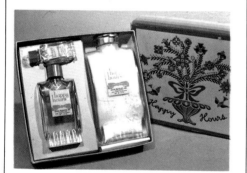

*1948 Happy Hours Set. Cologne 1 oz,
Talc 2¾ oz and Perfume $2* **MP $185**

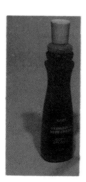

*1976 Body Splash
8 oz $5* **MP $1**

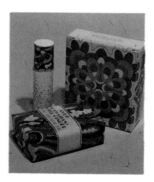

*1972 Floral Duet. Rollette
.33 oz and Soap 3 oz $3.25*
MP $13.50

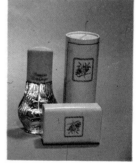

1980-83 Cologne Spray 1.5oz $6
MP $1 / *1983 As above, except 1oz
$6* **MP $4.50*** / *1980 Talc 3.5oz
$2.50* **MP $2*** / *1980 Soap 3oz
$1.75* **MP $1.50***

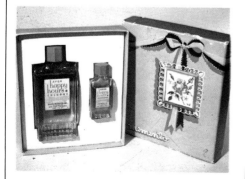

*1948 Memento Set. Cologne 1 oz and 3 drams
Perfume $1.50* **MP $150, $100 Perfume only**

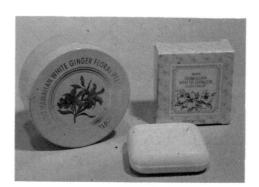

1983 Perfumed Skin Softener 2 oz $2.50 **MP $1.50***
1983 Guest Soap $1.50 **MP $1 boxed**

*Available from Avon at time of publication

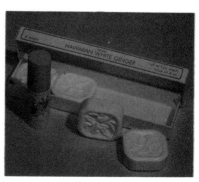

1983 Puff of Fragrance .4 oz $5 **MP $4***
*1983 Floral Boxed Soaps. Four 1 oz cakes
$5* **MP $4***

HER PRETTINESS

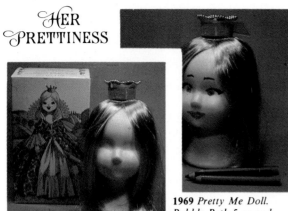

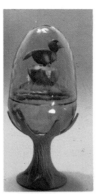

1969 *Pretty Me Doll. Bubble Bath 5 oz and 3 colored pencils for Doll's makeup* $6 **MP $12**

1969 *Enchanted Tree. Cologne Mist 3 oz* $5 **MP $8**

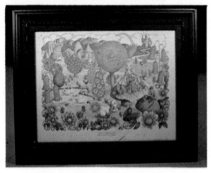

1969 *Art Reproduction (frame not included) 14x18. Free with any Her Prettiness purchase* **MP $9**

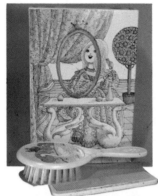

1969 *Brush and Comb Set. Brush 6½" long and Comb 5" long.* $3.50 **MP $7**

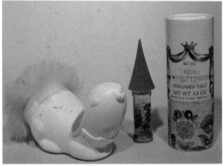

1969 *Bunny Puff & Talc 3½oz* $3.75 **MP $6**
1969 *Secret Tower Rollette .33oz* $1.75 **MP $4**
1970 *Talc 3½oz* $1 **MP $3**

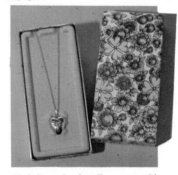

1969 *Love Locket Fragrance Glace* $4.50 **MP $12, $14 boxed**

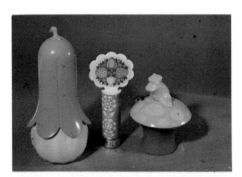

1969 *Flower Belle Cologne Mist 2 oz* $3.50 **MP $5**
1969 *Lip Kiss Pomades in Cherry, Peppermint and Chocolate* $1.95 **MP $4**
1969 *Magic Mushroom Cream Sachet* $3 **MP $4**

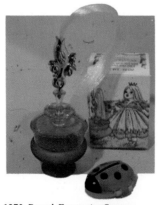

1970 *Royal Fountain Cream Sachet .66 oz* $3 **MP $6, $7 boxed**
1969 *Ladybug Solid Perfume Glace* $3 **MP $5**

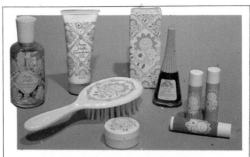

HELLO SUNSHINE

1979 *Cologne 2.5 oz* $3.50 **MP $1**
1979 *Hand Cream 1.5 oz* $2 **MP 50¢**
1979 *Nail Tint .5 oz* $2 **MP 75¢**
1979 *Lipkin Lip Balm .15 oz* $2 **MP 50¢**
1979 *Hairbrush 6½" long* $5.50 **MP $4**
1980 *Soild Perfume Compact .25oz* $3.50 **MP $1**

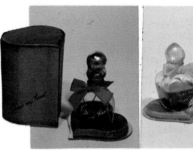

1946-48 *Gift Perfume ½ oz* $7.50 **MP $125, $160 boxed**

1948-50 *Gift Perfume ½ oz* $7.50 **MP $150, $195 boxed**

Here's my Heart

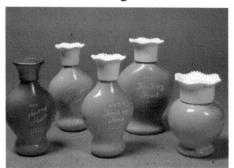

1958 *Lotion Sachet 1 oz (rare)* $2 **MP $19**
1958 *Lotion Sachet 1 oz* $2 **MP $13**
1959 *Lotion Sachet 1 oz* $2 **MP $7**
1958 *Powder Sachet 1 oz* $1.75 **MP $12**
1962 *Powder Sachet .9 oz* $1.75 **MP $10**

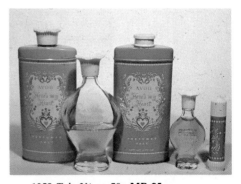

1958 *Talc 2¾ oz* 79¢ **MP $5**
1959 *Toilet Water 2 oz* $2.50 **MP $12**
1962 *Talc 2¾ oz* 79¢ **MP $2**
1969 *Half-ounce Cologne* $1.50 **MP $2**
1975 *DemiStik .19oz* $2 **MP $1**

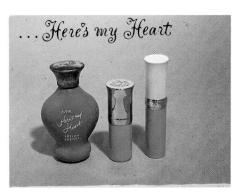

1958 *Lotion Sachet (rare) 1oz $2* **MP $19**
1958 *Spray Perfume 2 drams $3* **MP $15**
1963 *Perfume Mist 2 drams $3* **MP $7**

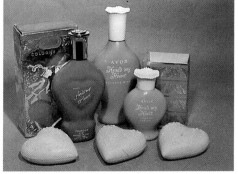

1957 *Cologne Mist 3oz $3* **MP $20, $30 boxed**
1958 *Cologne Mist 3oz $3* **MP $3**
1958 *Powder Sachet 1oz $1.75* **MP $12,
MP $25 in 1959 "Butterfly" Christmas box.**
(Also in 5 other fragrances.)
1966 *Soaps (box not shown) three 3oz $1.75*
MP $23 boxed

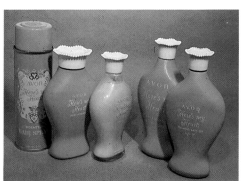

1966 *Hair Spray 7oz $1.50* **MP $5**
1961 *Body Powder 4oz $1.95* **MP $12**
1958 *Cream Lotion 4oz $1.10* **MP $8**
1960 *Perfumed Bath Oil 6oz $2.25* **MP $8**
1966 *Foaming Bath Oil 6oz $2.50* **MP $7**

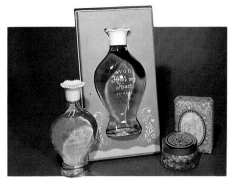

1961 *Cologne 2oz $1.75* **MP $4**
1960 *Cologne 4oz $3* **MP $10, $20 boxed**
1964 *Soap 3oz 39¢* **MP $5**
1975 *Cream Sachet .66oz $3* **MP $1**

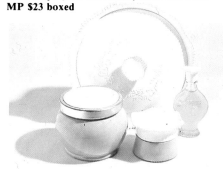

1958 *Beauty Dust 6oz $3* **MP $8**
1964 *Skin Softener 5oz $3* **MP $3**
1959 *Cream Sachet .66oz $2.50* **MP $2**
1964 *Perfume Oil ½oz $3.50* **MP $9**

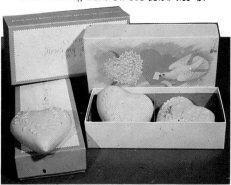

1962 *Left: two 4oz Boxed Soaps $1.29*
MP $25
1960 *Boxed Soaps. Two 4oz cakes $1.29*
MP $26

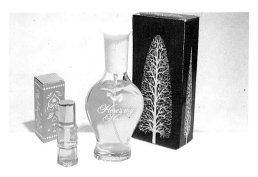

1979 *Purse Concentre .33oz $3* **MP $1**
1979 *Cologne Spray 1.8oz $6* **MP $1, $1.50**
in 1980 Xmas Box

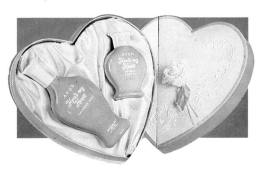

1958 *Sweethearts. Cologne Mist 3oz and choice of Lotion or Powder Sachet $5* **MP $47**

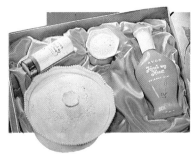

1959 *Heart O'Mine Set. Beauty Dust, Spray Perfume, Cream Sachet & Cologne Mist $11.95* **MP $55**

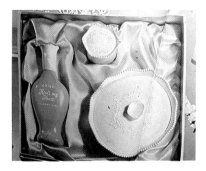

1960 *Romantic Mood. Cologne Mist, Cream Sachet & Beauty Dust $8.25* **MP $40**

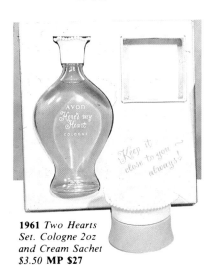

1961 *Two Hearts Set. Cologne 2oz and Cream Sachet $3.50* **MP $27**

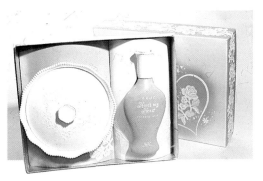

1963 *Remembrance Set. Beauty Dust 6oz & Cologne Mist 3oz $6.95* **MP $32**

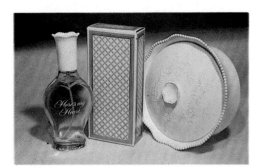

1976 *Cologne Spray 2.7oz $7* **MP $1**
1960's *Beauty Dust 6oz $3* **MP $15**
(with cream-colored lid)

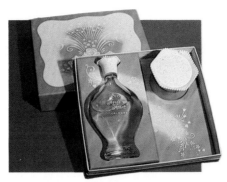

1964 *Heartfelt Set. Cologne 2oz and
Cream Sachet $3.50* **MP $26**

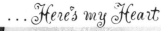

...Here's my Heart

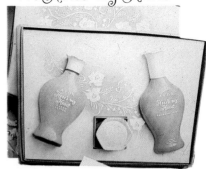

1964 *Hearts in Bloom. Cologne Mist 3oz,
Cream Lotion 4oz and Cream Sachet $6.50*
MP $35

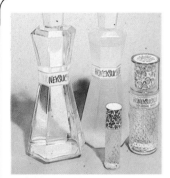

1966 *Bath Freshener 8oz
(glass) $3* **MP $2**
1972 *Bath Freshener 8oz
(plastic) $3.50* **MP $1**
1973 *Cologne Mist 2oz $4.25* **MP $1**
1972 *Rollette .33oz $2.50* **MP $1**

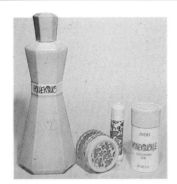

1966 *Foaming Bath Oil 8oz
$3* **MP $1**
1973 *Cream Sachet .66oz
$2.50* **MP $1**
1970 *DemiStik .19oz $1.50* **MP $1**
1978 *Cologne Ice 1oz $3.75* **MP $2**

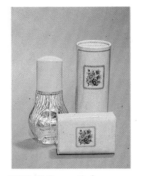

1980-83 *Spray Cologne
1.5oz $6* **MP $1**
1983 *As Above, except
1oz $6* **MP $4.50***
1980 *Talc 3.5oz $2.50* **MP $2***
1980 *Soap 3oz $1.75* **MP $1.50***

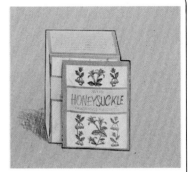

1967 *Fragrance Kwickettes, 14
per box $1.35* **MP $3**

HONEYSUCKLE

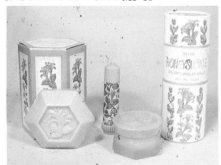

1968 *Boxed Soaps, 3 in box $3* **MP $10**
1968 *DemiStik $1.50* **MP $1**
1967 *Cream Sachet .66oz $2.50* **MP $2**
1966 *Talc 3½oz 98¢* **MP $1**

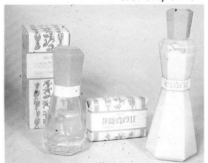

1971 *Cologne Mist 2oz $4.25* **MP $2**
1966 *Soap 3oz 49¢* **MP $1**
1969 *Cream Lotion 5oz $2* **MP $1**

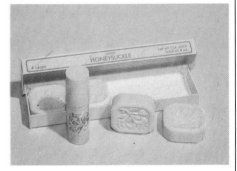

1983 *Puff of Fragrance .4oz $5*
MP $4*
1983 *Floral Boxed Soaps, four 1oz
cakes $5* **MP $4***

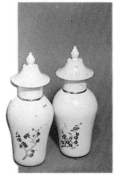

1973 *Cologne Mist
3oz $7.50* **MP $8**
(short issue)
1973 *Cologne Mist
3oz $7.50* **MP $3**

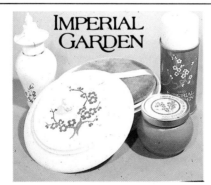

**IMPERIAL
GARDEN**

1973 *Beauty Dust 6oz $7.50* **MP $6**
1974 *Skin Softener 5oz $5* **MP $1**
1974 *Powder Mist 7oz $5* **MP $1**

*Available from Avon at time of publication

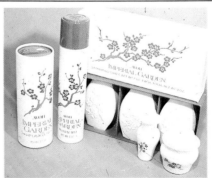

1975 *Talc 3½oz $2* **MP $1**
1974 *Emollient Mist 4oz $3.50* **MP $1**
1974 *Boxed Soap, three 3oz $4.50* **MP $8**
1973 *Rollette .33oz $4* **MP $2**
1973 *Cream Sachet .66oz $4* **MP $1**

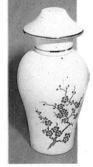

1973 *Ceramic
Vase with 18oz
peach-colored
bath crystals
$18* **MP $20**

——— *(See also Awards pg. 312 & Stockholder's Gifts pg. 330)* ———

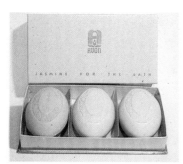

1934-36 *Jasmine Bath Soaps, 3 cakes*
$1.02 **MP $65**

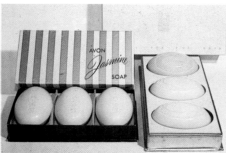

1954 only *Jasmine Bath Soaps, 3 cakes*
$1.69 **MP $65**
1937-46 *Jasmine Bath Soaps, 3 cakes*
$1.02 **MP $50**

JASMINE
*F*antasy Sets . . . .
heavenly com-
binations of fresh
Jasmine-scented
Bath Salts or
Toilet Water and
handsome ovals of
creamy Jasmine
Soap.

(Later named Royal
Jasmine and then Wild
Jasmine)

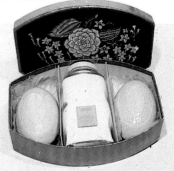

1944 *Fantasy in Jasmine. Bath Salts 9oz*
and 2 cakes Soap $1.60 **MP $100**

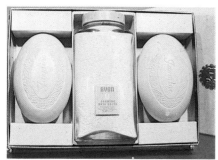

1939 *Fantasy in Jasmine. Bath Salts*
9oz and 2 cakes Soap $1.35 **MP $100,**
$40 Bath Salts only

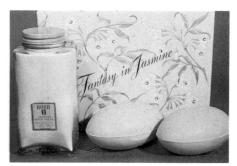

1940-43 *Fantasy in Jasmine. Bath Salts 9oz*
and 2 cakes Soap $1.35 **MP $100**

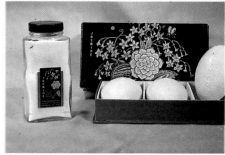

1945 *Bath Salts 9oz 69¢* **MP $45**
1948 *Boxed Soaps, 3 cakes $1.59* **MP $45**

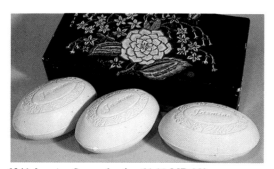

1946 *Jasmine Soaps, 3 cakes $1.85* **MP $50**

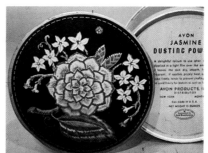

1947 *Dusting Powder 13oz $1.50* **MP $35**

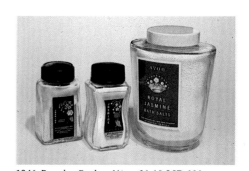

1946 *Powder Sachet 1¼oz $1.15* **MP $23,**
$28 boxed
1949 *Powder Sachet 1¼oz $1.19* **MP $35,**
$42 boxed
1954 *Bath Salts 8oz 89¢* **MP $30**

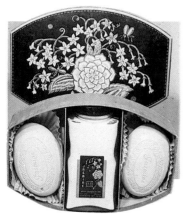

1945 *Fantasy in Jasmine. Bath Salts*
9oz and 2 cakes Soap $1.60 **MP $100**

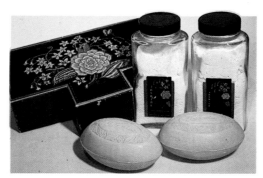

1946 *Fantasy in Jasmine. Bath Salts 9oz (left)*
& 2 cakes Soap $1.60 **MP $90**
1947 *Fantasy in Jasmine. Bath Salts (right)*
& 2 cakes Soap $2.25 **MP $90**

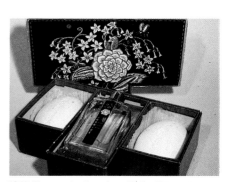

1948 *Fantasy in Jasmine. Toilet Water 2oz and*
2 cakes Soap $2.25 **MP $85**

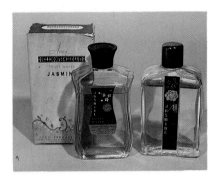

1950 *Toilet Water 2oz $1.25* **MP $38, $45 boxed**
1948-49 *Toilet Water 2oz $1.19* **MP $40, $50 boxed**

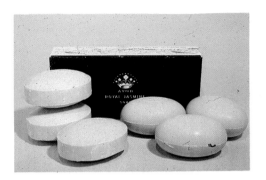

1954 *Royal Jasmine Boxed Soaps, 3 cakes, flat edges $1.69* **MP $30. With Round edges $40**

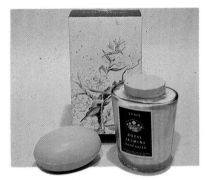

1954 *Royal Jasmine Set. Bath Salts 8oz and 1 cake Soap $1.39* **MP $50**

... JASMINE

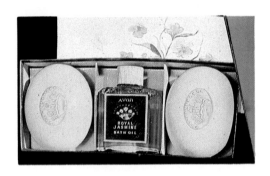

1955 *Fantasy in Jasmine. Bath Oil and 2 cakes Soap $1.95* **MP $50**

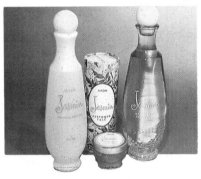

1966 *Foaming Bath Oil 8oz $2.50* **MP $3**
1964 *Talc 3½oz 89¢* **MP $2**
1964 *Bath Freshener 8oz $2.50* **MP $7**
1967 *Cream Sachet .66oz $2* **MP $2**

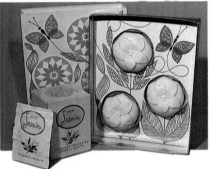

1966 *Fragrance Kwickettes, 14 per box $1.25* **MP $3**
1966 *Gift Soaps, three 2oz cakes $2* **MP $23**

WILD JASMINE

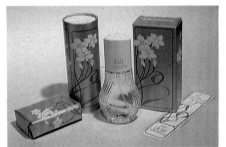

1980 *Soap 3oz $1.75* **MP $1**
1980 *Talc 3.5oz $2.50* **MP 25¢**
1980 *Spray Cologne 1.5oz $6* **MP $1**
1980 *Scented Book Mark. Free with Cologne Spray purchase, only C-17* **MP $1**

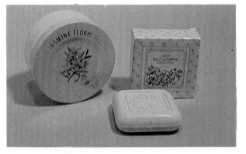

1983 *Floral Perfumed Skin Softener 2oz $2.50* **MP $1.50***
1983 *Fancy Floral Guest Soap 1oz $1.50* **MP $1 boxed**

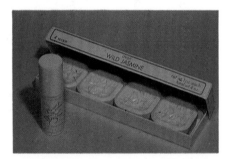

1983 *Puff of Fragrance .4oz $5* **MP $4***
1983 *Floral Boxed Soaps. Four 1oz cakes $5* **MP $4***

Lavender

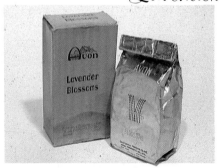

1934-37 *Lavender Blossoms 50¢ per bag* **MP $50, $60 boxed**

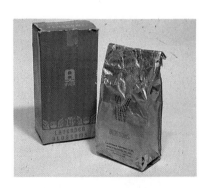

1937-38 *Lavender Blossoms 50¢ per bag* **MP $45, $55 boxed**

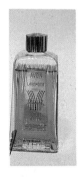

1934-37 *Lavender Toilet Water 4oz 78¢* **MP $50**

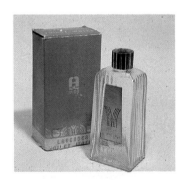

1937 *Lavender Toilet Water 4oz 78¢* **MP $50, $60 boxed**

*Available from Avon at time of publication

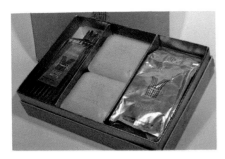

1934-37 *Lavender Ensemble. Toilet Water 4oz, 2 cakes Soap & Lavender Blossoms Sachet $1.50* **MP $155**
1934-37 *Toilet Water 4oz 78¢* **MP $50**

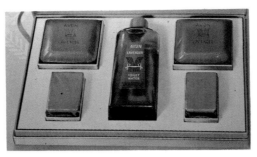

1938 only *Lavender Ensemble. Toilet Water 4 oz, 2 cakes Soap and 2 Sachet cakes $1.50* **MP $125**
1938 only *Toilet Water 4 oz 78¢* **MP $65**
1938 only *Sachet Cakes, 6 per pkg. 50¢* **MP $75**

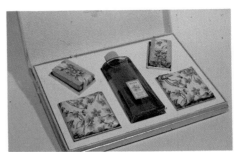

1939 only *Lavender Ensemble. Toilet Water 4 oz, 2 cakes Soap & 2 Sachet Cakes $1.50* **MP $125**
1939-44 *Toilet Water 4 oz 78¢* **MP $50**
1939-44 *Sachet Cakes, 6 per pkg. 50¢* **MP $45**

Lavender

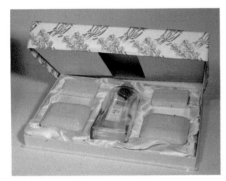

1944 only *Lavender Ensemble. Toilet Water 4 oz, 2 cakes Soap & 2 Sachet Cakes $1.95* **MP $120**

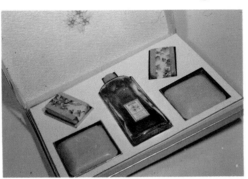

1939 only *Lavender Ensemble. Toilet Water 4 oz, 2 cakes Soap & 2 Sachet Cakes $1.50* **MP $125**
1939-44 *Toilet Water 4 oz 78¢* **MP $50**
1939-44 *Sachet Cakes, 6 per pkg. 50¢* **MP $45**

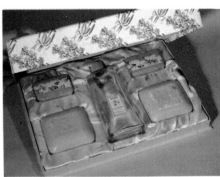

1940-43 *Lavender Ensemble. Toilet Water 4 oz, 2 cakes Soap & Sachet Cakes $1.75* **MP $120** *Toilet Water 78¢* **MP $40**

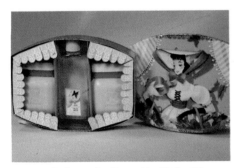

1945 only *Lavender Ensemble. Toilet Water 4 oz, 2 cakes Soap and 2 Sachet Cakes $1.95* **MP $100**
1944-45 *Sachet Cakes, 2 per pkg. 57¢* **MP $40**

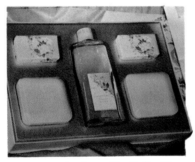

1946 *Lavender Ensemble. Toilet Water 4 oz, 2 Cakes Soap & 2 Sachet Cakes $1.95* **MP $95**

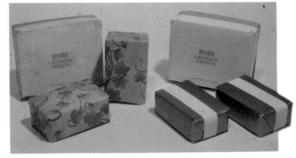

1947 *Sachet Cakes, 2 per pkg. 57¢* **MP $30**
1944-45 *Sachet Cakes, 2 per pkg. 57¢* **MP $40**

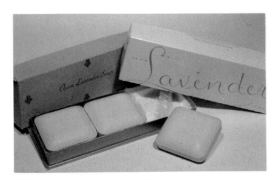

1934-43 *Lavender Soap, (left) 3 cakes 67¢* **MP $90**
1946 only *Lavender Soap, (right) 3 cakes 85¢* **MP $90**

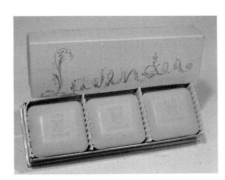

1945 *Lavender Soap, 3 cakes 85¢* **MP $90**

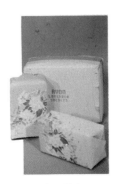

1946 *Sachet Cakes 2 wrapped 57¢* **MP $30**

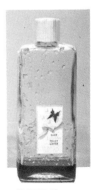

1945 *Toilet Water 4 oz 89¢* **MP $50**

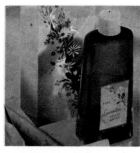

......Lavender

. . . enchanting and aristocratic. Never offered in perfume.

1946 only *Toilet Water 4oz 89¢* **MP $55, $65 boxed**

1961 *Powder Sachet .9oz (4-A design label) $2* **MP $10**
1965 *Above bottle with Xmas Carton, as shown* **MP $17**
1961 *Powder Sachet with .9oz on front label $2* **MP $14**

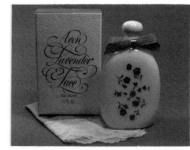

1970 *Lavender and Lace. Cologne 1.7oz and Lace-edged handkerchief $4.50* **MP $7. Bottle only MP $4.50**

Lemon Velvet

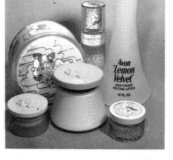

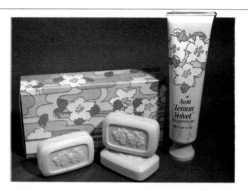

(rear)
1969 *Beauty Dust 6oz $3.50* **MP $4**
1972 *Cologne Mist 2oz $4.25* **MP $1**
1971 *Moisturized Friction Lotion (emb. flower on lid) 10oz $3* **MP $1 (1969** *not shown. As above w/plain lid* **MP $4**
(front)

1971 *Bath Mitt $1.50* **MP $2**
1972 *Powder Mist 7oz $4* **MP $1**
1971 *DemiStik .19 $1.75* **MP 75¢**
1972 *Rollette .33oz $2.50* **MP $2**

1971 *Cream Sachet .66oz $3* **MP $2**
1969 *Skin Softener 5oz $3.50* **MP $2**
1973 *Cream Sachet .66oz $2.50* **MP $1**

1969 *Boxed Soaps, three 3 oz cakes $3* **MP $7**
1971 *Cleansing Gel 6oz $3* **MP $1**

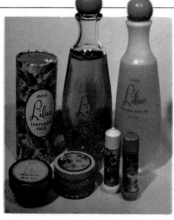

1963 *Perfumed Talc 3½oz 89¢* **MP $1**
1963 *Bath Freshener 8oz $2.50* **MP $7**
1966 *Foaming Bath Oil 8oz $2.50* **MP $3**
1967 *Cream Sachet .66oz $2* **MP $2**
1973 *Cream Sachet .66oz $2.50* **MP $1**
1970 *Perfumed Demi-Stik $1.75* **MP 75¢**
1968 *Perfumed Demi-Stik $1.50* **MP $2**

LILAC

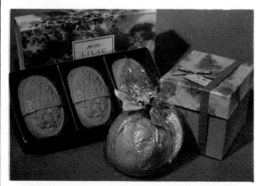

1968 *Boxed Soaps, three 3oz cakes $3* **MP $7**
1966 *Gift Soap, three 3oz cakes $2.50* **MP $18**
1966 *Kwickettes (not shown) 14 per box $1.25* **MP $3**

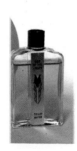

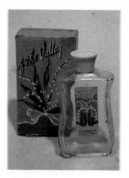

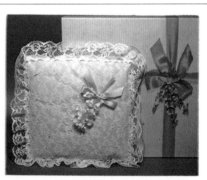

1934-39 *Toilet Water 2oz $1.04* **MP $45, $55 boxed**

1949 *Toilet Water 2oz $1.19* **MP $30, $40 boxed**

1979 *Fabric Scented Pillow w/spray of Lily of the Valley flowers 10x10" $15* **MP $11**

LILY OF THE VALLEY

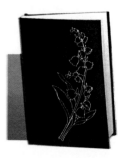

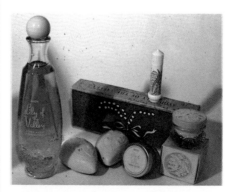

1963 *Bath Freshener 8oz $2.50* **MP $7**
1966 *Boxed Soaps, two 3oz cakes $2* **MP $20**
1967 *Cream Sachet .66oz $2* **MP $2**
1974 *Cream Sachet .66oz $2.50* **MP $2**
1974 *DemiStik .19oz $2* **MP 75¢**

1979 *Chateau of Flowers, a Harlequin novel exclusively for Avon. $1.99 with $7.50 purchase. U.S. only.* **MP $4**

Light Accents

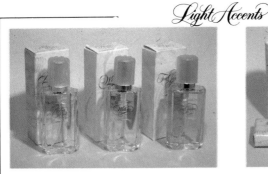
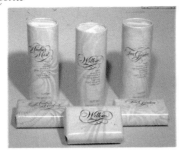

1983 *Cologne Spray. Amber Mist, Willow & Tea Garden 2oz $10 ea.* **MP $6 ea.***

1983 *Perfumed Talc. Amber Mist, Willow & Tea Garden 3.5oz $3.50 ea.* **MP $2 ea.***
1984 *Silky Soap. Amber Mist, Willow & Tea Garden 3oz $2.50 ea.* **MP $1.50 ea.***

Luscious

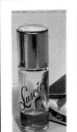
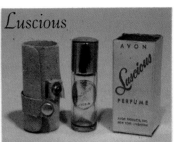

1950 *Luscious Perfume, the only 1 dram bottle issued with silk-screened label $1.75* **MP $15**

1950 *Luscious Perfume 1 dram. Issued with smooth gold cap in Leatherette wrapper $1.75* **MP $22 in wrapper, $25 boxed**

(See also Awards pg. 306)

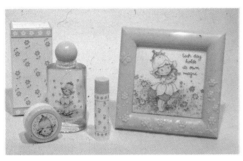
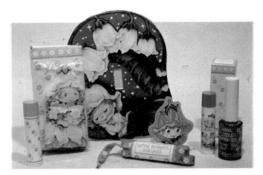
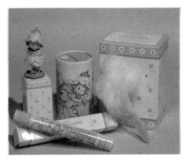

1981 *Cheeky Rose Blush .25oz $3* **MP 25¢**
1981 *Whisper Soft Cologne 1.5oz $5* **MP 50¢**
1981 *Cherriful Lip Tint .15oz $2* **MP 25¢**
1982 *Scented Picture Frame 4½"x4½" $8.50* **MP $3.50**

1982 *Finger Puppet with DemiStik .15oz $5* **MP $4***
1983 *Light Switch Cover $5.50* **MP $2.50**
1982 *Patch and Shoelaces $5* **MP $4***
1982 *Lip Tint, Orange or Strawberry .15oz $2* **MP $1***
1982 *Nail Tint, Orange or Strawberry .5oz $2* **MP $1***

1983 *Little Blossom Mini Doll 2¼" $5* **MP $4***
1983 *Dab O'Cologne .45oz $4* **MP $3***
1983 *Shaker Talc with Puff 2oz $5* **MP $4***

LITTLE BLOSSOM

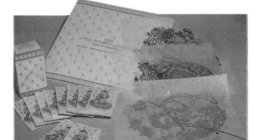
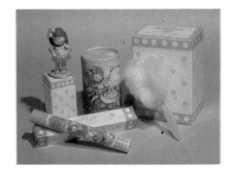

1983 *Bubble Bath Packets, 10 per carton .2oz ea. $3* **MP $1**
1983 *Iron-On Transfers, set of 3 69¢ with Little Blossom purchase in C-22 only* **MP $1**

1983 *Daisy Dreamer Mini Doll $5* **MP $4***
1983 *Dab O'Cologne .45oz $4* **MP $3***
1983 *Shaker Talc with Puff 2 oz $5* **MP $4***

1983 *Scamper Lily Mini Doll $5* **MP $4***
1983 *Dab O'Cologne .45oz $4* **MP $3***
1983 *Shaker Talc with Puff 2oz $5* **MP $4***

MARIONETTE

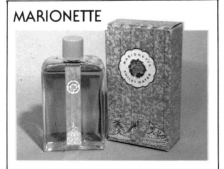

1938 *Marionette Toilet Water 2oz. Pre-introduction customer gift offered in C-16* **MP $45, $60 in gift box**

Mineral Spring

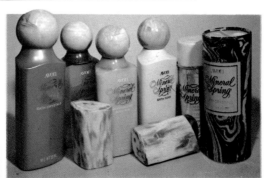

1972 *Bath Crystals 12oz $6* **MP $2**
1972 *Sparkling Freshener 8oz $4* **MP $1**
1972 *Body Rub 8oz $4* **MP $1**
1973 *Bathfoam 8oz $4* **MP $1**
1972 *Powder Mist 7oz $4* **MP $1**
1976 *Bath Crystals 12oz $5.50* **MP $2**
1972 *Boxed Soaps, two 4oz cakes $3.50* **MP $5**

*Available from Avon at time of publication

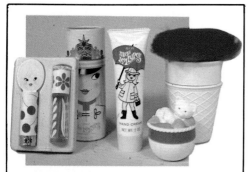

1968 *Miss Pretty Me. Lip Pop and Rollette*
$3.25 **MP $13**
1968 *Talc 3½oz $1* **MP $5**
1968 *Hand Cream (black boots) 2oz 75¢* **MP $5**
1967 *Cream Sachet .66oz $2* **MP $5**
1968 *Ice Cream Talc 3½oz $3* **MP $7**

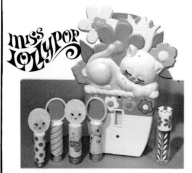

Lip Pops: 1967 *Cherry.* **1968** *Peppermint &*
Raspberry. **1969** *Cola. $1.50 ea.* **MP $4 ea.**
1968 *Rollette .33 oz $1.50* **MP $5**
1969 *Pretty Touch Switch Plate Cover 29¢*
MP $10

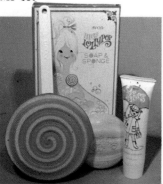

1967 *Sponge and Soap 4 oz $2.50*
MP $13
1968 *Hand Cream (white boots)*
2 oz 75¢ **MP $7**

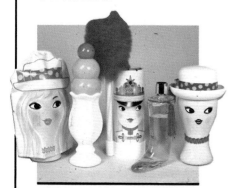

1968 *Bath Powder Mitt $2.50* **MP $7**
1968 *Double Dip Bubble Bath 5 oz $2* **MP $6**
1967 *Talc 3½ oz and Puff $2.50* **MP $12**
1967 *Boot Cologne 2 oz $2* **MP $8**
1967 *Cologne Mist 3 oz $3* **MP $8**

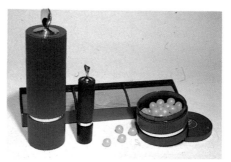

1972 *Boxed Soap, three 3 oz cakes $4* **MP $7**
1971 *Cologne Mist 3 oz $7.50* **MP $3**
1971 *Rollette .33 oz $4* **MP $1**
1972 *Bath Pearls, 75 capsules $5* **MP $6**

MOONWIND

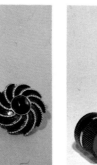 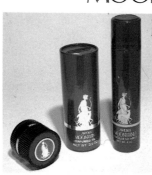

1972-73
Moonwind
Pin/Scarf
Holder $7
MP $10

1971 *Cream Sachet .66oz $4*
MP $1
1973 *Talc 3½oz $1.75* **MP $2***
1975 *Emollient Mist 4oz $4.50*
MP $2

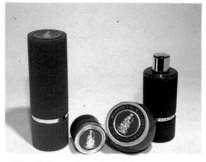

1976 *Cologne Mist 3 oz $8* **MP $1**
1975 *Cream Sachet .66 oz $4.50* **MP $1**
1973 *Skin Softener 5 oz $5* **MP $4***
1972 *Foaming Bath Oil 6 oz $5* **MP $2**

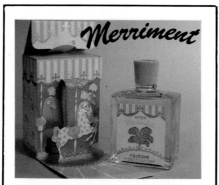

1955 *Merriment Cologne 4 oz (shown) or*
Bubble Bath 4 oz in Jolly Surprise Box
$1.50 **MP $50, $65 boxed**

*Available from Avon at time of publication

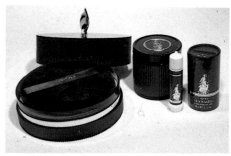

1971 *Beauty Dust 6 oz $7.50* **MP $6**
1972 *Skin Softener 5 oz $5* **MP $3**
1973 *DemiStik .19 oz $2.50* **MP $1**
1975 *Powder Sachet 1¼ oz $3.50* **MP $2**

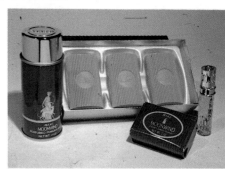

1972 *Powder Mist 7 oz $5* **MP $1**
1975 *Boxed Soap, three 3 oz cakes $6* **MP $6**
1976 *Rollette .33 oz $4.50* **MP $1**
1975 *Soap 3 oz $1.25* **MP $1**

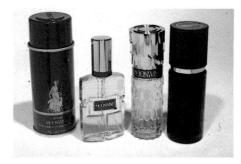

1979 *Powder Mist 4 oz $4.50* **MP 25¢**
1979 *Cologne Spray 1.8 oz $6* **MP 50¢**
1977 *Cologne Spray 1.8 oz $6.50* **MP $1**
1976 *Cologne Spray 2.7oz $8* **MP $8***

(See also Awards pg. 308)

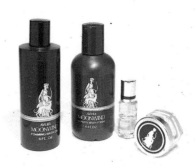

1977 *Foaming Bath Oil 6 oz $5.50* **MP $1**
1980 *Bath Foam 6 oz $5* **MP 50¢**
1979 *Purse Concentre .33 oz $3* **MP 25¢**
1979 *Creme Perfume .66 oz $3.50* **MP $4***

(See also Stockholder's Gifts pg. 330)

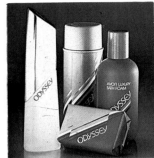

ODYSSEY

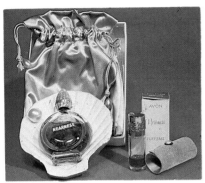

1955 *Gift Perfume ½oz. Satin Bag is gift wrap. $7.50* **MP $100 bottle only, $135 complete**
1955 *One dram Perfume in suedene wrapper $2.25* **MP $10, $17, $20 boxed**

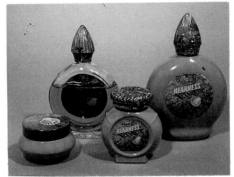

1955 *Cream Sachet .66oz $1.50* **MP $11**
1956 *Toilet Water 2oz $2* **MP $20**
1956 *Powder Sachet $1.50* **MP $12**
1957 *Cologne Mist 3oz $2.75* **MP $25**

1981 *Cologne Spray 1.8oz $10.50* **MP $7***
1981 *Powder Mist 4oz $5* **MP $3.50***
1981 *Bath Foam 6oz $5.50* **MP 25¢**
1981 *Soap 3oz $2.25* **MP $1.50***

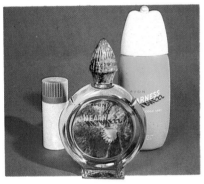

1956 *Cologne Stick $1.50* **MP $10**
1955 *Cologne 4oz $2.50* **MP $20**
1959 *Cologne Mist 3oz $2.95* **MP $24**

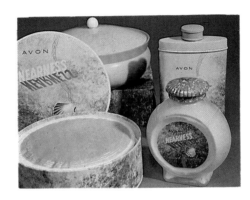

1956 *Beauty Dust $2.25* **MP $22**
1959 *Beauty Dust $2.95* **MP $20**
1957 *Talc in metal container 69¢* **MP $10**
1956 *Body Powder $1* **MP $16**

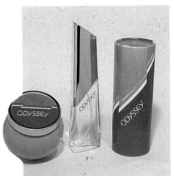

1982 *Perfumed Skin Softener 5oz $6* **MP $3***
1982 *Cologne Spray 1oz $9* **MP $7***
1982 *Talc 3.5oz $3.50* **MP $2***

(See also Awards pg. 310)

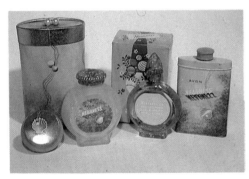

1956 *Two Pearls. Body Powder and Cream Sachet $2.50* **MP $50**
1957 *Nearness Charm. Toilet Water 2oz and Talc $2.50* **MP $45**

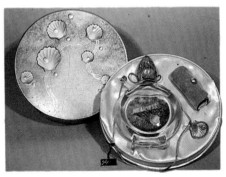

1956 *Always Near. Toilet Water 2oz, 1 dram Perfume & Shell Pendant $5.95* **MP $85, $35 Shell Pendant only**

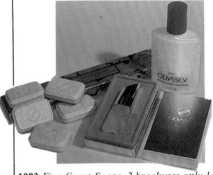

1983 *Five Guest Soaps, 2 brochures only 1oz ea. $6* **MP $4**
1983 *Light & Lavish Cologne 6oz $7.50* **MP $6***
1983 *Ultra Perfume .33oz $13* **MP $11***

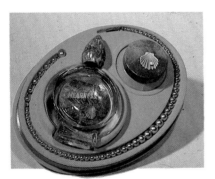

1957 *Circle of Pearls Toilet Water 2oz, Cream Sachet and Pearls $5.95* **MP $70**

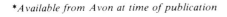
NEARNESS

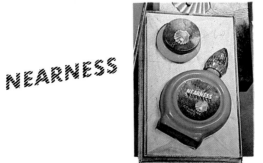

1958 *Sea Mist. Cologne Mist 3oz and Cream Sachet $3.95* **MP $60**

*Available from Avon at time of publication

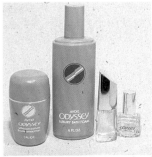

1982 *Ultra Sensation Body Smoother 3oz $6* **MP $5***
1982 *Luxury Bath Foam 6oz $6* **MP $4***
1982 *Fragrance Petite Cologne .33oz $4.50* **MP $2.50***
1981 *Classic Miniature Cologne .33 oz $4* **MP $1**

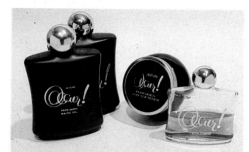

1964 *Perfumed Bath Oil 6oz $2.75* **MP $8**
1966 *Foaming Bath Oil 6oz $3* **MP $2**
1965 *Skin Softener (glass) 5oz $3.50* **MP $7**
1964 *Cologne 2oz $2.50* **MP $2**
1966 *Hair Spray (not shown) $1.50* **MP $3**

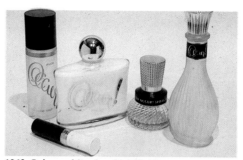

1963 *Cologne Mist 2oz $3* **MP $7**
1964 *Cream Lotion 4oz $1.75* **MP $6**
1967 *Spray Essence 1¼oz $4* **MP $3**
1966-68 *Cologne Silk 3oz $4* **MP $4**
1964 *Perfume Mist 2 drams $3.75* **MP $7**

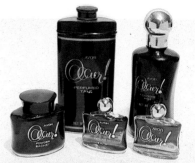

1963 *Powder Sachet .9oz $2.50* **MP $10**
1964 *Talc, metal, 2¾oz $1* **MP $1**
1964 *Perfume Oil ½oz $5* **MP $10**
1963 *Cologne Mist 3oz $5* **MP $3**
1969 *Cologne ½oz $1.50* **MP $2**

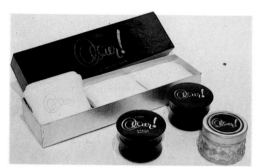

1965 *Boxed Soap, 3 cakes $2.25* **MP $18**
1963 *Cream Sachet .66oz $2.50* **MP $4**
1966 *Cream Sachet .66oz $2.50* **MP $1**
1975 *Cream Sachet .66oz $3* **MP $1**

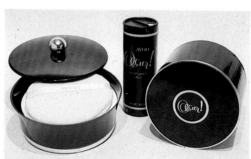

1963 *Beauty Dust 6oz $5* **MP $8**
1971 *Beauty Dust 6oz $4.50* **MP $7**
1975 *Talc 3½oz $2* **MP $2***

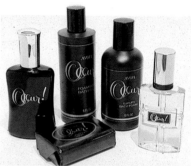

1976 *Cologne Spray 2.7oz $7* **MP $8***
1976 *Foaming Bath Oil 6oz $4.50* **MP $1**
1980 *Bath Foam 6oz $5* **MP 50¢**
1979 *Cologne Spray 1.8oz $6* **MP $1**
1965 *Soap 3oz 49¢* **MP $4**

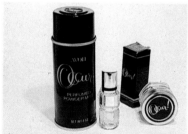

1979 *Powder Mist 4oz $4.50* **MP 50¢**
1979 *Perfume Concentre .33oz $3* **MP 50¢**
1979 *Creme Perfume .66oz $3* **MP $4***

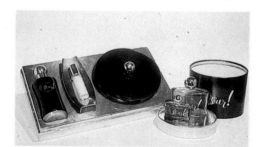

1963 *Sophisticate Set. Cologne Mist, Creme Rollette and Beauty Dust $12.95* **MP $40**
1964 *Fragrance Fortune Set. Perfume Oil ½oz and Cologne 2oz $6.25* **MP $30**

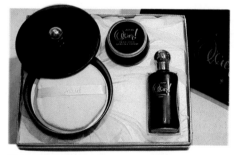

1965 *Deluxe Set. Beauty Dust, Skin Softener and Cologne Mist $13.95* **MP $40**

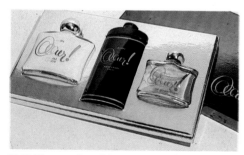

1964 *Elegance Set. Cream Lotion, Cologne 2oz and Talc $5.75* **MP $36**

Available from Avon at time of publication

Pavi Elle

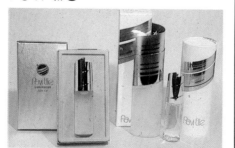

1983 *Ultra Perfume .33oz $13* **MP $11***
1983 *Cologne Spray 1.5oz $13* **MP $9***
1983 *Fragrance Petite Cologne .33oz $4.50* **MP $2.50***
1984 *Perfumed Talc 3.5oz $3.50* **MP $2***

Pearls & Lace

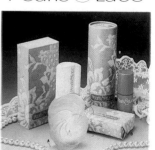

1984 *Cologne Spray 1.5oz $10.50* **MP $8***
1984 *Soft Talc 3.5oz $3.50* **MP $2***
1984 *Silky Powderscents .5oz $5* **MP $3***
1984 *Luscious Creme Soap 3oz $2.50* **MP $1.50***

PATCHWORK

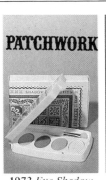
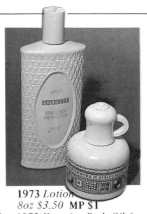

1973 *Eye Shadow Collection with applicator* $5 MP $8, $11 boxed
1973 *Lotion 8oz* $3.50 MP $1
1973 *Foaming Bath Oil 6oz* $5 MP $2

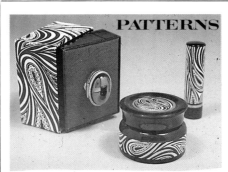

PATTERNS

1969 *Perfume Glace Ring* $6 MP $12
1969 *Cream Sachet .66oz* $3 MP $2
1969 *Lipstick, 3 shades* $1.50 MP $3

(See also Awards pg. 308)

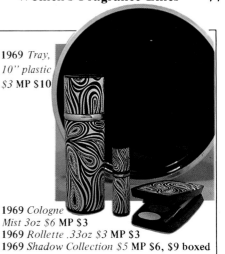

1969 *Tray, 10" plastic* $3 MP $10
1969 *Cologne Mist 3oz* $6 MP $3
1969 *Rollette .33oz* $3 MP $3
1969 *Shadow Collection* $5 MP $6, $9 boxed

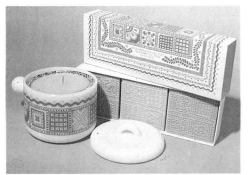

1973 *Perfumed Candle* $7 MP $7
1973 *Soaps, three 3oz cakes* $4.50 MP $8

(See also Awards pg. 312)

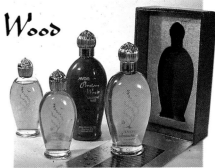

Persian Wood

1957 *Beauty Dust, glass* $3 MP $20
1956 *Cologne Mist 3oz* $3 MP $15
1958 *Powder Sachet, plastic 1¼oz* $2 MP $10
1958 *Lotion Sachet 1oz* $2 MP $11
1959 *Cream Sachet .66oz* $1.75 MP $10

1959 *Toilet Water 2oz* $2.50 MP $12
1961 *Cologne 2oz* $1.75 MP $4
1960 *Cologne Mist 3oz* $3.25 MP $6
1960 *Gift Cologne 4oz* $3 MP $10, $20 boxed

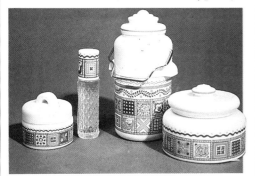

1973 *Cream Sachet .66oz* $4 MP $2
1973 *Rollette .33oz* $4 MP $2
1973 *Cologne Mist 3oz* $5 MP $3
1973 *Cologne Gelee 3oz* $5 MP $3

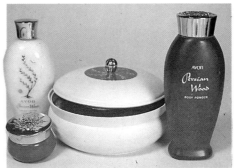

1959 *Cream Sachet .66oz* $1.75 MP $4
1961 *Cream Lotion 4oz* $1.25 MP $8
1961 *Beauty Dust, plastic 6oz* $3.25 MP $14
1961 *Body Powder 4oz* $1.95 MP $12

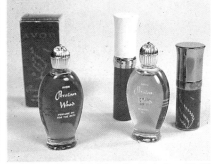

1963 *Perfumed Oil for the Bath ½oz* $3.50 MP $12
1963 *Perfume Mist 2 drams* $3.25 MP $7
1964 *Perfume Oil ½oz* $3.50 MP $9
1957 *Spray Perfume 2 drams* $3.25 MP $15

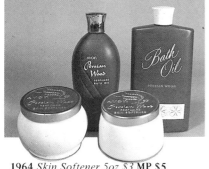

1964 *Skin Softener 5oz* $3 MP $5
1960 *Perfumed Bath Oil, plastic 6oz* $2.25 MP $8
1960 *Skin Softener 5oz* $3 MP $7
1962 *Bath Oil 6oz (from Bath Bouquet Set)* $2.79 MP $10 Bottle only

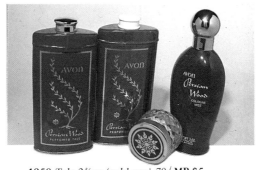

1958 *Talc 2¾oz (gold cap)* 79¢ MP $5
1962 *Talc 2¾oz (white cap)* 79¢ MP $3
1975 *Cream Sachet .66oz* $3 MP $1
1976 *Cologne Mist 3oz (smooth cap)* $7 MP $4

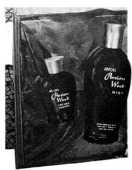

1958 *Persian Fancy. Cologne Mist and choice of Powder or Lotion Sachet* $5 MP $42

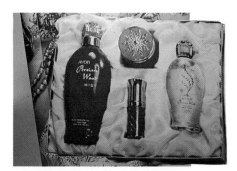

1959 *Persian Treasures. Cologne Mist, Cream Sachet, Spray Perfume & Toilet Water 2oz $10.75* **MP $62**

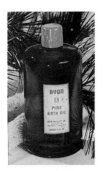

1940-51 *Bath Oil 6oz 85¢* **MP $30, $35** boxed

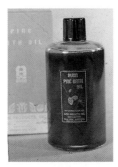

1941 only *Bath Oil 6oz 95¢* **MP $38, $43** boxed

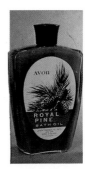

1957-60 *Royal Pine Bath Oil 8oz $1.95* **MP $25, $30** boxed

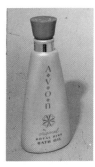

1961 *Original Royal Pine Bath Oil 8oz $2* **MP $8**

Pine

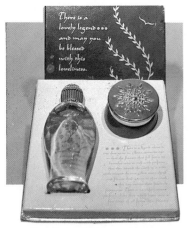

1961 *Persian Magic. Cologne 2oz & Cream Sachet $3.50* **MP $25**

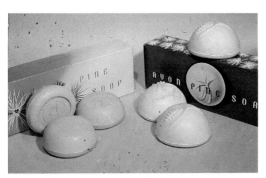

1939-58 *Boxed Soaps, 3 cakes 69¢* **MP $65**
1940 only *Boxed Soaps, 3 cakes (right) 69¢* **MP $80**

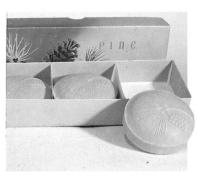

1959 *Royal Pine Soaps, 3 cakes $1.25* **MP $30**

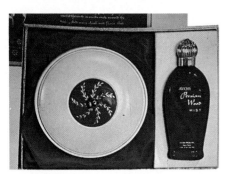

1961 *Persian Legend. Beauty Dust and Cologne Mist $6.50* **MP $40**

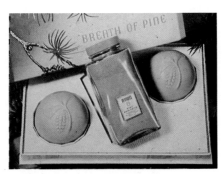

1939-42 *Breath of Pine. 2 cakes Soap & Bath Salts $1.25* **MP $70**

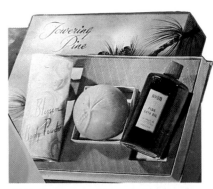

1941-42 *Towering Pine. Apple Blossom Body Powder, Pine Bath Oil 6oz & Soap $1.65* **MP $75**

...Persian Wood

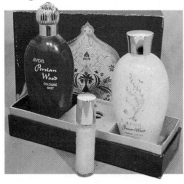

1963 *Persian Intrigue. .3oz Cologne Mist, 4oz Cream Lotion and Perfumed Cream Rollette $6.50* **MP $34**

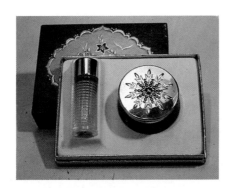

1964 *Persian Mood. One dram Perfume and Cream Sachet $4* **MP $28**

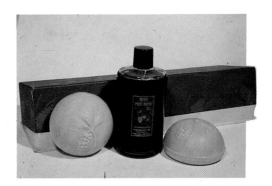

1941-43 *Royal Pine Set. Bath Oil 6oz and 2 Soaps $1.50* **MP $65**

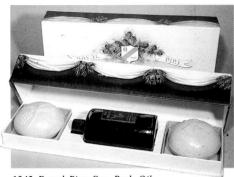

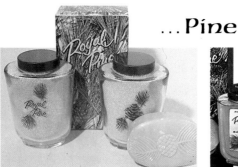

...Pine

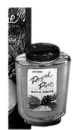

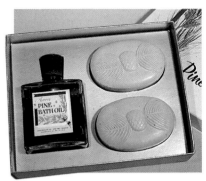

1943 *Royal Pine Set. Bath Oil 6 oz and 2 Soaps $1.60* **MP $65**
1945 *Same set as above, but issued in shorter box (shown closed) $1.60* **MP $65**

1954 *Royal Pine Set. Bath Salts 8oz and Soap $1.25* **MP $50** *(Shown with both issues of Bath Salts offered in Set)* **Either Bath Salts MP $35**

1957 *Bath Salts 8oz 89¢* **MP $25**

1956 *Pinehurst Set. Bath Oil 4oz and 2 cakes Soap $1.75* **MP $55** *Bath Oil* **MP $38**

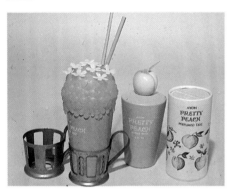

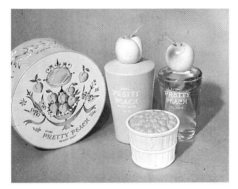

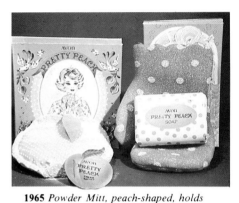

1964 *Cologne Mist (shown with both issues of holder) 2oz $2.50* **MP $16, Holder MP $4, Straws MP $2 each**
1964 *Bubble Bath 4oz $1.35* **MP $10**
1964 *Talc 2½oz 79¢* **MP $10**

1964 *Beauty Dust 4oz $2.50* **MP $15**
1964 *Lotion 4oz $1.35* **MP $10**
1964 *Cologne 2oz $1.50* **MP $10**
1964 *Cream Sachet .66oz $1.50* **MP $7**

1965 *Powder Mitt, peach-shaped, holds 2½oz Talc $1.50* **MP $9, $12 boxed**
1964 *Cream Sachet Sample, peach-shaped foil* **MP $2**
1966 *Peachy-Kleen sponge Bath Mitt and Soap 3oz $2.25* **MP $15, $18 boxed**

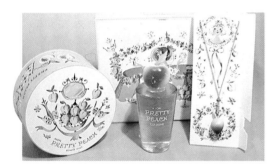

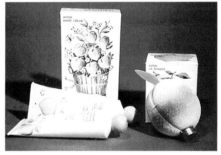

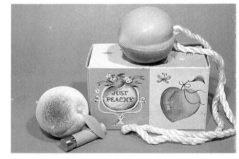

1965 *Peach Delight Set. Beauty Dust and Cologne 2oz & enameled "Peach" Necklace $5.95* **MP $60, $25 necklace only**

1964 *Peach Smooth Set. 2 tubes Hand Cream 1¾oz each $1.35* **MP $20**
1964 *Lip Pomade encased in styrofoam peach $1* **MP $20, $23 boxed**

1964 *Just Peachy. Peach Soap-On-A-Rope and Lip Pomade $2.35* **MP $42**

PRETTY PEACH

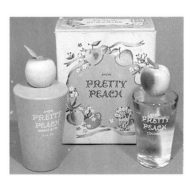

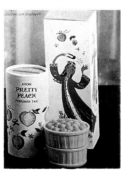

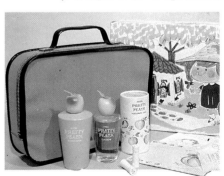

1964 *Soap, 2 halves and pit $1.50* **MP $18, $24 boxed**
1964 *Soap-On-A-Rope $1.35* **MP $12, $18 boxed**

1964 *Peach Surprise. Cologne 2oz, choice of 4oz Bubble Bath or Cream Lotion $2.35* **MP $26**

1965 *Pretty Peach Princess. Talc and Cream Sachet $2.25* **MP $23**

1964-65 *Miss Avon Set. Bubble Bath 4oz, Cologne 2oz, packages of Lip Dew Samples & Talc Samples (10 ea), descriptive product letter to "Miss Avon" & Case $7.50* **MP $95 complete $115 boxed. Lip Dew Samples MP $10, Talc Samples MP $10, "Miss Avon" Letter MP $25, Case MP $20**

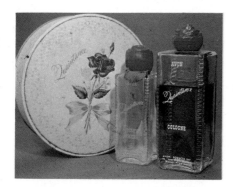
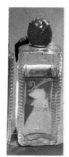
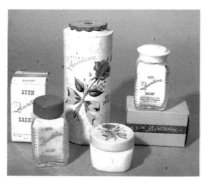
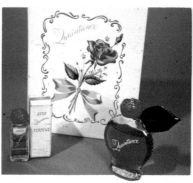

1948 Beauty Dust 6 oz $1.50 **MP $16**
1953 Toilet Water 2 oz $1.25 **MP $18**
1948 Cologne 4 oz $1.75 **MP $14**

*1948 Cologne
2 oz (sets only)*
MP $23

1949 Powder Sachet .9 oz $1.19 **MP $12,
$15 boxed**
1948 Body Powder 4½oz 75¢ **MP $16**
1952 Cream Sachet .66 oz $1.25 **MP $12**
*1949 Powder Sachet, 63rd Anniversary
Issue .9 oz 63¢* **MP $30, $40 boxed**

*1948 Perfume 1 dram
$1.50* **MP $75, $85 boxed**
1950 Perfume 3 drams $4 **MP $130,
$160 boxed**

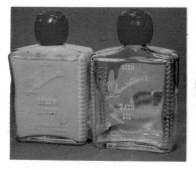
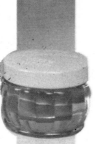
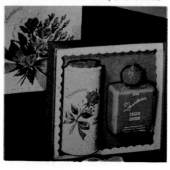
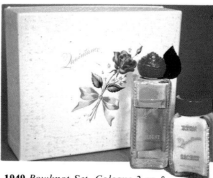

1948 Cream Lotion 4 oz 89¢ **MP $13**
1949 Bath Oil 4 oz $1.50 **MP $18**

*1950 Cream Sachet,
metal lid (rare)*
MP $40

*1949 Rosegay Set. Body Powder and
Cream Lotion $1.75* **MP $65**

*1949 Bowknot Set. Cologne 2 oz &
Powder Sachet $2.25* **MP $60**

Quaintance

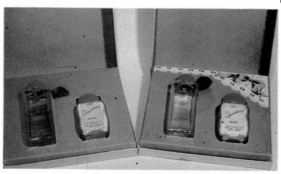
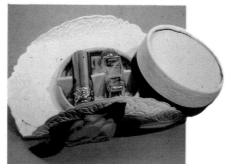
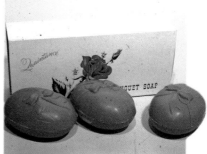

*1948 Quaintance Set. Cologne 2 oz and
Powder Sachet 1¼ oz $2.39* **MP $60**

*1948 Gay Bonnet. Hat-shaped box holds
Perfume ⅛ oz & Lipstick $2.35* **MP $110**

1954 Boxed Soap, 3 cakes $1.59 **MP $50**

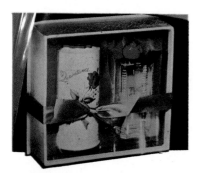
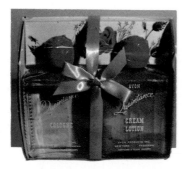
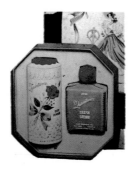
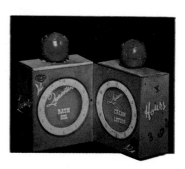

*1950 Harmony Set. Body Powder
and Cologne 2 oz $2.85* **MP $60**

*1952 Quaintance Harmony. Cologne
and Cream Lotion 4 oz each $2.75*
MP $55, $25 Cologne only
*1953 As above with Blue
Ribbon* **MP $55**

*1952 Miss Quaintance. Body
Powder and Cream Lotion
4 oz $1.95* **MP $60**

*1954 Leisure Hours. Bath Oil and
Cream Lotion 4 oz each $2.15*
MP $55

(See also Awards pg. 306)

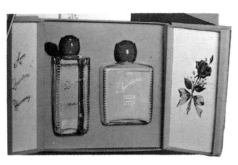

1954 *Harmony Set. Cologne 2 oz and Cream Lotion $2.25* **MP $57**

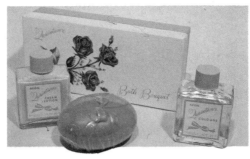

1955 *Bath Bouquet Set. Cream Lotion and Cologne 2 oz each, and Soap $1.95* **MP $60**

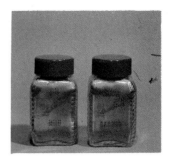

1948 only *Powder Sachets (different size labels) 1¼oz ea. $1.19* **MP $18 each**

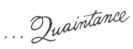

... Quaintance

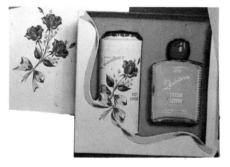

1954 *Rosegay Set. Body Powder and Cream Lotion $1.95* **MP $57**

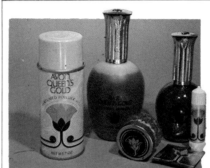

QUEEN'S GOLD

1975 *Fragrance Sample* **MP $1.50**

1975 *Powder Mist 7 oz $4.50* **MP $5**
1975 *Foaming Bath Oil 10 oz $7* **MP $8**
1975 *Cream Sachet .66 oz $3* **MP $4**
1975 *Cologne Mist 3 oz $7* **MP $5**
1975 *DemiStik .19oz $2* **MP $3**

(See also Bath Oil Gift pg. 309)

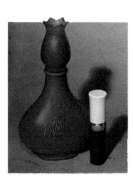

1965 *Perfumed Bath Oil 6 oz $2.75* **MP $7**
1964 *Perfume Mist 2 drams $3.75* **MP $7**

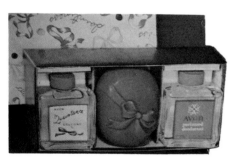

1955 *Daintiness Set. Cologne and Perfumed Deodorant 2 oz each, and Soap $1.95* **MP $55**

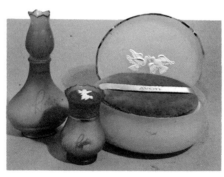

1965 *Cream Lotion 4 oz $1.75* **MP $4**
1964 *Powder Sachet .9 oz $2.50* **MP $10**
1964 *Beauty Dust 6 oz $5* **MP $12**

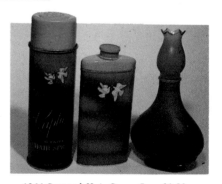

1966 *Scented Hair Spray 7 oz $1.50* **MP $3**
1965 *Talc 2¾ oz $1* **MP $1**
1966 *Foaming Bath Oil 6 oz $3* **MP $2**

(See also Awards pg. 308)

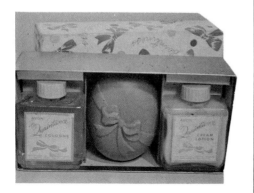

1956 *Daintiness Set. Cologne and Cream Lotion $1.95* **MP $57**

Rapture

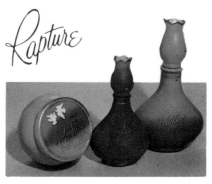

1965 *Skin Softener 5 oz $3.50* **MP $3**
1964 *Cologne 2 oz $2.50* **MP $3**
1964 *Cologne Mist 3 oz $5* **MP $2**

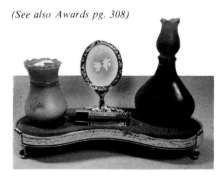

1964 *Rapture Rhapsody. Powder Sachet, Cologne 2 oz and 1 dram Perfume $10.95* **MP $52**

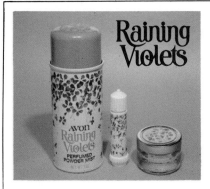

Raining Violets

1973 *Powder Mist 7 oz* **MP $1**
1974 *DemiStik .19 oz $1.75* **MP $1**
1975 *Cream Sachet .66 oz $3* **MP $1**

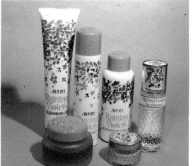

1973 *Cleansing Gel 6oz $3* **MP $2**
1973 *Emollient Mist 4oz $3* **MP $1**
1973 *Moisturizing Bath Oil 6oz $4* **MP $1**
1974 *Cologne Mist 2oz $4.25* **MP $2**
1973 *Cologne Gelee 3oz $4* **MP $2**
1974 *Cream Sachet .66oz $2.50* **MP $1**

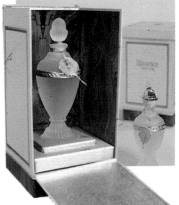

1966 *Perfume 1 oz $30* **MP $40,**
$55 boxed
1966 *Perfume ½ oz $15*
MP $25, $40 boxed

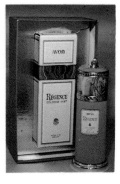

1966 *Cologne Mist*
3 oz in Presentation
Box **MP $35**

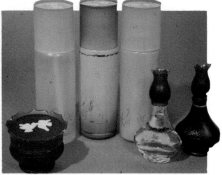

1964 *Cream Sachet .66oz $2.50* **MP $1**
1966 *Cologne Mist 2oz $3* **MP $9**
1966 *Cologne Mist 2oz $3* **MP $8**
1965 *Cologne Mist 2oz $3* **MP $7**
1969 *Half-ounce Cologne $1.50* **MP $3**
1964 *Perfume Oil ½oz $5* **MP $9**

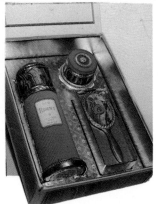

1966 *Gift Set. Cologne Mist,*
Cream Sachet & Purse Mirror
$12.50 **MP $45, mirror only $12**

RÉGENCE

(Say, "Ray-JAUNCE")

Packaging inspired by malachite, a rare stone treasured by European royal families for centuries

1968 *Perfumed Candle Container*
10½" $10 **MP $18**
1967 *Perfumed Candle Container*
$6 **MP $20**

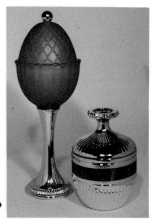

(See also Stockholder's Gifts pg. 330)

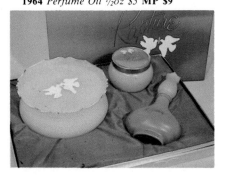

1965 *Deluxe Set. Beauty Dust, Skin*
Softener 5 oz and Cologne Mist 3 oz
$13.95 **MP $38**

Rapture

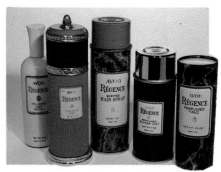

1966 *Cologne Mist Refill 3 oz $4* **MP $5**
1966 *Cologne Mist 3 oz $6* **MP $5**
1968 *Hair Spray 7 oz $1.50* **MP $3**
1967 *Powder Mist 7 oz $4* **MP $2**
1968 *Talc $1.25* **MP $1.50**

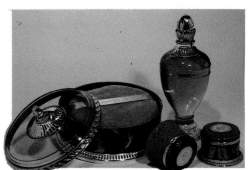

1966 *Beauty Dust with Malachite band 6 oz $6* **MP $10**
1966 *Beauty Dust, paper band (not shown) $6* **MP $13**
1967 *Skin-So-Soft Bath Oil 6 oz $5* **MP $6**
1968 *Cream Sachet .66 oz $3* **MP $3**
1966 *Cream Sachet .66 oz (Malachite band) $3* **MP $8**

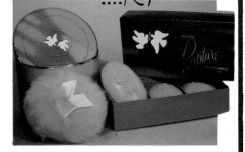

1971 *Beauty Dust non-refillable 6 oz $4.50*
MP $9
1965 *Boxed Soaps, 3 cakes $2* **MP $20**

(See also Awards pg. 308)
(See also Stockholder's Gifts pg. 330)

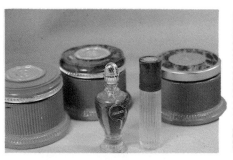

1967 *Skin Softener 5 oz $4* **MP $7**
1968 *Skin Softener 5 oz $4* **MP $5**
1967 *Perfumed Oil ½ oz $6* **MP $9**
1967 *Rollette .33 oz $3* **MP $2**
1971 *Skin Softener 5 oz $4* **MP $3**

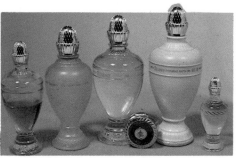

1967 *Cologne 2 oz $3* **MP $3**
1968 *Cologne Silk 3 oz $4.50* **MP $4**
1969 *Cologne 4 oz $6* **MP $3**
1967 *Perfume Glace .6 oz $5.50* **MP $7**
1969 *Foaming Bath Oil 6 oz $3.50* **MP $2**
1969 *Cologne ½ oz $1.75* **MP $3**

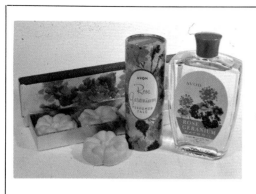
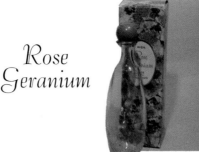
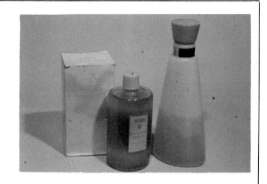

Rose Geranium

1966 *Boxed Soap, 4 cakes $2.25* **MP $25**
1964 *Talc 3½ oz 89¢* **MP $5**
1957-59 *Bath Oil 8 oz $1.95* **MP $30**

1963 *After Bath Freshener 8 oz $2.50* **MP $7**

1946-50 *Bath Oil 6 oz 95¢* **MP $25, $30 boxed**
1959-63 *Perfumed Bath Oil 8 oz $2* **MP $3**

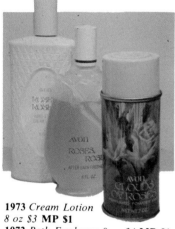
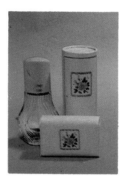
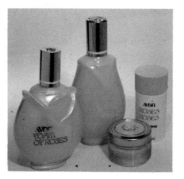
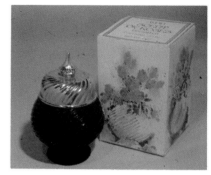

1973 *Cream Lotion 8 oz $3* **MP $1**
1972 *Bath Freshener 8 oz $4* **MP $1**
1972 *Powder Mist 7 oz $4* **MP $1**

1980 *Cologne Spray 1.5 oz $6* **MP $1**
1980 *Talc 3.5 oz $2.50* **MP $2***
1980 *Soap 3 oz $1.75* **MP $1.50***

1972 *Foam of Roses Bath Foam 5 oz $4* **MP $1**
1972 *Cologne Mist 3 oz $6* **MP $3**
1977 *Cream Sachet .66 oz $3* **MP $1**
1978 *Cologne Ice 1 oz $3.75* **MP $2**

1972 *Scent of Roses Cologne Gelee 6 oz $6* **MP $3, $4 boxed**

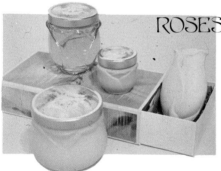
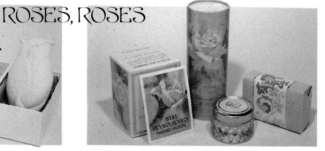
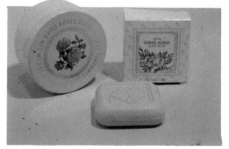

ROSES, ROSES

1972 *Cologne Gelee 3 oz $4* **MP $2**
1972 *Cream Sachet .66 oz $3* **MP $1**
1972 *Boxed Soap, three 3 oz cakes $3.50* **MP $6**
1973 *Skin Softener 5 oz $4* **MP $3**

1972 *Kwickettes, 14 per box $1.35* **MP $3**
1974 *Talc 3½ oz $1.50* **MP $1**
1975 *Cream Sachet .66 oz $3* **MP 75¢**
1974 & 75 *Xmas wrap Soap 3 oz $1.25* **MP $2**

1983 *Floral Perfumed Skin Softener 2 oz $2.50* **MP $1.50***
1983 *Fancy Floral Guest Soap 1 oz $1.50* **MP $1 boxed**

(See Bubble Bath Gelee pg. 165, Glow of Roses Candle pg. 203, Awards pg. 311)

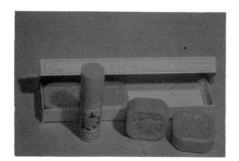
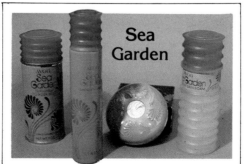
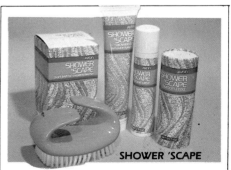

Sea Garden

SHOWER 'SCAPE

1983 *Puff of Fragrance .4 oz $5* **MP $4**
1983 *Floral Boxed Soaps. Four 1 oz cakes $5* **MP $4***

*Available from Avon at time of publication

1970 *Powder Mist 7oz $3.75* **MP $1**
1970 *Emollient Mist 4oz $3* **MP $1**
1970 *Shower Soap 6oz $2* **MP $6**
1970 *Emollient Bath Foam 5oz $4* **MP $3**

1980 *Soft Bristle Shower Brush $13* **MP $6**
1980 *Shower Gel 6 oz $5* **MP 50¢**
1980 *Moisture Mist 2.8 oz $4* **MP 50¢**
1980 *Smooth Talc 5 oz $4* **MP 50¢**

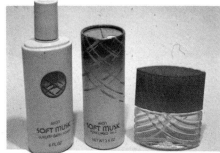

1983 *Body Smoother 3oz $5.50* **MP $4***
1982 *Bath Oil Pearls, 8 per pkg. $5.50*
MP $2.25

Skin-So-Soft

Avon's all-time favorite bath line, Skin-So-Soft bath products have been softening and smoothing skins for over 20 years.

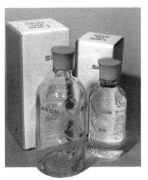

1964 *Emollient Bath Oil 8oz*
$4 **MP $2**
1961 *Emollient Bath Oil 4oz*
$2.25 **MP $3**

SOFT MUSK

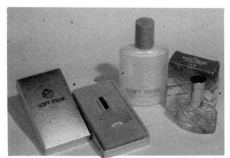

1983 *Luxury Bath Foam 6oz $6.50* **MP $4***
1982 *Talc 3.5oz $3.50* **MP $2***
1982 *Cologne Spray 1.5oz $10.50* **MP $9***

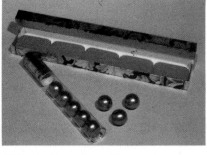

1982 *Fragrance Petite Cologne .33oz $4.50*
MP $2.50*
1982 *Essence of Soft Musk .33oz $5.50*
MP $4*
1983 *Perfumed Skin Softener 5oz $6* **MP $4***

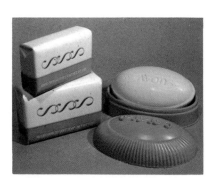

1964 *Soap 3oz 49¢* **MP $1.50***
1976 *Bath Soap 5oz $1.75* **MP $1.50**
1966 *Gift Soap 5¾oz in covered plastic*
Soap Dish $1.50 **MP $10. Dish only $5**

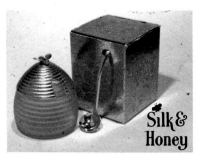

1983 *Perfume .33oz $13* **MP $11***
1983 *Light & Lavish Cologne 6oz $7.50*
MP $6*
1983 *Cologne Spray 1oz $9* **MP $6***

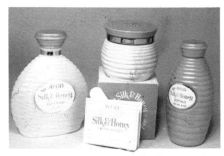

1983 *Five Guest Soaps (2 campaigns only)*
1oz each $6 **MP $4**
1983 *Bath Oil Pearls, 8 per pkg. 1.2oz*
$6.50 **MP $4***

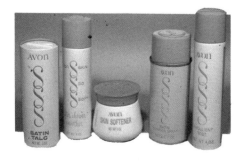

1968-76 *Talc 3oz $1.25* **MP 50¢**
1969 *After Shower Smoother 4oz $2.50*
MP 50¢
1973-79 *Skin Softener 5oz $4* **MP 50¢**
1973 *Powder Spray 7oz $4* **MP 75¢**
1975 *Emollient Mist 4oz $4* **MP $2**

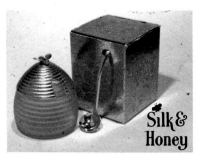
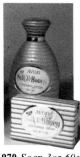

Silk & Honey

1969 *Silk & Honey Bath Gelee with golden ladle 4½oz $6* **MP $10 boxed,**
Ladle MP $4

1970 *Soap 3oz 60¢*
MP $2
1968 *Cream Lotion*
6oz $2.50 **MP $2**

1968 *Bath Foam 6oz $3* **MP $2**
1969 *Creamy Masque 3oz $2.50* **MP $2**
1968 *Softalc 3oz $1.50* **MP $2**

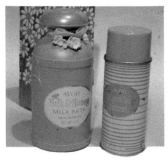

1970 *Milk Bath 6oz $5* **MP $5,**
$7 boxed
1970 *Powder Mist 7oz $3.75* **MP $3**

*Available from Avon at time of publication

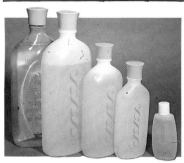
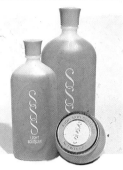
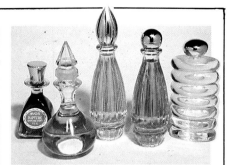
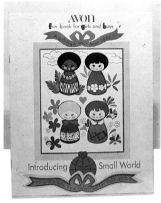

1972 *Bath Oil (clear) 16oz $7.50* **MP $1**
1972 *Bath Oil (frosted) 16oz $7.50* **MP $8***
1969 *Bath Oil 8oz $4* **MP $5***
1969 *Bath Oil 4oz $2.25* **MP 50¢**
1977 *Bath Oil 1oz trial size 25¢ with another purchase* **MP $1**
(as above, with aqua lid **MP 25¢***)*

1978 *Light Bouquet SSS Bath Oil 8oz $5* **MP $5***
1979 *As above, 16oz $8.50* **MP $8***
1980 *Skin Softener 5oz $5.50* **MP $3.50***

Scented SSS Miniatures (left to right)
1969 *1oz 8 fragrances $1.50* **MP $5**
1969 *2oz 9 fragrances $2.50* **MP $6**
1970 *2oz 8 fragrances $2.50* **MP $3**
1974 *2oz 5 fragrances $4* **MP $3**
1971 *2oz 5 fragrances $2.50* **MP $3**

1970 *Coloring Book sold only to Representatives and given to customer's children.* **MP $5**

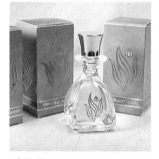
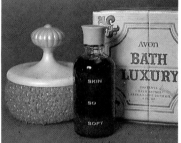
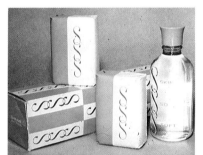
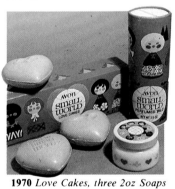

1966 *Fragrance Trio. Set of three 1oz miniatures in 9 fragrances* **MP $20** **complete with sleeve (not shown). Each bottle MP $5**

1966 *Bath Luxury. Sponge and SSS Bath Oil 4oz $4.50* **MP $13**

1964 *Bath Mates. SSS Bath Oil 4oz and two 3oz Soaps $3.23* **MP $10**

1971 *Fragrance Watch Glace .02oz $3.50* **MP $9**
1970 *Love Dove Cream Sachet .66oz $3* **MP $5**
1970 *Ali Barbara DemiStik $1.50* **MP $3**

. . . SKIN-SO-SOFT

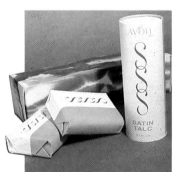
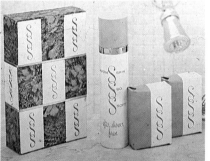
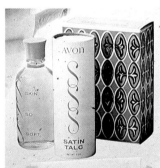

1967 *Skin-So-Soft Complements. Talc 3oz and two 3oz Soaps $2.50* **MP $11**

1965 *Shower Mates. After Shower Foam 4oz and two 3oz Soaps $3.20* **MP $14**

1968 *Skin-So-Soft Smoothies. SSS Bath Oil 4oz and Satin Talc 3oz $2.50* **MP $7**

1970 *Love Cakes, three 2oz Soaps $2* **MP $11**
1971 *Talc 3½oz $1.25* **MP $4**
1971 *Cream Sachet .66oz $2.50* **MP $5**

Small world

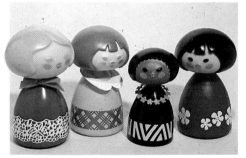
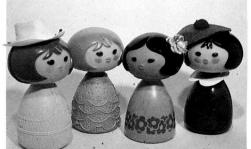
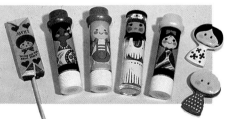

1970 *Heidi Cologne Mist 3oz $5* **MP $8**
1970 *Bubbly O'Bath Bubble Bath 5oz $3.50* **MP $10**
1970 *Splashu Cologne 2oz $3.50* **MP $8**
1970 *Poolu Non-tear Shampoo 5oz $3.50* **MP $8**

1971 *Wendy Cowgirl Cream Lotion 5oz $5* **MP $8**
1971 *English Girl Bubble Bath 5oz $3.50* **MP $8**
1971 *Senorita Non-tear Shampoo 5oz $3.50* **MP $8**
1971 *Gigi Cologne Mist 3oz $5* **MP $8**

*Available from Avon at time of publication

1970 *Lollipop given to Small World customers by Representatives* **MP $20**
1970 *Lipkin, Tropical Fruit $1.75* **MP $4**
1970 *Lipkin, Dutch Chocolate $1.75* **MP $4**
1971 *Rollette $1.75* **MP $5**
1970 *Lipkin, French Mint $1.75* **MP $4**
1970 *Polynesian Pin Pal .02oz $2.50* **MP $7**
1971 *Scandinavian Pin Pal .02oz $2.50* **MP $7**

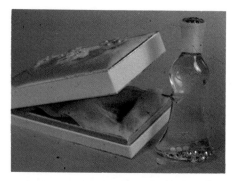

1961 *Perfume 1oz $20* **MP $65, $85 boxed**

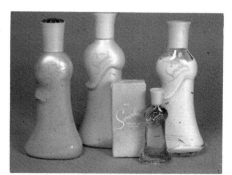

1961 *Cologne Mist 3oz $4* **MP $6**
1962 *Bath Oil, plastic 6oz $2.50* **MP $6**
1963 *Perfume Oil for Bath ½oz $4* **MP $12**
1962 *Cream Lotion 4oz $1.50* **MP $6**

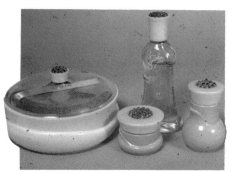

1961 *Beauty Dust 6oz $4* **MP $12**
1962 *Cream Sachet .66oz $2* **MP $5**
1961 *Cologne 2oz $2* **MP $6**
1962 *Powder Sachet .9oz $2* **MP $8**

Somewhere

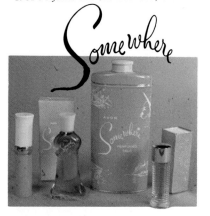

1963 *Perfume Mist 2 drams $3.25* **MP $7**
1964 *Perfume Oil ½oz $4* **MP $11**
1962 *Talc 2¾oz 89¢* **MP $4**
1962 *Perfume 1 dram $2.50* **MP $9**

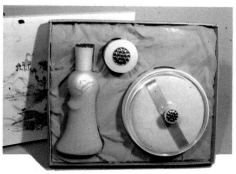

1962 *Unforgettable Set. Cologne Mist 3oz Cream Sachet .66oz and Beauty Dust 6oz $10.95* **MP $42**

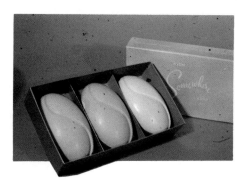

1962 *Boxed Soap, three 3oz cakes $1.50* **MP $25**

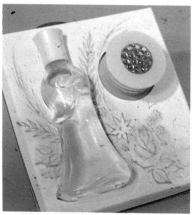

1964 *Dream Castle. Cologne 2oz and Cream Sachet $4* **MP $32**

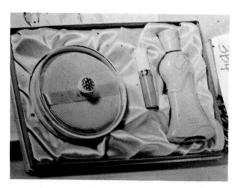

1964 *Dreams of Somewhere. Beauty Dust, Perfume Mist, Cream Lotion 4oz $9.25* **MP $42**

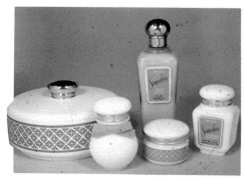

1966 *Beauty Dust 6oz $4* **MP $13**
1967 *Powder Sachet (rare) .9oz $2* **MP $26**
1966 *Cream Lotion 4oz $1.50* **MP $7**
1966 *Cream Sachet .66oz $2* **MP $2**
1966 *Powder Sachet .9oz $2* **MP $22**

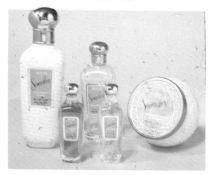

1966 *Cologne Mist 3oz $4* **MP $3**
1966 *Perfume Oil ½oz $4* **MP $8**
1966 *Cologne 2oz $2* **MP $3**
1969 *Cologne ½oz $1.50* **MP $3**
1966 *Skin Softener 5oz $3.25* **MP $2**

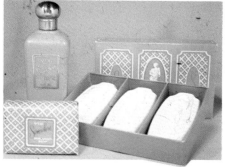

1966 *Bath Oil 6oz $2.75* **MP $3**
1966 *Soap 3oz 49¢* **MP $4**
1966 *Boxed Soap, three 3oz cakes $2* **MP $16**

(See also Awards page 307)

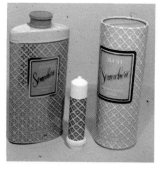

1966 *Talc 2¾oz $1* **MP $1**
1975 *DemiStik .19oz $2* **MP $1**
1974 *Talc 3½oz $1.50* **MP 75¢**

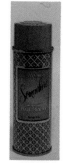

1966 *Scented Hair Spray 7oz $1.50* **MP $3**

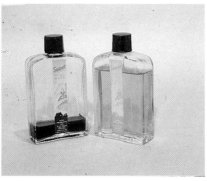

1941 *Toilet Water 2oz in "green dress", Founder's Day customer offer in July 1941 only. 20¢* **MP $40, $55 boxed**
1940 *Toilet Water 2oz in "yellow dress" introductory bottle $1.19* **MP $40, $55 boxed**

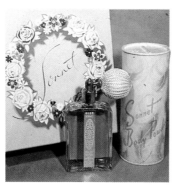

1941 *Sonnet Set. Toilet Water 2oz Atomizer and Body Powder 5oz $2* **MP $75**

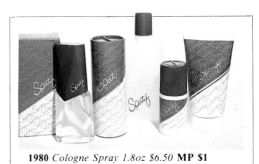

1980 *Cologne Spray 1.8oz $6.50* **MP $1**
1980 *Talc 3.5 oz $3* **MP 50¢**
1980 *Moisturizing Body Splash 8oz $5* **MP 75¢**
1980 *Roll-On Deodorant 2oz $1.89* **MP 50¢**
1980 *Fresh & Foaming Body Cleanser 6oz $5.50* **MP 75¢**

(See also Awards pg. 307)

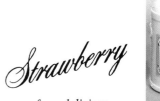
Sportif

Sonnet

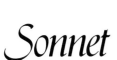

*. . . as eloquent
as a love poem . . .*

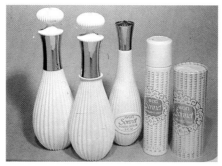

1972 *Cologne Mist 3oz $7.50* **MP $5**
1972 *Cologne Mist 3oz (with ring below neck) $7.50* **MP $1**
1973 *Foaming Bath Oil 6oz $5* **MP $2**
1975 *Emollient Mist 4oz $4.50* **MP $1**
1973 *Talc 3½oz $1.75* **MP $50¢**

Strawberry

. . . for a delicious, fragrance-filled experience . . .

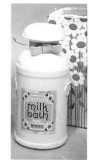

1968 *Milk Bath Strawberry Scented 6oz $4* **MP $6**

(See also Awards pg. 309)

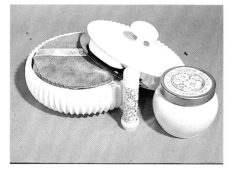

1973 *Beauty Dust 6oz $7.50* **MP $5**
1973 *DemiStik, .19oz $2.50* **MP $1**
1973 *Skin Softener 5oz $5* **MP $1**

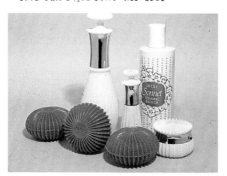

1972 *Boxed Soaps, three 3oz $5* **MP $10**
1977 *Cologne Spray 2.7oz $7.50* **MP $1**
1972 *Rollette .33oz $4* **MP $1**
1977 *Foaming Bath Oil 6oz $4.50* **MP $1**
1972 *Cream Sachet .66oz $4* **MP $1**

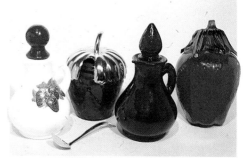

1969 *Strawberries and Cream. Strawberry scented Bathfoam 4oz $3.50* **MP $7**
1971 *Bath Gelee 4½oz with golden ladle $7* **MP $9**
1971 *Bath Foam Pitcher 4oz $4* **MP $7**
1973 *Big Berry Strawberry Bathfoam 10oz $5* **MP $5**

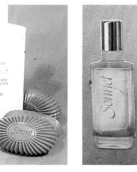

1975 *Powder Sachet 1¼oz $3.50* **MP $1**
1973 *Powder Mist 7oz $5* **MP $1**
1973 *Cream Lotion 8oz $3.50* **MP $1**
1973 *Boxed Soap, three 3oz $5* **MP $8**

1975 *Cologne 2oz $5* **MP $1**

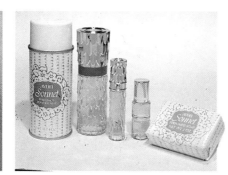

1979 *Powder Mist 4oz $4.50* **MP $1**
1974 *Cologne Mist 2oz $6* **MP $2**
1976 *Rollette .33oz $4.50* **MP $2**
1979 *Purse Concentre .33oz $3* **MP $1**
1975 *Soap 3oz $1.25* **MP $1**

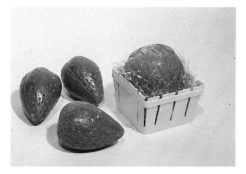

1971 *Strawberry Guest Soap, 3 in box, 2oz each $3* **MP $15 boxed (box not shown)**
1969 *Strawberry Fair. Plastic Soap Dish holds cellophane 'straw' and 5oz Strawberry scented soap $3* **MP $8, $11 boxed**

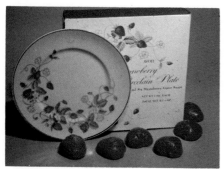

1978 *Strawberry Porcelain Plate, hand decorated with 22k gold trim. Six 1oz strawberry scented soaps $17.50* **MP $18. Plate MP $13**

Strawberry

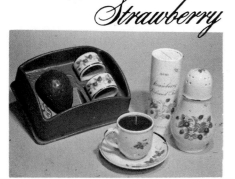

1978 *Strawberry Porcelain Napkin Rings, ea. 2" diam & one Strawberry scented 5oz soap $11* **MP $11**
1978 *Strawberry Porcelain Demi-Cup Fragrance Candlette, Strawberry scent. Saucer 4" diam $15* **MP $11**
1979 *Strawberry Porcelain Sugar Shaker & Talc 3.5oz $16* **MP $12, Talc MP $2**

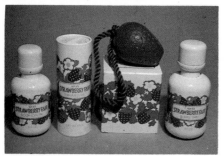

1979 *Strawberry Fair Body Lotion 6oz $4.50* **MP $1**
1979 *Strawberry Fair Talc 3.5oz $2.50* **MP $1**
1979 *Strawberry Fair Shower Soap $5.50* **MP $5**
1979 *Bubble Bath 8oz $4.50* **MP $1**

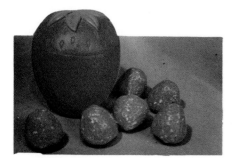

1974 *Pick-A-Berry plastic soap container holds six 1oz Strawberry Scented Soaps $6* **MP $7**

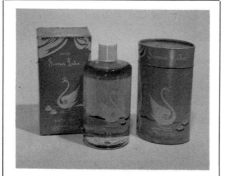

1947 *Bath Oil 6oz $1.25* **MP $55, $70** boxed
1947 *Bath Salts 85¢* **MP $38**

Swan Lake

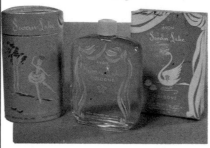

1947 *Body Powder 9oz 85¢* **MP $38**
1947 *Cologne 4oz $1.35* **MP $55, $70 boxed**

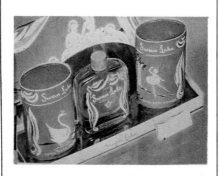

1947 *Three Piece Set. Body Powder 9oz, Cologne 4oz and Bath Salts $3.25* **MP $150**

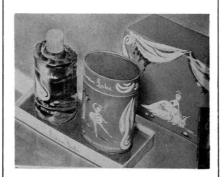

1947 *Two Piece Set. Bath Oil 6oz and Body Powder 9oz $2.29* **MP $120**

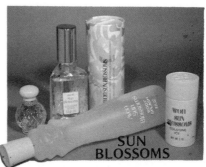

SUN BLOSSOMS

1978 *Cologne .5oz $2* **MP $1**
1978 *Cologne Spray 1.8oz $5* **MP $1**
1978 *Talc 3.5oz $2* **MP $1**
1978 *Body Splash 8oz $5* **MP $1**
1978 *Cologne Ice 1oz $3.75* **MP $2**

Sweet Honesty

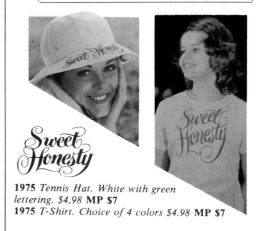

1975 *Tennis Hat. White with green lettering. $4.98* **MP $7**
1975 *T-Shirt. Choice of 4 colors $4.98* **MP $7**

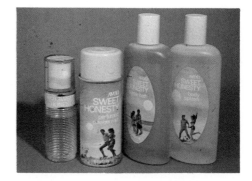

1973 *Cologne Mist 2oz $4.50* **MP $1**
1974 *Powder Mist 7oz $3.75* **MP $1**
1976 *Bubble Bath 10oz $4.50* **MP 50¢**
1976 *Body Splash 10oz $5* **MP 50¢**

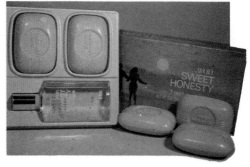

1977 *Gift Set. Two cakes Soap, 3oz each and Cologne 2oz $9* **MP $6**
1978 *Boxed Soap, three 3oz cakes $6.50* **MP $6**

Tasha

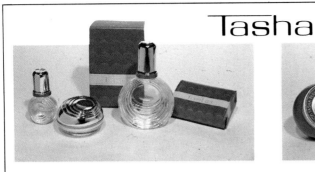

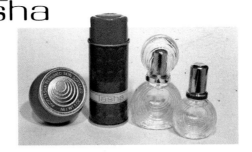

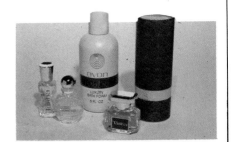

1980 *Purse Concentre .33oz $4* **MP 50¢**
1980 *Creme Perfume .66oz $4.50* **MP 50¢**
1979 *Cologne 2oz $7* **MP 50¢**
1980 *Soap 3oz $1.75* **MP $1.50**

1980 *Skin Softener 5oz $6* **MP 50¢**
1980 *Powder Mist 4oz $5* **MP 50¢**
1979 *Cologne Spray 1.8oz $8* **MP $1**
1979 *Cologne 2oz $7* **MP $1**

1979 *Cologne .33oz $3* **MP $1**
1980 *Cologne .33oz $3.50* **MP 50¢**
1980 *Bath Foam 6oz $5.50* **MP 50¢**
1979 *Light Perfume .5oz $7* **MP $1**
1980 *Talc 3.5oz $3.50* **MP 50¢**

(See also Awards pg. 310)

.....SWEET HONESTY

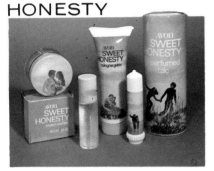

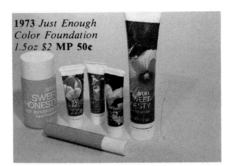

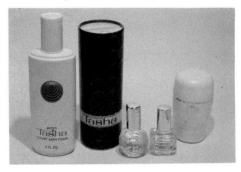

1973 *Cream Sachet .66oz $3* **MP $1**
1973 *Rollette .33oz $3* **MP $1**
1974 *Cologne Gelee 1.5oz $2.50* **MP $1**
1974 *DemiStik .19oz $2* **MP $1**
1974 *Talc 3½oz $1.50* **MP $1**

1973 *Just Enough Color Foundation 1.5oz $2* **MP 50¢**

1973 *Bright & Shining Eye Shadow .25oz $1.50* **MP 50¢**
1974 *Lip Color .2oz 4 shades $1.75* **MP 50¢**
1973 *Very Real Blush ¼oz $1.75* **MP 50¢**
1974 *Face Beamer 1.5oz $2* **MP 50¢**
1973 *Wide Eyes Mascara .15oz $2* **MP 50¢**

1982 *Luxury Bath Foam 6oz $6* **MP $50¢**
1982 *Bonus Size Talc 5¼oz (1 camp. only) $3.50* **MP $1**
1982 *Fragrance Petite Cologne .33oz $4.50* **MP $75¢**
1981 *Classic Miniature Cologne .33oz $4* **MP $1**
1982 *Ultra Sensation Body Smoother 3oz $6* **MP $50¢**

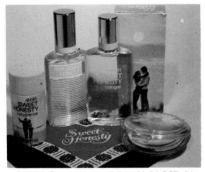

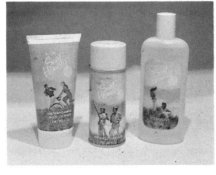

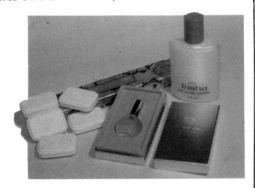

1977 *Cologne Spray 1.8oz $5.50* **MP $1**
1977 *Cologne Ice 1oz $3.75* **MP $2**
1977 *Cologne 2oz $5* **MP $1**
1973 *Translucent Powder Compact .5oz $3.50* **MP $1**
1978 *Scarf, with Avon purchase $1. Value $3.50* **MP $4**

1981 *Fresh & Foaming Bath Cleanser 6oz $6* **MP $1**
1981 *Powder Mist 4oz $4.50* **MP $1**
1981 *Body Splash 10oz $6* **MP $1**

1983 *Five Guest Soaps (2 campaigns only) 1oz each $6* **MP $4**
1983 *Light & Lavish Cologne 6oz $7.50* **MP 50¢**
1983 *Ultra Perfume .33oz $13* **MP $3 boxed**

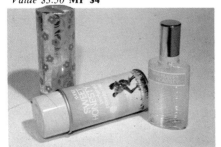

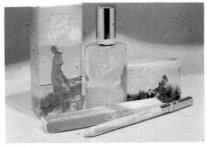

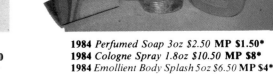

1979 *Christmas Canister Talc 3.5oz $2.50* **MP $1.50**
1979 *Powder Mist 4oz $4.50* **MP $2, short issue**
1976 *Cologne Spray 1.8oz $5.50* **MP $1**

1981 *Cologne Spray 1.8oz $8* **MP $2**
1982 *Perfumed Soap 3oz $2.25* **MP $1.50**
1982 *A Stroke of Fragrance Pencil .08oz $5.50* **MP $1**

1984 *Perfumed Soap 3oz $2.50* **MP $1.50***
1984 *Cologne Spray 1.8oz $10.50* **MP $8***
1984 *Emollient Body Splash 5oz $6.50* **MP $4***

**Available from Avon at time of publication*

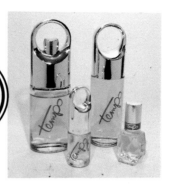

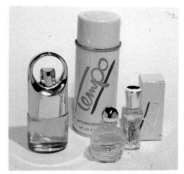

1979 *Skin Softener 5oz $6* **MP 50¢**
1979 *Body Satin 6oz $5* **MP 50¢**
1978 *solid Perfume Compact .2oz $3.75*
MP $1
1979 *Creme Perfume .66oz $4.50* **MP 50¢**

(See also Awards pg. 310)

1978 *Cologne Spray 1.8oz $7.50* **MP $1**
1978 *Cologne 2oz $6.50* **MP $1**
1979 *Purse Concentre .33oz $4* **MP 50¢**
1978 *Ultra Cologne .33oz $3* **MP $1**

1979 *Cologne Spray 1oz $7* **MP $1**
1979 *Powder Mist 4oz $5* **MP 50¢**
1980 *Cologne .33oz $3.50* **MP 75¢**
1979 *Cologne .33oz $3* **MP $1**

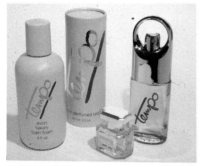

1979 *Bath Foam 6oz $5.50* **MP 50¢**
1979 *Talc 3.5oz $3* **MP 25¢**
1979 *Light Perfume .5oz $7* **MP $1**
1980 *Light Spray Cologne, sold only to
Reps. Bottle and carton have special
labels. 1.8oz $2.75* **MP $4, $6 boxed**

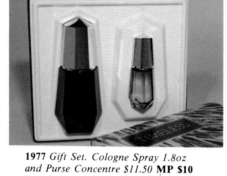

1977 *Gift Set. Cologne Spray 1.8oz
and Purse Concentre $11.50* **MP $10
(same set as 1976 but with different
box cover)**

Timeless
. . .for all your Timeless tomorrows

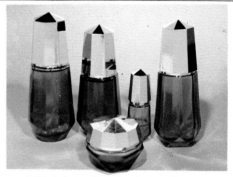

1974 *Cologne Mist 2oz $7.50* **MP $1**
1977 *Cologne 2oz $6.50* **MP $1**
1974 *Rollette .33oz $5* **MP $1**
1976 *Cologne Spray 1.8oz $7.50* **MP $9***
1974 *Creme Perfume .66oz $5* **MP 50¢**

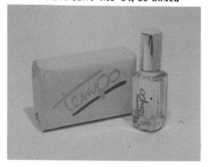

1979 *Perfumed Soap 3oz $1.50* **MP $1**
1979 *"Thanks America" Cologne Try-it
Size (2 campaigns only) .33oz 75¢* **MP $2**

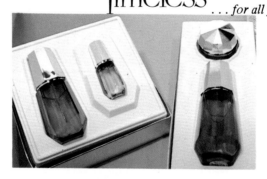

1976 *Gift Set. Cologne Spray and Rollette
$12.50* **MP $10**
1975 *Gift Set. Cologne Mist 2oz and Creme
Perfume $13.50* **MP $8**

(See also Awards pg. 309)

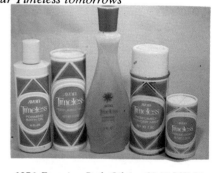

1976 *Foaming Bath Oil 6oz $5.50* **MP $1**
1975 *Talc 3½oz $2.50* **MP $2***
1975 *Foaming Bath Oil 6oz $5.50* **MP $1**
12oz, not shown, $8.50 **MP $2**
1975 *Powder Mist 7oz $5* **MP $1**
1976 *Powder Sachet 1¼oz $3.50* **MP $1**

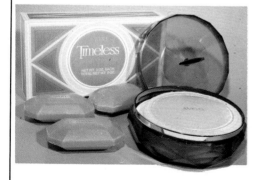

1975 *Boxed Soaps, three 3oz cakes $6* **MP $5**
1977 *Beauty Dust 6oz $9.50* **MP $3**

Available from Avon at time of publication

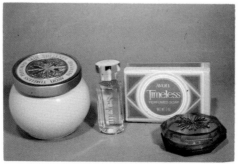

1975 *Skin Softener 5oz $5.50* **MP $3***
1977 *Cologne .33oz $3* **MP $1**
1976 *Soap 3oz $1.25* **MP $1.50***
1978 *Solid Perf. Compact .2oz $3.75* **MP $1**

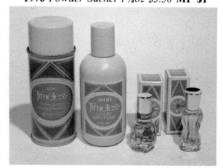

1979 *Powder Mist 4oz $5* **MP $3***
1979 *Bath Foam 6oz $5.50* **MP 50¢**
1978 *Cologne .33oz $3* **MP $1**
1979 *Cologne .33oz $3* **MP $1**

TOCCARA

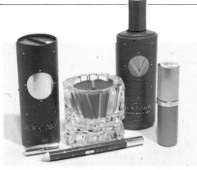

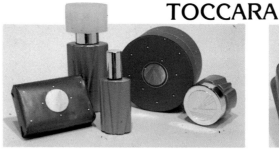

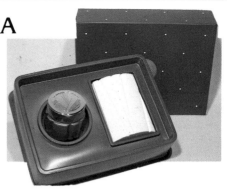

1983 *Perfumed Talc 3.5oz $3.50* **MP $1**
1982 *special Edition Fragrance Candle (2 campaigns only) $18* **MP $10**
1982 *Luxury Bath Foam 6oz $6* **MP $1**
1982 *Special Edition Purse Spray .5oz $10.50* **MP $1**
1982 *A Stroke of Fragrance Pencil .08oz $6* **MP $2**

1982 *Perfumed Soap 3oz $2.25* **MP $1.50**
1981 *Renewable Cologne Spray 1.25oz $12* **MP $1**
1981 *Renewable Perfume Lustre .5oz $8* **MP $1**
1981 *Dusting Powder 3oz $11* **MP $1**
1981 *Creme Cologne 1oz $9.50* **MP $1**
(See also Awards page 307)

1982 *Deluxe Gift Set. Creme Cologne 1oz and Sculptured Soap 3.5oz (2 campaigns only) $13* **MP $6**

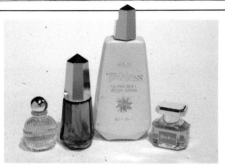

1980 *Cologne .33oz $3.50* **MP 75¢**
1979 *Cologne Spray 1oz $7* **MP $6***
1979 *Body Satin 6oz $5* **MP 50¢**
1979 *Light Perfume .5oz $7* **MP $1**

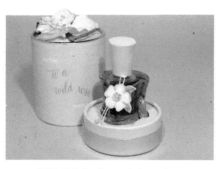

1950 *Gift Perfume. 2 dram $4.50*
MP $85, $120 boxed

To a Wild Rose

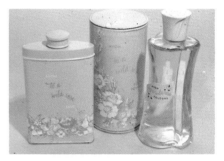

1954 *Talc 2¾oz 49¢* **MP $11**
1950 *Body Powder 5oz 85¢* **MP $20**
1950 *Cologne 4oz $2* **MP $23**

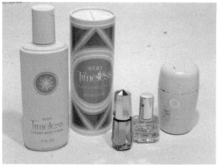

1982 *Luxury Bath Foam 6oz $6* **MP $4***
1982 *Bonus Size Talc 5¼oz (1 campaign only) $3.50* **MP $1**
1982 *Fragrance Petite Cologne .33oz $4.50* **MP $2.50***
1981 *Classic Minature Cologne .33oz $4* **MP $1**
1982 *Ultra Sensation Body Smoother 3oz $6* **MP $5***

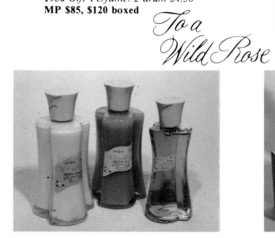

1953 *Cream Lotion 4oz 89¢* **MP $23**
1953 *Bath Oil 4oz $1.25* **MP $23**
1950 *Toilet Water 2oz $1.50* **MP $23**

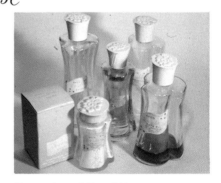

Rare embossed Rose Lids:
Powder Sachet 1¼oz, Cologne 4oz, Toilet Water 2oz, Cream Lotion 4oz and Bath Oil 4oz. For embossed lid add **$5** *to bottle* **MP**

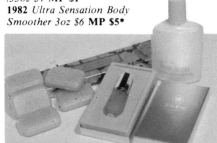

1983 *Five Guest Soaps (2 campaigns only) 1oz each $6* **MP $4**
1983 *Light & Lavish Cologne 6oz $7.50* **MP $6***
1983 *Ultra Perfume .33oz $13* **MP $11***

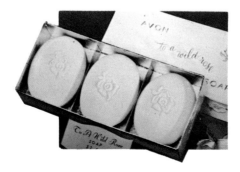
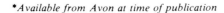

1953-55 *Boxed Soap, 3 cakes $1.50*
MP $30

*Available from Avon at time of publication

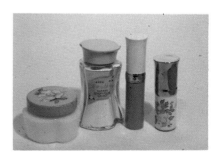

1950 *Cream Sachet $1.25* **MP $13**
1951 *Powder Sachet 1¼oz $1.19* **MP $17**
1963 *Perfume Mist, 2 drams $3* **MP $7**
1960 *Spray Perfume 2 drams $2.95*
MP $12, $16 boxed

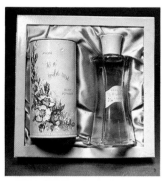

1950 *Gift Set. Body Powder 5oz and Cologne 4oz $2.85* **MP $55**

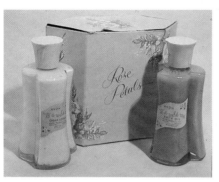

1953 *Rose Petals. Cream Lotion and Bath Oil 4oz each $2.15* **MP $55**

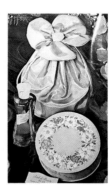

1950 *Petal of Beauty. Cologne and Beauty Dust. Drawstring silk bag $5.25* **MP $75, bag only $25**

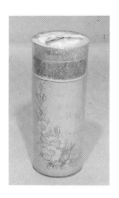

1952 *Wild Roses. Body Powder & Cream Sachet $1.95* **MP $48**

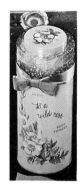

1953 *Wild Roses. Body Powder and Cream Sachet $1.95* **MP $46**

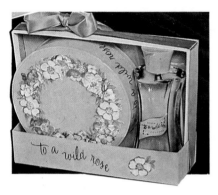

1954 *Petal of Beauty. Beauty Dust and Cologne $3.75* **MP $60**

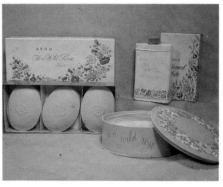

1960 *Boxed Soap, 3 cakes $1.98* **MP $20**
1954 *Talc 3oz 59¢* **MP $7.** *As shown with*
1960 *Christmas carton 69¢* **MP $13**
1950 *Beauty Dust $1.75* **MP $23**

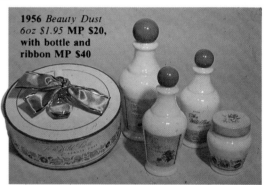

1956 *Beauty Dust 6oz $1.95* **MP $20, with bottle and ribbon MP $40**

1956 *Cream Lotion 4oz 95¢* **MP $18**
1957 *Cologne 2oz (sets only)* **MP $18**
1955 *Toilet Water 2oz $1.50* **MP $15**
1955 *Powder Sachet 1¼oz $1.25* **MP $12**

...To a Wild Rose

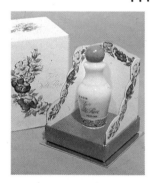

1956 *Gift Perfume ½oz $5* **MP $75, $110 boxed**

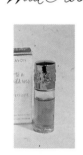

1950 *One Dram Perfume $1.50* **MP $12, $15 boxed**

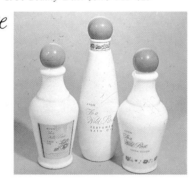

1956 *Bath Oil 4oz $1.35* **MP $13**
1959 *Perfumed Bath Oil 8oz $2.25* **MP $9**
1965 *Cream Lotion 4oz $1.25* **MP $9**

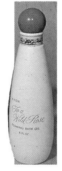

1966 *Foaming Bath Oil 6oz $2.50* **MP $5**

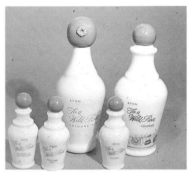

1963 *Perfume Oil for the Bath ½oz $3.50* **MP $12**
1964 *Perfume Oil ½oz $3.50* **MP $9**
1958 *Cologne Mist 3oz $2.50* **MP $25**
1969 *Cologne ½oz $1.50* **MP $3**
1955 *Cologne 4oz $2* **MP $20**

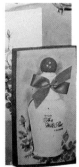

1960 *Gift Cologne 4oz $2.50* **MP $28**

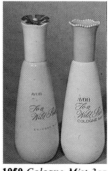

1959 *Cologne Mist 3oz $2.95* **MP $2** *(w/o oz on front)*
1975 *Cologne Mist 3oz $7* **MP $3** *(lid change)*

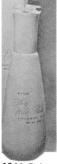

1966 *Cologne Mist 3oz $3.25* **MP $3** *(with oz on front)*

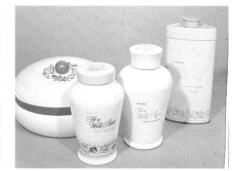

1964 *Beauty Dust 6oz $3.25* **MP $10**
1955 *Body Powder (paper band) $1* **MP $17**
1961 *Body Powder 4oz (plastic) $1.79* **MP $12**
1962 *Talc 2¾oz $1* **MP $2**

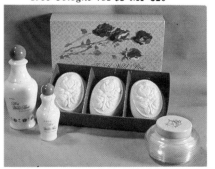

1961 *Cologne 2oz $1.50* **MP $3**
1956 *Toilet Water ½oz from Special Date Set* **MP $25**
1968 *Boxed Soaps, three 3oz $3* **MP $7**
1960 *Cream Sachet .66oz $1.25* **MP $3**
Above shown in 1960 Plastic Holder, special purchase 50¢ **MP $9**

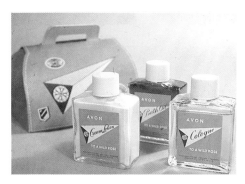

1951 *Miss Coed. Cream Lotion, Bath Oil and Cologne 2 oz each $2.35* **MP $85 complete. Each bottle $20**

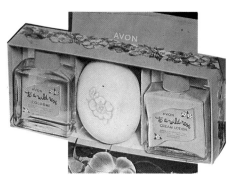

1954 *Bath Bouquet. Cologne, Cream Lotion 2oz each and Soap $1.95* **MP $56. Each bottle MP $18**

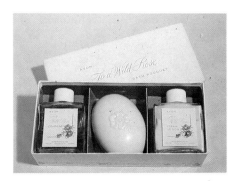

1955 *Bath Bouquet. Cologne and Cream Lotion 2oz each and 1 cake Soap $1.95* **MP $55. Each bottle MP $18**

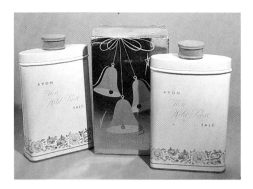

1955 *Pink Bells. 2 Talc 2¾oz each $1* **MP $30**

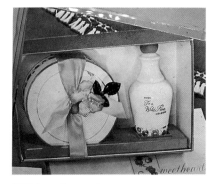

1955 *Sweethearts. Beauty Dust and Cologne $3.95* **MP $51**

. . . To a Wild Rose

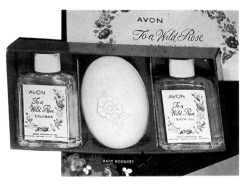

1956 *Bath Bouquet. Cologne, Bath Oil 2oz each and 1 cake Soap $2.25* **MP $56. Each bottle MP $18**

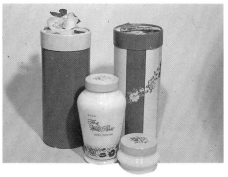

1955 *Adorable Set (left) Body Powder and Cream Sachet $2.25* **MP $36**
1956 *Adorable Set (right) Body Powder and Cream Sachet $2.25* **MP $36**

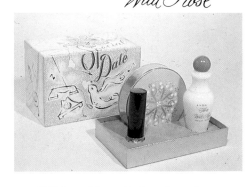

1956 *Special Date. Fashion Lipstick, Powder Pak and Toilet Water ½oz $2.50* **MP $50**

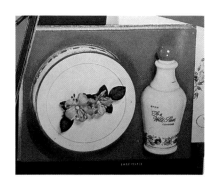

1956 *Sweethearts. Beauty Dust and Cologne $3.95* **MP $50**

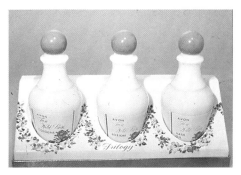

1957 *Trilogy. Cologne, Cream Lotion, Bath Oil 2oz each $2.95* **MP $65**

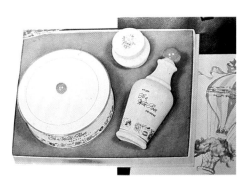

1957 *Roses Adrift. Beauty Dust, Cream Sachet and Cologne $4.95* **MP $56**

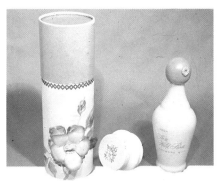

1958 *A Spray of Roses. Cologne Mist 3oz & Cream Sachet $3.95* **MP $40**

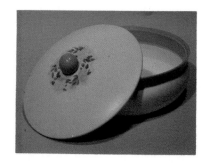

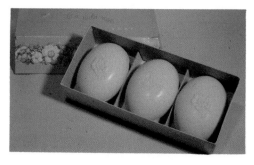

1960-63 *Beauty Dust 6oz $2.95* **MP $12**

1955-59 *Boxed Soaps, three 3oz cakes $1.59* **MP $25**

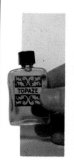

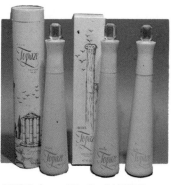

1935 *Customer Gift, March 5-25 honoring the McConnells' Golden Anniversary* **MP $80**

1959 *Cologne Mist 3oz $4* **MP $1, $5 in round box**
1969 *Cologne Mist, as above, boxed* **MP $3**
1971 *Cologne Mist, 3oz $5* **MP $1**

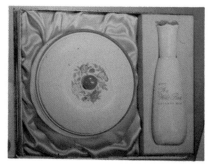

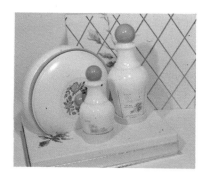

1961 *Spray of Roses. Beauty Dust and Cologne Mist 3oz $5.90* **MP $30**

1963 *Holiday Roses Beauty Dust, Cream Lotion 4oz and Cologne 2oz $6.50* **MP $55**

Topaze

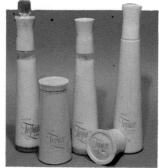

1959 *Cream Lotion 4oz (rare jeweled closure) $1.50* **MP $12**
1961 *Talc, tin 2¾oz $1* **MP $10**
1960 *Cream Lotion 4oz $1.50* **MP $3**
1965 *Cream Sachet .66oz $2.50* **MP $1**
1966 *Foaming Bath Oil 6oz $2.75* **MP $1**

...To a Wild Rose

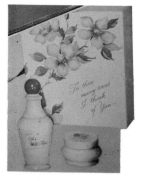

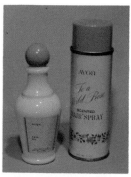

1961 *Lovely As A Rose. Cologne 2oz and Cream Sachet $3* **MP $30**

1964 *Wild Roses. Cologne 2oz and Cream Sachet $3.50* **MP $27**

1950's *Bath Oil (rare label) 4oz $1.35* **MP $15**
1966 *Scented Hair Spray 7oz $1.50* **MP $3**

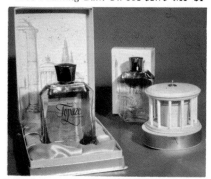

1959 *Cologne 4oz $3.75* **MP $15, $25 boxed**
1960 *Cologne 2oz $2* **MP $2, $3 boxed**
1960 *Temple of Love Holder for .75oz Topaze Cream Sachet 75¢* **MP $16, $20 boxed. Cream Sachet .75oz $2* **MP $8**

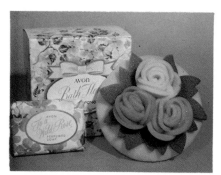

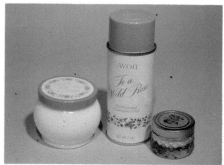

1965 *Bath Flower 3oz Soap and Bath Sponge $2.50* **MP $21**

1971 *Skin Softener* **(lid change)** *5oz $3.50* **MP $3**
1971 *Powder Mist 7oz $3.75* **MP $4 (label change)**
1975 *Cream Sachet .66oz $3* **MP $1**

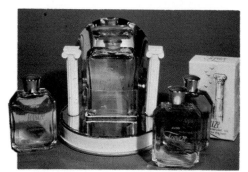

1969 *Cologne ½oz $1.50* **MP $3**
1959 *Perfume 1oz $20* **MP $105, $140 boxed**
1963 *Perfume Oil for the Bath ½oz $4* **MP $50, $60 boxed**
1964 *Perfume Oil ½oz $4* **MP $9, $10 boxed**

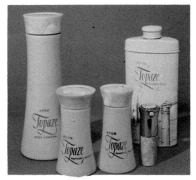

1961 *Body Powder 4oz $2.25* **MP $12**
1959 *Powder Sachet .9oz $2* **MP $6**
1961 *Powder Sachet .9oz (right) $2* **MP $10**
1959 *Spray Perfume 2 dram $3.75* **MP $12**
1962 *Talc 2³/₄oz $1* **MP $2**

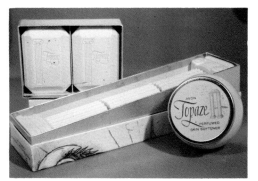

1961 *Boxed Soap, 2 cakes $1.50* **MP $25**
1965 *Column of 3 Soaps $1.75* **MP $30**
1964 *Skin Softener 5oz $3.25* **MP $3**

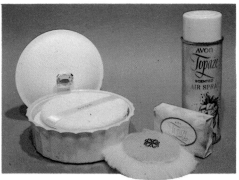

1961 *Beauty Dust 6oz $4* **MP $4**
1960 *Beauty Dust as above
but with yellow lamb's wool puff $4* **MP $15**
1964 *Soap 3oz 39¢* **MP $4**
1966 *Hair Spray 7oz $1.50* **MP $3**

...*Topaze*

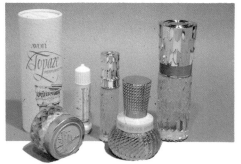

1974 *Talc 3¹/₂oz $1.50* **MP $1**
1975 *Cream Sachet .66oz $3* **MP $1**
1975 *DemiStik .19oz $2* **MP $1**
1977 *Purse Concentre .33oz $3* **MP $1**
1967 *Spray Essence 1¹/₄oz $3.50* **MP $3**
1977 *Cologne Spray 1.8oz $5.50* **MP $1**

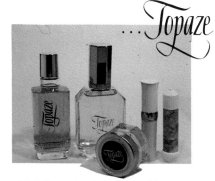

1975 *Cologne 2oz $4* **MP $1 with
Christmas carton MP $3**
1976 *Cologne Spray 2.7oz $8* **MP $8.50***
1977 *Cream Sachet .66oz $4.50* **MP $1**
1963 *Perfume Mist 2 drams $3.25* **MP $7**
1977 *DemiStik .19oz $2.50* **MP $1**

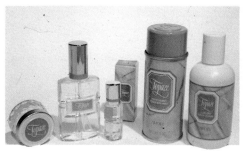

1979 *Creme Perfume .66 oz $3.50* **MP $4***
1979 *Cologne Spray 1.8oz $6* **MP $5**
1979 *Purse Concentre .33oz $3* **MP 50¢**
1979 *Powder Mist 4oz $4.50* **MP 50¢**
1980 *Bath Foam 6oz $5* **MP 50¢**

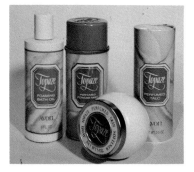

1977 *Foaming Bath Oil 6oz $5.50* **MP $1**
1977 *Powder Mist 7oz $5* **MP $1**
1977 *Skin Softener 5oz $5.50* **MP $3***
1977 *Talc 3¹/₂oz $2.50* **MP $2***

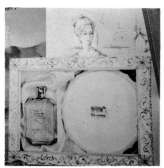

1960 *Topaze Treasure. Cologne 2oz
and Beauty Dust 6oz $5.95* **MP $33**

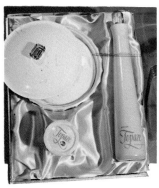

1960 *Golden Topaze. Beauty
Dust, Cologne Mist 3oz and
Cream Sachet .75oz $9.95*
MP $40

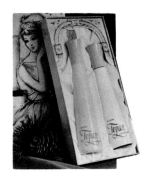

1964 *Topaze Princess.
Cologne Mist and
Cream Lotion $5.95*
MP $25

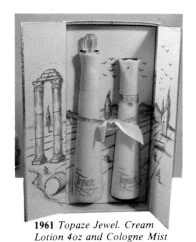

1961 *Topaze Jewel. Cream
Lotion 4oz and Cologne Mist
$4.95* **MP $31**

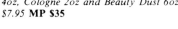

1963 *Topaze Elegance. Cream Lotion
4oz, Cologne 2oz and Beauty Dust 6oz
$7.95* **MP $35**

*Available from Avon at time of publication

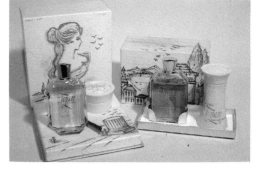

1961 *Golden Gem. Cologne 2oz and Cream Sachet
.75 oz $4* **MP $25**
1964 *Topaze Setting. Cologne 2oz and
Powder Sachet $4* **MP $25**

(See also Awards pg. 307)

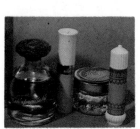
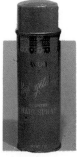
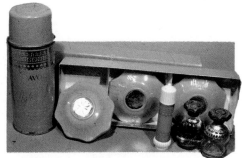
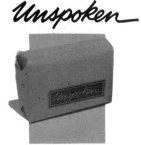

Unspoken

1966 *Cologne 2oz $2.50* **MP $3**
1965 *Perfume Mist 2 drams $3.75* **MP $7**
1975 *Cream Sachet .66oz $3* **MP $1**
1975 *DemiStik .19oz $2* **MP $1**

1966 *Scented Hair Spray 7oz $1.50* **MP $3**

1968 *Powder Mist 7oz $3.75* **MP $1**
1965 *Boxed Soap, three 3oz cakes $2* **MP $22**
1975 *DemiStik .19oz $2* **MP $1**
1969 *Cologne ½oz $1.50* **MP $3**
1965 *Perfume Oil ½oz* **MP $8**

1979 *Perfumed Soap 3oz $1.50* **MP $1**

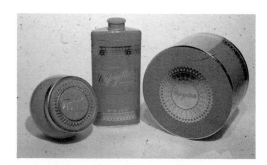
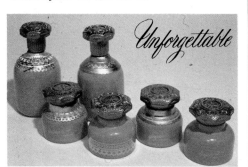
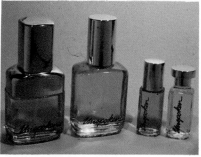

Unforgettable

1965 *Beauty Dust 6oz $5* **MP $6**
1966 *Cream Lotion 4oz $1.75* **MP $6**
1966 *Foaming Bath Oil 6oz $3* **MP $3**
1966 *Cream Sachet .66oz $2.50* **MP $1**

1965-76 *Cologne Mist 3oz with open filigree trim, $5* **MP $1.** *With solid filigree trim 3oz $5* **MP $6**
1965 only *Powder Sachet .9oz $2.50* **MP $15**
1966-67 *Powder Sachet .9oz $2.50* **MP $3**
1965 *Powder Sachet .9oz $2.50* **MP $2**
1968-69 *Powder Sachet .9oz $2.50* **MP $2**

1975 *Cologne Spray 1.8oz $7.50* **MP $1**
1977 *Cologne 2oz $6.50* **MP $2**
1975 *Rollette .33oz $5* **MP $1** *(name changed to Purse Concentre in 1979* **MP 50¢**)
1977 *Cologne .33oz $3* **MP $1**

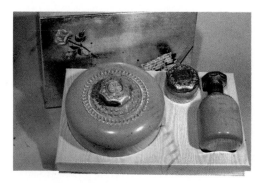
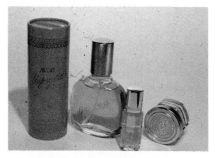
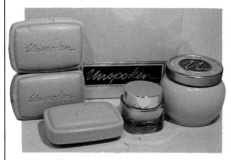

1965 *Skin Softener 5oz $3.50* **MP $1**
1966 *Talc 2¾oz $1* **MP $2**
1971 *Beauty Dust, cardboard, 6oz $4.50* **MP $10**

1974 *Talc 3½oz $1.50* **MP 50¢**
1976 *Cologne Spray 2.7oz $7* **MP $1**
1979 *Purse Concentre .33oz $3* **MP $1**
1979 *Creme Perfume .66oz $3.50* **MP $1**

1975 *Boxed Soap, three 3oz cakes $6* **MP $50**
1975 *Creme Perfume .66oz $5* **MP $1**
1976 *Skin Softener 5oz $5.50* **MP $3**

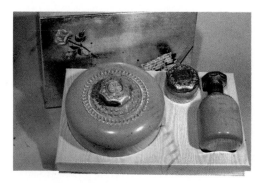
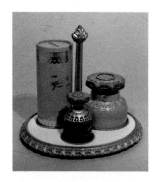
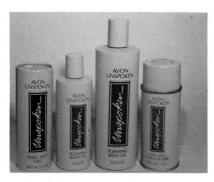

1965 *Deluxe Set. Beauty Dust 6oz, Cream Sachet .66oz and Cologne Mist 3oz $12.95* **MP $38**

1965 *Heirloom Set. Talc 1½oz, Powder Sachet .9oz and Perfume Oil ½oz $10.95* **MP $52, $62 boxed, tray $22**
1966 *As above, except Powder Sachet issued without gold collar (see 1966 Sachet)* **MP $40, $50 boxed**

1976 *Talc 3½oz $2.50* **MP 50¢**
1976 *Foaming Bath Oil 6oz $5.50* **MP $1**
1976 *Foaming Bath Oil 12oz $8.50* **MP $2**
1977 *Powder Mist 7oz $5* **MP $1**

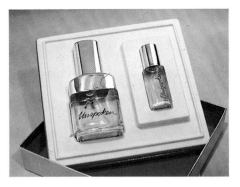

1976 Gift Set. Cologne Spray 1.8oz and Rollette .33oz $12.50 **MP $12**

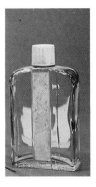

1947 Toilet Water 2oz $1.19 **MP $40**

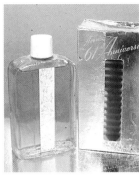

1947 Toilet Water 2oz 61¢ for one campaign honoring 61st Anniversary. **MP $60 in Anniversary Box**

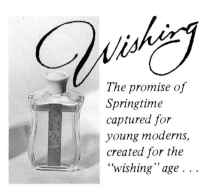

Wishing

The promise of Springtime captured for young moderns, created for the "wishing" age . . .

1947 Toilet Water 2oz $1.19 **MP $40**

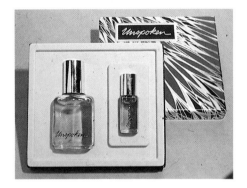

1977 Gift Set. Cologne 2oz and Rollette .33oz $10.50 **MP $10**

. . . Unspoken

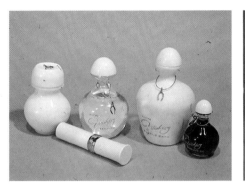

1964 Powder Sachet .9oz $1.75 **MP $10**
1963 Cologne 2oz with Wishbone $1.78 **MP $9**
1963 Bubble Bath 4oz $1.35 **MP $6**
1964 Perfume Oil ½oz w/Wishbone $3.50 **MP $12**
1965 Perfume Mist 2 dram $3 **MP $7**

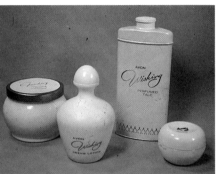

1965 Skin Softener 5oz $3 **MP $4**
1963 Cream Lotion, plastic 4oz $1.35 **MP $6**
1963 Talc 2¾oz 79¢ **MP $4**
1963 Cream Sachet .66oz $1.75 **MP $2.50**

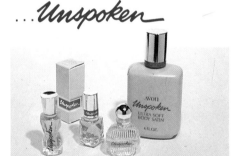

1979 Cologne .33oz $3 **MP $1**
1978 Cologne .33oz $3 **MP $1**
1980 Cologne .33oz $3.50 **MP 50¢**
1979 Body Satin 6oz $5 **MP 50¢**

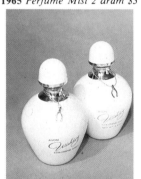

1963 Cologne Mist 2½oz $2.95 **MP $4**
1968 Cologne Mist 2½oz $3.50 **MP $6**

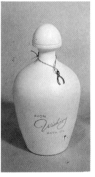

1964 Bath Oil 6oz $2.25 **MP $12 with Wishbone**

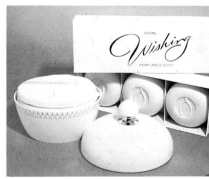

1963 Beauty Dust 4oz $2.95 **MP $13**
1963 Boxed Soap, 3 cakes $1.35 **MP $25**

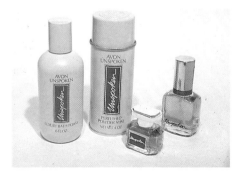

1979 Bath Foam 6oz $5.50 **MP 50¢**
1979 Powder Mist 4oz $5 **MP 50¢**
1979 Light Perfume .5oz $7 **MP $1**
1979 Cologne Spray 1oz $7 **MP $1**

(See also Awards pg. 309)

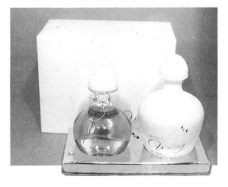

1963 Wish Come True. Cologne 2oz and Bubble Bath 4oz $3.10 **MP $28**

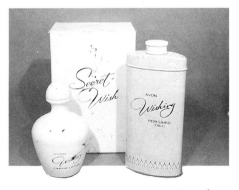

1963 Secret Wish. Cream Lotion 4oz and Talc 2¾oz $2.14 **MP $21**

(See also Awards pg. 307)

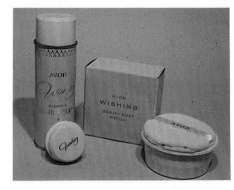

1966 *Scented Hair Spray 7oz $1.50* **MP $3**
1970 *Cream Sachet .66oz $2.50* **MP $25**
1963 *Beauty Dust Refill 4oz $1.75* **MP $6**

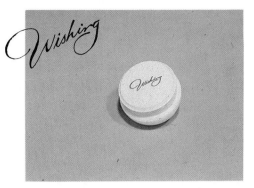

Wishing

1970 *Cream Sachet .66oz $2.50* **MP $25**

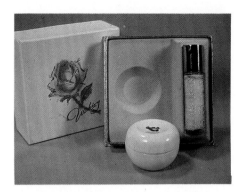

1964 *Wishing Duette. Cream Rollette and Cream Sachet .66oz $3.50* **MP $20**

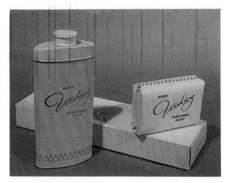

1964 *Perfumed Pair. Talc and Soap 3oz $1.18* **MP $20**

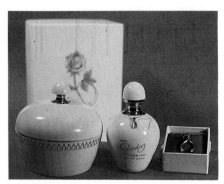

1964 *Charm of Wishing. Beauty Dust, Cologne Mist and Wishbone Charm Necklace $8.50* **MP $65. Necklace $20, $30 boxed**

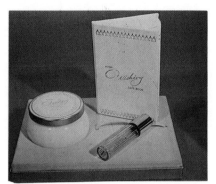

1965 *Wishing Date Set. Rollette, Skin Softener and Date Book $6* **MP $35. Date Book MP $15**

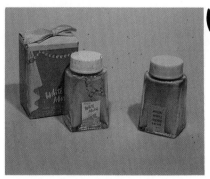

White Moiré

1946 *Powder Sachet in 60th Anniversary Box 1¼oz $1.15* **MP $45 boxed**
1946 *Powder Sachet 1¼oz $1.15* **MP $40**

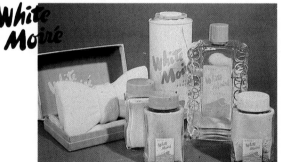

1946 *French Milled Soap 8½oz bar $1.15* **MP $55**
1946 *Body Powder, plastic sifter 65¢* **MP $26**
1946 *Cologne 6oz $1.75* **MP $85**
1949 *Powder Sachet 1¼oz $1.19* **MP $21**
1947 *Powder Sachet 1¼oz $1.19* **MP $25**
1946 *Powder Sachet, white cap 1¼oz $1.15* **MP $30**

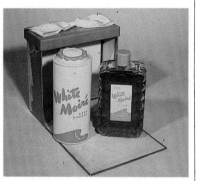

1945 *White Moire Set. Body Powder 5oz and Cologne 6oz $2.50* **MP $145**

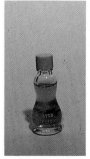

1952 *Perfume (sets only) 1 dr* **MP $65 Bottle**

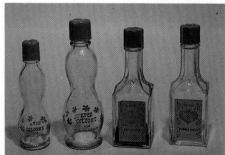

1952 *Cologne (sets only) ½oz* **MP $35**
1952 *Cologne (sets only) 1oz* **MP $35**
1954 *Cologne (sets only) 1oz* **MP $30**
1954 *Bubble Bath (sets only) 1oz* **MP $30**

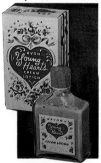

1954 *Cream Lotion 50¢* **MP $20, $25 boxed**

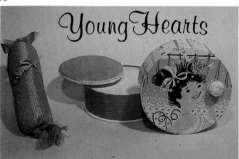

Young Hearts

1946 only *Sachet issued in Young Hearts Set* **MP $25** *(See Set p. 107)*
1954 *Beauty Dust $1.19* **MP $25**

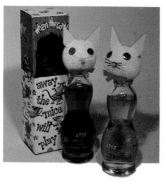

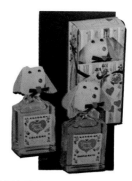

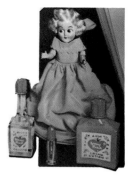

.....Young Hearts

. . . it was only the Young Hearts packaging that was exclusive to little girls, the fragrance was Cotillion.

1952 *Bubble Bath 2oz $1.10* **MP $50 with head, $65 boxed**
1952 *Cologne 2oz $1.25* **MP $50 with head, $65 boxed**

1954 *Kiddie Kologne $1.25* **MP $45 with head, $55 boxed**
1954 *Kiddie Bubble Bath $1.10* **MP $45 with head, $55 boxed**

1954 *Little Doll Set. Cologne, Pomade Lipstick and Cream Lotion $2.95* **MP $125, $40 Doll**

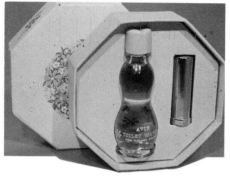

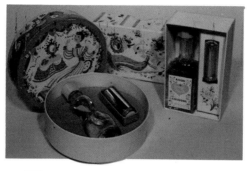

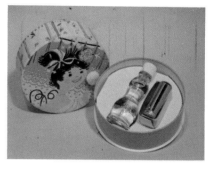

1952 *Honey Bun. Toilet Water ½oz and Pomade Lipstick $1.19* **MP $55, $35 Toilet Water**

1953 *Honey Bun. Toilet Water ½oz and Pomade Lipstick $1.19* **MP $55**
1954 *Honey Bun. Cologne 1oz and Pomade Lipstick $1.19* **MP $55**

1954 *Honey Bun Set (short issue) Toilet Water ½oz and Pomade Lipstick $1.19* **MP $65**

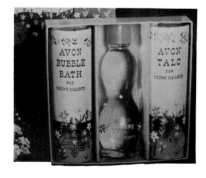

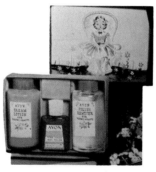

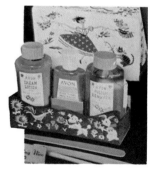

1952 *Young Hearts Set. Bubble Bath, Cologne and Talc $1.65* **MP $90 Bubble Bath and Talc MP $20 each**

1952 *'N Everything Nice. Cream Lotion, Nail Polish, Polish Remover, Orange Stick and 2 Emery Boards $1.50* **MP $70 Polish Remover MP $25**

1953 *'N Everything Nice. Cream Lotion 2oz, Nail Polish .5oz, Polish Remover 2oz, Orange Stick and 2 Emery Boards $1.50* **MP $70**

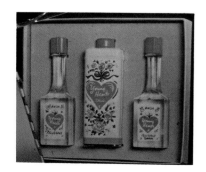

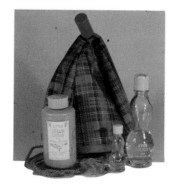

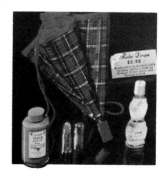

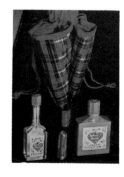

1954 *Young Hearts Set. Cologne 1oz, Talc and Bubble Bath $1.95* **MP $100, $25 Talc, $30 each bottle**

1952 *Rain Drops. Umbrella Handbag holds Cream Lotion, 1 dram Perfume and 2oz Cologne $2.95* **MP $160, $25 Cream Lotion, $35 Handbag only**

1953 *Rain Drops. Cream Lotion, Pomade Lipstick and Cologne $2.95* **MP $110, $7 Pomade, $35 Umbrella Handbag**

1954 *Rain Drops. Umbrella Handbag holds Cologne 1oz, Pomade Lipstick and Cream Lotion $3.25* **MP $110, $35 Umbrella Handbag**

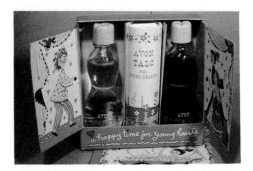

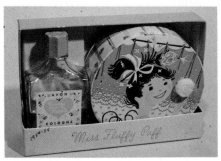

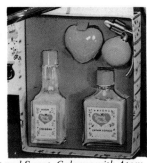

...Young Hearts

1953 *Young Hearts Set. Cologne, Talc and Bubble Bath* $1.75 **MP $110**

1954 *Miss Fluffy Puff. Cologne and Beauty Dust* $2.35 **MP $70**

1955 *Neat and Sweet. Cologne with Atomizer, Cream Lotion and heart shaped Soap* $2.50 **MP $95**
1954 *Neat and Sweet (not shown) Same as above, but without atomizer* $2.10 **MP $85**

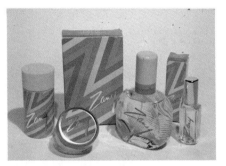

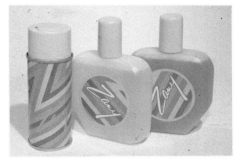

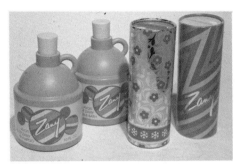

1979 *Cologne Ice 1oz* $4 **MP $1.50**
1979 *Creme Perfume .66oz* $3.50 **MP 50¢**
1979 *Cologne Spray 1.8oz* $5.50 **MP $1**
1979 *Try-It-Size Cologne .33oz* 75¢ *in C-17 & C-18 only* **MP $1.50, $2 boxed**

1979 *Powder Mist 4oz* $2.25 **MP 50¢**
1979 *Body Splash 10oz* $5 **MP 50¢**
1979 *Bubble Bath 10oz* $4.50 **MP 50¢**

(The Zany Radio and Disco Bag, a prize in the Zany Sweepstakes, is shown on page 310)

1979 *Jug of Shampoo 10oz* $6 **MP $2**
1979 *Jug of Bubble Bath 10oz* $6 **MP $2**
1979 *Xmas Canister Talc* $2.50 **MP $1**
1979 *Talc 3.5oz* $2.50 **MP 50¢**
1979 *Purse Concentre (not shown)* .33oz $3 **MP $1**

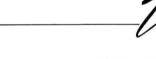

Zany

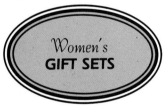

Women's
GIFT SETS

Gertrude Recordon

In 1927 the California Perfume Company engaged the services of Gertrude Recordon, a graduate cosmetician and well-known authority on beauty problems. She served in an advisory capacity, giving helpful information to Representatives and answering customer questions on skin care products and cosmetics.

The Gertrude Recordon Facial Treatment Set was manufactured according to her formulae and under her personal supervision.

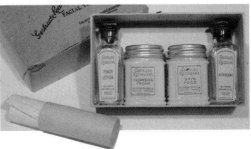

1927-29 *Gertrude Recordon Introductory Facial Set, trial-size containers of Peach Lotion, Cleansing Cream, Skin Food and Astringent and roll of Facial Tissues.* $1. **MP $330.** *complete set,* **$85 each bottle, $55 each jar**

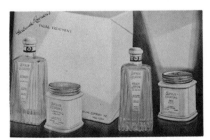

1927-29 *Gertrude Recordon Facial Set. Peach Lotion, Astringent, Cleansing Cream and Skin Food* $4 **MP $285 complete set, $80 each bottle, $50 each jar**

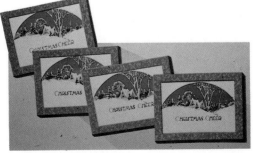

1928 *Christmas Cheer Set. Four boxes of Sachet Powder with Greeting Card and Mailing Carton* $1.40 **MP $175 complete, $35 each box**

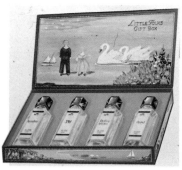

1931 *Little Folks Gift Box. Vernafleur, "391", Trailing Arbutus and Ariel Perfumes 90¢* **MP $240, $45 each bottle**

LITTLE FOLKS SETS

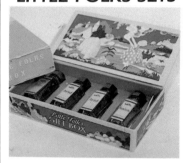

1932 *Little Folks Gift Box. Vernalfeur, "391", Arbutus and Ariel Perfumes 90¢* **MP $230, $45 each bottle**

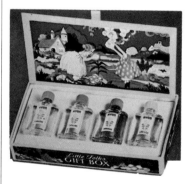

1937 *Little Folks Gift Box. Cotillion, Gardenia, Narcissus and Trailing Arbutus Perfumes 94¢* **MP $155, $30 each bottle**

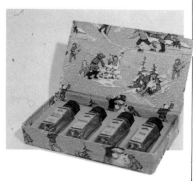

1933 *Little Folks Xmas Gift Box. Trailing Arbutus, Vernafleur, Ariel and "391" Perfumes 90¢* **MP $250**

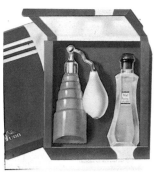

1930-31 *Atomizer Set No. 6A. Atomizer Bottle and Ariel Perfume 1oz $1.75* **MP $160** *Set 6B issued with Vernafleur Perfume $2* **MP $160, $85 atomizer bottle only**

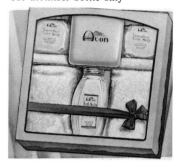

1931-33 *Assortment No. 8. Dusting Powder, Bath Salts, 2 Vernafleur Toilet Soaps, Cannon Bath Towel 45x22½, 2 Washcloths $3.50* **MP $165**

GIFT SETS OF THE 1930's

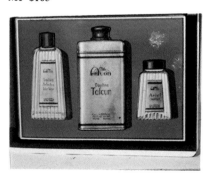

1934 *Avon Trio. Trailing Arbutus Toilet Water, Daphne Talcum and Ariel Sachet Powder $1.60* **MP $140**

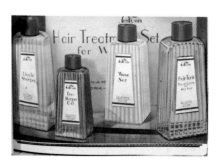

1931-35 *Hair Treatment Set for Women. Liquid Shampoo 6oz, Pre-Shampoo Oil 2oz, Wave Set 4oz and Hair Tonic Eau de Quinine 6oz for dry or oily hair $3* **MP $185**

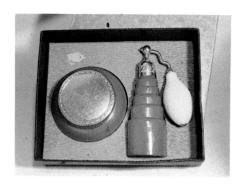

1930's *Atomizer Set. Powder Box and Atomizer Bottle* **MP $400**

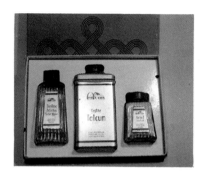

1935 *Avon Trio. Trailing Arbutus Toilet Water, Daphne Talcum and Ariel Sachet Powder $1.60* **MP $140**

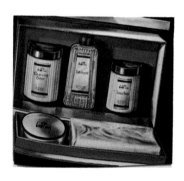

1934 *Facial Set. Cleansing Cream, Astringent, Tissue Cream, Ariel Face Powder and Cleansing Tissues $1.68* **MP $155**

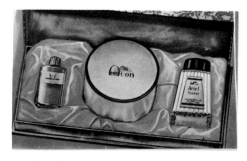

1935-37 *Gift Set D. Ariel Perfume Flaconette and Sachet, Ariel or Vernafleur Face Powder $2.34* **MP $135**

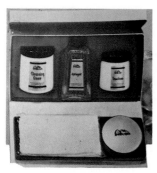

1935 *Facial Set. Cleansing Cream, Tissue Cream, Astringent, Ariel Face Powder and Cleansing tissues $1.68* **MP $150**

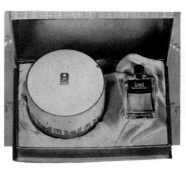

1936 *Gift Set A. Face Powder and Gardenia Perfume Flaconette $1.30* **MP $97**

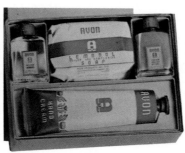

1938-39 *Beauty Kit for Fingers. Nail Polish, Polish Remover, Lemonol Soap, Hand Cream $1.35* **MP $90**

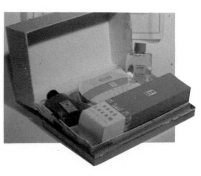

Beauty Kit for Fingers shown in substitute box $1.35 **MP $90**

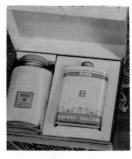

1939 *Bath Duet. Daphne Talc and Bath Salts in choice of Pine, Vernafleur, Ariel or Jasmine $1* **MP $60**

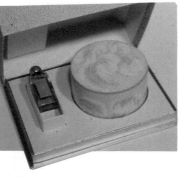

1943 *Colonial Set. Perfume 1 dram and Face Powder $1.45* **MP $65**

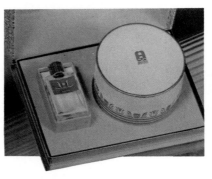

1939 *Colonial Set. Gardenia Perfume 1 dram and Face Powder $1.30* **MP $95**

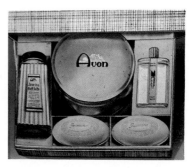

1935 *Bath Ensemble. Jasmine Bath Salts and 2 Cakes Soap, Dusting Powder 13oz and Trailing Arbutus Toilet Water 2oz $3.50* **MP $180**

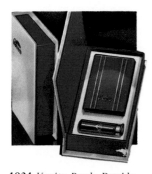

1934 *Vanity Book. Double Compact and Lipstick $2.27* **MP $65**

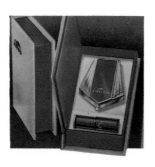

1931-32 *Vanity Book. Double Fan Compact and Lipstick $2.50* **MP $75**

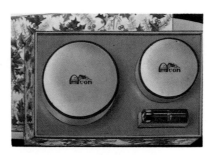

1933-35 *Gift Set No. 21. Face Powder, Dressing Table Rouge and Lipstick $1.56* **MP $77**

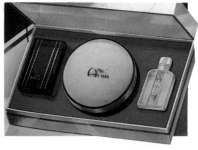

1934-45 *Avon Threesome. Double Compact, Face Powder and Bolero Perfume Flaconette $3.57* **MP $150**

COSMETIC SETS OF THE 1930's.....

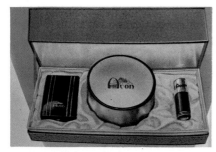

1935 *Gift Set F. Double Compact, Ariel or Vernafleur Face Powder and Lipstick $2.80* **MP $92**

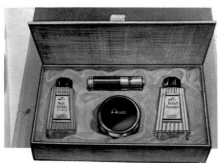

1935 *Gift Set W. Nail Polish, Polish Remover, Rouge Compact and Lipstick $1.67* **MP $100**

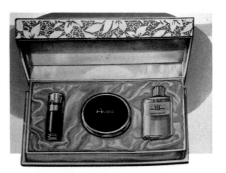

1935 *Gift Set B. Lipstick, Rouge Compact and Trailing Arbutus Perfume Flaconette $1.56* **MP $115**

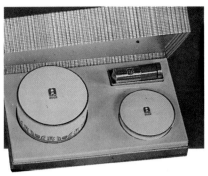

1936 Gift Set No. 21. Ariel or Vernafleur Face Powder, Dressing Table Rouge and Lipstick $1.56 **MP $52**

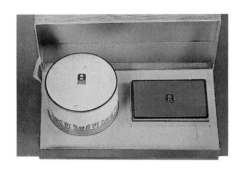

1936-37 Powder-Compact Set (named Aristocrat in 1938) Ariel or Vernafleur Face Powder and Double Compact $2.50 **MP $56**

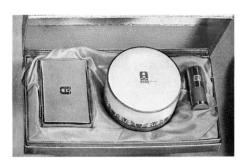

1936-37 Gift Set F (named Mastercraft in 1938) Double Compact, Ariel or Vernafleur Face Powder and Lipstick $3.05 **MP $65**

....COSMETIC SETS OF THE 1930's

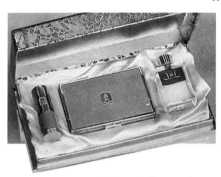

1936-37 Gift Set K (named Empress in 1938) Lipstick, Double Compact and Gardenia Perfume $2.79 **MP $125**

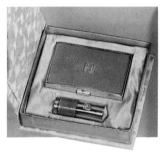

1936-38 Vanity Book (named The Sportwise in 1939) Double Compact and Lipstick $2.27 **MP $53**

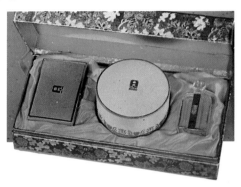

1936-38 Threesome Set (named Mayfair in 1939) Double Compact Ariel or Vernafleur Face Powder and Bolero Perfume Flaconette $3.57 **MP $140**

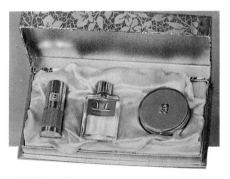

1936-37 Gift Set B. Lipstick, Rouge Compact and Trailing Arbutus Perfume Flaconette $1.56 **MP $110**

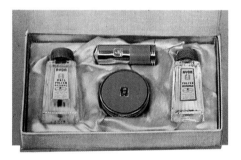

1936-37 Gift Set W. (named Cosmopolitan in 1938) Nail Polish, Polish Remover, Rouge Compact and Lipstick $1.67 **MP $90**

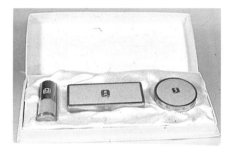

1938-41 Charmer Set. Lipstick, Mascara and Rouge Compact $2.15 **MP $63**

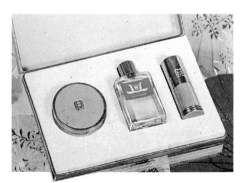

1939 Spectator Set. Rouge Compact, Trailing Arbutus Flaconette and Lipstick $1.56 **MP $110**

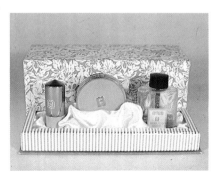

1939 Orchid Set. Lipstick, Rouge Compact and Cream Polish $1.50 **MP $60**

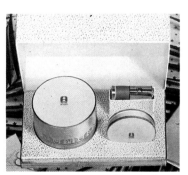

1939-41 Makeup Ensemble. Ariel or Vernafleur Face Powder, Lipstick and Dressing Table Rouge $1.56 **MP $52**

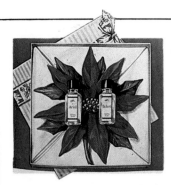

1934-36 *Perfume Handkerchief Set in Xmas Box. Ariel & Bolero Perfumes 99¢* **MP $135**
1933-34 *As above, but with Ariel & "391" Perfumes 85¢* **MP $150**

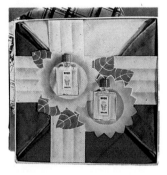

1936-39 *Perfume Handkerchief Set. 4 Handkerchiefs, Cotillion and Gardenia Perfumes 1/8oz $1* **MP $100, $20 each bottle**

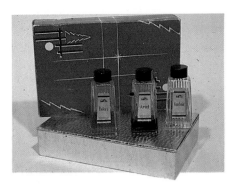

1934-36 *Bolero, Ariel & Gardenia Perfumes shown in Xmas Box $1.46* **MP $165**
1933-34 *As above, with Ariel, "391" & Vernafleur Perfumes $1.46* **MP $185**

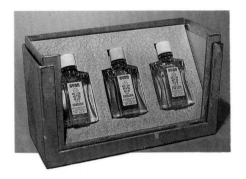

1939-40 *Cotillion, Gardenia and Trailing Arbutus Perfumes $1.25* **MP $100, $25 ea. bottle (label change)**

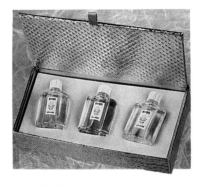

1937-38
Cotillion, Narcissus and Gardenia Perfumes 1/8oz $1.25 **MP $105, $25 each bottle**

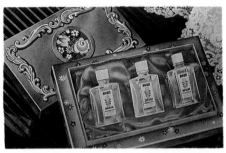

1940-43 *Gardenia, Cotillion and Trailing Arbutus Perfumes $1.35* **MP $95 $25 each bottle**

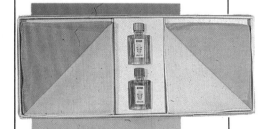

1939 only *Perfume Handkerchief Set. Four Handkerchiefs, Cotillion and Gardenia Perfumes 1/8oz $1* **MP $90, $20 ea. bottle**

PERFUME HANDKERCHIEF SETS

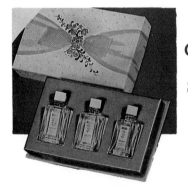

1944 *Gardenia, Cotillion and Trailing Arbutus Perfumes $1.50* **MP $95, $22 each bottle**

GOLD BOX SETS

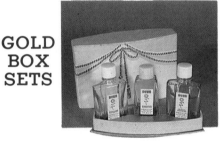

1945 *Gardenia, Cotillion and Trailing Arbutus Perfume $1.50* **MP $90, $22 each bottle**

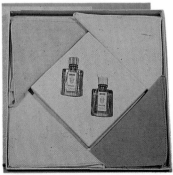

1939-42 *Perfume Handkerchief Set. 4 Handkerchiefs, Cotillion and Gardenia Perfumes 1/8oz $1* **MP $85, $18 each bottle**

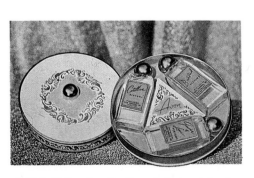

1947 *Gold Box Set. Cotillion, Ballad and Garden of Love Perfumes 1 dram $2.50* **MP $85, $20 each bottle**

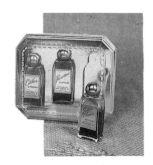

1949 *Gold Box Set. Cotillion, Flowertime and Golden Promise Perfumes 1 dram $2.25* **MP $85, $20 each bottle**

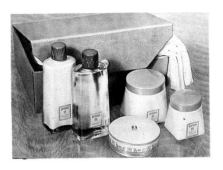

1937-39 *Facial Set for Dry or Oily Skin. Lotus Cream, Skin Freshener or Astringent, Tissue Cream, Cleansing Cream, Face Powder & Tissue $1.89* **MP $95**

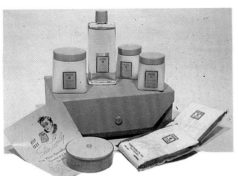

1940 only *Facial Set for Dry, Normal or Oily Skin. Cleansing Cream, Night Cream, choice of Skin Freshener or Astringent, choice of Foundation Cream or Finishing Lotion, Face Powder, Facial Tissues & Folder $1.89* **MP $95**

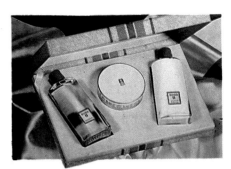

1939 *Wings to Beauty. Skin Freshener and Lotus Cream 2oz and Face Powder $1* **MP $65**

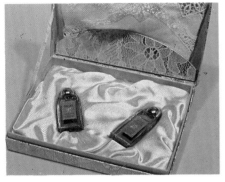

1940-41 *Milady Set. White Linen Handkerchief and 1 dram Ballad & Gardenia Perfumes $2.25* **MP $100**

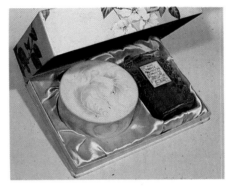

1942 *Petal of Beauty. Orchard Blossoms Cologne 6oz and Beauty Dust $2.20* **MP $140**

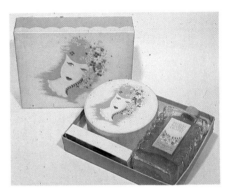

1946 *Petal of Beauty. Orchard Blossoms Cologne 6oz and Beauty Dust $2.20* **MP $110**

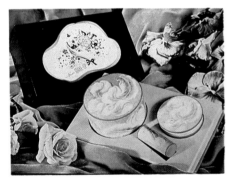

1943 *Make-Up Ensemble. Face Powder, Rouge and Lipstick $1.75* **MP $55**

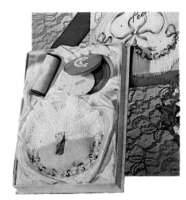

1944 *Peek-a-Boo Set. Lipstick, Rouge and Sachet Pillow $2.50* **MP $76**

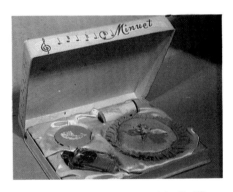

1944 *Minuet Set. Rouge, Lipstick, Cotillion Perfume and Sachet Pillow $3.95* **MP $100**

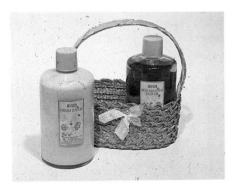

1947-48 *Beauty Basket. Cream Lotion and Rose Geranium Bath Oil 6oz each $2* **MP $100**

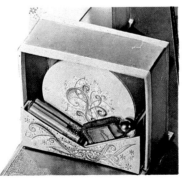

1949 *Flower Cluster. Face Powder, Lipstick & 1 dram Perfume $3* **MP $52**

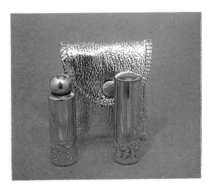

1949 *Golden Duet. Purse holds 1 dram Golden Promise Perfume and Lipstick $2.50* **MP $50**

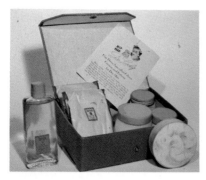

1941-42 *Facial Set for dry, normal or oily skin. Cleansing Cream 1¾oz, Night Cream ⅞oz, Foundation Cream ⅞oz or Finishing Lotion, Skin Freshener or Astringent 2oz, Face Powder, Facial Tissues and Folder $1,89* **MP $80**

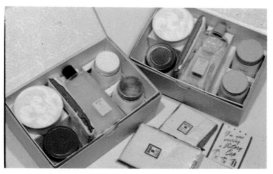

1943-44 *Facial Sets. Same contents 1940-1942 Sets (see left) except for Wartime packaging of substitute lids. $1.98 each set.* **MP $100 w/Wartime packaging**

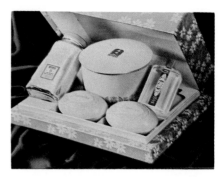

1940-43 *Bath Ensemble. Jasmine Bath Salts and 2 Bath Soaps, Dusting Powder and Jasmine Toilet Water $3.50* **MP $140**

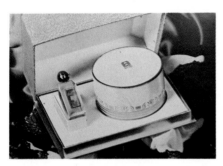

1940 *Colonial Set. Face Powder and 1 dram Garden of Love Perfume $1.25* **MP $66**

GIFT SETS
OF THE 1940's

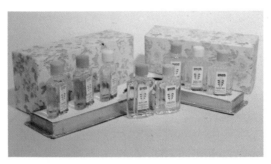

1939 *Fair Lady. Cotillion, Gardenia, Trailing Arbutus & Sweet Pea Perfume ⅛oz each 94¢* **MP $125,** **$25 each bottle**
1940-42 *As above (note smaller bottles) 94¢* **MP $125,** **$25 each bottle**

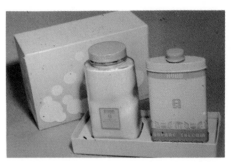

1940-41 *Bath Duet. Daphne Talcum and Bath Salts in choice of Jasmine, Pine, Ariel or Vernafleur $1* **MP $55**

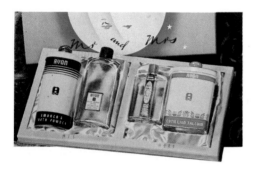

1940-42 *Mr. and Mrs. Smoker's Tooth Powder, After Shaving Lotion, Cotillion Toilet Water 2oz and Cotillion Talcum $2.50* **MP $128**

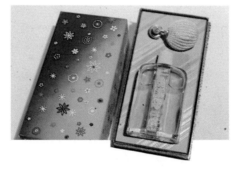

1941-42 *Fragrant Mist. Toilet Water in Marionette, Sonnet, Jasmine, Cotillion or Apple Blossom $1.50* **MP $60**

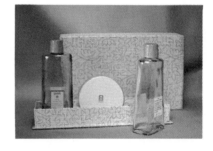

1941 *Wings to Beauty. Skin Freshener and Lotus Cream, 2oz each and Face Powder (also issued with cardboard Feather Face Powder) $1* **MP $55**

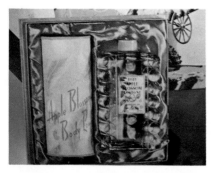

1942 *Flower Time. Apple Blossom Body Powder and Cologne 6oz $1.65* **MP $110**

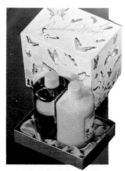

1942-44 *Rainbow Wings. Cream Lotion and Rose Geranium Bath Oil 6oz each $2* **MP $75**

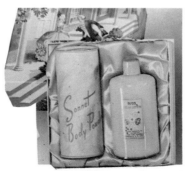

1942 *Colonial Days. Sonnet Body Powder 5oz and Cream Lotion 6oz $1.60* **MP $70**

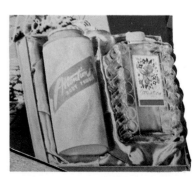

1943 *Flower Time. Attention Body Powder 5oz and Attention Cologne 6oz $1.65* **MP $110**

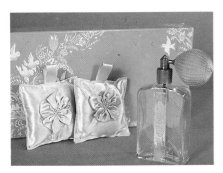

1943 *Scentiments Set. 2 Pillow Sachets and Attention Toilet Water 2oz (Set did not include atomizer as shown) $1.85* **MP $70**

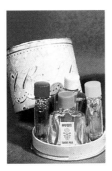

1945 *Fair Lady. 4 Perfumes 1/8oz each $1* **MP $125,** **$25 each bottle**

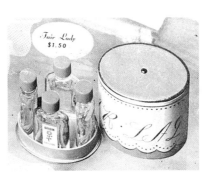

1946 *Fair Lady. Lily of the Valley, Gardenia, Cotillion & Garden of Love Perfume 1/8oz $1.50* **MP $115, each bottle MP $22**

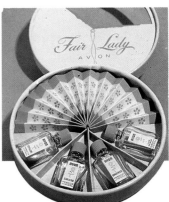

1948 *Fair Lady. 4 Perfumes 1/8oz each $1.50* **MP $115,** **$22 each bottle**

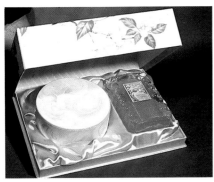

1943 *Petal of Beauty. Orchard Blossoms Cologne 6oz and Beauty Dust $2.20* **MP $130.**

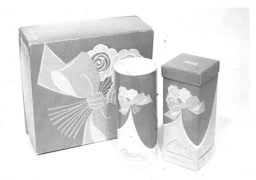

1943 only *Pink Ribbon Set. Attention Bath Salts 9oz and Attention Body Powder 5oz $1.61* **MP $75, each item MP $25**

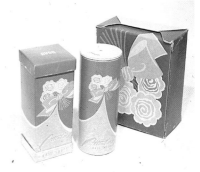

1944-45 *Pink Ribbon Set. Attention Bath Salts 9oz and Attention Body Powder 5oz in wartime fold-out box $1.61* **MP $75, $25 each item**

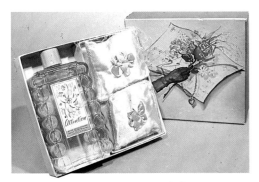

1945 *Scentiments. Attention Cologne 6oz and 2 Sachet Pillows $2.50* **MP $125**

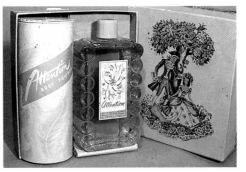

1945 *Flower Time. Attention Body Powder 5oz and Attention Cologne 6oz $1.65* **MP $105**

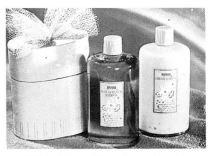

1945 *Rainbow Wings. Rose Geranium Bath Oil and Cream Lotion 6oz each $2* **MP $75**

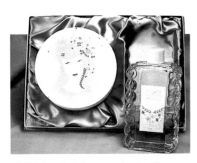

1945 *Petal of Beauty. Apple Blossom Beauty Dust and Orchard Blossoms Cologne 6oz $2.20* **MP $125**

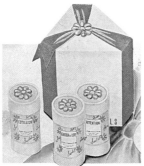

1944 *Little Jewels. Cotillion, Garden of Love & Attention Powder Sachet $3.25* **MP $80, $22 each Sachet**

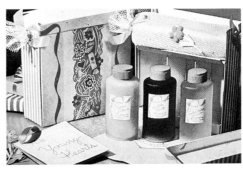

1945 *Young Hearts Set. Sachet Powder, Cream Lotion, Toilet Water and Bubble Bath, all 2oz, Cotillion Fragrance $3.75* **MP $80, $20 each bottle**

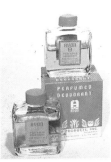

1949 *Perfumed Deodorant Set 98¢* **MP $22**

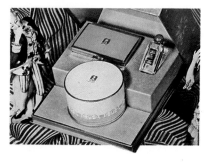

1940 *Mayfair Set. Double Compact, Face Powder and 1 dram Cotillion Perfume* $3.35 **MP $95**

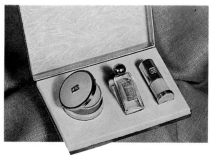

1940 *Spectator Set. Rouge Compact, Lipstick and Garden of Love Perfume, 1 dram $1.56* **MP $80**

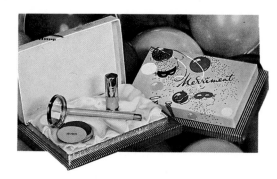

1940-41 *Merriment. Rouge Compact, Eyebrow Pencil and Lipstick $1.50* **MP $55**
1942 *(not shown) As above, except Lipstick Case is gold Bamboo $1.60* **MP $50**

COSMETIC SETS OF THE 1940's

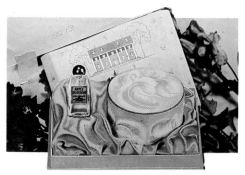

1941 *Colonial Set. Apple Blossom Perfume 1 dram and Face Powder $1.25* **MP $65**

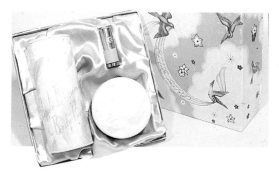

1941 *Blue Bird Set. Apple Blossom Body Powder, Face Powder and Lipstick $2.25* **MP $65**

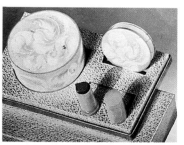

1942 *Make-Up Ensemble. Face Powder, Rouge and Lipstick, plastic $1.75* **MP $50**

(See Cosmetic Sets also page 105)

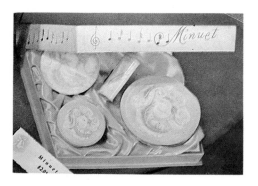

1942 *Minuet. Powder Compact, Rouge Lipstick & Face Powder $2.95* **MP $70**

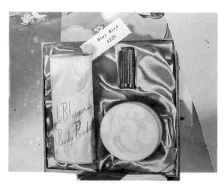

1942 *Blue Bird. Apple Blossom Body Powder, Face Powder and Lipstick $2.25* **MP $75**
1943 *(not shown) same as above, except Lipstick case is blue plastic* **MP $80**

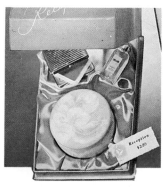

1941-42 *Reception Set. Face Powder, Compact and Cotillion Perfume 1 dram $2.95* **MP $75**

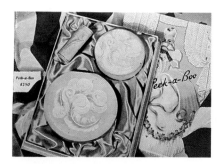

1942-43 *Peek-a-Boo Set. Lipstick, Rouge and Face Powder, all cardboard $2.50* **MP $65**

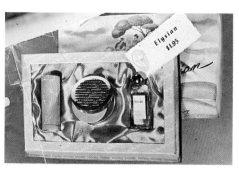

1942 *Elysian Set. Lipstick, Rouge Compact and Cotillion Perfume 1 dram $1.95* **MP $80**

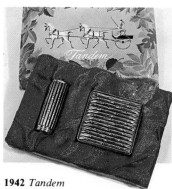

1942 *Tandem Set. Lipstick and Single Compact $1.95* **MP $50**
1941 *As above, except Lipstick is blue & gold $1.75* **MP $55**

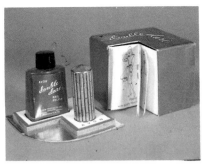

1946 *Double Dare Set. Double Dare Nail Polish ½oz and Lipstick $2.95* **MP $52**

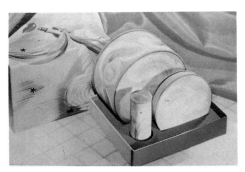

1945 *Make-Up Ensemble. Face Powder, Rouge and Lipstick $1.75* **MP $45**

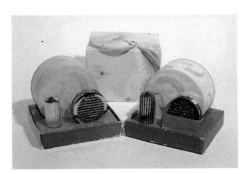

1946 *Make-Up Ensembles. Face Powder, Rouge Compact and Lipstick $1.75* **MP $50 each**

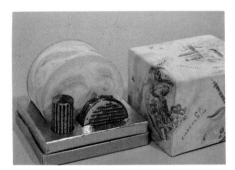

1947 *Make-Up Ensemble. Face Powder, Rouge Compact and Lipstick $2.35* **MP $50**

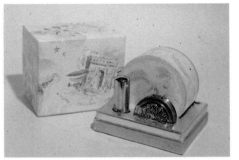

1948 *Make-Up Ensemble. Face Powder, Rouge Compact and Lipstick $2.35* **MP $40**

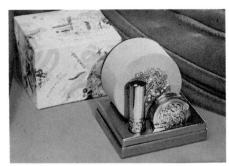

1949 *Make-Up Ensemble. Face Powder, Rouge and Lipstick $2.35* **MP $40**

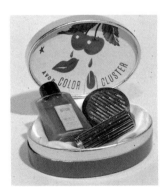

1946 *Color Cluster. Lipstick, Rouge Compact and ½oz Nail Polish $2* **MP $50**

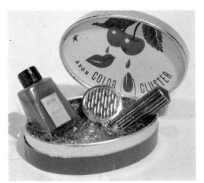

1947 *Color Cluster. Lipstick, Rouge Compact and ½oz Nail Polish $2* **MP $50**

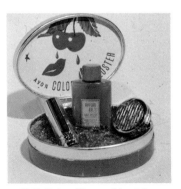

1948 *Color Cluster. Lipstick, Rouge Compact and ½oz Nail Polish $2* **MP $45**

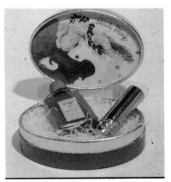

1948 *Beauty Mark. Lipstick and ½oz Nail Polish $1.35* **MP $40**

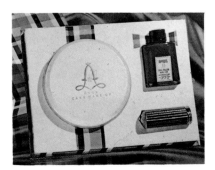

1947 *That's For Me. Cake Make-Up, Nail Polish and Lipstick $2* **MP $42**

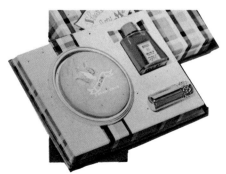

1949 *That's For Me. Cake Make-Up, Nail Polish and Lipstick $2* **MP $40**

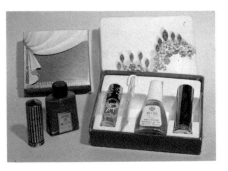

1946 *Leading Lady. Lipstick and Nail Polish $1* **MP $45**
1957 *Avon Jewels. Liquid Rouge, Nail Polish and Lipstick $2.50* **MP $25**

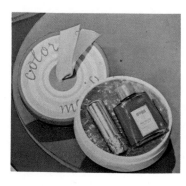

1949 *Color Magic. Nail Polish and Lipstick $1.35* **MP $35**

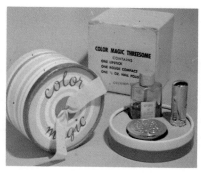

1949 *Color Magic Threesome. Nail Polish, Lipstick and Purse Rouge $2.19* **MP $45**, **$55 boxed**

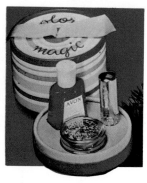

1950 *Color Magic. Nail Polish, Lipstick and Purse Rouge $2.15* **MP $40**

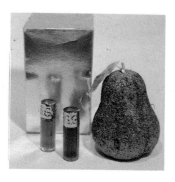

1953 *Precious Pear. Two 1 dram Perfumes, choice of fragrances $2.75* **MP $90**

(See also 1940's Cosmetic Sets p. 105)

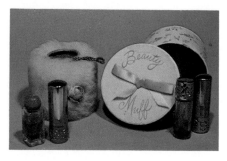

1949 *Beauty Muff Set. Muff holds 1 dram Quaintance Perfume and Lipstick $2.35* **MP $115**
1950 *Beauty Muff Set. Muff holds choice of 1 dram Perfume and Lipstick $2.39* **MP $100**

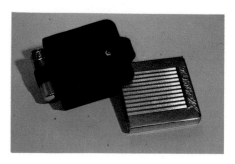

1949 *Gay Look. Taffeta Snap-Case holds Deluxe Lipstick and Compact $5* **MP $32**

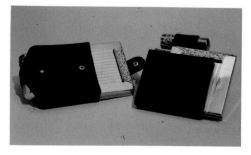

1950 *Gay Look. Taffeta Snap-Case holds Deluxe Lipstick and Compact $5.75* **MP $32**
1953 *Gay Look. Faille covered case holds Deluxe Lipstick and Compact $5.75* **MP $32**

COSMETIC SETS OF THE 1950's.....

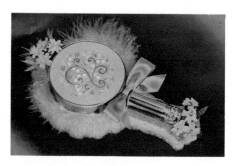

1950 *Adorable Set. Powder Pak 7/8oz and Lipstick $2.15* **MP $50**

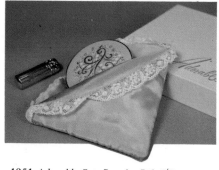

1951 *Adorable Set. Powder Pak 7/8oz, Lipstick and Sachet Packet $2.95* **MP $60**, **$65 boxed**

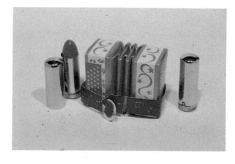

1954 *Concertina. Two Fashion Lipsticks $1.10* **MP $40**

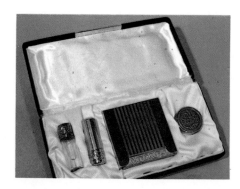

1950 *High Fashion. Black faille box holds 1 dram Perfume, Deluxe Compact and Lipstick, Compact Rouge $10* **MP $60**

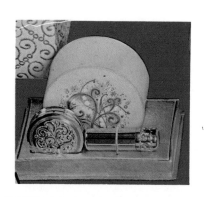

1952-53 *Make-Up Ensemble. Face Powder, Purse Rouge and Lipstick $2.75* **MP $35**

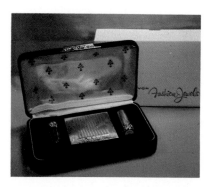

1954 *Fashion Jewels. Gold Compact, jeweled Lipstick and Perfume 1 dram $10.50* **MP $45**, **$50 boxed**

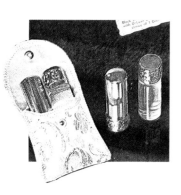

1950 *Avonette. Lipstick and 1 dram Perfume $2.50* **MP $50**

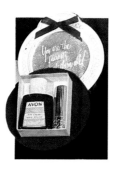

1950 *Lady Fair. Nail Polish and Lipstick $1.65* **MP $30**

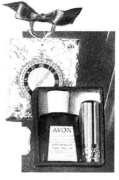

1952 *Time For Beauty. Nail Polish and Lipstick $1.65* **MP $30**

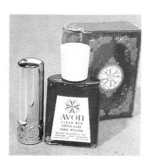

1954 *Beauty Pair. Deluxe Lipstick and Nail Polish $1.50* **MP $25**

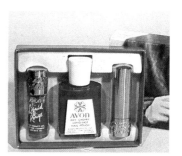

1956 *Top Style. Liquid Rouge, Nail Polish and Deluxe Lipstick $1.95* **MP $30**

COSMETIC SETS OF THE 1950's

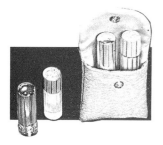

1952 *Avonette. Lipstick and 1 dram Perfume $2.65* **MP $45**

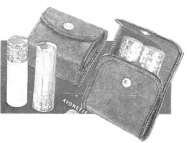

1953 *Avonette. Lipstick and 1 dram Perfume $2.65* **MP $45**

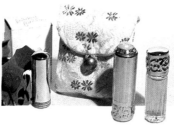

1953 *Holiday Fashion. 2 brass Lipsticks $1.10* **MP $30**
1954 *Charmer. Brocade Case holds jeweled Lipstick and 1 dram Perfume $3* **MP $38**

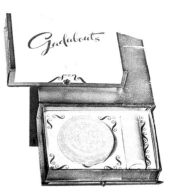

1953 *Gadabouts. Compact and Cologne Stick $2.25* **MP $28**

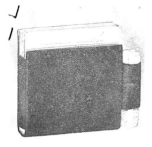

1955 *Gay Look. Faille Case holds Deluxe Lipstick and Compact $5.75* **MP $30**

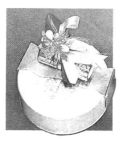

1955 *Color Corsage. Face Powder and Lipstick $1.89* **MP $25**

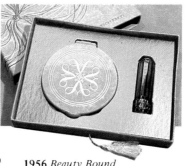

1956 *Beauty Bound Powder Compact and jeweled Lipstick $2.50* **MP $22**

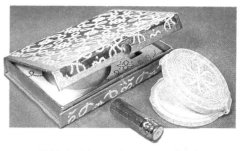

1954 *Gadabouts. Compact and Deluxe Lipstick $2.10* **MP $26**

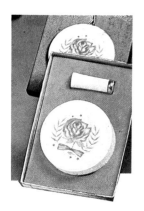

1958 *Makeup Mates. Face Powder and Lipstick $1.98* **MP $20**

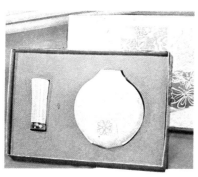

1958 *Touch of Paris. Powder Compact and Lipstick $2.10* **MP $20**

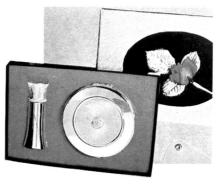

1958 *Classic Style. Deluxe Lipstick and Compact $5* **MP $25**

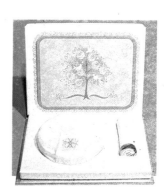

1959 *Pearl Favorites. Powder-Pak Compact and Lipstick $2.19* **MP $2**

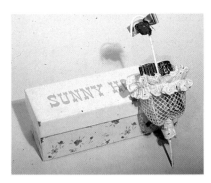

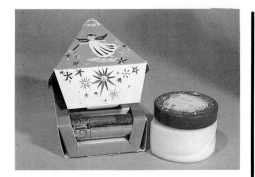

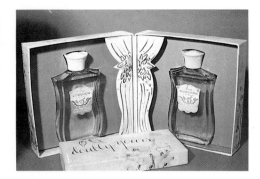

1952 *Sunny Hours. White net umbrella holds 1 dram Perfume and gold Lipstick $2.50* **MP $40, $48 boxed**

1953-55 *Christmas Angels. Cream Sachet .66oz in choice of Forever Spring (shown), To A Wild Rose, Quaintance, Cotillion and Golden Promise and Deluxe Lipstick $2* **MP $32**

1950 *Doubly Yours. Cotillion and Flower Time Colognes 2oz each $2.10* **MP $75**

GIFT SETS OF THE 1950's.....

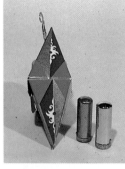

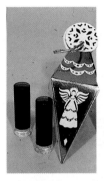

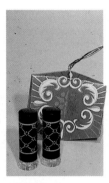

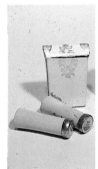

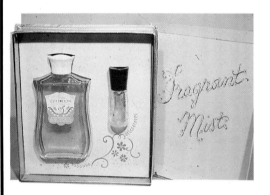

1955 *Two Loves. 2 gold Lipsticks $1.10* **MP $36**

1956 *Two Loves. 2 Fashion Lipsticks $1.49* **MP $36**

1957 *Beauty Pair. 2 Fashion Lipsticks $1.49* **MP $36**

1958 *Fashion First. Two Fashion Lipsticks $1.69* **MP $25**

1951 *Fragrant Mist. Toilet Water 2oz and 1 dram Perfume in 4 fragrances $2.35* **MP $55**

.....COSMETIC SETS OF THE 1950's

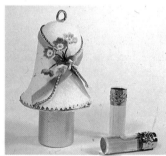

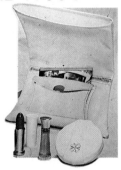

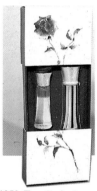

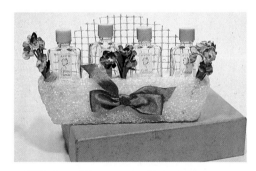

1954 *Lady Belle. Two 1 dram Perfumes in choice of Cotillion, To A Wild Rose, Golden Promise, Quaintance and Forever Spring $3* **MP $90**

1959 *Pak-Purse. Crushed Leather purse holds Fashion Lipstick, 1 dram Top-Style Perfume and Powder-Pak Compact $8.95* **MP $42**

1959 *Top Style Beauty. Top Style Lipstick and 1 dram Perfume $2.95* **MP $28**

1950 *Avon Blossoms. Cotillion, Quaintance, Golden Promise & Luscious Perfumes ⅝oz ea. $2* **MP $100, $120 boxed, $18 each bottle**

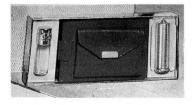

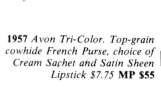

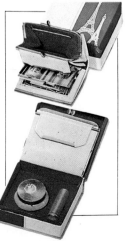

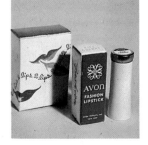

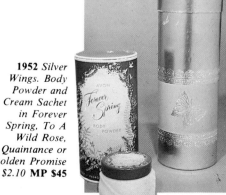

1956 *Lady Fair. Genuine Leather Wallet, choice of Long Life or Deluxe Lipstick and any 1 dram Perfume $5.95* **MP $60**

1957 *Avon Tri-Color. Top-grain cowhide French Purse, choice of Cream Sachet and Satin Sheen Lipstick $7.75* **MP $55**

1959 *Two Lips. 2 Fashion Lipsticks $1.69* **MP $24**

1952 *Silver Wings. Body Powder and Cream Sachet in Forever Spring, To A Wild Rose, Quaintance or Golden Promise $2.10* **MP $45**

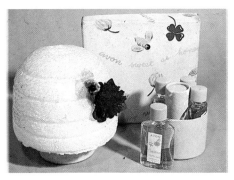

1951 *Sweet as Honey. Foam beehive holds Quaintance, Golden Promise, Luscious and Cotillion Perfumes $2.50* **MP $100, $125 boxed**

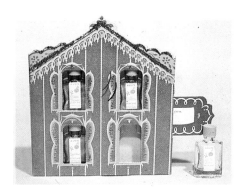

1952-53 *House of Charm. Lily of the Valley, Cotillion, Golden Promise and Quaintance ⅝oz each. $1.95* **MP $120, $18 each bottle**

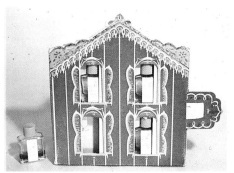

1954 *House of Charm. Same fragrance as 1952 Set (left) ⅝oz each. $1.95* **MP $120, $18 each bottle.**

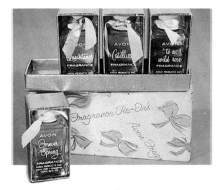

1953 *Fragrance Tie-Ins. Four ½oz bottles of Fragrance: Forever Spring, Quaintance, Cotillion and To A Wild Rose $2.50* **MP $75**

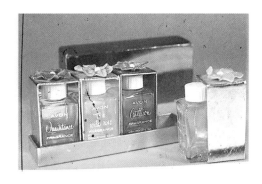

1954 *Fragrance Rainbow. Four ½oz bottles of Fragrance: Cotillion, To A Wild Rose, Forever Spring, Quaintance $2.50* **MP $75**

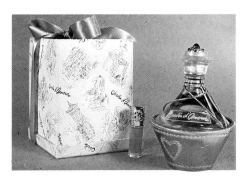

1954 *Perfume Set. 1½oz & 1 dram $15* **MP $200 complete**

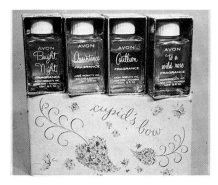

1955 *Cupid's Bow. Four ½oz bottles of Fragrance: Bright Night, Quaintance, Cotillion and To A Wild Rose $2.50* **MP $75**

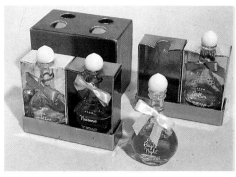

1956 *Fragrance Rainbow. Four 3 dram bottles of Fragrance: Nearness, Bright Night, Cotillion and To A Wild Rose $2.75* **MP $75**

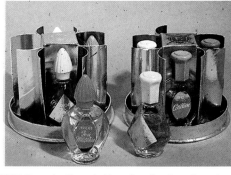

1957 *Gems in Crystal. Four ½oz bottles of Bright Night, Cotillion, To A Wild Rose and Nearness (Two different bottles used) $2.95* **MP $78 either set**

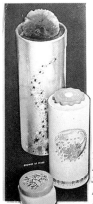

GIFT SETS OF THE 1950's

1955 *Shower of Stars. Body Powder 4½oz and Cream Sachet .66oz in Golden Promise, Quaintance or Forever Spring $2.10* **MP $45**

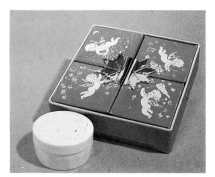

1956 *Cream Sachet Petites. 4 individually colored plastic jars hold Cream Sachet in Cotillion (pink), Bright Night (white), Nearness (blue) and To A Wild Rose (rose). Each separately boxed and issued in gold Gift Box $3.25* **MP $60, $10 each boxed jar**

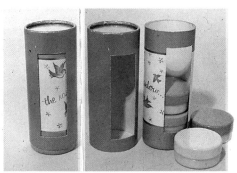

1957 *Somewhere Over the Rainbow. Four .3 oz Cream Sachets in To A Wild Rose, Cotillion, Bright Night and Nearness $3.25* **MP $60 complete, $10 each jar**

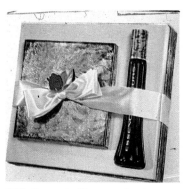

1958 *Dramatic Moments Set. Essence de Fleurs Spray 1oz and Beauty Dust in 6 fragrances $5 to $5.50* **MP $45**

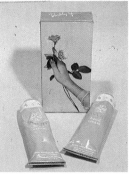

1954 *Doubly Yours. Two 2½oz Hand Cream $1.18* **MP $25**

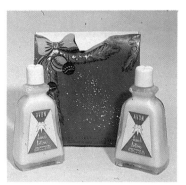

1951 *Special Set. Two 4oz Hand Lotion $1.18* **MP $42**

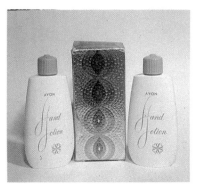

1965 *Double Pak. Two 4oz Hand Lotion $1.29* **MP $15**

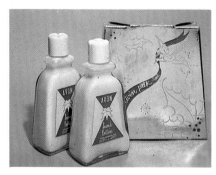

1952-53 *Twin Pak. Two 4oz Hand Lotion $1.10* **MP $40**

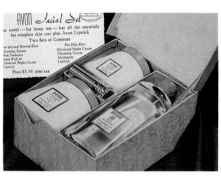

1953 *Facial Set.* **For Dry Skin:** *Fluffy Cleansing Cream, Dry Skin Cream, Skin Freshener & Lipstick...***For Normal Skin:** *Fluffy Cleansing Cream, Skin Freshener, Super Rich or Ozonized Night Cream & Lipstick...***For Oily Skin:** *Cleansing Cream, Ozonized Night Cream, Astringent & Lipstick. Each set $3.39* **MP $50 each Set**

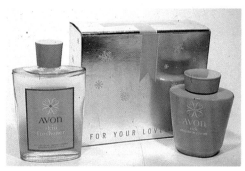

1954 *For Your Loveliness. Rich Moisture Cream 3½oz & choice of Skin Freshener or Hand Lotion 4oz $2.75* **MP $23**

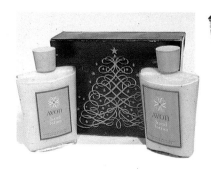

1954 *Hand Beauty. Two 4oz Hand Lotion $1.10* **MP $20**

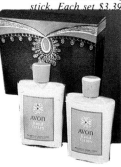

1955 *Hand Beauty. Two 4oz Hand Lotion $1.18* **MP $20** -

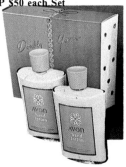

1956 *Doubly Yours. Two 4oz Hand Lotion $1.19* **MP $20**

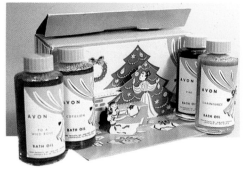

1956 *That's For Me. Four 2oz Bath Oils: To A Wild Rose, Cotillion, Pine and Quaintance $1.95* **MP $100, $20 each bottle**

BATH AND SKIN CARE SETS OF THE 1950's . .

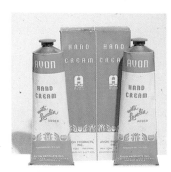

1953 *Hand Cream Duo. Two 2½oz Hand Cream $1.10* **MP $18 boxed**

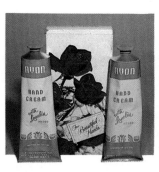

1954 *For Beautiful Hands. 2 Hand Creams with Lanolin added 2½oz each $1.10* **MP $25 boxed**

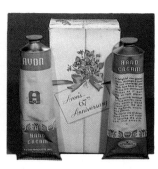

1953 *Two Hand Cream 2½oz each in 67th Anniversary Box $1.10* **MP $26 boxed**

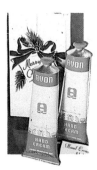

1953 *Hand Cream Duo. Two 2½oz Hand Cream $1.10* **MP $26 Xmas boxed**

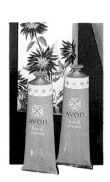

1954 *Hand Cream Duo. Two 2½oz Hand Cream $1.10* **MP $25 Xmas boxed**

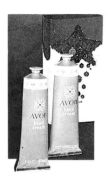
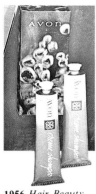
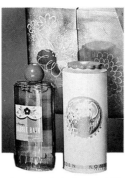
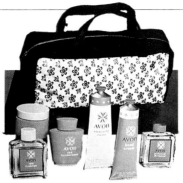
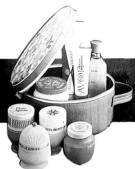

1955 *Doubly Yours. 2 tubes Hand Cream $1.18* **MP $25 Xmas boxed**

1956 *Hair Beauty. Two tubes Creme Shampoo $1* **MP $25 Xmas boxed**

1955 *Bath Delights. Bubble Bath 4oz and Body Powder 4½oz in Golden Promise, Quaintance, Forever Spring $2.10* **MP $50 Xmas boxed**

1954 *Happy Traveler. Rich Moisture Cream, Cleansing Cream, Hand Cream, Skin Freshener, Deodorant, Pack of Tissues and empty plastic jar $5.95* **MP $60 complete**

1956 *Women's Travel Kit. Zippered bag holds tube of Hand Cream and Cream Deodorant, Skin-So-Soft 4oz, Cleansing Cream and choice of one Night Cream $12.95* **MP $60 complete**

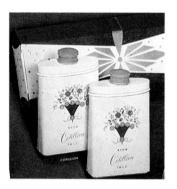
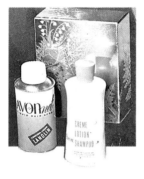
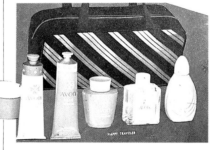

AVON TRAVEL KITS

1957 *Modern Mood. Two Talc in a choice of 4 fragrances $1.29* **MP $24 Xmas boxed**

1955 *Foam 'N Spray. Creme Lotion Shampoo 6oz and Hair Spray $2.19* **MP $30 Xmas boxed**

1955-56 *Traveler. Cleansing Cream, Hand Cream, Rich Moisture Cream, Skin Freshener, Deodorant and empty plastic jar $5.95* **MP $60 complete**

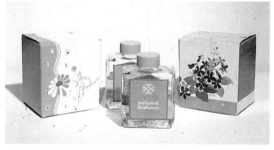

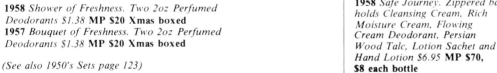
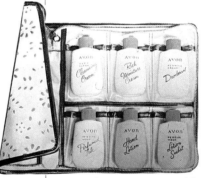
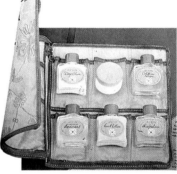

1958 *Shower of Freshness. Two 2oz Perfumed Deodorants $1.38* **MP $20 Xmas boxed**
1957 *Bouquet of Freshness. Two 2oz Perfumed Deodorants $1.38* **MP $20 Xmas boxed**

(See also 1950's Sets page 123)

1958 *Safe Journey. Zippered bag holds Cleansing Cream, Rich Moisture Cream, Flowing Cream Deodorant, Persian Wood Talc, Lotion Sachet and Hand Lotion $6.95* **MP $70, $8 each bottle**

1957 *Beautiful Journey. Plastic zipper bag holds refillable containers of Cleansing Lotion, Rich Moisture Cream, Cotillion Cologne, Perfumed Deodorant, Hand Lotion and Skin Freshener $5.95* **MP $85, $15 Cotillion Cologne, $10 each container**

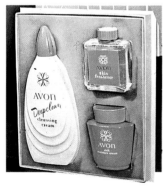
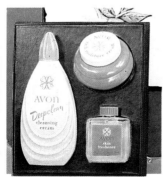
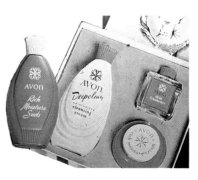
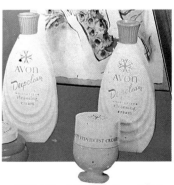

1956 *For Your Beauty. Deep Clean Cleansing Cream, Skin Freshener & Rich Moisture Cream $2.95* **MP $30**

1957 *A Thing of Beauty. Deep Clean Cleansing Cream, Rich Moisture Cream & Skin Freshener $3.50* **MP $25**

1958 *Beautiful You. Skin Freshener, Rich Moisture Cream & choice of Deep Clean Cleansing Cream or Rich Moisture Suds $3.50* **MP $25**

1959 *Gift of Beauty. Deep Clean Cleansing Cream & choice of Vita Moist or Rich Moisture Cream $3.50 & $3.95* **MP $22**

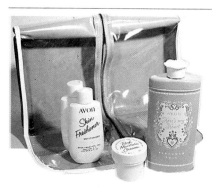

1959 *On The Wing. Skin Freshener and Cleansing Lotion 2oz each, Talc 2³⁄₄oz and choice of Rich Moisture or Vita Moist Cream 1¹⁄₂oz $6.25* **MP $45**

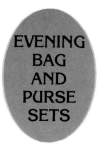

EVENING BAG AND PURSE SETS

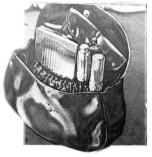

1949 *Evening Charm. Black Satin Evening Bag with Coin Purse, Deluxe Compact and Lipstick and 1 dram Perfume $10* **MP $65**

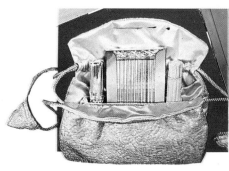

1952 *Evening Charm. Evening Bag contains Deluxe Compact, Lipstick and 1 dram Perfume $10.95* **MP $60**

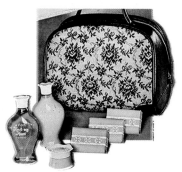

1962 *Tote Along. Tapestry design bag with Cream Lotion 4oz, Cologne 4oz, Cream Sachet .66oz. Choice of 6 fragrances (Somewhere issued with two 2oz Colognes) $12.95* **MP $43**

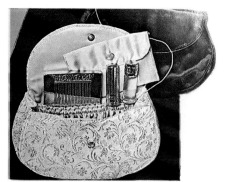

1950 *Evening Charm. Brocade Evening Bag with coin purse contains Deluxe Compact, Lipstick and 1 dram Perfume $10.95* **MP $60**

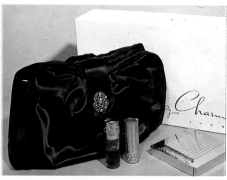

1950 *Evening Charm, Black Satin Evening Bag contains Deluxe Compact, Lipstick, 1 dram Perfume and Coin Purse $10.95* **MP $60**

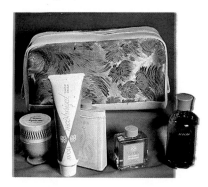

1963 *Women's Travel Kit. Choice of Night Cream, Moisturized Hand Cream, Talc, Perfumed Deodorant and Skin-So-Soft 4oz $11.95* **MP $42**

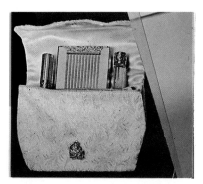

1953 *Evening Charm. Brocade Evening Bag contains Deluxe Compact, Lipstick and 1 dram Perfume $10.95* **MP $55**

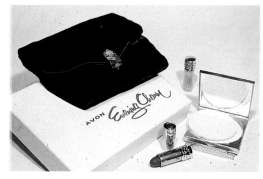

1953 *Evening Charm. Black Velvet Bag with Deluxe Compact and Lipstick and 1 dram Perfume $10.95* **MP $55**

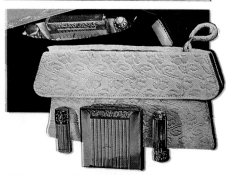

1954 *Evening Charm. Brocade Evening Bag (shown) or Black Velvet Bag contains Deluxe Compact, jeweled Lipstick and 1 dram Perfume $12.50* **MP $55**

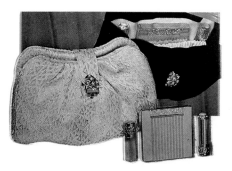

1955 *Evening Charm. Brocade or Black Satin Evening Bag contains Deluxe Compact, jeweled Lipstick and 1 dram Perfume $12.50* **MP $55**

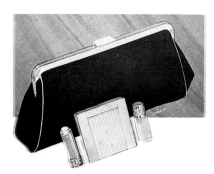

1955 *Dress-Up. Black Faille bag contains Deluxe Compact, jeweled Lipstick and 1 dram Perfume $10.95* **MP $55**

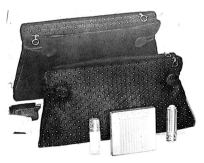

1956 Dress-Up. Reversible Bag contains Deluxe Compact, jeweled Lipstick and 1 dram Perfume $12.50 **MP $52**

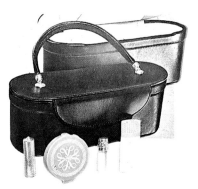

1956 Around Town. Polished calf leather Bag contains Cologne Stick and 1 dram Perfume (choice of frag.) Long Life Lipstick and Powder-Pak Compact $12.50 **MP $55**

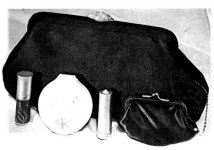

1957 In Style. Brushed Satin Bag with attached coin purse contains Persian Wood Spray Perfume, Powder Pak Compact and Satin Sheen Lipstick $12.95 **MP $52**

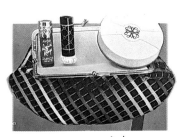

1957 Make-Up Tuck-In. Cosmetic purse contains Liquid Rouge, Fashion Lipstick and Powder-Pak $3.50 **MP $35**

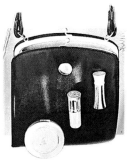

1958 On The Avenue. Leather Bag contains Top Style Compact and Lipstick and Persian Wood Spray Perfume $12.95 **MP $52**

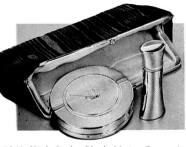

1960 High Style. Black Moire Cosmetic Purse contains Top Style Compact and Lipstick $5.95 **MP $30**

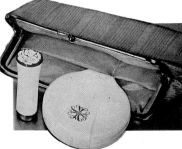

1960 Going Steady. Grey Moire Cosmetic Purse contains Pearlescent Compact and Fashion Lipstick $3.50 **MP $25**

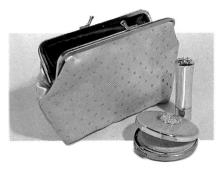

1961 Champagne Mood. Satin Bag contains Compact Deluxe and Lipstick Deluxe $6.50 **MP $25**

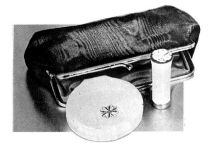

1961 Fashion First. Cosmetic Bag contains Pearlescent Compact and Fashion Lipstick $3.95 **MP $20**

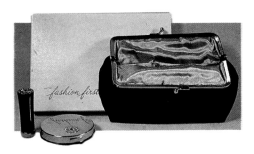

1962 Fashion First. Cosmetic Bag contains Fashion Compact and Lipstick $3.95 **MP $25, $28 boxed**

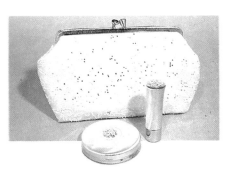

1963 Modern Mood. Acetate Satin Cosmetic Bag with pockets to hold Compact Deluxe and Lipstick $7 **MP $23**

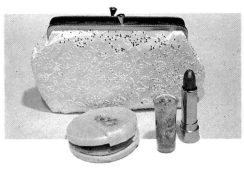

1963 Modern Mood. Acetate Satin Cosmetic Bag with pockets to hold Pink Pearl Compact and Fashion Lipstick $4.50 **MP $20**

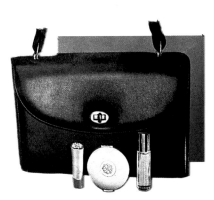

1964 Beauty Bound. Simulated Calfskin Handbag contains Compact Deluxe, Lipstick Deluxe, Creme Rollette in choice of 9 frag. $14.95 **MP $45**

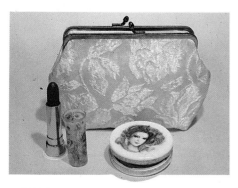

1964 *Purse Companions. Cameo Compact and Fashion Lipstick $6.50* **MP $25**

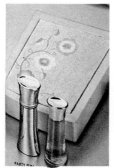

1960 *Party Fun. Top Style Lipstick and 1 dram Perfume $3.75* **MP $26**

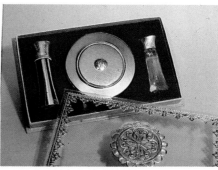

1960 *Classic Harmony. Lipstick, Compact and 1 dram Perfume, all Top Style $6.95* **MP $35**

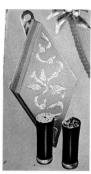

1962 *Color Trick. Two Fashion Lipsticks $1.96* **MP $25**

COSMETIC SETS

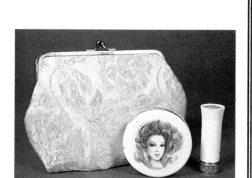

1965 *Purse Companions. Brocade Purse with Cameo Compact and Lipstick $6.50* **MP $25**

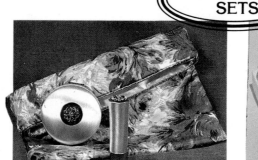

1962 *Deluxe Twin Set. Taffeta Clutch Bag, Compact Deluxe and Lipstick Deluxe $7.50* **MP $20, $7 bag only**

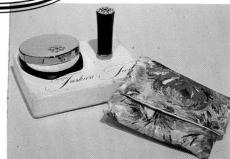

1962 *Fashion Twin Set. Fashion Compact and Lipstick $3.50* **MP $30, $7 bag only**

. . . EVENING BAG AND PURSE SETS

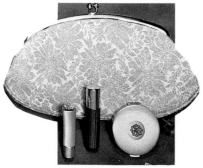

1965 *Evening Lights. Brocade Evening Bag contains Compact Deluxe, Lipstick Deluxe, Creme Rollette, choice of 9 frag. $14.95* **MP $30**

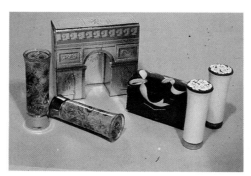

1964 *Golden Arch. 2 floral Fashion Lipsticks $1.96* **MP $26**
1960 *Golden Rings. 2 Fashion Lipsticks $1.79* **MP $26**

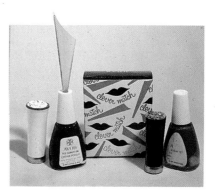

1961 *Clever Match (left) Lipstick and Cream or Pearl Nail Polish $1.67 & $1.83* **MP $18 boxed**
1962 *Clever Match (right) Lipstick and Cream or Pearl Nail Polish $1.67 & $1.83* **MP $18 boxed**

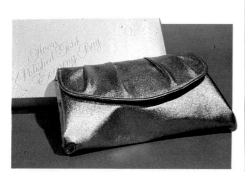

1978 *Evening Bag. Gold leather-like 10x6" $6.50 with $15 purchase* **MP retail value $15**

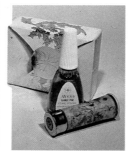

1963 *Color Note. Fashion Lipstick and Cream or Silver Notes Nail Polish $1.67 and $1.83* **MP $18**

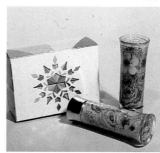

1963 *Fashion Star. 2 Fashion Lipsticks $1.69* **MP $25**

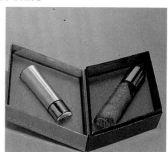

1963 *Touch-Up Twins. Lipstick Deluxe and Creme Rollette in a choice of Here's My Heart, Persian Wood, To A Wild Rose $3.10. Somewhere, Topaze, Cotillion $3.35. Occur! $3.85* **MP $23**

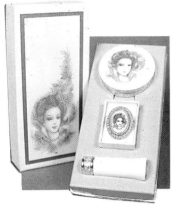

1965 *Cameo Set. Compact, Lipstick and Brooch $6.50* **MP $45, Brooch MP $18**

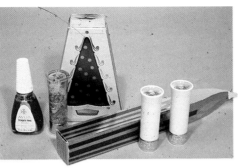

1964 *Pair Tree. Nail Polish and Fashion Lipstick $1.83* **MP $18**
1965 *Fashion Twins. 2 Cameo Lipsticks $1.65* **MP $22**

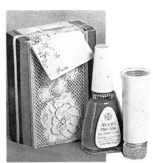

1965 *Color Compliments. Cameo Lipstick and Pearl or Satin Nail Polish $1.80 with Cream Nail Polish $1.65* **MP $18**

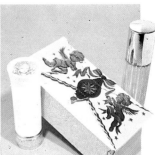

1965 *Touch-Up Twins. Cameo Lipstick and Rollette in choice of Here's My Heart, Persian Wood, Wishing, To A Wild Rose $2.70, Somewhere, Topaze, Cotillion $2.95, Occur!, Rapture $3.45* **MP $16**

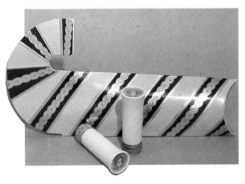

1966 *Candy Cane Twins. 2 Fashion Cameo Lipsticks $1.96* **MP $23**

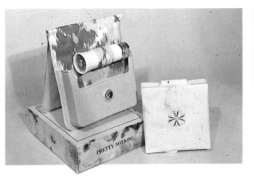

1965 *Pretty Notions. Vinyl Case holds Fashion Award Compact, Cameo Lipstick $4.50* **MP $26**

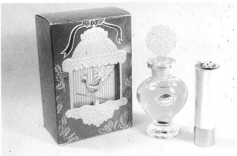

1965 *Star Attractions. Lipstick Deluxe and Cologne 1/2oz in 9 frag. $2.50* **MP $20**

. . .COSMETIC SETS OF THE 1960's

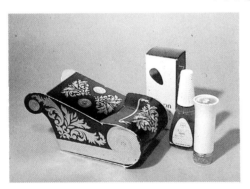

1966 *Sleigh Mates. Cameo Lipstick and Satin Nail Enamel $1.83, with Pearl Nail Enamel $1.93* **MP $22**

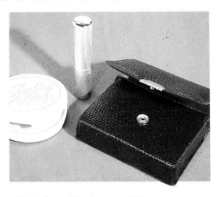

1966 *Avon Blushmates. Telescopic make-up brush, Avon Blush or Sparkling Blush $5.50 and $6* **MP $16**

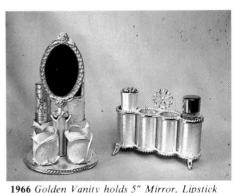

1966 *Golden Vanity holds 5" Mirror, Lipstick and Rollette $10* **MP $34 complete, $18 holder only, $5 mirror only**
1964 *Vanity Showcase, 3" h. Lipstick Deluxe and 1 dram Perfume $5* **MP $25, $10 holder only**

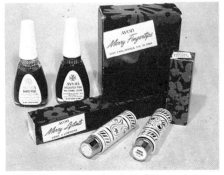

1967 *Merry Fingertips. 2 Nail Enamels in velvetized Gift boxes $1.70* **MP $12**
1967 *Merry Liptints. 2 Encore Lipsticks in velvetized Gift boxes $2.20* **MP $12 boxed and with sleeve**

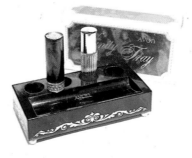

1968 *Vanity Tray. Fashion Lipstick and Perfumed Rollette .33oz $6* **MP $19 complete, tray only MP $9**

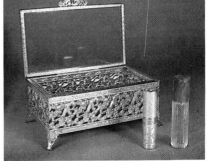

1968 *Golden Heirloom Jewel Box. Deluxe Lipstick and Rollette $15* **MP $40, $30 box only**

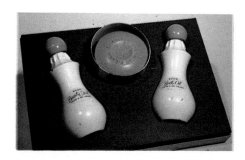

1960 *Modern Simplicity. Bath Oil 4oz, Beauty Dust 3oz and Soap in Cotillion, To A Wild Rose or Here's My Heart* $3.98 **MP $47**

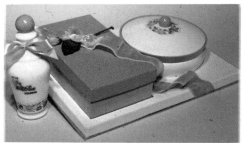

1960 *A Lady's Choice. Beauty Dust and Splash Cologne 4oz in To A Wild Rose (shown), Here's My Heart, Cotillion and Persian Wood* $5.45 **MP $43** *(See Cotillion & Persian Wood Sets p. 123)*

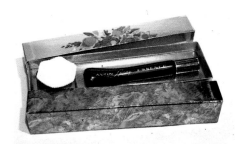

1960 *Beguiling. Cream Sachet and Spray Essence in Bright Night, Nearness, To A Wild Rose, Cotillion* $4.50, *Here's My Heart and Persian Wood* $5 **MP $26**

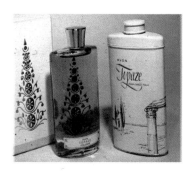

1962 *Refreshing Hours. Talc 2¾oz and Cologne 2½oz in To A Wild Rose* $2.25, *Here's My Heart and Persian Wood* $2.50, *Somewhere, Topaze and Cotillion* $2.75 **MP $30**

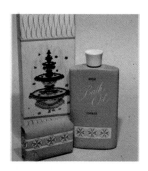

1962 *Bath Bouquet. Bath Oil 6oz and Soap 3oz in 10 fragrances* $2.79 & $2.98 **MP $20, bottle only MP $10**

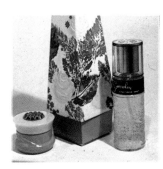

1963 *Floral Enchantment. Cologne Mist 2 oz and Cream Sachet .66oz in 7 frag.* $4 *to* $5.50 **MP $19**

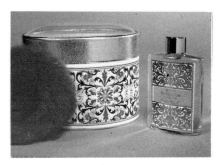

1962 *Bath Classic. Cologne 1½oz and Bath Powder 5oz in 6 frag.* $4.50 to $5 **MP $38**

GIFT SETS OF THE 1960's . .

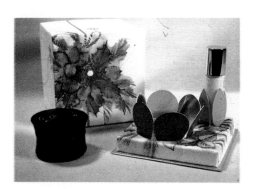

1963 *Flower Fantasy. Cream Sachet .66oz and Creme Rollette .33oz in Here's My Heart, Persian Wood, To A Wild Rose* $3.50 *and Cotillion, Somewhere, Topaze* $4 *and Occur! (shown)* $5 **MP $19**

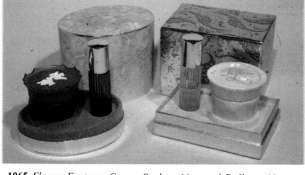

1965 *Flower Fantasy. Cream Sachet .66oz and Rollette .33oz in 7 frag. (Rapture shown)* $5 **MP $17**
1967 *Two Loves. Rollette .33oz and Cream Sachet .66oz in 8 frag. (Topaze shown)* $5 **MP $15** *(See Rapture p. 122)*

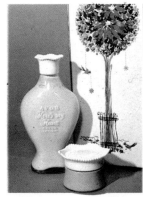

1962 *Fragrance Gems. Cream Lotion 4oz & Cream Sachet .66 oz· in 6 frag.* $2.60 *to* $3.50 **MP $17**

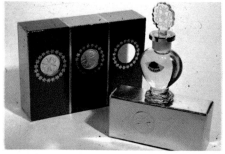

1964 *Fragrance Gold. Three ½oz Colognes in 9 frag* $3.50 **MP $25** *with sleeve, each bottle* $5, $6 **boxed**

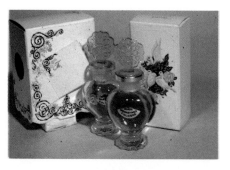

1965 *Fragrance Gold Duet. Two ½oz Colognes in a choice of 9 frag.* $2.30 **MP $19** *with sleeve, each bottle* $5, $6 **boxed**

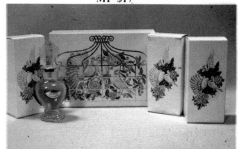

1965 *Fragrance Favorites. Three ½oz Colognes in 10 frag.* $3.50 **MP $24** *with sleeve*

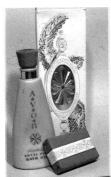

1963 *Bath Bouquet. Royal Jasmine, Rose Geranium or Royal Pine (shown) Bath Oil 8oz & 3oz Soap $2.39* **MP $18**

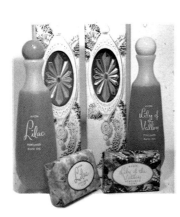

1963 *Bath Bouquet. Perfumed Bath Oil 8oz & 3oz Soap Lilac or Lily of the Valley $2.89* **MP $18**

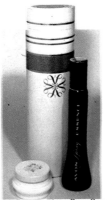

1964 *Decoration Set. Spray Essence 1oz & Cream Sachet .66oz in Here's My Heart, Persian Wood, To A Wild Rose $5.50; Topaze, Cotillion, Somewhere $6* **MP $22**

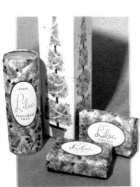

1964 *Flower Bath Set. Talc 3½oz & two 3oz Soaps in Lily of the Valley, Lilac, Jasmine or Rose Geranium $1.67* **MP $20**

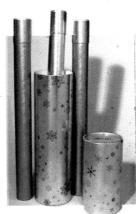

1965 *Bath Sparklers. Powdered Bubble Bath, set of 3 frag. 5oz each in tubes $2.50* **MP $30, $7 each tube**

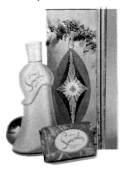

1964 *Bath Bouquet. Bath Oil 6oz and Soap 3oz in 6 fragrances $2.64 & $2.89* **MP $18**

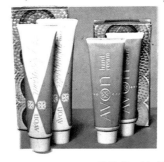

Christmas 1965 *Double Paks —*
2 Moisturized Hand Cream 3¾oz each, $1.75 **MP $12**
2 Avon Hand Cream 3oz each $1.35 **MP $12**
2 Hand Lotion 4oz each, $1.55 **MP $15**
2 Silicone Glove 2¼oz each, $1.55 **MP $12**

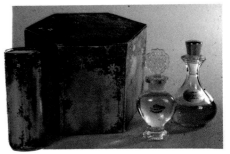

1965 *Bath Bouquet. Cologne ½oz Bath Oil 2oz and Talc 1½oz in Here's My Heart, To A Wild Rose, Wishing $4; Somewhere, Cotillion, Topaze $4.25; Rapture & Occur! $4.50* **MP $40**

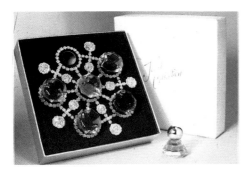

1964 *Jewel Collection. Six ⅝oz dram flacons of Perfume Oil: Somewhere, Topaze, Cotillion, Persian Wood, Here's My Heart and To A Wild Rose $5.95* **MP $62, $8 each bottle**

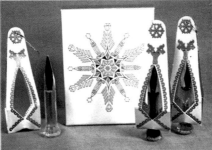

1965 *Fragrance Ornaments. 3 bottles Perfume Oil ⅝ dram: Set A, Wishing, Somewhere & Occur!; Set B, Rapture, To A Wild Rose & Topaze; Set C, Unforgettable, Here's My Heart & Cotillion $4.50 set* **MP $60 boxed set of 3, $15 each bottle in cut-out ornament, $11 each bottle only**

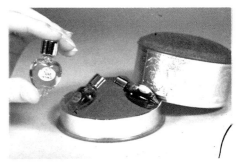

1966 *Perfume Oil Petites. Three ⅝ dram bottles in Set A, B and C (same frag. as those in 1965 Fragrance Ornaments) $4.50* **MP $55 in re-usable pin-cushion box. MP $13 each bottle**

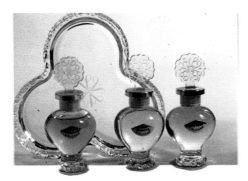

1966 *Colognes ½oz (sold individually) in 10 frag. $1.25* **MP $5, $6 boxed**
1966 *Fragrance Vanity Tray (glass) $1.25* **MP $9, $15 boxed**

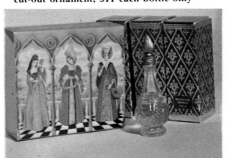

1966 *Renaissance Trio. ½oz Colognes in a choice of 9 frag. $1.75 each or 3/$3.50* **MP $5 each, $19 boxed set of 3 in sleeve**

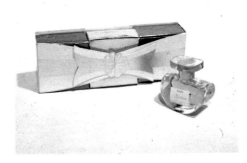

1960 *Gift Magic Set. 3½oz Colognes in choice of Topaze, Persian Wood, Here's My Heart, To A Wild Rose, Cotillion, Nearness & Bright Night, each in a different colored foil box. $2.98* **MP each $8 boxed, $30 boxed set of 3 in sleeve**

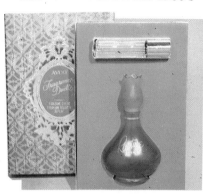

1966 *Fragrance Duette. Cologne 2oz and Rollette in Rapture, Unforgettable and Occur! $5* **MP $16**

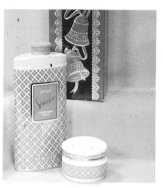

1966 *Fragrance Chimes. Talc 2³/₄oz and Cream Sachet in Here's My Heart, Wishing and To A Wild Rose $2.54; Somewhere, Topaze, Cotillion $2.89; Unforgettable, Rapture and Occur! $3.50* **MP $14**

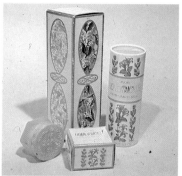

1967 *Floral Medley. Cream Sachet & Talc Honeysuckle (shown), Jasmine, Lily of the Valley $3.48* **MP $14**

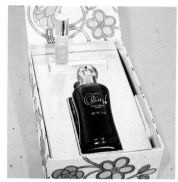

1967 *Keepsakes. Cologne Mist 3oz and Rollette in Occur!, Rapture and Unforgettable $8.50* **MP $16**

. . . SETS OF THE 1960's

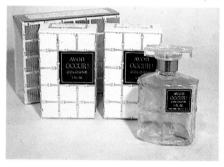

1967 *Cologne Gems in 8 frag. Choice of 2, 1oz each $3.50* **MP $15 complete, $5 each bottle, $6 each boxed**

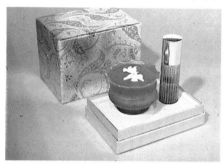

1967 *Two Loves. Cream Sachet and Rollette in 8 frag. (Rapture shown) $3.50 $4 & $5* **MP $15** *(See also Topaze p. 120)*

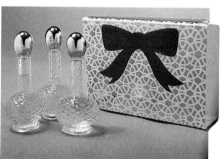

1968 *Fragrance Fling Trio. Cologne in 3 frag. ¹/₂oz $4* **MP $14 with sleeve, $3 each bottle, $3.50 boxed**

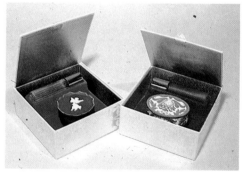

1968 *Scentiments Set. Cream Sachet & Rollette in Somewhere, Topaze, Cotillion $4; Rapture, Unforgettable, Occur! $5; Brocade & Regence $6* **MP $14**

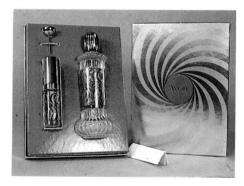

1968 *Splash 'N' Spray Set. Cologne in 5 frag. 2¹/₂oz Purse Spray bottle and funnel $6.50 to $7* **MP $32, $6 funnel only**

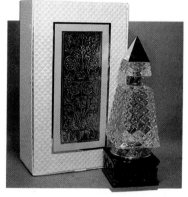

1969 *Pyramid of Fragrance. Cream Sachet .66oz, Cologne 2oz and Perfume ¹/₈oz in 3 frag. $12.50* **MP $25 boxed, $9 Perfume, $6 Sachet and Cologne**

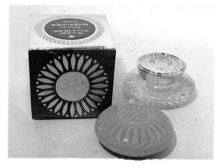

1969 *Scentiments. Cream Sachet ¹/₂oz and Soap 3oz in Occur!, Rapture, Topaze, Unforgettable, Somewhere and Cotillion $3.50* **MP $13**

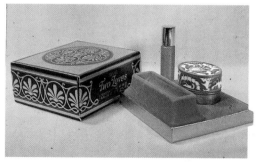

1969 *Two Loves Set. Rollette .33oz and Cream Sachet .66oz in Brocade (shown), Charisma and Regence $6* **MP $13**

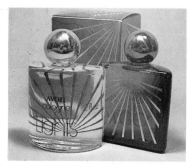

1969 *Lights and Shadows. Lights Cologne in clear bottle, Shadows Cologne in shadowed bottle, each 2oz. Set $4* **MP $6**

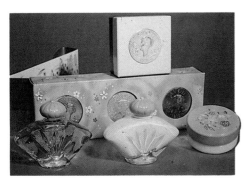

1958 *Wishing Set. ½oz Cologne, Lotion Sachet and jar of Cream Sachet in choice of fragrances. Any combination of 3 $2.50* **MP $55 complete, $15 each item boxed**

FRAGRANCE MAGIC SETS

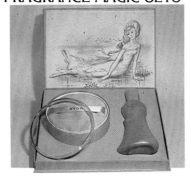

1962 *Fragrance Magic Set. Cologne Mist 3oz and Beauty Dust 5oz in choice of 6 fragrances (Somewhere shown) $8* **MP $38**

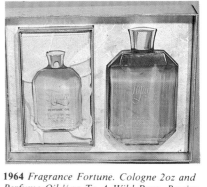

1964 *Fragrance Fortune. Cologne 2oz and Perfume Oil ½oz To A Wild Rose, Persian Wood, Here's My Heart $5.50 and Topaze (shown) Cotillion, Somewhere $6.25* **MP $30**

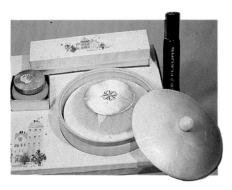

1959 *Paris Mood Set. Spray Essence 1oz, Beauty Dust 6oz and Cream Sachet. Choice of 6 fragrances $7.95* **MP $50**

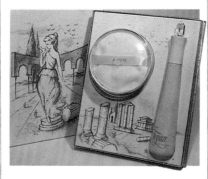

1962 *Fragrance Magic Set. Cologne Mist 3oz and Beauty Dust 5oz (Topaze shown) $8* **MP $38**

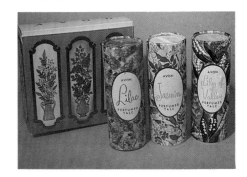

1965 *Floral Talc Trio: Lily of the Valley, Lilac and Jasmine 3½oz each $2.65* **MP $18**

LADY'S CHOICE SETS

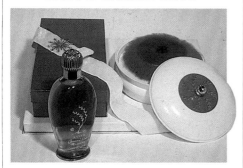

1960 *A Lady's Choice. Beauty Dust and Splash Cologne 4oz in choice of 4 fragrances (Persian Wood shown) $6.25* **MP $50**

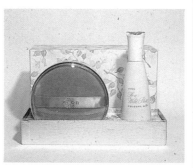

1962 *Fragrance Magic Set. Cologne Mist 3oz and Beauty Dust 5oz (To A Wild Rose shown) $6* **MP $38**

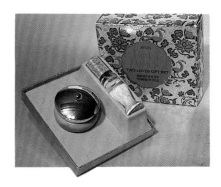

1970 *Two Loves Set. Rollette .33oz and Cream Sachet .66oz in Bird of Paradise, Elusive and Charisma $6* **MP $13**

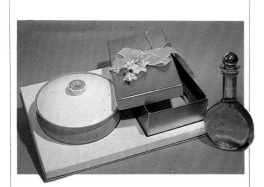

1960 *A Lady's Choice. Beauty Dust and Splash Cologne 4oz in 4 fragrances (Cotillion shown) $5.45* **MP $50**

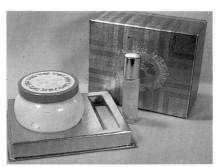

1964 *Beauty Scents. Skin Softener 5oz and Creme Rollette in 6 frag. $4.75 to $5.25* **MP $16**

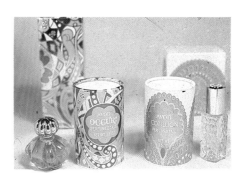

1971 *Precious Pair. Cologne ½oz and Talc 1½oz in 7 frag. $4* **MP $5**
1972 *Fragrance Fancy. Talc 1.5oz and Rollette .33oz in 7 frag. $4* **MP $5**

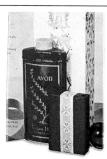
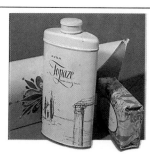
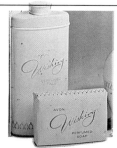

1962 *To A Wild Rose $1.08; Here's My Heart, Persian Wood $1.18; Somewhere, Topaze, Cotillion $1.28* **MP $20**

1963 *Persian Wood, Here's My Heart, To A Wild Rose $1.18; Somewhere, Topaze, Cotillion $1.28* **MP $18**

1964 *Here's My Heart, Persian Wood, To A Wild Rose $1.18; Somewhere, Topaze, Cotillion $1.28* **MP $16**

1964 Wishing **MP $20** *(left)*
1966 *Here's My Heart, To A Wild Rose, Wishing $1.28; Cotillion, Somewhere, Topaze $1.38; Unforgettable, Rapture, Occur! $1.49* **MP $14**

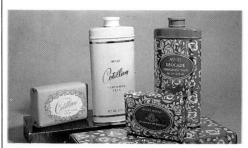

1967 *(left) Here's My Heart, To A Wild Rose $1.39; Somewhere, Topaze, Cotillion $1.49; Unforgettable, Rapture, Occur! $1.59* **MP $12**
1968 *(right) Honeysuckle, Hawaiian White Ginger, Unforgettable, To A Wild Rose $1.79; Brocade, Regence $1.98* **MP $10**

PERFUMED PAIRS

Each set contains one Talc 2¾oz and one matched Soap 3oz

(See 1974 Perfumed Pair page 125)

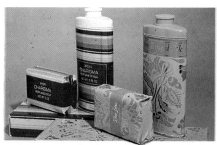

1970 *(left) Honeysuckle, Hawaiian White Ginger, Elusive, Blue Lotus, Bird of Paradise, Charisma $2.25* **MP $8**
1969 *(right) Honeysuckle, Hawaiian White Ginger, Blue Lotus, To A Wild Rose $2; Brocade, Charisma $2.25* **MP $10**

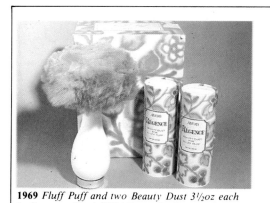

1969 *Fluff Puff and two Beauty Dust 3½oz each in Regence, To A Wild Rose, Cotillion and Unforgettable $5.50* **MP $22**
1967 *Fluff Puff, long-handled (not shown) and one 3½oz Talc. Carton designed and fragrances same as above. White with pink puff only.* **MP $22**

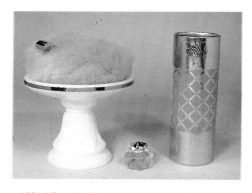

1970 *Ultra Fluff Set. 3½oz Beauty Dust, Lamb's Wool Puff and ⅛oz Perfume in Charisma, Brocade and Regence $10* **MP $17**

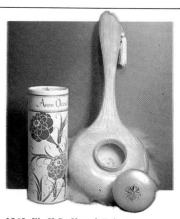

1969 *Fluff Puff and Talc 3½oz Occur! (shown), Unforgettable and Rapture $6* **MP $13**

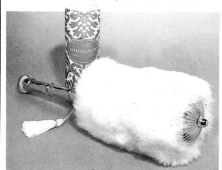

1969 *Roll-A-Fluff. Roll-on dispenser and Talc 3½oz. Brocade in white; Charisma, red; Regence, green $13.50* **MP $20**

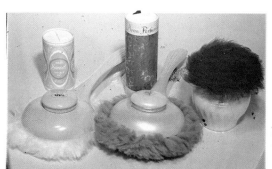

1976 *Fluff Puff and 2oz Talc (left) in Sonnet or Roses. Roses $7.50* **MP $5**

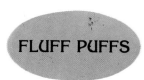

FLUFF PUFFS

1968 *Fluff Puff and Talc (center) 3½oz. Shown in Somewhere. Also in Here's My Heart (blue), Honeysuckle (yellow) and To A Wild Rose (pink) $6* **MP $15**
1970 *Powder Puffery Beauty Dust (right) 5oz in Charisma, Brocade, Cotillion and To A Wild Rose $5* **MP $7**

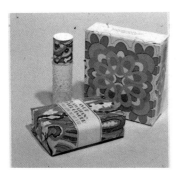

1972 *Floral Duet. Rollette .33oz and Soap 3oz in Hawaiian White Ginger (shown) and Honeysuckle $3.25* **MP $13**

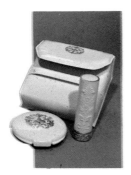

1971 *Sheer Companions. Vinyl carrying case holds Ultra Sheer Pressed Powder Compact ½oz and Lipstick $6* **MP $10**

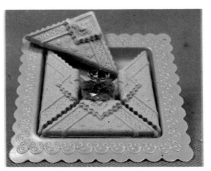

1972 *Fragrance and Frills. Perfume ⅛oz and four 1½oz Soaps in Field Flowers or Bird of Paradise $6.75* **MP $10 boxed**

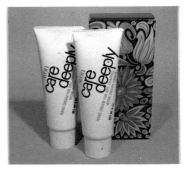

1974 *Care Deeply Hand Cream Set. Two 4oz tubes $3* **MP $4 Xmas boxed**

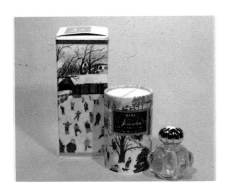

1973 *Minuette Duet. Cologne ½oz and Talc 1½oz in 6 frag. $4* **MP $5**

SETS OF THE 1970's

1974 *Fragrance Treasures. Cream Sachet .66oz & Soap 3oz in Sonnet, Charisma or Moonwind $5* **MP $6**
1974 *Perfumed Pair. Cologne ½oz and Talc 1½oz in choice of 6 fragrances $4* **MP $5**

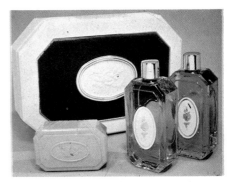

1973 *Treasure Chest. Cologne 4oz, Skin-So-Soft 4oz and Soap 5oz all in Sonnet or Moonwind $25* **MP $42**

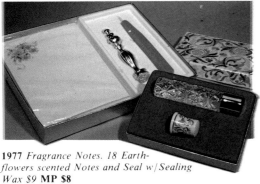

1977 *Fragrance Notes. 18 Earth-flowers scented Notes and Seal w/Sealing Wax $9* **MP $8**
1978 *Fragrant Notions. Needle Holder bottle with .33oz Ariane or Timeless Cologne and Porcelain Thimble $8.50* **MP $8**

SETS OF THE 1980's

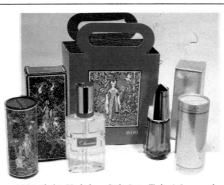

1981 *(left) Holiday Gift Set. Talc 1.5oz and Cologne Spray 1.8 oz in 6 fragrances (Charisma shown) $9.50* **MP $5**
1981 *Ultra Holiday Gift Set. Cologne Spray 1oz and Talc 1.5oz in 5 Ultra fragrances (Timeless shown) $9.50* **MP $5**

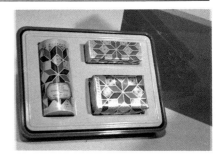

1982 *Country Christmas Collection. Talc 1.5oz, Ultra Cologne .33oz and Soap 3oz in Odyssey, Foxfire, Timeless, Candid, Ariane or Tasha $14.50* **MP $8**

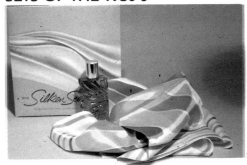

1980 *Silken Scents Scarf & Cologne. Vanity bottle of Candid or Timeless Cologne 1.75oz & Polyester Scarf 25x25" $15* **MP $10**

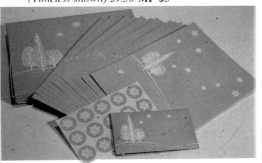

1980 *Scent With Love. 15 Fragranced Postalettes, 15 gummed Seals and packet of Unforgettable Sachet .18oz $6.50* **MP $5 complete**

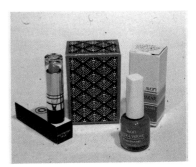

1980 *The Duo. Colorcreme Lipstick and Ultra Wear Creme or Pearl Nail Polish $6* **MP $3 boxed**

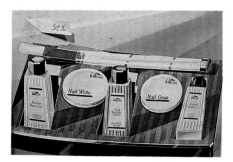

1930-36 *Manicure Set No. 2. Polish Remover, Nail White, Nail Polish, Nail Cream and Cuticle Softener, Orangewood Stick, Cotton, Emery Boards $2.50* **MP $122**

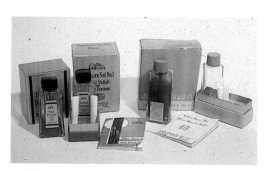

1930-36 *Manicure Set No. 1. Nail Polish and Polish Remover, booklet "What Story Do Your Hands Tell?" $1* **MP $75. $10 booklet**
1937 *Manicure Set No. 1. Nail Polish and Polish Remover, booklet "What Story Do Your Hands Tell?" $1* **MP $75, $10 booklet**

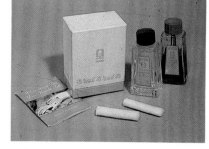

1936 *Manicure Set No. 1. Polish Remover, Nail Polish, 2 Cotton Rolls and Booklet "What Story Do Your Hands Tell?" 52¢* **MP $70**

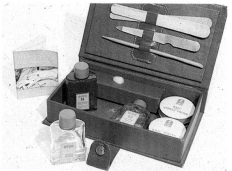

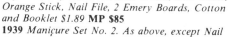

1938 *Manicure Set No. 2. Nail Polish, Cuticle Softener, Oily Remover, Nail Cream, Nail White, Orange Stick, Nail File, 2 Emery Boards, Cotton and Booklet $1.89* **MP $85**
1939 *Manicure Set No. 2. As above, except Nail & Cuticle Cream replaces Nail Cream $1.89* **MP $80**

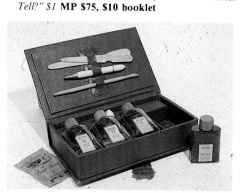

1940-42 *Manicure Set Deluxe. (with Aqua lids) Nail Polish, Oily Remover, Cuticle Softener, Cuticle Oil, Nail White Pencil, 5" Orangewood Stick, 2 Emery Boards, Cotton and Booklet $2.25* **MP $65**
1943 *As above, with Black lids $2.35* **MP $75**

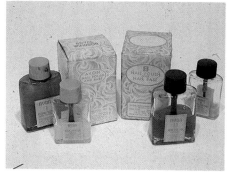

1941-43 *Combination Set. Nail Base and choice of Nail Polish (shown in Royal Windsor shade) 52¢* **MP $38**
1944-45 *Combination Set. Nail Polish and choice of Base or Top Coat 59¢* **MP $40**

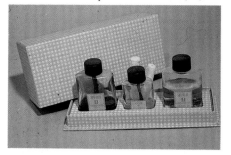

1942 *Nail Polish Threesome. Nail Polish, Nail Base, Oily Remover and Booklet 85¢* **MP $43**

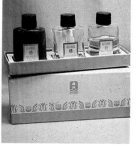

1943 *Nail Polish Threesome. Nail Polish, Oily Remover, Nail Base, 2 rolls Cotton and Booklet 85¢* **MP $46, $10 Booklet**

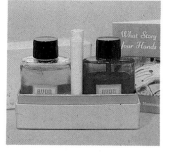

1943 *Nail Polish Twosome. Nail Polish, Oily Remover, 2 rolls Cotton and Booklet 59¢* **MP $31**

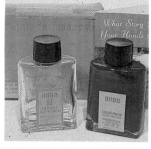

1944 *Nail Polish Twosome. Nail Polish and Cuticle Softener ½oz each, 2 rolls cotton and Booklet 59¢* **MP $31**

— MANICURE SETS —

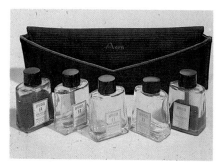

1944 *Deluxe Manicure Set. Nail Polish, Nail Base, Top Coat, Cuticle Softener, Oily Remover and Nail White Pencil $3.25* **MP $60**
1945 *Manicure Set Deluxe. As above, except bottles have Aqua lids $3.25* **MP $55**

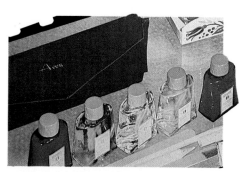

1947 *Deluxe Manicure Set. 2 bottles Nail Polish, Cling-Tite, Oily Remover, Cuticle Softener, Nail White Pencil, Orange Stick and 2 Emery Boards $3.50* **MP $52**

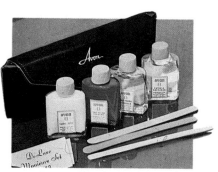

1948 *Deluxe Manicure Set. Nail Polish, Cling-Tite, Oily Remover, Cuticle Softener, Orange Stick and 2 Emery Boards $3.50* **MP $47**

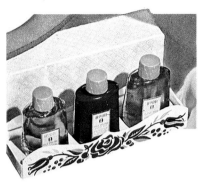

1947-49 *Manicure Threesome. Nail Polish, Cling-Tite, Oily Remover $1* **MP $28**

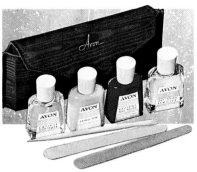

1950 *Deluxe Manicure Set. Cuticle Softener, Cling-Tite, Nail Polish, Oily Remover, Orange Stick and 2 Emery Boards $2.50* **MP $36**

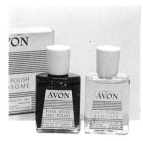

1950 *Nail Polish Twosome. Nail Polish and Oily Remover 98¢* **MP $17**

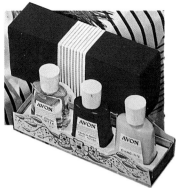

1950 *Manicure Threesome. Oily Remover, Nail Polish, Cling-Tite $1.29* **MP $30**

.....MANICURE SETS

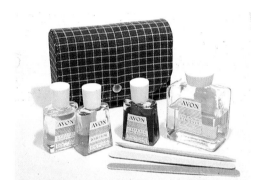

1953 *Deluxe Manicure Set. Cuticle Softener, Double Cote, Nail Polish, Oily Remover 2oz, Orange Stick and 2 Emery Boards $2.50* **MP $35**

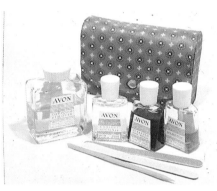

1954 *Deluxe Manicure Set. Oily Remover 2oz, Cuticle Softener, Nail Polish, Double Cote, Orange Stick and 2 Emery Boards $2.65* **MP $35**

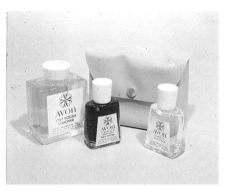

1955 *Little Favorite. Nail Polish, Oily Remover, Cuticle Softener $1.50* **MP $21**

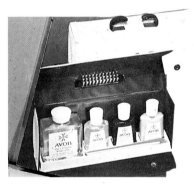

1955 *Deluxe Manicure Set. Oily Remover, Cuticle Softener, Nail Polish, Silvery Base Coat, Nail Brush & Emery Boards $2.95* **MP $35**

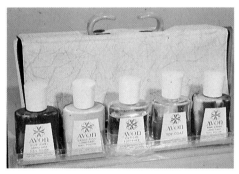

1956 *Deluxe Manicure Set. Removable tray holds Polish, Polish Remover, Cuticle Softener, Silvery Base, Top Coat, Emery Boards, Nail Brush. Handle seen through top of case. $3.25* **MP $33**

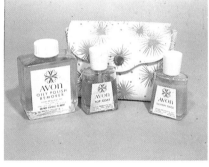

1957 *Color Changes. Oily Remover 2oz, Top Coat ½oz and Nail Enamel ½oz $1.95* **MP $21**

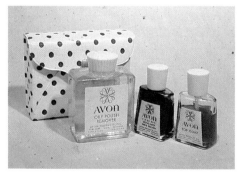

1956 *Polka Dot. Nail Polish, Oily Remover 2oz and Top Coat $1.69* **MP $21**

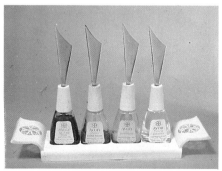

1958 *Color Bar. Set of 4: Nail Polish, Silvery Base, Top Coat and Cuticle Softener $3* **MP $20, $8 Tray only**

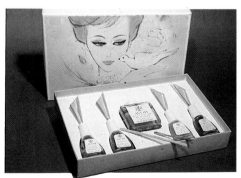

1959 *Manicure DeLuxe. Cuticle Softener, Silvery Base, Top Coat, Cream Polish, Oily Remover 2oz, Emery Board & Orangewood Stick $3.95* **MP $25**

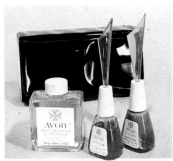

1960 *Manicure Petite. Oily Remover, Nail Enamel, Top Coat $2.98* **MP $17**

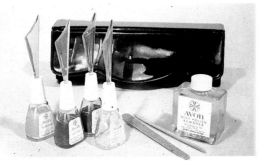

1960 *De Luxe Manicure Set. All vinyl Case holds Oily Remover, Silvery Base, Top Coat, Nail Enamel, Cuticle Softener, Orangewood Stick and Emery Board $4.98* **MP $26**

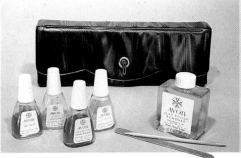

1961 *Deluxe Manicure Set. Moire plastic Case holds Silvery Base, Cuticle Softener, Nail Enamel, Top Coat, Oily Remover, Orange Stick and Emery Board $4.98* **MP $26**

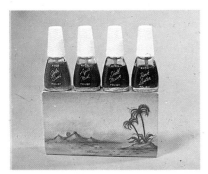

1962 *Hawaiian Delights. 4 bottles Nail Polish. Aqua, Pink, Shell and Gold $2.98* **MP $20, $4 each bottle**

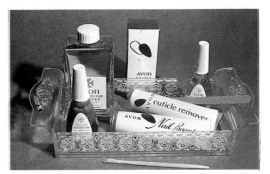

1962 *Manicure Complete. Nail Beauty, Cuticle Remover, Oily Remover, Double Coat, Nail Polish, Orange Stick and Emery Board $3.98* **MP $25 boxed, $10 Tray only**

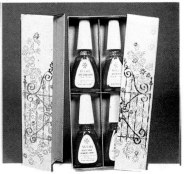

1964 *Color Garden. 4 bottles Nail Polish. Cream $2.76, Pearl $3.40* **MP $18**

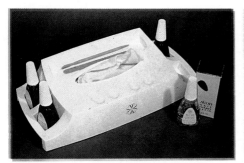

1965 *Manicure Tray. Long-Last Base Coat, 3 Nail Enamels, Orange Stick, Emery Board and Tissues $5* **MP $18, $9 Tray only**

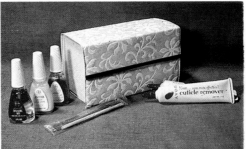

1966 *Manicure Kit. Nail Enamel, Nail Beauty, Cuticle Remover, Base Coat, Enamel Set, 10 Remover Pads, Orange Stick, Emery Board $8.50* **MP $22 boxed, $8 Case only**

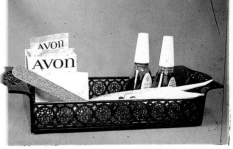

1967 *Manicure Complete. Tray 10¼" long, Nail Polish, Double Coat, Cuticle Cream, Nail Beauty, 10 Remover Pads, Emery Board and Orange Stick $5* **MP $18, $8 Tray only**

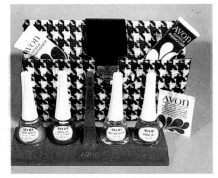

1968 *Manicure Beauti-Kit. Long-Last Top Coat, Enamel Set, Cuticle Conditioner, Enamel Remover Pads (10), Cuticle Remover, 2 Nail Enamels and Emery Board $12* **MP $22, $8 Case only**

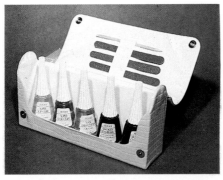

1978 *Nail Care Kit. Simulated alligator Kit, sold only in U.S., holds .5oz Super Strengthener, Base Coat, Top Coat and 2 Nail Enamels, 3 Emery Boards and Cuticle Stick $10* **MP $7.50**

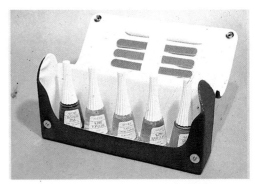

1979 *Nail Care Kit. Simulated alligator Kit, sold only in U.S. Issued with same items as 1978 Kit (left) Retail value $12* **MP $6.50**

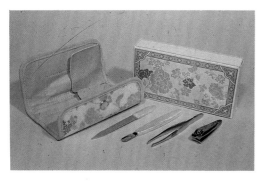
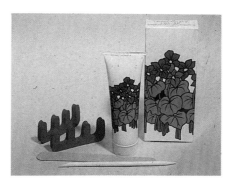
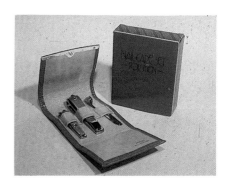

1984 *Pastel Bouquet Manicure Set. Nail clipper, tweezer, cuticle pusher and nail file $16* **MP $14**

1983 *Fabulous Foot Care Kit. 1oz Fancy Feet Cream, emery board, orange stick and pair of toesies $4.50* **MP $4**

1984 *Nailcare Set for Men. Small nail clipper, large nail clipper and folding nail file in leather-like case $16* **MP $14**

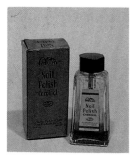
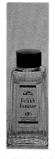
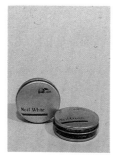
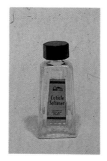
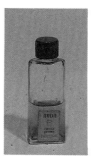
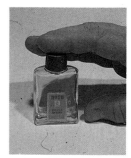

1930-36 *Nail Polish 50¢* **MP $25, $30 boxed**

1930 *Polish Remover 50¢* **MP $25, $30 boxed**

1931-36 *Nail White 25¢* **MP $12**
1931-36 *Nail Cream 25¢* **MP $12**

1931-36 *Cuticle Softener 50¢* **MP $25**

1937 *Cuticle Softener 26¢* **MP $27**

1938 *Cuticle Softener 29¢* **MP $8**

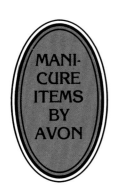

MANI-CURE ITEMS BY AVON

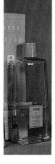
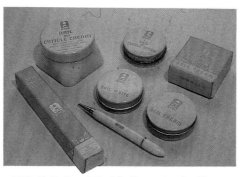
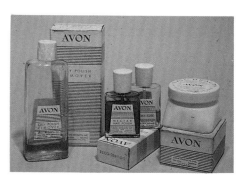

1936-37 *Oily Polish Remover 2oz 43¢* **MP $25, $30 boxed**

1940-49 *Nail and Cuticle Cream 1oz jar 37¢* **MP $8, $10 boxed**
1939 *Nail & Cuticle Cream (top) 26¢* **MP $10**
1937 *Nail White 26¢* **MP $4, $9 boxed**
1937-39 *Nail Cream 26¢* **MP $4, $9 boxed**
1941 *Nail White Pencil 52¢* **MP $4, $8 boxed**

1950-54 *Oily Remover 2oz 49¢* **MP $8, $12 boxed**
1950 *Nail Polish 49¢* **MP $6, $8 boxed**
1950 *Double-Cote 49¢* **MP $6, $8 boxed**
1950 *Nail & Cuticle Cream 49¢* **MP $7, $10 boxed**

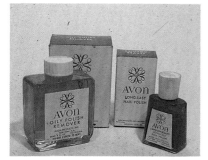
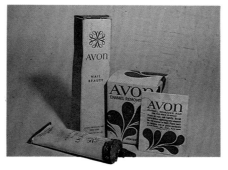
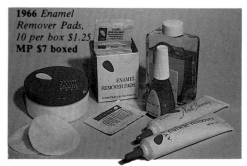

1955 *Oily Remover 2oz 49¢* **MP $4, $6 boxed**
1954 *Long-Last or Pearlescent Nail Polish 59¢ & 75¢* **MP $4, $6 boxed**

1957 *Nail Beauty 1oz tube 59¢* **MP $5, $6 boxed**
1967 *Enamel Remover Pads, 10 per box 90¢* **MP $7 boxed**

1966 *Enamel Remover Pads, 10 per box $1.25* **MP $7 boxed**

1963-66 *Nail Polish Remover, 20 pads 98¢* **MP $11**
1962 *Nail Polish 85¢* **MP $3**
1962 *Oily Remover 3oz 69¢* **MP $3.50**
1962 *Nail Beauty 69¢* **MP $4**
1962 *Cuticle Remover 69¢* **MP $4**

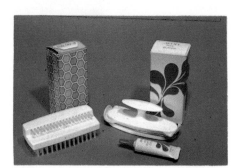

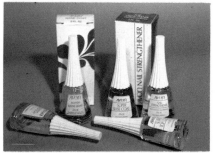

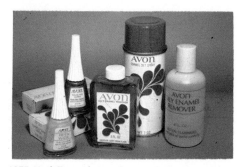

1970 *Nail Brush $2.50* **MP $2, $3 boxed**
1973 *Nail Buffer 3½" long $2.50* **MP $3,**
$4 boxed
1973 *Nail Buffing Cream ¼oz $1.25* **MP $2**

1969 *Enamel Fling Nail Enamel in Mauvelous or Sunspin .5oz $1.25* **MP $3 each**

1975 *Super Top Coat .5oz $1.75* **MP 50¢**
1977 *Super Top Coat .5oz $1.29* **MP 50¢**
1975 *Super Base Coat .5oz $1.75* **MP 50¢**
1977 *Super Base Coat .5oz $1.29* **MP 50¢**
1977 *Nail Strengthener .5oz $1.39* **MP 50¢**

. . . MANICURE ITEMS

1977 *Nail Enamel .5oz Cremes & Pearls, 32 shades $2.25* **MP 50¢**
1974 *Nail Enamel .5oz Cremes, Satins & Pearls $1.10 & $1.20* **MP 50¢**
1968 *Oily Enamel Remover 3oz 90¢* **MP 75¢**
1971 *Enamel Set Spray 7oz $2* **MP $2**
1977 *Oily Enamel Remover 4oz $1.19* **MP 25¢**

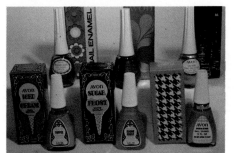

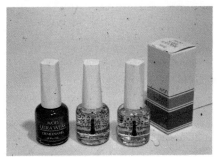

1968 *Tinsel Topping Nail Enamel, Silver or Copper .5oz $1.25* **MP $4 each**
1971 *Skylighters Nail Enamel, 3 shades .5oz $1.25* **MP $4 each, $6 boxed**
1966 *Iced Cream Nail Enamel, 6 shades .5oz $1.25* **MP $4 each, $6 boxed**
1966 *Sugar Frost Matte Overlay .5oz $1.25* **MP $4**
1966 *Chic Sparklers Nail Enamel .5oz $1.25* **MP $4 each, $6 boxed**

1980 *Super Nail Mend & Wrap Kit. Mending Liquid ½oz, Mending Tissues & Cuticle Stick $4.75* **MP 50¢**
1980 *Super Strengthener for Nails ½oz $1.65* **MP 25¢**
1980 *Super Nail Dry ½oz $2* **MP 25¢**

1980 *Ultra Wear Creme or Pearl Enamel ½oz $2.75* **MP 25¢**
1980 *Ultra Wear Base Coat ½oz $1.65* **MP 25¢**
1980 *Ultra Wear Top Coat ½oz $1.65* **MP 25¢**

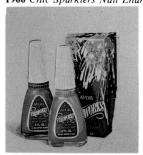

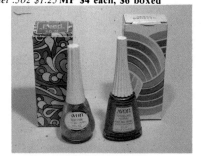

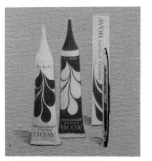

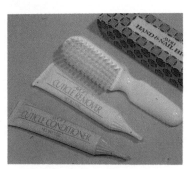

1967 *Fireworks Base Coat .5oz $1.25* **MP $4, $6 boxed**
1967 *Fireworks Nail Enamel .5oz $1.25* **MP $4, $6 boxed**

1960 *Satin Nail Enamel .5oz $1* **MP $2, $6 in Xmas carton**
1979 *Color-Up America Gift Box & Nail Enamel $2.25* **MP 50¢, $3 boxed** *(incorrect bottle shown, see 1977 Nail Enamel above)*

1968 *Cuticle Conditioner 1oz 90¢* **MP $3**
1968 *Cuticle Remover 1oz 90¢* **MP $3**
1970 *Cuticle Trainer $1.50* **MP $2.50, $3 boxed**

1977-82 *Cuticle Conditioner 1oz $1.19* **MP 75¢**
1977-82 *Cuticle Remover 1oz $1.19* **MP 75¢**
1973-76 *Hand & Nail Brush $2.50* **MP $2, $2.50 boxed**

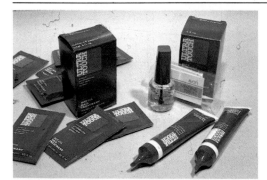

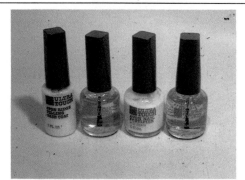

ULTRA TOUCH

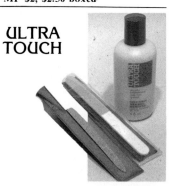

1982 *Hot Oil Nail Treatment, 8 packets per box $3.50* **MP $3 boxed**
1982 *Mend and Wrap Kit. Mending Liquid .5oz, mending tissues, cuticle stick $5.50* **MP $3 complete**
1982 *Cuticle Remover 1oz $2.50* **MP $1.50***
1982 *Cuticle & Nail Conditioning Cream 1oz $2.50* **MP 50¢**

1984 *Ridge-Filling Base Coat .5oz $2.50* **MP $1.50***
1982 *Super Base Coat .5oz $2.50* **MP 25¢**
1982 *Nail Fortifier .5oz $2.50* **MP 25¢**
1982 *Shiny Top Shield .5oz $2.50* **MP 25¢**

**Available from Avon at time of publication*

1982 *Professional Nail File in vinyl sleeve, 1 campaign only 99¢* **MP $3**
1982 *All-In-One Nail Buffer $5* **MP $4***
1982 *Oily Nail Enamel Remover 4oz $2.75* **MP $1.50***

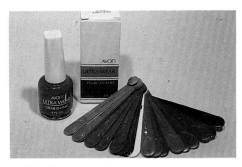

1980 *Ultra Wear Creme or Pearl Enamel .5oz $2.75* **MP 25¢**
1983 *Ultra Wear Nail Enamel Shade Selector* **MP $3.25***

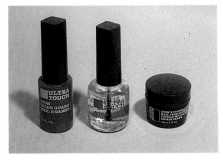

1984 *Ultra Touch Color Guard Nail Enamel .5oz $4* **MP $2***
1982 *Ultra Touch Quick Nail Dry .5oz $2.50* **MP 25¢**
1984 *Ultra Touch Cuticle Repair Cream .5oz $2.50* **MP $1.49***

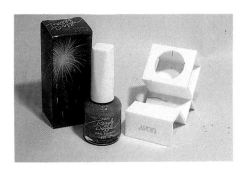

1983 *Razzle Dazzle Nail Enamel, 6 shades .5oz $3.50* **MP 25¢**
1984 *Manicure Rest and Nail Care Book 49¢ with Ultra Touch purchase* **MP $3**

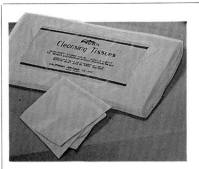

1930 *Cleansing Tissues, package of 135 wrapped in Cellophane 50¢* **MP $65**

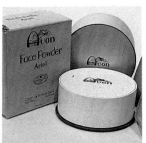

1930-36 *Face Powder, Ariel or Vernafleur 8 shades 75¢* **MP $25, $37 boxed**

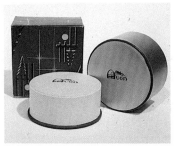

1930-36 *Face Powder, Ariel or Vernafleur, 8 shades 75¢* **MP $45 Xmas boxed**

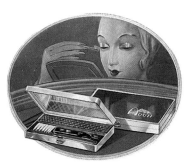

1933-36 *Mascara Compact, brown or black shades $1.04* **MP $38**

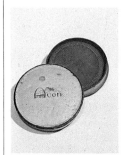

1930 *Purse Size Face Powder, Ariel 50¢* **MP $30**

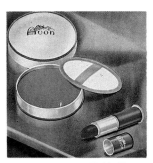

1930-33 *Dressing Table Rouge 45¢* **MP $32**
1931-32 *Lipstick 65¢* **MP $16**

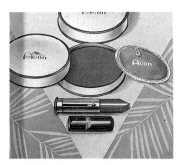

1933-35 *Dressing Table Rouge (redesigned puff), 3 shades 47¢* **MP $30**
1933-34 *Lipstick, push-up mechanism, 3 shades 52¢* **MP $15**
1934-38 *Lipstick (not shown) See 1935 Gift Sets B, F & W p. 102 52¢* **MP $15**

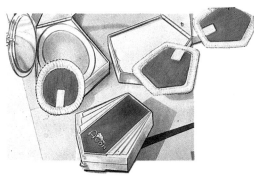

1931-32 *Double Fan Compact with Mirror, Powder and Rouge, refillable $1.50* **MP $50**

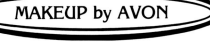

MAKEUP by AVON

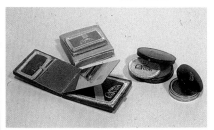

1933-36 *Double Compact with Mirror, Powder and Rouge $1.75* **MP $40**
1934 *Compact Rouge Refill 52¢* **MP $15**
1934-36 *Rouge Compact 52¢* **MP $30**
1930-36 *Cream Rouge 78¢* **MP $25**

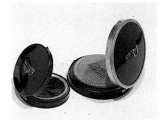

1931-33 *Eyelash Cream, Brown or Blue-Gray $1* **MP $30**
1934-36 *Rouge Compact 52¢* **MP $30**

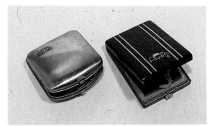

1930-32 *Double Compact $1.85* **MP $50**
1933-36 *Double Compact $1.75* **MP $40**

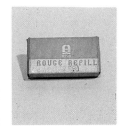

1936-42 *Rouge Refill 52¢* **MP $7**

*Available from Avon at time of publication

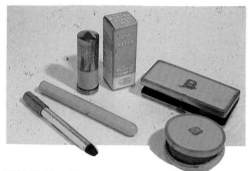

1936-41 *Lipstick 52¢* **MP $12, $15 boxed**
1936-41 *Mascara Compact, brown or black $1.04* **MP $18**
1940 *Eyebrow Pencil in brown or black, Metal Case 35¢* **MP $10**
1937-41 *Cream Rouge Compact 78¢* **MP $18**

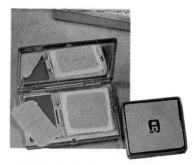

1936-41 *Double Compact for Loose Powder and Rouge $1.75* **MP $20**
1936-41 *Single Compact for Loose Powder $1.25* **MP $18**

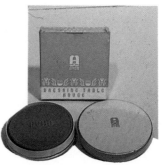

1936-41 *Dressing Table Rouge 47¢* **MP $10, $12 boxed**

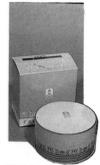

1936-41 *Face Powder, Ariel or Vernafleur 78¢* **MP $15, $20 boxed**

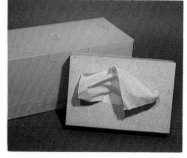

1937 *Facial Tissues, 360 per box 50¢* **MP $45**
1965 *Facial Tissues, issued with 1965 Manicure Tray* **MP $8**

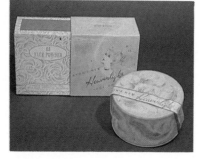

1946-49 *Heavenlight Face Powder, one texture 89¢* **MP $10** *(must say* **Heavenlight** *on packaging),* **$15 boxed, $20 with sleeve**

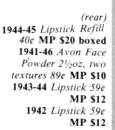

(rear) **1944-45** *Lipstick Refill 40¢* **MP $20 boxed**
1941-46 *Avon Face Powder 2½oz, two textures 89¢* **MP $10**
1943-44 *Lipstick 59¢* **MP $12**
1942 *Lipstick 59¢* **MP $12**

(front) **1943** *Mascara 69¢* **MP $20**
1941-47 *Dressing Table Rouge 47¢* **MP $10**
1943-45 *Rouge Compact, single feather 59¢* **MP $15**
1946-48 *Above Compact issued with Eye Shadow 79¢* **MP $15**

. . . . MAKEUP BY AVON

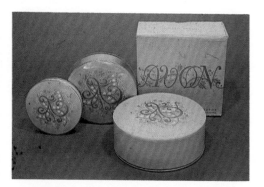

1949 *Dressing Table Rouge ½oz 59¢* **MP $6**
1949 *Powder-Pak 89¢* **MP $6**
1949 *Face Powder 2½oz 89¢* **MP $9**

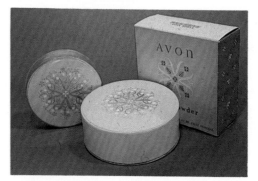

1955 *Powder-Pak 95¢* **MP $5**
1955 *Face Powder 2½oz 95¢* **MP $8, $10 boxed**

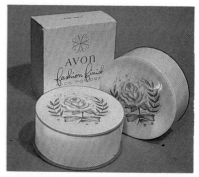

1960 *Fashion Finish Face Powder 2½oz $1.25* **MP $5, $7 boxed**
1958 *Sheer Mist Face Powder 2½oz $1.10* **MP $7**

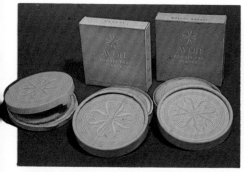

1954-56 *Powder-Pak Compact w/Mirror $1.10* **MP $6**
1954 *Powder-Pak Plaque 69¢* **MP $5, $7 boxed**
1958 *Powder-Pak Plaque 79¢* **MP $4, $6 boxed**

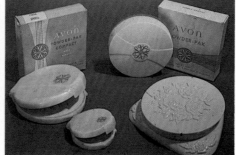

Compacts —
1957 *Powder-Pak $1.25* **MP $3, $5 boxed**
1957 *Dressing Table Powder-Pak .7oz 95¢* **MP $3, $5 boxed**
1959 *Cake or Cream Rouge w/Mirror $1* **MP $3**
1965 *Dressing Table Powder-Pak .7oz $1.25* **MP $4**

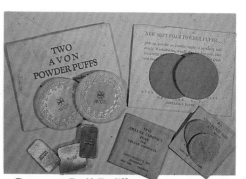

Compact Puff Refills —
1960's *Compact and Powder-Pak 2/20¢* **MP $2 each, $5 envelope of 2**
1960's *Foam 2/20¢* **MP $2, $5 envelope of 2**
1940's *For Double Compacts 2/5¢* **MP $3 each**
1950's *For Deluxe Compact 10¢ ea.* **MP $3 in env.**
1940's-50's *Rouge Compact 2/10¢* **MP $2, $5 in env.**

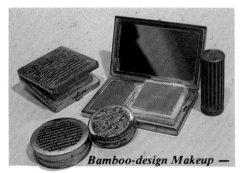

Bamboo-design Makeup —

1941-42, then 46-48 *Single Compact $1.25*
MP $20
1941-42, 1946-48 *Double Compact $1.75* **MP $26**
1942, 1946-48 *Lipstick 59¢* **MP $11**
1942, 1946-48 *Cake Rouge Compact 59¢* **MP $10**
1941-42, 1946-48 *Cream Rouge Compact 78¢*
MP $10

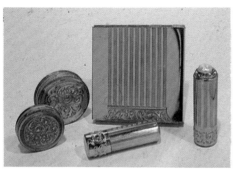

1949-57 *Cream Rouge Compact 69¢* **MP $6**
1949-57 *Cake Rouge Compact 79¢* **MP $6**
1949-57 *Deluxe Compact $3.50* **MP $13**
1954 *Jeweled Lipstick (right) 95¢* **MP $12**
1949-57 *Jewel-Etched Deluxe Lipstick (front)*
89¢ **MP $8**

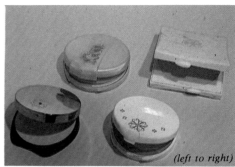

(left to right)

1962-63 *Powder-Pak Fashion Compact .5oz $2*
MP $6
1963 *Pink Pearl Compact .7oz $2.50* **MP $4**
1963 *Petti-Pat Compact, non refillable .5oz*
$1.10 **MP $5**
1965 *Fashion Award Compact (square) .7oz*
$1.75 **MP $6**

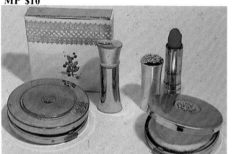

1958-61 *Top Style Compact .5oz $3.50* **MP $9,**
$11 boxed
1958-61 *Top Style Lipstick $1.50* **MP $8**
1961-65 *Compact Deluxe .5oz $3.50* **MP $7**
1961-65 *Lipstick Deluxe $1.35* **MP $6**

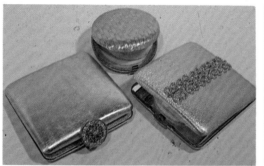

1965-67 *Imperial Jewel Compact .5oz $6* **MP $10**
1966 *Competite Compact .25oz $4.50* **MP $8**
1967 *Imperial Deluxe Compact .5oz $7* **MP $9**

COMPACTS and LIP MAKEUP

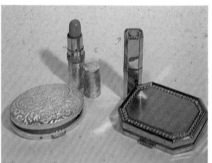

1967 *Deluxe Oval Compact .5oz $5.50* **MP $8**
1967 *Deluxe Lipstick $2* **MP $5**
1968 *Jeweled Lipstick, refillable $6* **MP $6**
1968 *Jeweled Compact .5oz $10* **MP $10**

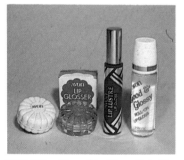

1973 *Ultra Sheer Lip Gloss Pot .10oz*
2 shades $2.25 **MP $1**
1973 *Lip Glosser .10oz $2* **MP $1**
1978 *Lip Lustre .30oz $3.50* **MP 50¢**
1978 *Good and Glossy Roll-On Lip*
Gloss .33oz in Natural, Mint & Straw-
berry flavors $3 **MP $1**

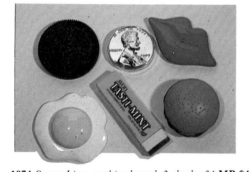

1974 *Sweet Lips, cookie shaped, 2 shades $4* **MP $4**
1976 *Lucky Penny .14oz, 2 shades $4* **MP $2**
1976 *Kiss 'N Makeup .20oz, 2 shades $4* **MP $2**
1978 *Sunnyshine Up .14oz, 2 shades $5* **MP $2**
1978 *Tasti-Mint .14oz, 2 shades $5* **MP $2**
1977 *Funburger .20oz, 2 shades $4.50* **MP $2**

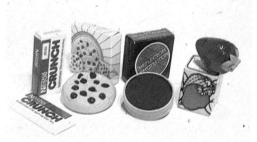

1980 *Nestle Crunch Lip Gloss Compact .14oz $5.50*
MP $1.50
1979 *Chocolate Chiplick Lip Gloss Compact .15oz*
$5.50 **MP $1.50**
1980 *Reflector Protector Lip Gloss Compact .14oz*
$6 **MP $1.50**
1979 *Berry Nice Lip Gloss Compact .14oz $5.50*
MP $1.50

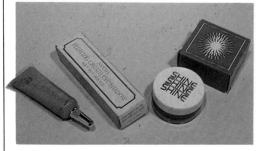

1970-75 *Flowing Cream Shadow .25oz $1.50* **MP 75¢,**
$1 boxed
1981 *Shine, Shine, Shine Lip Color, 6 shades .25oz*
$3.50 **MP 50¢ boxed**

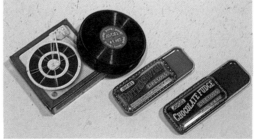

1981 *#1 Hit. Lip Gloss Compact .14oz $6.50* **MP $1**
1982 *Lip Toppings. Butterscotch or Chocolate Fudge*
2oz $2 **MP 50¢**

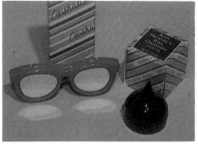

1983 *Lip Shades lip gloss, 2 shades .12 oz*
$6.50 **MP $1**
1983 *Hershey's Kiss. Chocolate lip gloss*
.15oz $4.50 **MP $1**

COMPACTS and LIP MAKEUP

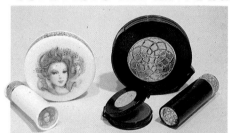

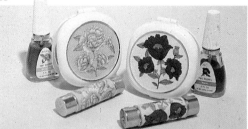

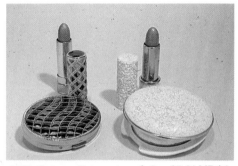

1965 *Fashion Cameo Lipstick 98¢* **MP $5**
1964 *Cameo Compact .5oz $2.50* **MP $6**
1967 *Fashion Compact .7oz $2.25* **MP $3**
1967 *Fashion Glace Compact, 8 fragrances,*
$2.50 & $3 **MP $3**
1967 *Fashion Lipstick $1.35* **MP $2**

1967-68 *Flower Prints Coordinates in flowered Fabric Cases—*
Lipsticks *and* **Nail Enamels** *issued in shades of Pink in Poppy design, Red in Daisy design, Mauve in Carnation design and Peach in Sunflower design. Compacts, issued in a choice of Flower design and Powder-Pak shade.*
—Compacts .5oz $2.50 **MP $5**   *—Lipsticks $1.50* **MP $4**   *—Nail Enamels .5oz $1.25 each* **MP $4**

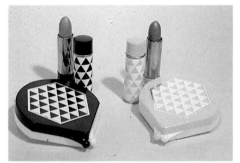

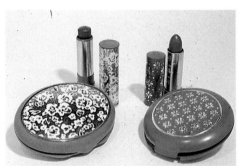

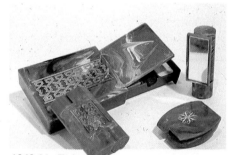

1969 *Gadabouts Compact .5oz in black and white or yellow and white checked pattern $2.50* **MP $5**
1969 *Gadabouts Lipstick, 6 shades in choice of patterned Case $1.50* **MP $4**

1968 *Festive Fancy Oval Compact .5oz $3* **MP $4**
1968 *Festive Fancy Lipstick, 6 shades $1.75* **MP $3**
1968 *Festive Fancy Demistik (not shown) in Rapture, Occur! or Unforgettable $2.50* **MP $3**
1968 *Encore Lipstick $1.25* **MP $2**
1969 *Encore Compact .5oz $2* **MP $3**

1969 *Empress Compact, oval .5oz $7.50* **MP $6**
1969 *Empress Lipstick $3* **MP $3**
1969 *Deluxe Compact "Carved Ivory" .5oz $4* **MP $4**
1969 *Deluxe Lipstick "Carved Ivory" Refillable $2.50* **MP $4**

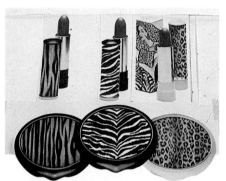

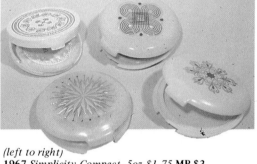

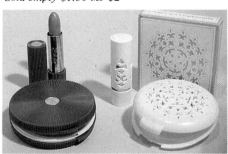

1969 *Captivator Lipsticks—$1.75 each* **MP $3** *each, $4 boxed*
Tiger with Jungle Red or Instant Mocha Zebra with Sultry Coral or Desert Dawn Leopard with Wild Amber or Persimmon
1969 *Captivator Compacts, Tiger, Zebra or Leopard design in choice of powder shades $3.50* **MP $4** *each, $5 boxed*

(left to right)
1967 *Simplicity Compact .5oz $1.75* **MP $3**
1971 *Simplicity Compact .5oz $2.75* **MP $4**
1973 *Designers Accent-in-Mauve Compact .5oz. Sold empty $1.50* **MP $2**
1973 *Designers Accent-in-Yellow Compact .5oz. Sold empty $1.50* **MP $2**

1969 *Lip Twins. Mirrored Case with 2 Lipsticks $4* **MP $5**
1969 *Blushmaker Compact. Highlighter, Blush .3oz each and 2" long Brush in mirrored Case with drawer. $5* **MP $6**
1974 *Looking Pretty Mirrored Lipstick, 4 shades $3* **MP $4**
1970 *Powder Shadow Duet .06oz $2.25* **MP $1**

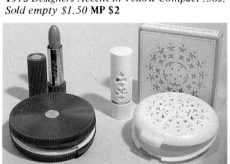

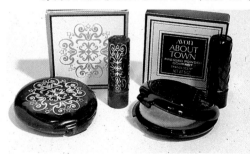

1969 *Enamel Fling in Mauvelous and Sunspin .5oz $1.25* **MP $3** *each*
1969 *Swing Fling Compact .5oz $3* **MP $4**
1969 *Ring Fling Lipstick in Jazzberry with pale and dark pink adjustable Ring. $3* **MP $9, $5 Ring only (see also p. 135)**

1971 *Encore Compact .5oz $3.50* **MP $3**
1971 *Encore Lipstick .13 oz $1.35* **MP $2**
1972 *Fashion Lace Compact .5oz $3.50* **MP $3**
1972 *Fashion Lace Lipstick .13oz $1.50* **MP $1**

1974 *About Town Compact .5oz $3.50* **MP $2, $3 boxed**
1974 *About Town Lipstick .13oz $1.50* **MP $1**
1976 *About Town Compact .5oz Translucent only $3.75* **MP $2**
*(**1977** Available in 7 shades $3.50 **MP $2**)*

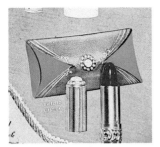

1956 *Jewelled Deluxe Lipstick in Christmas Wrap $1.50* **MP $18, $12 Lipstick only**

LIP MAKEUP

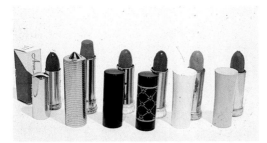

1954 *Fashion Lipstick 95¢* **MP $12, $17 boxed**
1956 *Long Life Lipstick $1.10* **MP $10**
(1958 *Above Lipstick called Satin Sheen $1.10* **MP $10**)
1956 *Fashion Lipstick 79¢* **MP $12**
1957 *Fashion Lipstick 79¢* **MP $12**
1957 *Fashion Lipstick 89¢* **MP $12**
1958 *Fashion Lipstick, honey beige cap 89¢* **MP $11**

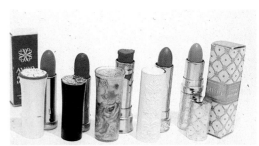

1960-61 *Fashion Lipstick 98¢* **MP $10, $13 boxed**
1962 *Fashion Lipstick 98¢* **MP $10**
1963 *Fashion Lipstick 98¢* **MP $9**
1966 *Ultra Sheer Lipstick $1.75* **MP $1**
1966 *Lipstick Refillable $2* **MP $8, $10 boxed**

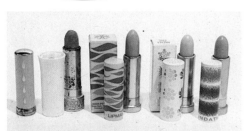

1962 *Lip Dew $1.25* **MP $3**
1966 *Lip Toner in Mocha, Plum and Lime $1.25* **MP $3**
1969 *Lipmaker in Warm Tone or Cool Tone $1.50* **MP $3, $5 boxed**
1969 *Lip Dew $1.50* **MP $2, $3 boxed**
1971 *Lip Foundation in Fair or Deep .15oz $1.50* **MP $1, $1.50 boxed**

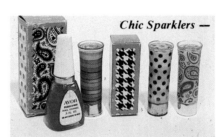

Chic Sparklers —

1966 *Nail Enamel in Yum Plum, Comin' Up Rose, Polk-A-Lily and Peach-A-Boo (shown) $1.25* **MP 4, $6 boxed**
1966 *Yum Plum Lipstick $1.25* **MP $4**
1966 *Peach-A-Boo Lipstick design shown on box $1.25* **MP $4, $6 boxed**
1966 *Polk-A-Lily Lipstick $1.25* **MP $4**
1966 *Comin' Up Rose Lipstick $1.25* **MP $4**

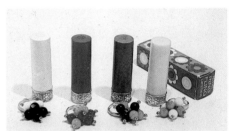

1969 *Ring Fling Lipsticks with Adjustable Ring $3 each* **MP $9, $5 Ring only, $12 boxed**
Glazed Copper with White & Black Ring
Iced Cantaloupe with Coral & Orange Ring
Iced Watermelon with Aqua & Navy Ring
Put-on Pink with Lime & Green Ring
Nectar (not shown) in yellow Case with Yellow & Orange Ring (see Jazzberry p. 134)

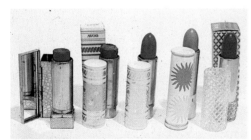

1967 *Applique Lipstick with snap-open Mirror $3.50* **MP $8**
1966-67 *Encore Lipstick, also used as refill $1.10* **MP $6, $8 boxed**
1967-68 *Encore Lipstick, also used as refill $1.10* **MP $6**
1970 *Sunseekers Lipstick in 4 shades $2* **MP $3**
1972 *Encore Lipstick $1.35* **MP $1**

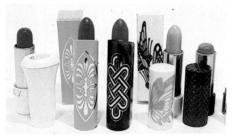

1971 *Lipstick a la Mode .13oz. Flip-open lid on top holds .02oz Perfume Glace in choice of 5 fragrances. Both refillable. $4.50* **MP $7**
1972 *Pop-Top Lipstick .13oz $2* **MP $3, $4 boxed**
1973 *Pop-Top Lipstick .13oz, 4 shades $2* **MP $2**
1974 *Color Magic Lipstick .13oz of blue or green turns to pink or peach on lips $2* **MP $4, $6 boxed**
1975 *Windsor Lipstick $2* **MP 50¢**

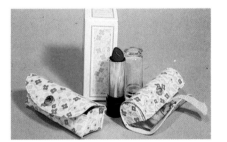

1978 *Colorcreme Lipstick $2.25* **MP $2.50***
1978 *Lipstick Case, with any Avon purchase C-16 only 99¢ (2 styles, round or square ends)* **MP $4**

*Available from Avon at time of publication

(See Patterns pg. 77; Petit Point pg. 191)

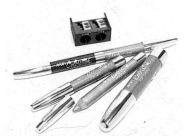

Colorsticks (top to bottom) —
1979 *Sharpener for Lip and Eye Lining $1.25* **MP $1**
1979 *Duo for Eyes .10oz $5* **MP $2**
1979 *Lip Lining .03oz $3* **MP $1.50**
1979 *Eye Lining .03oz $3* **MP $1.50**
1979 *Cheeks .15oz $4.50* **MP $1.50**

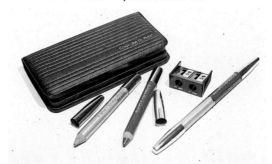

1981 *Colorcase by Avon. Mirrored vinyl case to hold 4 Colorsticks, with 2 Colorsticks purchase* **MP $4**
1982 *Colorstick for Eye Lining .03oz $3.50* **MP $1**
1982 *Colorstick for Lip Lining .03oz $3.50* **MP $1**
1982 *Colorstick Duo for Eyes .10oz $6* **MP $2**
1982 *Sharpener for Lip and Eye Lining $1.25* **MP $1**

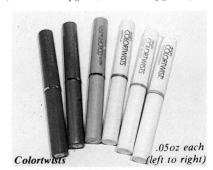

Colortwists .05oz each (left to right)
1981 *Lipstick $6* **MP $1**
1981 *Cheek Blush $6* **MP $1**
1981 *Eye Shadow $6* **MP $1**
1983 *Lipstick $6* **MP $4***
1983 *Cheek Blush $6* **MP $4***
1983 *Eye Shadow $6* **MP $4***

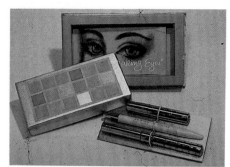
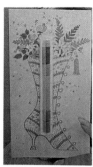
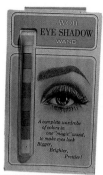
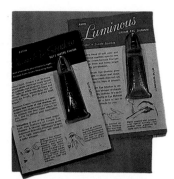

EYE MAKEUP BY AVON

1960 *Making Eyes. Curl 'n Color Mascara, Eyebrow Pencil and Eye Shadow Stick $3.95* **MP $20**

1965 *Eye Shadow Wand on Xmas Card $1.35* **MP $6 on card**

1964 *Eye Shadow Wand in plastic holder, 7 shades $1.35* **MP $2, $4 on card**

1963-66 *Cream Eye Shadow, 7 shades $1.25* **MP $2, $3 on card**
1963-66 *Luminous Cream Eye Shadow, 5 shades $1.25* **MP $2, $3 on card**

1959-63 *Curl 'n Color Mascara, 6 shades $2* **MP $4, $6 on card** *(below left)*

1962-66 *Eyebrow Pencil, 5 shades $1* **MP $2, $3 on card** *(below left)*

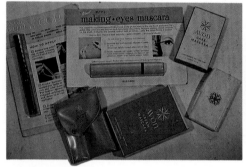
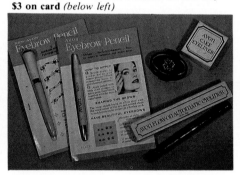
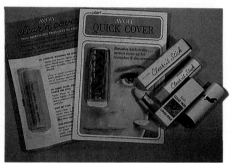

1963-70 *Making Eyes Mascara, 5 shades $1.35* **MP $1, $2 on card**
1959-66 *Cake Mascara with Brush, 2 shades $1* **MP $2, $4 boxed**
1959-66 *Cream Mascara with Brush in plastic case 69¢* **MP $4, $6 boxed**

1960-62 *Eyebrow Pencil, 4 shades $1* **MP $3, $5 on card**
1967-74 *Cake Eyeliner, 7 shades $1.50* **MP $1 boxed**
1972 *Flow-On Automatic Eyeliner, 4 shades $4.50* **MP $2 boxed**

1963-66 *Clear 'n' Cover Stick 89¢* **MP $3, $6 on card**
1968-73 *Quick Cover, 3 shades $1.50* **MP $3, $5 on card**
1959-63 *Clear-it Stick 89¢* **MP $5, $8 boxed**
1970-72 *Clear Skin Cover Stick $1.75* **MP $1, $2 boxed**

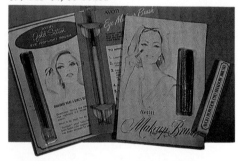
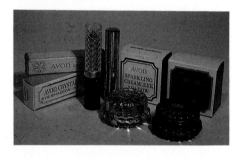
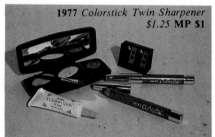

1965-66 *Gold Satin Eye Highlight Brush $1.50* **MP $5, $7 in plastic case on card**
1962-67 *Eye Makeup Brush $1* **MP $5 as shown**
1965-68 *Makeup Brush in gold Telescopic Case $2.25* **MP $7 on card, $5 brush only**

1970-75 *Crystal Shadows .07oz, 4 shades $2* **MP $1**
1957-66 *Eye Shadow Stick, 5 shades $1* **MP $4**
1968 *Sparkling Cream Eye Shadow, 4 shades $1.75* **MP $1 boxed**
1970 *Eye Gleam .06oz $1.50* **MP $1, $2 boxed**

1977 *Colorstick Twin Sharpener $1.25* **MP $1**
1972 *Certain Look Eye Shine $1.50* **MP 25¢**
1969 *Flatter Eyes Compact, 2 Eye Shadows, Eyeliner & Brush $4.50* **MP $1**
1977 *Colorstick for Lips .05oz, 7 shades $3.50* **MP $1.50**
1977 *Colorstick for Eyes .06oz, 7 shades $3.50* **MP $1.50**

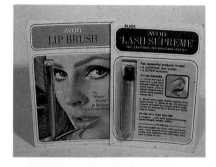
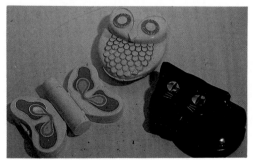
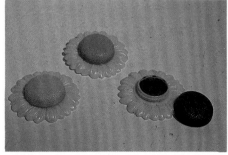

1959-65 *Lip Brush $1.50* **MP $4, $6 on card**
1966-72 *Lash Supreme refill $1.25* **MP $2, $3 on card**

1970 *Butterfly Collection. Lipstick and 4 Eye Shadows $7.50* **MP $7.50**
1972 *Owl Collection. Lip Gloss, Lip Conditioner and 3 Powder Eye Shadows $8* **MP $7**
1973 *Honey Cat Makeup Collection. Lip Gloss, Lip Conditioner, 4 Eye Shadows $8* **MP $7**

1980 *Blue-Eyed Susan, Green-Eyed Susan and Brown-Eyed Susan Eye Shadow Compacts .15oz $6* **MP $3**

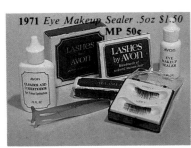

1969-75 Cleaner and Conditioner for False Eyelashes .75oz $1.50 **MP 50¢**
1969-73 Eyelash Applicator $1.50 **MP $1, $1.50 boxed**
1970 Natural Full Lashes $6.50 or Fluffy Lashes $7 and Adhesive **MP each $6, $7 boxed**
1969 Demi-Lashes and Adhesive $6 **MP $5, $6 boxed**

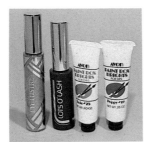

1980-81 Soft Powder Eye Lustre 5 shades .13oz $4.50 **MP 50¢**
1980 Lots O'Lash Mascara 2 shades .33oz $4 **MP $3.50***
1980 Paint Box Brights for Eyes 3 shades .30oz $2 **MP 50¢**
1980 Paint Box Brights for Lips 3 shades .25oz $2 **MP 50¢**

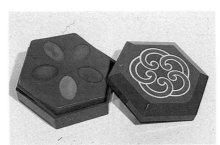

1980-81 Sensational Eyes Collection. Five eye shadows in reusable container .15oz $11 **MP $7**

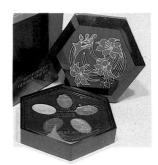

1982 China Fantasy Collection. Five eye shadows in reusable container, 2 campaigns only .15oz $9 **MP $4**

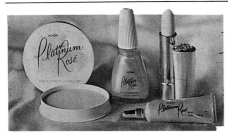

1963-66 Platinum Rose — Complexion Highlight .07 oz $1.35 **MP $**
Fingertip Highlight .5oz $1.35 **MP $4**
Lip Highlight $1.35 **MP $7**
Eye Highlight $1.35 **MP $4**

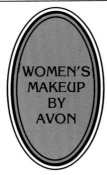

WOMEN'S MAKEUP BY AVON

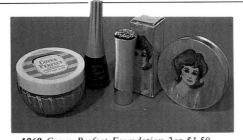

1969 Cover Perfect Foundation 2oz $1.50 **MP $1**
1969 Liquid Eyeliner 1/4oz $2 **MP $1**
1965 Gold Satin Lip Highlight $1.75 **MP $7, $9 boxed**
1965 Gold Satin Complexion Highlight .8oz $1.75 **MP $5**

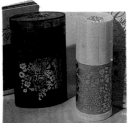

1971 Go Togethers. Foundation Stick 1/2oz and Blush Stick .3oz $6 **MP $3**
1972 Creme Stick Foundation .85oz $3.50 **MP $2**

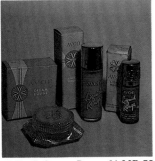

1961-67 Cream Rouge $1 **MP 75¢, $1 boxed**
1959-66 Liquid Rouge 2 dram 89¢ **MP $3, $5 boxed**
1956-59 Liquid Rouge No. 1 thru No. 5 1/4oz 69¢ **MP $5, $8 boxed**

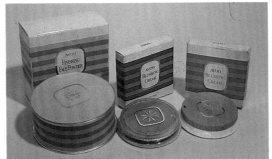

1967-69 Finishing Face Powder 2.5oz $1.50 **MP $4, $6 boxed**
1968-70 Blushing Cream 3 shades 1/4oz $2 **MP $4, $6 boxed**
1970-75 Blushing Cream 3 shades 1/4oz $1.50 **MP $1, $2 boxed**

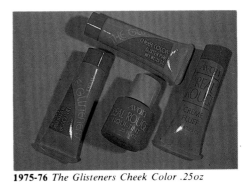

1975-76 The Glisteners Cheek Color .25oz Coral or Pink $1.75 **MP 50¢**
1975-76 The Glisteners Lip Color .25oz Coral or Pink $1.75 **MP 50¢**
1976 Real Rouge Liqui-Tint .25oz $2 **MP 25¢**
1976 Real Rouge Creme Fluff .25oz $2.50 **MP 25¢**

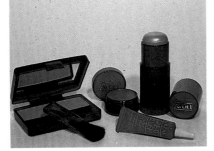

Great Blush —
1976-79 Powder Compact .40oz & Brush, 4 shades $4.50 **MP $2**
1978-79 Creme Cheek Pot .25oz $3 **MP 50¢**
1976-78 Soft Creme 3 shades .25oz $2.50 **MP 50¢**
1976-79 Frost Stick .85oz $4.50 **MP 50¢**

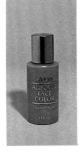

1979-80 All-Over Face Color 1oz $3.50 **MP $1**

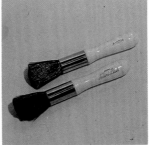

1965 only Makeup Brush (top) $2 **MP $8**
1965 only Brush for Natural Blush $2 **MP $10**

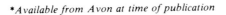

Available from Avon at time of publication

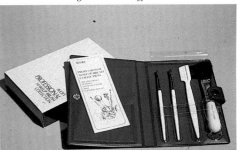

1980 Professional Makeup Collection. Vinyl Kit and instruction booklet $15 **MP $20** Holds: (see below)
1981 Lip Brush $4 **MP $4***
1981 Eye Shadow Brush $4 **MP $4***
1981 Brow/Lash Brush $4 **MP $4***
1981 Blush Brush $6.50 **MP $5***

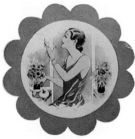

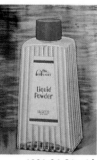

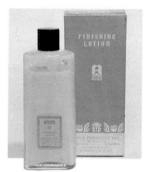

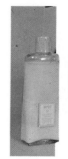

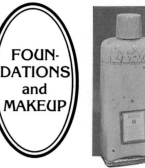

Tinted lotion, specially designed for the oily skin, was Liquid Powder in the 1930's, renamed Finishing Lotion in the 1940's and then Foundation Lotion in the 1950's.

1931-36 *Liquid Powder 4oz $1* **MP $60**

1944 *Finishing Lotion 2oz 59¢* **MP $20 with black lid, $26 boxed**

1938-50 *Finishing Lotion 2oz 52¢* **MP $15**

FOUN-DATIONS and MAKEUP

1950-52 *Foundation Lotion 2oz 59¢* **MP $24**

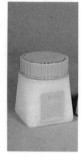

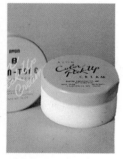

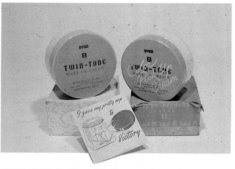

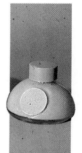

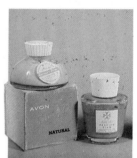

1943-46 *Twin-Tone Makeup 1⅞oz 89¢* **MP $12**

1946-52 *Color Pick-Up Cream 1⅞oz 89¢* **MP $10**
1952-53 *As above except smaller size 1oz 75¢* **MP $15**

1944-45 *Twin-Tone Makeup with wartime cardboard lid 89¢* **MP $20**
1946 *Color Pick-Up Cream stamped over Twin-Tone Makeup lid, issued during name change period* **MP $14 as shown**

1946-48 *Color Pick-Up Liquid 1oz 59¢* **MP $10**

1952-53 *Fashion Film Liquid 1oz 75¢* **MP $9, $12 boxed**
1954-58 *Fashion Film Liquid 1oz 95¢* **MP $8**

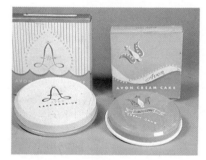

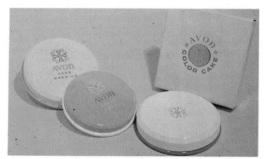

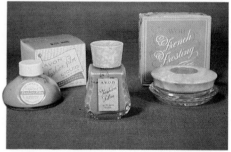

1946-54 *Cake Make-Up, 5 shades 1¾oz $1.25* **MP $5, $8 boxed**
1948-54 *Cream Cake, 6 shades .6oz 89¢* **MP $5, $8 boxed**

1954-56 *Cake Make-Up, 8 shades 1¾oz $1* **MP $6**
1954-56 *Cream Cake, 8 shades .6oz 95¢* **MP $6**
1961-65 *Color Cake 2oz $1.25* **MP $4, $5 boxed**

1953-54 *Fashion Film 1oz 75¢ (smooth lid)* **MP $9, $12 boxed**
1958-61 *Fashion Film 1oz $1.10* **MP $8**
1957-64 *French Frosting 1oz $1.25* **MP $7**

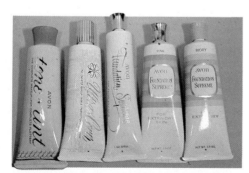

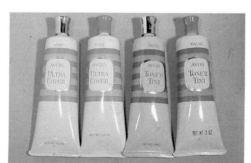

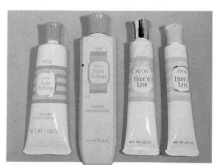

1963-67 *Tone 'N' Tint 2oz, 10 shades $1.35* **MP $3**
1965-67 *Ultra Cover, 11 shades 2oz $1.35* **MP $3**
1965-67 *Foundation Supreme, 11 shades 1½oz $1.35* **MP $3**
1967 only *Foundation Supreme* **(gold lid)** *8 shades 1.9oz $1.50* **MP $5**
1967-68 *Foundation Supreme, 8 shades 1.9oz $1.50* **MP $3**

1967 only *Ultra Cover, 8 shades 2.1oz $1.75* **MP $5 with gold lid**
1967-69 *Ultra Cover, 8 shades 2.1oz $1.75* **MP $2**
1967 only *Tone 'N' Tint, 8 shades 2oz $1.50* **MP $5 with gold lid**
1967-76 *Tone 'N' Tint, 8 shades 2oz $1.50* **MP 50¢**

1970-73 *Satin Supreme, 8 shades 1½oz $1.50* **MP $1**
1968-70 *Satin Supreme 1⅛oz $1.50* **MP $1.50**
1966-68 *Hide 'N' Lite .75oz $1.50* **MP $3 with gold lid**
1968-69 *Hide 'N' Lite .75oz $1.50* **MP $2**

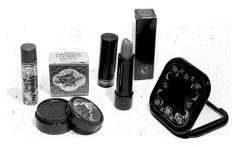

1982 Oriental Classics DemiStik, Sweet Honesty .15 oz $3 MP 50¢
1982 Oriental Classics Lip Gloss .25oz $3 MP 50¢
1982 Elegant Touches Lipstick $3.50 MP 50¢
1982 Elegant Touches Double Mirror Compact $7.50 MP $3

MAKEUP LINES

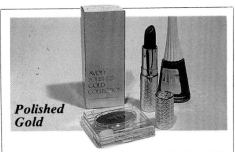

Polished Gold

1978 Creamy Eye Shadow .12oz, 2 shades $3 MP $1.50
1978 Lipstick .13oz 3 shades $4 MP $1.50
1978 Nail Enamel .5oz 3 shades $2.25 MP $1.50   (See Evening Bag p. 118)

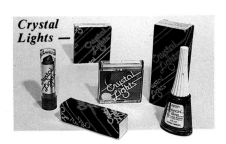

Crystal Lights —

1979 Moisture Lipstick, 3 shades .13oz $3 MP $1, $1.50 boxed
1979 Eye Shadow, 4 shades .10oz $4 MP $1, $1.50 boxed
1979 Pearl Nail Enamel, 3 shades .5oz $2.50 MP $1, $1.50 boxed

Eventone

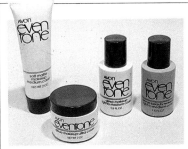
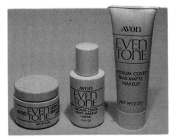
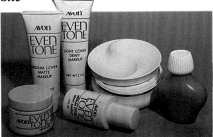
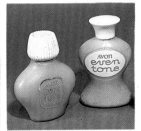

1982 Medium Cover Soft Matte 2oz $3 MP 50¢
1982 Ultra Cover Dewy 2oz $3.50 MP 50¢
1982 Light to Medium Cover Dewy 1.5oz $3 MP 50¢
1982 Bronze Beauty 1.5oz $3 MP 50¢

1978 Ultra Cover Dewy 2oz $2.75 MP 50¢
1978 Medium Cover Dewy 1.5oz $2.25 MP 50¢
1978 Medium Cover Semi-Matte 2oz $2.25 MP 50¢

1976 Ultra Cover Dewy or Matte 2oz $2.75 MP 50¢ each
1976 Medium Cover Matte 2oz $2.25 MP 50¢
1976 Light Cover Dewy 2oz $2.25 MP 50¢
1976 Fin. Face Powder & Puff 1.5oz $3 MP $1
1976 Medium Cover Dewy 1.5oz $2.25 MP 50¢
1970 Liquid Foundation 1.5oz $1.50 MP 50¢

1966-70 Foundation 1½oz $1.50 MP $1
1962-66 Foundation 1½oz $1.35 MP $1
(1961 not shown, as above, with gold lid $1.35 MP $4)

Beautiful Reflections

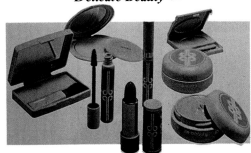

1980 Reflective Nail Glaze, 2 shades .5oz $3 MP $1
1980 Reflective Lipstick .13oz $3.50 MP $1
1980 Soft Reflections Body Glow, 2 shades 1½oz $6.50 MP $1
1980 Dazzle Dust Highlighting Powder, 3 shades .05oz $6.50 MP $1

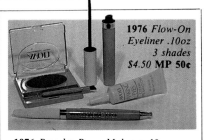

1976 Flow-On Eyeliner .10oz 3 shades $4.50 MP 50¢

1976 Powder Brow Makeup .10oz 3 shades $3 MP 75¢
1976 Cream Eye Shadow .25oz 5 shades $2 MP 50¢
1976 Brow & Liner Pencil, 3 shades $2.50 MP 50¢

Ultra Sheer —

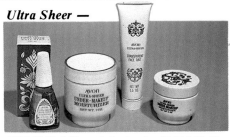

1967-68 Nail Tints, 3 shades .5oz $1.50 MP $3
(1968-74 Nain Tints, not shown, new issue with gold lid MP 50¢)

1968-74 Nail Tints, not shown, new issue with gold lid MP 50¢
1969-74 Under-Makeup Moisturizer, 3 shades 2oz $3.50 MP 75¢
1971-74 Transparent Face Tint, 4 shades 1.5oz $2.50 MP 50¢
1974-76 Under-Makeup Moisturizer, 3 shades 2oz $3.50 MP $1

Delicate Beauty —

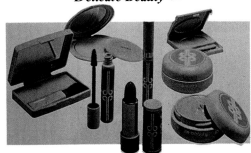

1976 Blush Compact .4oz $5 MP 50¢
1974 Pressed Powder Compact ½oz $3.50 MP $1
1976 Powder Eye Shadow .1oz $3.50 MP 50¢
1975 Automatic Mascara .15oz $3.50 MP 50¢
1975 Automatic Eyeliner .1oz $5 MP 50¢
1974 Under-Makeup Moisturizer 2oz $5 MP 50¢
1974 Lipstick .13oz $2.25 MP 25¢
1974 Cream Foundation 2oz $5 MP 50¢
1975 Powder Shadow Duet (not shown) $3.50 MP $1
1977 Liquid Makeup (not shown) 2oz $5 MP 75¢

Making Eyes

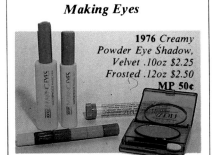

1976 Creamy Powder Eye Shadow, Velvet .10oz $2.25 Frosted .12oz $2.50 MP 50¢

1977 Waterproof Mascara .43oz 2 shades $2.75 MP $2
(1976 Waterproof Mascara .12oz not shown $2.50 MP $2)
1978 Waterproof Mascara .20oz 2 shades $2.75 MP 50¢
1976 Frosted or Velvet Eye Shadow Wand 5 colors .05oz ea. $2.75 MP 75¢

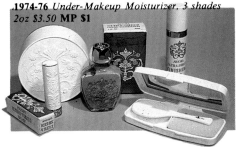

1966-75 Lipstick $1.75 MP 25¢
1966-75 Face Powder 1 shade 1¾oz $2.50 MP $1
1966-75 Natural Veil 2 shades 1oz $2.25 MP 50¢
1967-74 Finishing Glo ¾oz $2.50 MP 50¢
1966-74 Pressed Powder with Puff .5oz $3 MP $2
(See Lip Gloss Pot, p. 133)

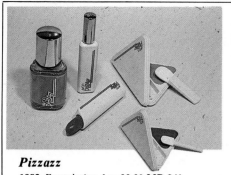

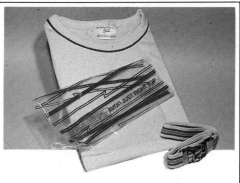

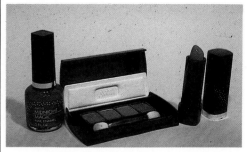

Pizzazz
1982 *Foundation 1oz $5.50* **MP $4***
1982 *Mascara .25oz $4.50* **MP $3***
1982 *Lip Tint .13oz $4.50* **MP $3***
1982 *Blush .25oz $5.50* **MP $4***
1982 *Eye Shadow .75oz $4.50* **MP $3***

1982 *"Just Right" Top $3.99 with purchase* **MP $10**
1982 *"Just Right" Belt, free with purchase* **MP $5**

Midnight Magic
1983 *Nail Enamel, 4 shades .4oz $4* **MP 50¢**
1983 *Eye Shadows Case $9* **MP $2**
1983 *Lipstick, 4 shades .13oz $5* **MP 50¢**

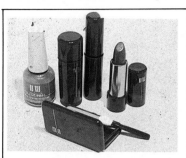

Ultra Wear
1982 *Nail Enamel .5oz $4* **MP $2***
1983 *Blush Stick .25oz $6* **MP $4***
1983 *Mascara .33oz $5* **MP $3***
1983 *Lipstick .13oz $4* **MP $2***
1982 *Eye Shadow .10oz $5* **MP $3***

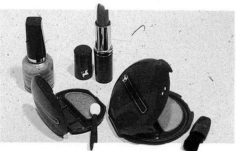

Opulent Collection
(2 campaigns only)
1981 *Nail Enamel, 3 shades .5oz $3.50* **MP $1**
1981 *Lipstick, 3 shades .13oz $4.50* **MP $1**
1981 *Eye Shadow, 3 shades .10oz $5.50* **MP $1**
1981 *Powder Blush .25oz $6* **MP $1**

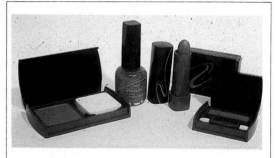

Versatilities
1983 *Powder Blush .15oz $7* **MP $5***
1983 *Nail Color .5oz $3.50* **MP $2***
1983 *Lip Color .10oz $5* **MP $3.50***
1983 *Eye Shadow .06oz $5* **MP $3.50***

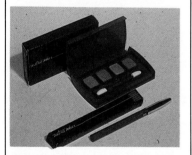

1983 *Eye Shadow Boutique .12oz $8*
MP $5*
1983 *Eyelining Pencil .03 oz $3.50*
MP $2*

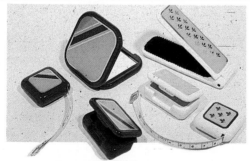

Purse Portables
1981 *Tape Measure $6* **MP $5**
1981 *Double Mirror Compact $7* **MP $6**
1981 *Pill Box $5* **MP $4**
1982 *Pill Box $5* **MP $4**
1982 *Lint Brush $6* **MP $5**
1982 *Tape Measure $6* **MP $5**

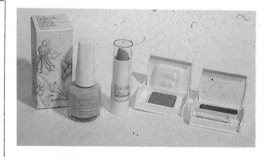

Delicate Pales
1984 *Nail Enamel .5oz $3.50* **MP 50¢**
1984 *Lipstick .13oz $3.50* **MP 25¢**
1984 *Powder Blush .06oz $5.50* **MP 50¢**
1984 *Eye Shadow .06oz $4.50* **MP 50¢**

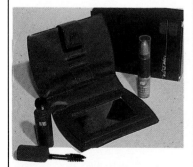

1984 *Trial-size Mascara .10oz 49¢*
MP 50¢
1983 *Case for Eyes to carry Mascara,
Eyelining Pencil & Eyeshadow, with
product purchase, 1 campaign only*
MP $5
1983 *Lip 'N Nail Duo. Matched
Lipstick and Nail Enamel, 2 campaigns
only $5* **MP $2**

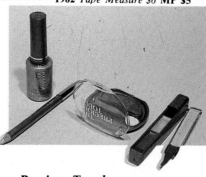

Precious Touch
1982 *Nail Enamel .5oz $3.50* **MP $1**
1982 *Eye Lining Colorstick .04oz $3.50*
MP 50¢
1982 *Eye Shadow .10oz $5* **MP $1**
1982 *Brush-On Lip Duo .08oz $6* **MP $1**

Available from Avon at time of publication

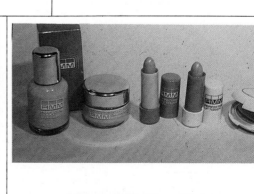

Advanced Moisture Makeup
1984 *Liquid Makeup 1oz $5.50* **MP $4***
1984 *Creme Makeup 1oz $5.50* **MP $4***
1984 *Concealing Stick .13oz $4.50* **MP $3***
1984 *Lip Toner .13oz $4.50* **MP $3***
1984 *Pressed Face Powder .5oz $6.50* **MP $5***

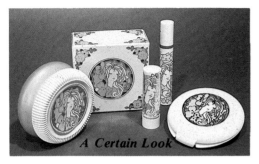

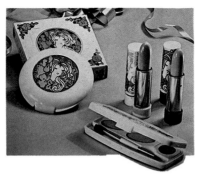

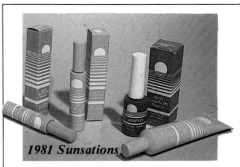

1972-75 Dew Glow $\frac{1}{4}$oz $3.50 **MP $3,**
$3.50 boxed
1970-74 Lipstick .13oz $1.50 **MP $1.50**
1972-75 Lash-Long Mascara .15oz $2 **MP $1**
1970-74 Blushpetite and Brush .19oz $3 **MP $2**
(See Eye Shine pg. 136)

1970-74 Blushpetite .19oz $3 **MP $3 boxed**
1970-74 Lipstick $1.50 **MP $1.50**
1970-74 Lip Beamer .13oz $1.50 **MP $1.50**
1970-74 Shadow and Liner Trio. Cake
Eyeliner .02oz, 2 Eye Shadows .08oz and
double-tipped Brush $4.50 **MP $3**

Sun Sheer Eye Shadow .20oz $5 **MP $1**
Sun Sheer Lip Gloss .25oz $5 **MP $1**
Sun Sheer Nail Enamel .5oz $3.50 **MP $1**
Sun Sheer Face Color 1.5oz $4 **MP $1**

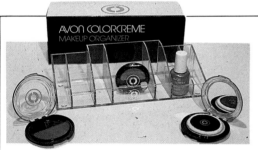

1977 Colorworks —

Oil-Free Makeup 1.5oz $3 **MP 50¢**
Supershine Lip Gloss .15oz $2.50 **MP 50¢**
Oil-Free Cheekblush .20oz $3 **MP 50¢**
Lasting Color Eye Shadow .15oz $2.50
MP 50¢
Lashes, Lashes Mascara .25oz $2.75 **MP 50¢**
1978 Oil-Absorbing Pressed Powder Compact
.5oz $3.75 **MP $1**
1977 Canvas Bag. Free with purchase **MP $12**

(See Candid, Patterns & Sweet Honesty in Fragrance Line section)

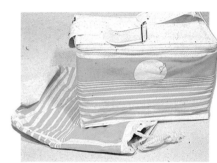

1981 Summertime Cooler 10½x7½x6½",
1 campaign only, $2.99 with purchase
MP $5
1981 Convertible Pillow/Tote, free with
Sunsations purchase **MP $5**

1980 Colorcreme

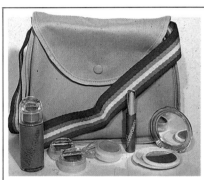

Makeup Organizer 10x3½" with purchase, U.S. only
$3.99 **MP $6**
Creamy Powder Blush .25oz and Brush $5 **MP $1**
Creamy Powder Eye Shadow .10oz $4 **MP $1**
All-Over Face Color 1oz $3.50 **MP 50¢**
Colorsetter Powder Compact .5oz $5 **MP $1**

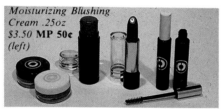

Moisturizing Blushing
Cream .25oz
$3.50 **MP 50¢**
(left)

Cream Eye Shadow .25oz $3.50 **MP 50¢**
Blush-Up Stick .25oz $5 **MP 50¢**
Moisture Lipstick .13oz $2.50 **MP 50¢**
Waterproof Mascara .20oz $3.50 with silver
lid **MP 50¢**
Waterproof Mascara .20oz $3.50 (white lid)
MP 50¢

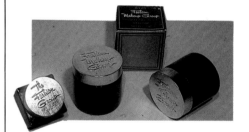

1971 Hi-Lite Cream .5oz $2.50 **MP $1**
1975-81 Cremelucent Foundation 2oz $5
MP $1, $1.50 boxed
1977-80 Under-Makeup Moisturizer 2oz $5
MP $1.50, $2 boxed

Fashion Makeup Group

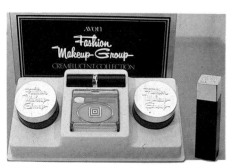

1977 Cremelucent Collection $16 **MP $20 set**
Under-Makeup Moisturizer 2oz $5 **MP $1.50**
Cremelucent Lipstick .13oz $2.50 **MP 50¢**
Powder Eye Shadow .10oz $3.50 **MP 75¢**
Cremelucent Foundation 2oz $5 **MP $1**
1971 Blushing Stick .75oz $4 **MP $1**

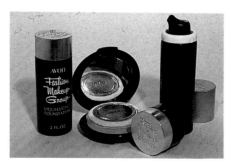

1975 Liqui-lucent Foundation 2oz 1 shade $4
MP $1
1976 Pressed Powder Compact 5oz, Translucent
$5.50 **MP $1**
1978 Cremelucent Moisture Blush 5oz $3.75 **MP $1**
1971 Under-Makeup Moisture Veil 2oz Aerosol $5
MP $1

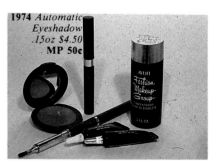

1974 Automatic
Eyeshadow
.15oz $4.50
MP 50¢

1975 Creamy Rouge Compact .20oz $4 **MP $1**
1971 Brushstick for Lips .05oz $4.50 **MP $1**
1975 Eye Color Creme .25oz (white cap)
$2.50 **MP 25¢**
1973 Eye Color Creme .25oz (gold cap)
$2.50 **MP $1**
1973 Moisture Droplets 2oz $4 **MP 50¢**

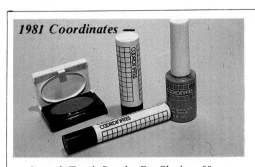

1981 Coordinates —
Smooth Touch Powder Eye Shadow .08oz
$4.50 **MP 75¢**
Full Color Lipstick .13oz $3 **MP 50¢**
Quick Dry Nail Enamel .5oz $2.50 **MP 50¢**
Roll-On Lash Color .15oz $3.50 **MP 50¢**

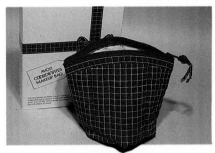

1982 Coordinates Makeup Bag $1.99 with
purchase **MP $6, $6.50 boxed**

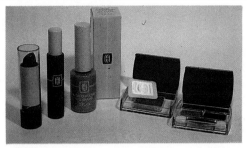

1983 Coordinates —
Lipstick .13oz $3.50 **MP $2***
Mascara .15oz $4 **MP $2***
Nail Enamel .5oz $3.50 **MP $2***
Powder Blush .06oz $5.50 **MP $3***
Highlight 'N Shadow Powders .06oz $5.50 **MP $3.50***

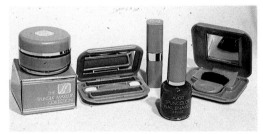

Spunsilks —
1980 *Spunfinish Cream Makeup 1oz $6.50* **MP $1**
1980 *Spunpowder Eye Shadow Duo .20oz $8* **MP $1**
1980 *Spuncolor Lipstick .13oz $4.50* **MP 75¢**
1980 *Spuncolor Nail Enamel .5oz $4* **MP 75¢**
1980 *Spuncolor Blush .20oz $8* **MP $1**

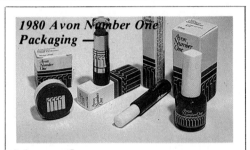

1980 Avon Number One
Packaging —
Colorcreme Cream
Eyeshadow .25oz $4.50 **MP $3, $4 boxed**
Colorcreme Lipstick .13oz $3.50 **MP $2, $3 boxed**
Colorcreme Mascara .20oz $4 **MP $2, $3 boxed**
Ultra Wear Nail Enamel .25oz $2.75 **MP $2,**
$3 boxed

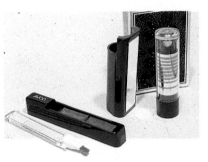

1982 Colorcreme Brush-On Lip Duo .08oz
$6 **MP $1**
1981 Beautiful Images. Mirrored
Colorcreme Lipstick .13oz $7 **MP $2**

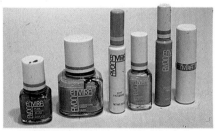

1979 Envira —
Pure Color Blush .33oz $4 **MP 50¢**
Conditioning Makeup 1oz $4 **MP 50¢**
Soft Eye Definer .25oz $4.50 **MP 50¢**
Gentle Eye Color .25oz $4 **MP 50¢**
Conditioning Mascara .25oz $4 **MP 50¢**
Pure Color Lipstick .13oz $2.75 **MP 50¢**

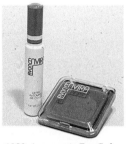

1982 Automatic Eye Color
.25oz $5 **MP $3.50***
1982 Cream Blush .15oz
$4 **MP $3***

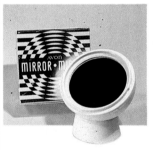

1971 Mirror, Mirror
$3.50 **MP $5,**
$7 boxed

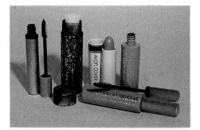

1973 Lash Supreme .15oz $2 **MP $1**
1971 Shine Down Stick .6oz $2.50 **MP $4**
1977 Cover-All Concealing Stick $3.25
MP 25¢
1978 Lash Supreme .25oz $2.75 **MP 25¢**
1977 Lash Supreme .5oz $2.75 **MP $1**

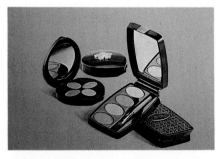

1969 Sparkling Cream Shadow Collection
$3.50 **MP $10**
1967 Silvery Powder Shadow Collection
$5 **MP $12**

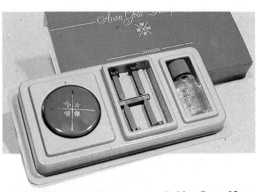

1982 Gold Stamps Kit. 4 stamps, Golden Dust .05oz
and Gentle Fixative .2oz $7 **MP $6 complete**

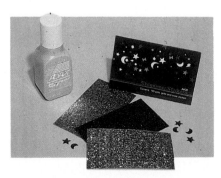

1983 Adapt Makeup 1.5oz $6 **MP $4***
1983 Shimmer Stickers. 189 decals in pink,
gold & silver $3.50 **MP $2 complete**

*Available from Avon at time of publication

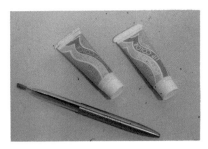

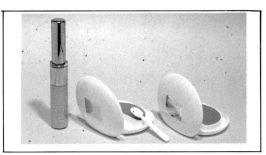

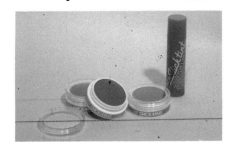

1966-74 *Lip Brush $1.75* **MP $3**
1973-76 *Softshine Lip Color .2oz*
$1.50 **MP 75¢**

Accolade —
1982 *Concealing Cream .33oz $5* **MP $4***
1982 *Eye Shadow .10oz $5* **MP $4***
1982 *Blush .22oz $5* **MP $4***

1983 *Stack 'M MS. Lip, Eye and Cheek*
stackable pots .06oz each $3.50 each **MP 25¢**
1983 *Slick Tint .15oz $3* **MP $2***

. . . WOMEN'S MAKEUP

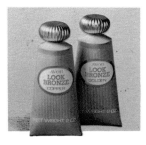

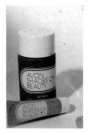

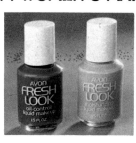

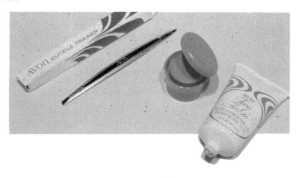

1969 *Look Bronze in*
Copper or Golden 2oz
$2.50 **MP 75¢**

1975 *Shades of*
Beauty Liquid
Foundation
1.5oz $2 **MP 50¢**
1975 *Shades of*
Beauty Creamy Blush
.25oz $2 **MP 25¢**

1979-82 *Fresh Look Makeup,*
Oil-control 1.5oz or
Moisturizing $2.50 **MP 50¢**

1970 *Cuticle Trainer $1.50* **MP $2.50, $3 boxed**
1975 only *Two-To-Go. Blusher .10oz and Foundation 1oz*
$4 **MP $3**

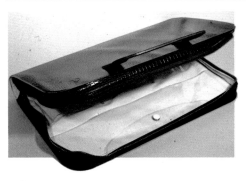

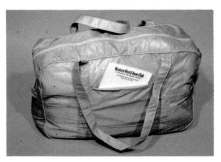

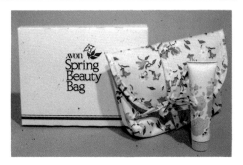

1976 *Sunny Griffin Makeup Case. First a Sales*
Prize and then sold to Representatives **MP $13**
with Award Certificate, $8 without

1980 *Sportin' Tote. Nylon bag with $5*
purchase in C-17 only $6.99 **MP $8.50**

1981 *Spring Beauty Bag, 7¼x5"*
fabric with $8.50 purchase in C-6 only. Take-
Along Hand Cream inc. free $1.99 **MP $6,**
$7 boxed (U.S. only)

COSMETIC BAGS and SKIN CARE LINES BY AVON

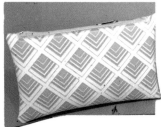

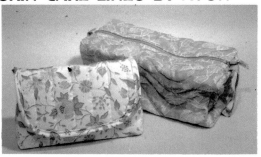

Tracy —

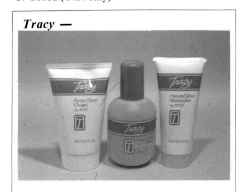

1977 *Zippered Cosmetic Case $1 with*
specified purchase. Designed
exclusively for Avon, the Deco-inspired vinyl case is
approximately 8x5". Included, a pamphlet of makeup
tips from Sunny Griffin on how to make yourself
more beautiful. One campaign only. Retail value over
$3 **MP $5**

1983 *Country Flowers Beauty Bag. 7x4½"*
$2.99 with purchase **MP $8**
1984 *Victorian Rose Traveler 9x4x4" with*
$10 purchase or $2.99 with $5 purchase in
C-6 only **MP $9**

1981 *Deep Clean Cream 4oz $4* **MP $1**
1981 *Twice-A-Day Lotion 6oz $4* **MP $1**
1981 *Moisturizer 3oz $4* **MP $1**

*Available from Avon at time of publication

Perfect Balance, Dry Skin —

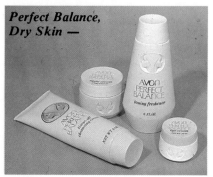

1974 *Tissue-Off Cleansing Cream 4oz $3* **MP 50¢**
1974 *Night Cream 2½oz $4* **MP 50¢**
1974 *Toning Freshener 6oz $3* **MP 50¢**
1974 *Eye Cream ¾oz $3.50* **MP 50¢**

Perfect Balance, Oily Skin —

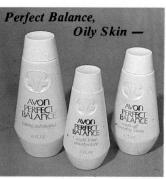

1974 *Toning Astringent 6oz $3* **MP 50¢**
1974 *Night Time Moisturizer 3oz $4* **MP 50¢**
1974 *Wash-Off Cleansing Lotion 4oz $3*
MP 50¢

SKIN CARE LINES

Summer Dew —

1973 *Moisturizing Body Fluff 4oz $5*
MP $4.50
1973 *Moisturizing Body Creme 5oz $5*
MP $4.50

DEW KISS

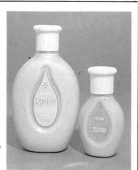

1975 *Dew Kiss 5oz $4.50* **MP $1**

1972 *Dew Kiss 1.5oz $1.50* **MP 50¢**

1966 *Dew Kiss (left) 1½oz $1.25* **MP $3**
(1967 *As above, 3½oz $2.50* **MP $3**)
1960 *Dew Kiss 1½oz $1.25* **MP $5 with Tag**

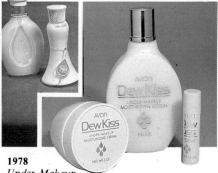

1978
Under-Makeup Moisturizing Cream 3oz $3.50 **MP 50¢**
1978 *Under-Makeup Moisturizing Lotion 5oz (shown) $4.50* **MP 50¢**,
1.5oz $2 **MP $1**, *3.5oz $3.50* **MP $1**
1978 *Lip Dew .15oz $1.75* **MP 50¢**

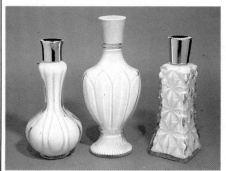

1973 *Vanity Decanter 4oz $4* **MP $5**
1974 *Vanity Decanter 4oz $5* **MP $4**
1974 *Vanity Decanter 4oz $5* **MP $3**

Prima Natura —

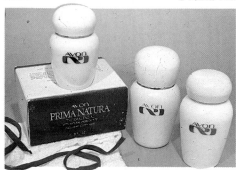

1971 *Thermal Facial and Mask 3oz $6.50*
MP $7 complete
1971 *Cleansing Formula 4oz $5.50* **MP $6**
1971 *Moisturizing Freshener 4oz $3.50* **MP $6**

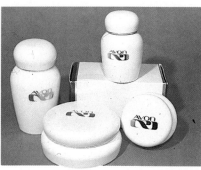

1971 *Toning Freshener 4oz $3.50* **MP $6**
1971 *Creme of Soap 5oz $4.50* **MP $7**
1971 *Night Veil Concentrate 2½oz $6*
MP $6
1971 *Eye Cream Concentrate ¾oz $4* **MP $6**

Delicate Beauty

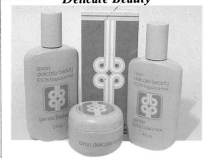

1976 *Gentle Freshener 5oz $4* **MP 50¢**
1976 *Whipped Nightcreme 3oz $5* **MP 50¢**
1976 *Lotion Cleanser 4oz $4* **MP 50¢**

Skinplicity

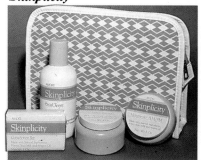

1978 *Tote Bag. Free with purchase of 3 Skinplicity items in C-12* **MP $7**
1978 *Complexion Bar 3oz $1.50* **MP $1.50**
1978 *Facial Toner 6oz $3* **MP 50¢**
1978 *Cream Cleanser 4oz $3* **MP 50¢**
1978 *Moisturizer AM/PM 3oz $4* **MP 50¢**

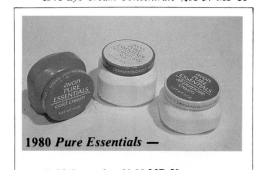

1980 Pure Essentials —

Cold Cream 3oz $1.89 **MP 50¢**
Petroleum Jelly Plus 4oz $1.89 **MP 50¢**
All-Purpose Cream 3oz $1.89 **MP 50¢**

Moisture Secret —

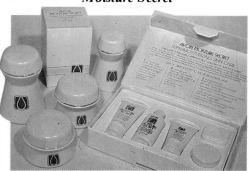

1975 *Enriched Freshener 5oz $5* **MP 50¢**
1977 *Daytime Moisturizer 3oz $5* **MP 50¢**
1975 *Cremegel Cleanser 4oz $5* **MP 50¢**
1975 *Night Concentrate 3oz $6* **MP 50¢**
1978 *4-Day Difference Kit: $2.50* **MP $6 boxed**

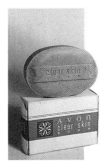 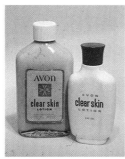 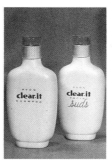 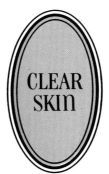 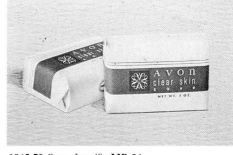

1957-65 *Soap 3¼oz*
49¢ **MP $9 boxed**

1957 *Lotion 6oz $1*
MP $10
1963-70 *Lotion 3oz 79¢*
MP $1

1960 *Clear-It
Shampoo 6oz $1.25*
MP $5
1961 *Clear-It Suds
6oz $1.25* **MP $5**

1965-70 *Soap 3oz 49¢* **MP $4**

. . . SKIN CARE LINES

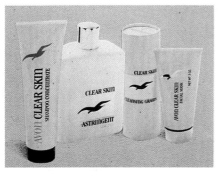 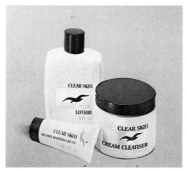 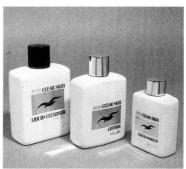 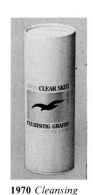

1970-74 *Shampoo Concentrate 5oz $1.50*
MP $2
1971 *Astringent 12oz $3* **MP $1**
1970-73 *Cleansing Grains 4.5oz $1.75*
MP $1
1971-73 *Facial Mask 3oz $1.75* **MP $2**

1973 *Oil-Free Blotting Cream .65oz*
$1.50 **MP $1**
1973 *Lotion 4oz $1.50* **MP 75¢**
1973-74 *Cream Cleanser 5oz $1.75*
MP $1

1973 *Liquid Cleanser 5oz $2* **MP 50¢**
1970-73 *Lotion 4oz $1.50* **MP $1**
1970 *Liquid Makeup 2oz $1.75* **MP $1**

1970 *Cleansing
Grains 4½oz*
$1.75 **MP 75¢**

1978 *Med. Astringent 12oz $2.99* **MP 50¢**
(rear) **1978** *Medicated Liquid Cleanser 10oz*
$2.99 **MP 50¢**

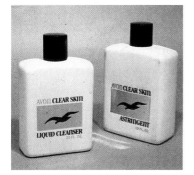 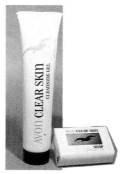 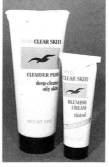 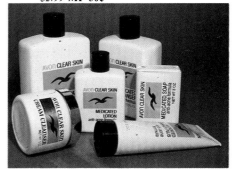

1974 *Liquid Cleanser 10oz $3.50*
MP 50¢
1973 *Astringent 12oz $3* **MP 50¢**,
6oz $1.75 **MP 50¢**

1973 *Cleansing Gel
6oz $3* **MP $1**
1970 *Soap 3oz 70¢*
MP $2.50

1976 *Cleanser Plus
3oz $1.79* **MP 50¢**
1977 *Blemish Cream
1oz $1.29* **MP 75¢**

1970 *Cream Cleanser 5oz jar $1.50* **MP $1**
1978 *Medicated Lotion 4oz $1.89* **MP 50¢**
1978 *Medicated Soap 3oz 99¢* **MP $1.50**
1978 *Medicated Cleanser Plus 3oz*
$1.99 **MP 50¢**

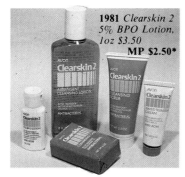 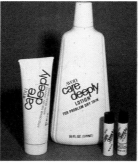 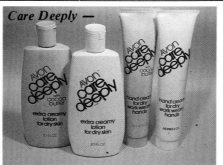 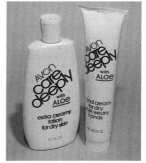

1981 *Clearskin 2
5% BPO Lotion,
1oz $3.50*
MP $2.50*

1982 *Cleansing Lotion 8oz $4.75*
MP $4*
1982 *Cleansing Scrub 2.5oz $3.75*
MP $3*
1982 *Cleansing Cake 3oz $2*
MP $1.25*

Care Deeply —

1973 *Hand Cream 4oz $1.35*
MP 50¢, *6oz $1.79* **MP 50¢**
1974 *Lotion 16oz shown $2.99*
MP $3*, *8oz $1.99* **MP 50¢**
1975 *Lip Balm .15oz $1.10* **MP 25¢**
1977 *Lip Balm with Sunscreen .15oz*
79¢ **MP 25¢**

1982 *Lotion with Cocoa Butter
10oz $3.49* **MP $3***
1982 *Lotion 10oz $3.49* **MP 50¢**
1982 *Hand Cream with Cocoa
Butter 6oz $2.79* **MP $2.50***
1982 *Hand Cream 6oz $2.79*
MP $2.50*

1983 *Lotion with Aloe 10oz
$3.49* **MP $3.50***
1983 *Hand Cream with Aloe
6oz $2.79* **MP $2.25***

*Available from Avon at time of publication

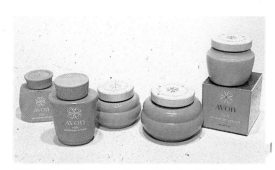

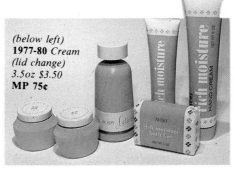

(below left)
1977-80 *Cream (lid change) 3.5oz $3.50* **MP 75¢**

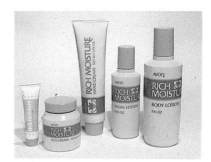

1953-54 only *Cream, embossed lid, 2oz $1.50* **MP $15**
1954-57 *Cream 2oz (shown) & 3½oz $1.50 & $2.50* **MP $6 each**
1957-61 *Cream 2oz $1.50* **MP $3**
1957-61 *Cream 3½oz $2.50* **MP $4**
1961-72 *Cream 2oz $1.50* **MP $1, $1.50 boxed**

1973-75 *Cream 3.5oz $3* **MP 75¢**
1965 *Lotion 8oz $3* **MP $1**
1969-75 *Hand Cream 3.75oz 89¢* **MP 50¢**
1974-75 *Hand Cream 6oz $2* **MP $2**
1972-78 *Bath Bar 5oz $1.50* **MP $2.50**

1979 *Trial Size Hand Cream .5oz with purchase 35¢* **MP 50¢**
1980 *Face Cream 3.5oz $3.50* **MP $3***
1980 *Hand Cream 3.75oz $2* **MP $1***
1980 *Facial Lotion 4oz $3.75* **MP 50¢***
1980 *Body Lotion 8oz $3.50* **MP $3***

Vita-Moist

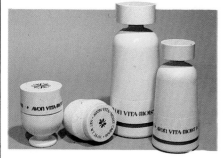

1959 *Cream 2oz $3* **MP $2**
1961 *Cream 1oz (not shown) $1.75* **MP $4**
1974-80 *Cream 3.5oz $3.50* **MP 50¢**
1974-80 *Lotion 16oz $5.50* **MP 75¢**
1969-80 *Lotion 8oz (new design) $3* **MP 25¢**

1980 *Body Lotion 8oz $3.50* **MP $3***
1980 *Hand Cream 3.75oz $2* **MP $1***
1980 *Face Cream 3.5oz $3.50* **MP $3***

Rich Moisture

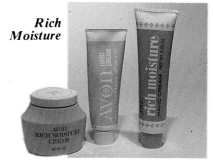

1975-76 *Cream 2oz $2* **MP $1**
1970-73 *Hand Cream 3oz 79¢* **MP $2**
1969-75 *Rich Moisture Hand Cream 3.75oz 89¢* **MP 50¢**

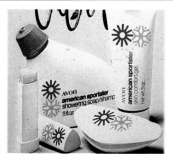

1970 American Sportster —
Super Stick 1/3oz $2.50 **MP $4**
Showering Soap/Shampoo 8oz $2.50 **MP $5**
Skin Comfort Gel 3oz $2.50 **MP $4**
Outdoor Shield .9oz $2.50 **MP $4**

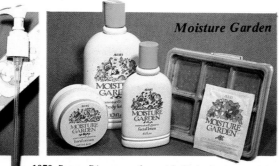

Moisture Garden

1979 *Pump Dispenser, free with Body Lotion in C-3 only* **MP $1.50 boxed**
1979 *Hand Cream 4oz $1.59* **MP 50¢**
1979 *Body Lotion 10oz $2.99* **MP 50¢**
1979 *Facial Lotion 4oz $2.59* **MP 50¢**
1979 *Rosea Vinca Collection Seed Starter Kit $1 with purchase in C-3 only* **MP $2**

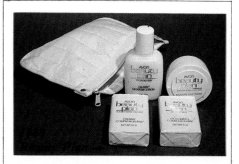

Beauty Plan Bag with purchase only in C-13 $2.99 **MP $4**
Oil-Free Moisture Lotion 3oz $4 **MP 50¢**
Moisture-Full Cream 3oz $4 **MP 50¢**
Creamy Complexion Bar 3oz $1.75 **MP $1.50**
Oil-Control Complexion Bar 3oz $1.75 **MP $1.50**

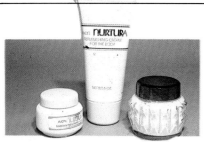

Nurtura —

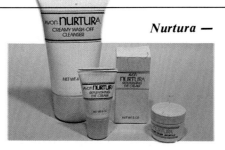

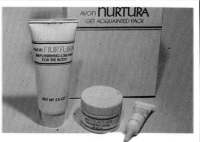

1979 *Replenishing Cream 2oz $5.50* **MP $6***
1980 *Replenishing Cream for the Body 5oz $5.50* **MP $6***
1980 *Vanity Jar 4oz $8* **MP $4**

1983 *Wash-Off Cleanser 4oz $7.50* **MP $5**
1981 *Eye Cream .5oz $6.50* **MP $4**
1982 *Replenishing Cream, trial size 69¢* **MP 25¢**

1982 *Nurtura Get Acquainted Kit with try-it sizes of Replenishing Cream for the Body, Replenishing Face Cream and Eye Cream $2* **MP $1 complete**

*Available from Avon at time of publication

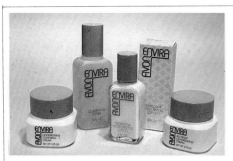

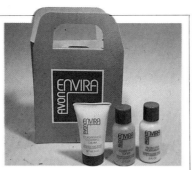

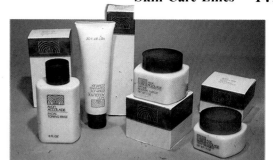

1980 Envira —
Conditioning Cleansing Cream 3.75oz $5 **MP $6***
Clarifying Toner 5oz $5 **MP $6***
Protective Moisturizing Lotion 2oz $5 **MP $6***
All-Night Conditioning Cream 3.75oz $6 **MP 50¢**

1982 Envira Beauty Discovery Kit.
*Replenishing Cream .5oz, Toner .5oz
and Moisturizing Lotion .5oz $2*
MP $5*

1981 Accolade —
Facial Toning Rinse 4oz $7.50 **MP $7***
Complete Cleansing Complex 3oz $7.50 **MP $7***
Daytime Moisture Support 3oz $7.50 **MP $7***
Night Treatment 1.75oz $8.50 **MP $8***

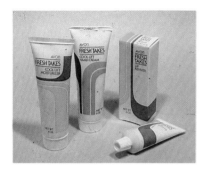

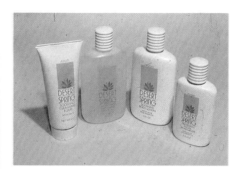

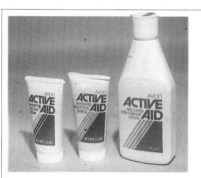

Fresh Takes —
1981-83 *Moisturizer 1oz $1.75* **MP 50¢**
1981-83 *Hand Cream 1oz $1.75* **MP 50¢**
1981-83 *Lip Reviver .5oz $2.25* **MP 75¢**

Desert Spring —
1983 *Cleansing Foam 3oz $4* **MP 50¢**
1983 *Skin Tonic 5oz $4* **MP 50¢**
1983 *Body Lotion 5oz $4* **MP 50¢**
1983 *Facial Moisturizer 3oz $4* **MP 50¢**

Moisture Therapy —
1983 *Body Lotion 7oz $6* **MP $5***
1983 *Bath Oil 7oz $7.50* **MP $5.50***
1983 *Hand Cream 3oz $3.75* **MP $3***
1983 *Hand Cream, trial size 39¢* **MP 59¢***

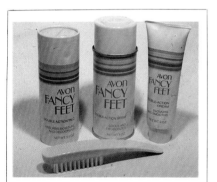

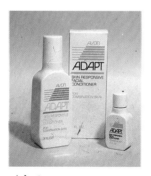

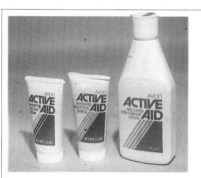

Fancy Feet — 1981 —
Talc 3.5oz $3 **MP $2***
Foot Spray 4oz $3.75 **MP $3***
Cream 3oz $3 **MP $2***
Brush 6" long $3.75 **MP $3***

Adapt —
1983 *Facial Conditioner 3oz
$8* **MP $6**
1983 *Facial Conditioner, trial
size .5oz 39¢* **MP 59¢***

Active Aid — 1981 —
Antiseptic Cream 1.5oz $2.49 **MP $2***
Medicated Protective Shield 1.5oz $2.49 **MP 25¢**
Medicated Lotion 8oz $2.99 **MP 50¢**
Antiseptic Spray 3oz $2.99 **MP $3***

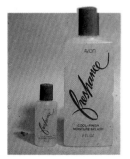

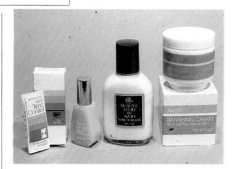

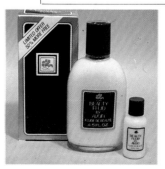

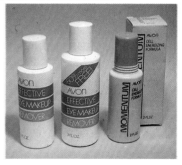

Freshance —
1983 *Moisture Splash
1oz 39¢* **MP 59¢***
1983 *Moisture Splash
8oz $6.50* **MP $5***

1980 *Time Control .75oz $7.50* **MP 25¢**
1980 *Beauty Fluid 3oz $5* **MP $4***
1981 *Banishing Cream 3oz $6.50* **MP $6***

*Available from Avon at time of publication

1982 *Beauty Fluid, Bonus Size
4.5oz $5.50* **MP $1, $1.25 boxed**
1981 *Beauty Fluid, trial size
.5oz 79¢* **MP 79¢***

1981 *Effective Eye Makeup Remover
2oz $3* **MP $2***
1982 *Effective Eye Makeup Remover,
Bonus Size 3oz $3* **MP 75¢**
1982 *Momentum 2oz $7* **MP $8***

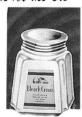

1930-34 *Bleach Cream
3oz 75¢* **MP $46**

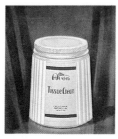

1930-34 *Tissue Cream
2oz 75¢* **MP $46**

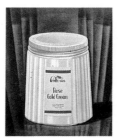

1932-34 *Rose Cold
Cream 2oz 52¢* **MP $46**
1930-32 only *Rose Cold
Cream (not shown) 4oz
75¢* **MP $55**

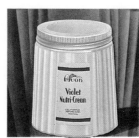

1930-32 *Violet Nutri-Cream
4oz $1* **MP $55**
1932-34 *As above (not
shown) 2oz 65¢* **MP $46**

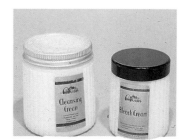

1931-34 *Cleansing Cream 4oz $1*
MP $55
1934-35 *Bleach Cream 2oz 52¢*
MP $40

CREAMS
AND
LOTIONS

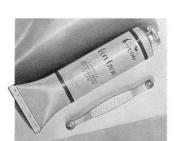

1930-34 *Pore Cream 75¢*
MP $30
1930 *Blackhead Remover 15¢*
MP $10

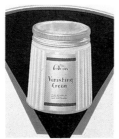

1932-34 *Vanishing
Cream 2oz 52¢* **MP $46**

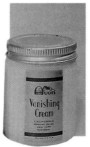

1930-32 *Vanishing
Cream 4oz 75¢*
MP $55

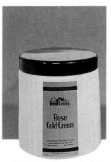

1934-36 *Rose Cold
Cream 4oz 78¢*
MP $40

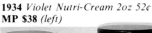

1934 *Violet Nutri-Cream 2oz 52¢*
MP $38 *(left)*

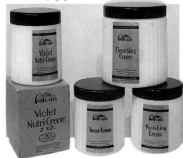

1934-36 *Cleansing Cream 4oz 78¢*
MP $40
1934-36 *Tissue Cream 2oz 52¢* **MP $40**
1934-36 *Vanishing Cream 2oz 52¢*
MP $40
Above jars, boxed, MP add $8

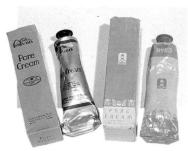

1934-36 *Pore Cream 78¢* **MP $25,
$33 boxed**
1936 *Pore Cream 1¼oz 78¢*
MP $12, $18 boxed

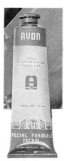

1940 *Special
Formula
Cream 1¼oz
78¢* **MP $12**

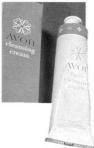

1956 only
*Cleansing Cream
2½oz 59¢* **MP $9,
$12 boxed**

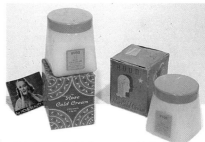

1941 *Rose Cold Cream in gift box
1¾oz 52¢* **MP $20 as shown**
1940 *Rose Cold Cream in gift box 2oz
52¢* **MP $20 as shown**

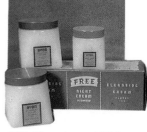

1951 *Cleansing and Night
Cream Set. 2 large jars,
1 medium size $1.78*
MP $35 set

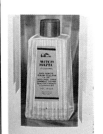

1930-34 *Witch Hazel
Extract 4oz (shown)
8oz & 16oz 50¢, 85¢
and $1.45* **MP $45,
$55 & $75**

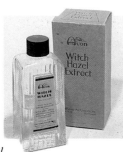

1934-36 *Witch Hazel
Extract 4, 8 and 16oz
33¢, 57¢ and $1.04*
MP $40, $50 & $70

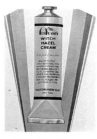

1930-34 *Witch
Hazel Cream 75¢*
MP $30

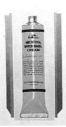

1930-34 *Menthol
Witch Hazel
Cream 50¢*
MP $30

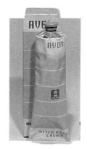

1936-39 *Witch
Hazel Cream
52¢* **MP $13,
$18 boxed**

Witch
Hazel

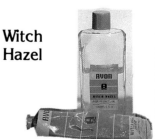

1937 *Witch Hazel Extract 4oz
37¢, 8oz 63¢, 16oz $1.04*
MP $25
1939-41 *Witch Hazel Cream,
tube 52¢* **MP $12, $15 boxed**

Night Cream 1³/₄oz each (add $4 to MP for box) — Cleansing Creams 3¹/₂oz (add $4 to MP for box) —

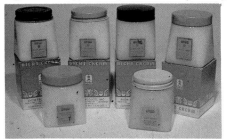

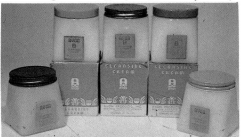

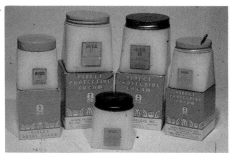

1944-45 *For Normal skin 89¢* **MP $10 w/black lid**
1951-54 *Ozonized 89¢* **MP $9, $20 ("Distributor")**
1941-51 *Normal Skin 78¢* **MP $8**
1944-45 *Dry Skin 89¢* **MP $10 w/black or white lid**
1941-46 *Dry Skin 78¢* **MP $8**
(1940-41 Dry, Normal or Oily, not shown,
2oz 78¢ **MP $10)**

1944-45 *Dry Skin 89¢* **MP $10 w/metal lid**
1941-46 *Oily Skin 78¢* **MP $8**
1944-45 *Oily Skin 89¢* **MP $10 w/metal lid**
1941-46 *Dry Skin 78¢* **MP $8**
1944-45 *Dry Skin 89¢* **MP $10 w/white lid**
(1937-41 Dry, Normal or Oily, not shown, 4oz
78¢ **MP $10)**

1937-41 *Violet Nutri Cream 2oz 52¢ (shown)*
& 4oz 78¢ **MP $12**
1941-45 *Violet Protective (formerly Nutri)*
Cream 3¹/₂oz 78¢ **MP $9**
1944-45 *Violet Protective 3¹/₂oz 89¢* **MP $11**
w/metal lid
1941-45 *Violet Protective 1³/₄oz 52¢* **MP $9**
1944-45 *Violet Protective 1³/₄oz 59¢* **MP $11**
w/black lid

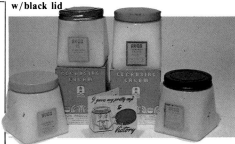

DATING GUIDE FOR JARS FROM 1937 THROUGH 1954

Catalogs often did not reflect the changes in labels. Original product pictures were often seen in subsequent catalogs. Jar size, contents and label information all aid in dating these Cream Jars.
1937-38 *Jar labels appeared with name of product, tulip-A and Avon.*
1939 *Avon Products, Inc., Div. N.Y.-Montreal was added to the labels.*
1939-47 *Labels were changed to read Avon Products, Inc., Dist. N.Y.-Montreal.*
1947-51 *Labels were changed to Avon Products, Inc., Dist. N.Y.-Pasadena and the tulip-A was dropped from the label.*
1951-54 *Labels were changed to read Avon Products, Inc., N.Y.-Pasadena (Dist. was dropped).*
Jar Sizes: 1937-41 *Shown in catalogs as: Medium (2oz) and Large (4oz)*
1941-54 *Medium (1³/₄oz) and Large (3¹/₂oz). Small jar sizes were issued in sets only.*

1939-46 *Makeup creams were issued only in ⁷/₈oz size jars — Foundation Cream, Color Pick-Up and Twin-Tone.*
Regular Pricing:
1937-42 *52¢ (Medium) and 78¢ (Large).*
1942-54 *59¢ (Medium) and 89¢ (Large).*
Name Changes:
1940 *Tissue Cream re-named Complexion Cream, discontinued in* **1949**
1941 *Violet Nutri-Creme re-named Violet Protective, discontinued* **1945**
1943 *Foundation Cream re-named Twin-Tone, changed in* **1946** *to Color Pick-Up.*
1947 *Night Cream for Dry Skin re-named Special Dry Skin, changed in* **1950** *to Super Rich.*
1951 *Night Cream for Normal Skin re-named Ozonized Night Cream.*
1953 *Rose Cold Cream re-named All-Purpose Cream, discontinued in* **1954** *in this jar design.*

Cleansing Creams 3¹/₂oz (add $4 to MP for box) —
1941-46 *Normal Skin 78¢* **MP $8**
1944-45 *Normal Skin 89¢* **MP $11 with metal lid and Victory folder**
1947-54 *Fluffy type 89¢* **MP $8**
1947-54 *Fluffy type 89¢* **MP $8**
(1937-41 For Dry, Normal or Oily, not shown, 4oz 78¢ **MP $10)**

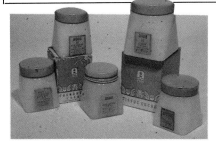

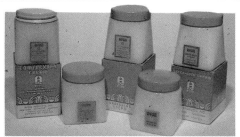

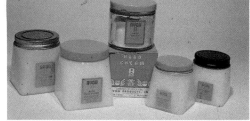

1946 only *Color Pick-Up Cream ⁷/₈oz 89¢*
MP $20
1939-43 *Foundation Cream ⁷/₈oz 52¢* **MP $10**
1943 *Foundation Cream ⁷/₈oz 59¢* **MP $12**
1937-40 only *Tissue Cream 2oz 78¢* **MP $13**
1936-39 *Tissue Cream ⁷/₈oz (in Facial sets only)*
MP $15
(add $4 to MP for box)

1943 *Complexion Cream (formerly Tissue) 1³/₄oz 59¢* **MP $12**
1940-49 *Complexion Cream 2oz 52¢* **MP $8**
1941-45 *Vanishing Cream 1³/₄oz 59¢* **MP $9**
1937-41 *Vanishing Cream 2oz 52¢* **MP $12**
1951-54 *Super-Rich Cream (formerly Special Dry Skin Cream) 1³/₄oz 89¢* **MP $9**
$20 ("Distributor" on label)
(add $4 to MP for box)

1944-45 *Rose Cold Cream 3¹/₂oz 89¢* **MP $10 w/metal lid**
1941-53 *Rose Cold Cream 3¹/₂oz 78¢* **MP $8**
1943-45 *Hand Cream 3-1/3oz $1.78* **MP $20 in wartime pkg., Boxed $25**
1946-51 *Special Formula Cream 1³/₄oz 89¢* **MP $9**
1945 *As above w/black lid* **MP $11**

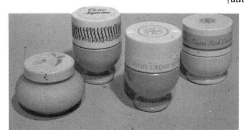

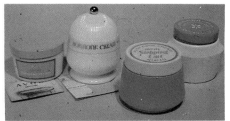

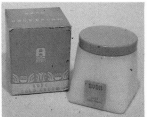

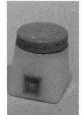

1957-61 *Strawberry Cooler 3³/₄oz $1.50* **MP $6**
1961-69 *Creme Supreme 2¹/₄oz $3* **MP $3**
1969-74 *Creme Supreme 2¹/₄oz $3* **MP $2**
1968-69 *Super Rich Cream 2¹/₄oz $3* **MP $4**
1965-68 *Super Rich (not shown) as above but lid label in script and 4-A gold design* **MP $3**

1954-61 *Hormone Cream 1³/₄oz $2* **MP $4**
1965-74 *Hormone Cream 2¹/₄oz $3* **MP $1**
1969-74 *Stepping Out Foot Care Cream 4oz $2*
MP 50¢
1976-80 *Cold Cream 3.1oz $1.39* **MP 25¢**

1936-41 *Rose Cream 4oz 78¢* **MP $12**

1936-41 *Bleach Cream 2oz 52¢* **MP $12**

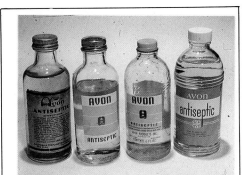

1930-37 *Antiseptic 6oz 35¢* **MP $35**
1933-37 *12oz (not shown) 62¢* **MP $40**
1936-41 *Antiseptic 6oz 36¢* **MP $18**
1936-41 *12oz (not shown) 62¢* **MP $23**
1941-54 *Antiseptic 6oz 36¢* **MP $10**
1941-54 *12oz (not shown) 62¢* **MP $14**
1954-61 *Antiseptic 7oz 49¢* **MP $5**

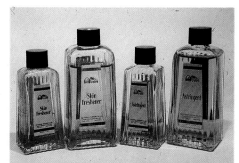

1935-36 *Skin Freshener 2oz 45¢* **MP $50**
1930-36 *Skin Freshener 4oz 75¢* **MP $45**
1935-36 *Astringent 2oz 45¢* **MP $50**
1930-36 *Astringent 4oz 75¢* **MP $45**

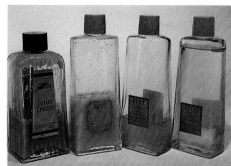

1930-36 *Lotus Cream 4oz 75¢* **MP $45**
1936-44 *Lotus Cream 4oz 52¢* **MP $18**
1936-54 *Skin Freshener 4oz 78¢* **MP $15**
1936-54 *Astringent 4oz 78¢* **MP $15**

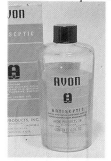
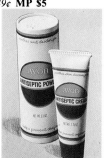

1945-46 *Antiseptic (war issue) 6oz 36¢* **MP $45, $55 boxed**

ANTISEPTICS
(See also pg. 157)

1970-72 *Antiseptic Powder 3.5oz $1* **MP 50¢**
1970-72 *Antiseptic Cream 1.75oz $1* **MP 50¢**

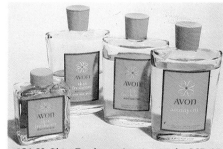

1954-58 *Skin Freshener 2oz (sets only)* **MP $5**
1965-66 *Skin Freshener for Dry or Normal Skin 4oz $1.25* **MP $7**
1957-65 *Skin Freshener or Astringent, Moisturized 4oz $1* **MP $4**
1954-57 *Astringent (shown) or Skin Freshener (pink lotion) 4oz $1* **MP $5**

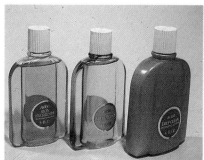

1969-73 *Skin Freshener 4oz $1.25* **MP $1**
1969-73 *Astringent 4oz $1.25* **MP $1**
1970-73 *Cleansing Lotion 6oz $1.50* **MP $1**

SKIN CARE

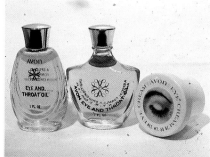

1967 *Eye & Throat Oil 1oz (Rare, issued during glass strike) $2.50* **MP $10**
1965 *Eye & Throat Oil 1oz $2.50* **MP $3**
1960 *Eye Cream .58oz $1.75* **MP $2**

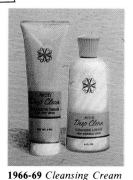

1966-69 *Cleansing Cream for Dry Skin 4oz $1.25* **MP $2**
1968-69 *Cleansing Lotion for Normal Skin 6oz $1.25* **MP $5**

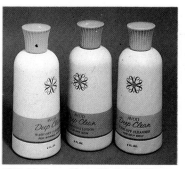

1966-69 *Deep Clean Wash-Off Cleanser for Normal Skin 6oz $1.25* **MP $3**
1966-69 *Deep Clean Cleansing Lotion for Dry Skin 6oz $1.25* **MP $3**
1966-69 *Deep Clean Wash-Off Cleanser for Oily Skin 6oz $1.25* **MP $3**

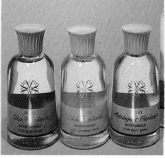

1968-69 *Skin Freshener, Moisturized: (left to right) Dry, Normal, Oily Skin 4oz $1.25* **MP $3, $4 boxed** *(1966-68 As above, except labels read: For Dry, Normal or Oily Skin followed by the word Moisturized* **MP $4)**

Insect Repellant —

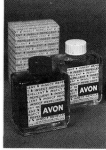

1959 *(red cap) 2oz 59¢* **MP $8**
1960 *(white cap) 2oz 59¢* **MP $7**

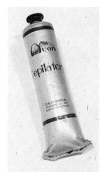

1930-31 *Depilatory Cream 78¢* **MP $50**

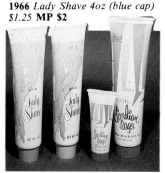

1966 *Lady Shave 4oz (blue cap) $1.25* **MP $2**
1971 *Lady Shave 4oz (pink cap) $1.25* **MP 50¢**
1971 *Fashion Legs Leg Makeup Trial 1oz 50¢ with purchase* **MP 75¢**
1968 *Fashion Legs Leg Makeup 6oz $3* **MP 50¢**

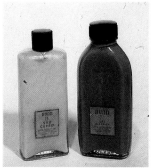

1943-45 *Sun Cream 4oz (black lid) 85¢* **MP $20**
1943-45 *Leg Makeup 4oz (black lid) 69¢* **MP $20**

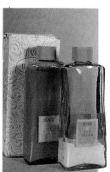

1945-49 *Leg Makeup 4oz 49¢* **MP $20, $25 boxed**
1945-47 *Sun Cream 4oz 85¢* **MP $20**

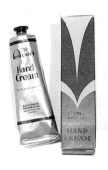 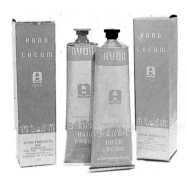 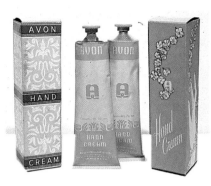 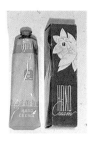 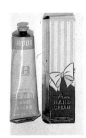

1940 *Hand Cream*
52¢ **MP $18 boxed**

1942 *Hand Cream*
59¢ **MP $17 boxed**

1934-35 *Hand Cream 52¢*
MP $30, $38 boxed

1938-54 *Hand Cream 2½oz 52¢*
MP $8, $12 boxed

1939 *Hand Cream 52¢* **MP $20 boxed**
1941 *Hand Cream 52¢* **MP $17 boxed**

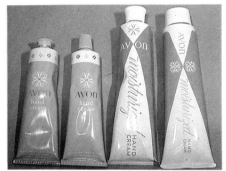 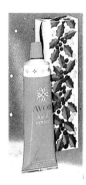

HAND
CREAMS
AND
FACIALS

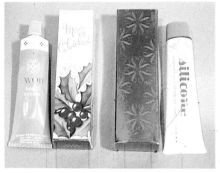

1955-57 *Hand Cream 59¢* **MP $6 (Pasadena)**
1957-59 *Hand Cream 59¢* **MP $5 (Pasadena)**
1958-62 *Moisturized Hand Cream 79¢* **MP $4**
1962-68 *Moisturized Hand Cream 3¾oz*
89¢ **MP $3**

1957 *Hand Cream,*
Xmas boxed 59¢
MP $8

1959 *Hand Cream, Xmas boxed 59¢* **MP $7**
1962 *Silicone Glove, Xmas boxed 2½oz 79¢*
MP $5

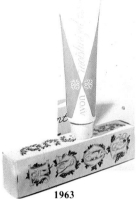 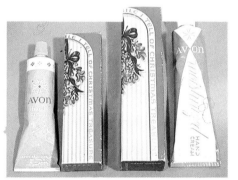 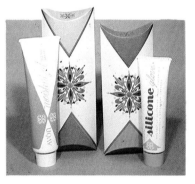 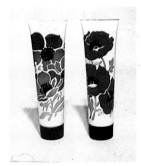

1963
Moisturized Hand Cream,
Xmas boxed 3¾oz **MP $5**

1960 *Hand Cream, Xmas boxed 69¢* **MP $6**
1960 *Moisturized Hand Cream, Xmas boxed*
89¢ **MP $6**

1964 *Moisturized Hand Cream. Xmas*
boxed 89¢ **MP $5**
1964 *Silicone Glove. Xmas boxed 79¢*
MP $4

1980 *Take-Along Hand*
Cream in Vita-Moist (red) or
Rich Moisture (blue) 1oz
$1.29 each **MP 75¢**

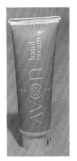 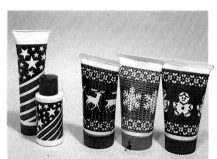 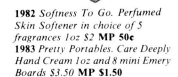 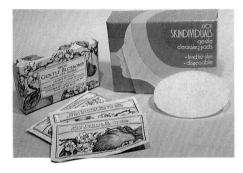

1962-70 *Hand*
Cream 3oz
69¢ **MP $3**

1982 *Stars 'N Stripes to Go After Tan*
Moisturizer and Sun Tan Lotion 1oz each
$2 ea. **MP 50¢ ea.**
1982 *Seasonal Smoothers 1.5 oz each (left*
to right) Top Condition Hand Cream, Rich
Moisture Hand Cream, Hello Sunshine
Hand Cream $2 ea. **MP 50¢ ea.**

1982 *Softness To Go. Perfumed*
Skin Softener in choice of 5
fragrances 1oz $2 **MP 50¢**
1983 *Pretty Portables. Care Deeply*
Hand Cream 1oz and 8 mini Emery
Boards $3.50 **MP $1.50**

1983 *Gentle Blossoms Rinse-Off Masks. 3 one-*
treatment masks in Peach, Cherry and Orange
fragrances .6oz $2.50 **MP $2* complete**
1982 *Skindividuals. 14 gentle cleansing pads per*
box $3.50 **MP $3***

*Available from Avon at time of publication

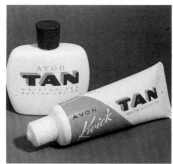

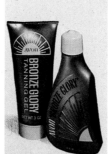

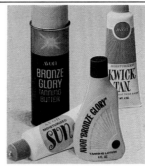

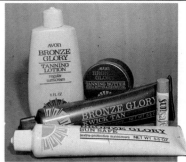

1949-57 Sun Lotion 4oz 98¢ **MP $13**

1958 Tan Moisturized Suntan Lotion 4oz 98¢ **MP $3**

1979 Sun Seekers — *(rear)*
Tanning Oil 4oz $2.29 **MP 25¢**
Sunsafe Lotion 4oz $2.29 **MP 25¢**
Tanning Lotion 4oz $2.29 **MP 25¢**

1962 Kwick Tan for Quickest Tan 4oz $1.10 **MP $1.50**

Bronze Glory —
1970 Tanning Gel 3oz $1.75 **MP 50¢**
1968 Tanning Oil 4oz $1.75 **MP 50¢**

1973 Bronze Glory Tanning Butter 7oz $2.50 **MP 25¢**
1966 Kwick Tan 4oz $1.50 **MP 50¢**
1965 Sun Safe 4oz $1.75 **MP 75¢**
1972 Bronze Glory Lotion 4oz $2 **MP 25¢**

1975 Tanning Lotion 6oz $3 **MP 25¢**
1977 Tanning Butter 1.75oz $1.49 **MP 50¢**
1975 Kwick Tan 5.5oz tube $3 **MP 25¢**
1975 Sun Safe 5.5oz tube $3 **MP 25¢**
1973 Sun Safe Stick .15oz 89¢ **MP 25¢**

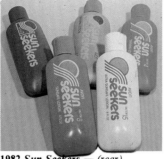

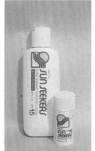

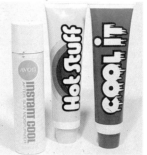

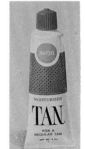

(front)
Tan Saver Moisturizing Lotion 4oz $2.29 **MP 25¢**
1980 Ultra Sunsafe Lotion 4oz $3.75 **MP 25¢**
1980 Tanning Butter 1.75oz $3 **MP 25¢**

1982 Sun Seekers — *(rear)*
Tanning Oil 4oz $4.50 **MP 25¢**
Tanning Lotion 4oz $4.50 **25¢**
Water-Resistant Tanning Lotion 4oz $5.50 **MP 25¢**
Sunsafe Lotion 4oz $4.50 **MP 25¢**
Ultra Sunsafe Lotion 4oz $5 **MP 25¢**

Sun Seekers —
1984 Ultra Sunsafe Tanning Lotion 4oz $5.50 **MP $4***
1983 Protective Stick .5oz $5.50 **MP $4***

1971 Instant Cool After Sun Moisturizer 4oz $2.50 **MP $1**
1981 Hot Stuff Tanning Lotion 3.75oz $3 **MP 25¢**
1981 Cool It Moisturizing Lotion 3.75oz $3 **MP 25¢**

1966 Tan 4oz $1.50 **MP 50¢**

A

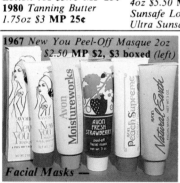

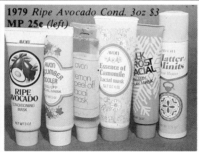

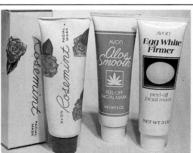

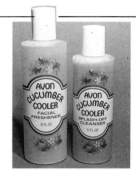

1967 New You Peel-Off Masque 2oz $2.50 **MP $2, $3 boxed** *(left)*

Facial Masks —
1977 Moistureworks Creamy 3oz $3 **MP 50¢**
1978 Fresh Strawberry Peel-Off 3oz $3 **MP 50¢**
1973 Peach Supreme Creamy 3oz $2 **MP $1**
1977 Natural Earth 3oz $3 **MP 50¢**

1979 Ripe Avocado Cond. 3oz $3 **MP 25¢** *(left)*

1976 Cucumber Cooler Peel-Off 3oz $3 **MP 50¢**
1977 Lemon Peel-Off 3oz $3 **MP 50¢**
1975 Essence of Camomile 4oz $2 **MP 75¢**
1978 Milk Frost 3oz $3 **MP 50¢**
1971 Matter of Minits, Aerosol 3.75oz $2.50 **MP $2**

1962 Rosemint 3oz $1.25 **MP $3, $5 boxed**
1980 Aloe Smooth Peel-Off 3oz $3 **MP $2.50***
1981 Egg White Firmer Peel-Off 3oz $3.50 **MP $2.50***

1978 Cucumber Cooler Facial Freshener 8oz $3.50 **MP 75¢**
1978 Cucumber Cooler Splash-Off Cleanser 6oz $3.50 **MP 75¢**

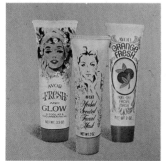

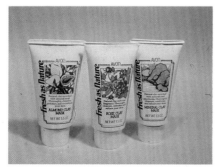

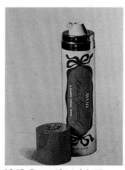

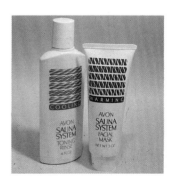

1968 Fresh and Glow 3.5oz $1.50 **MP 75¢**
1973 Herbal Scented 2oz $1.25 **MP 75¢**
1974 Orange Fresh Peel-Off 2oz $2.50 **MP 50¢**

1982 Fresh as Nature Clay Mask *(left to right)*
Almond 1.5oz $2.50 **MP $1.50***
Rose 1.5oz $2.50 **MP $1.50***
Mineral 1.5oz $2.50 **MP $1.50***

1965 Beautifacial 3.75oz $2.50 **MP $2**

1982 Sauna System Toning Rinser 4oz $4 **MP $3***
1982 Sauna System Warming Facial Mask 3oz $4 **MP $3***

**Available from Avon at time of publication*

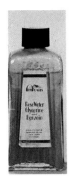

1930-36 *Rose Water, Glycerine & Benzoin 4oz 75¢ MP $45*

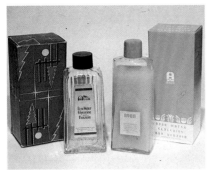

1936 *Rose Water, Glycerin & Benzoin 4oz Xmas boxed 78¢* **MP $60**
1937-41 *Rose Water, Glycerin & Benzoin 4oz 78¢* **MP $20, $25 boxed**

LOTIONS

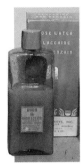

1941-47 *Hand Lotion, Rose Water, Glycerine & Benzoin 4oz 52¢* **MP $17, $21 boxed**

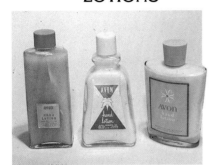

Hand Lotion —
1948-50 *4oz 59¢* **MP $17**
1950-53 *4oz 59¢* **MP $16**
1953-58 *4oz 69¢* **MP $6**

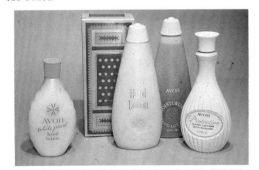

1958-62 *White Pearl Hand Lotion 6oz 98¢* **MP $4**
1966-70 *Hand Lotion 10oz $1.50* **MP $3, $6 as shown in 1966 Xmas box**
1970-74 *Moisturized Hand Lotion 10oz $1.50* **MP $2**
1969-74 *Protective Hand Lotion with Silicone 7.75oz $1.50* **MP $2**

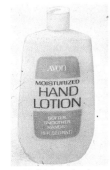

1979 *Moisturized Hand Lotion 16oz $2.99* **MP 50¢**

Available from Avon at time of publication

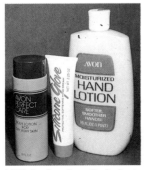

1975 *Perfect Care Body Lotion for Dry, Ashy Skin 6oz $3* **MP 50¢**
1970 *Silicone Glove 2.25oz 79¢* **MP $1.25*, 4.5oz $1.35 MP $2.50***
1976 *Moisturized Hand Lotion 16oz $2.69* **MP 75¢**

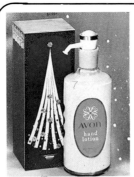

1956 *Hand Lotion 8oz $1.39* **MP $16, $23 as shown in 1957 Xmas box**

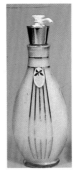

1963 *Gift Hand Lotion 8oz $2.50* **MP $11**

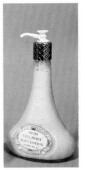

1965 *Gift Body Lotion. Rich Moisture or Vita Moist Lotion 8oz $3.50* **MP $8**

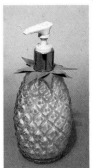

1973 *Pineapple Decanter with Moisturized Hand Lotion 10oz $6* **MP $9**

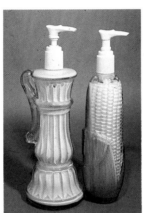

1974 *Country Pump with Rich Moisture or Vita Moist Lotion 10oz $6* **MP $6**
1977 *Golden Harvest Moisturized Hand Lotion 10oz $8.50* **MP $6**

1971 *Lovely Touch with Rich Moisture or Vita Moist Lotion 12oz $6* **MP $7**
1972 *Lovely Touch with Rich Moisture or Vita Moist Lotion 12oz $6* **MP $8**

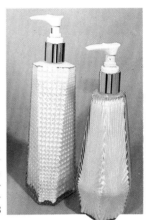

LOTION and SOAP DISPENSERS

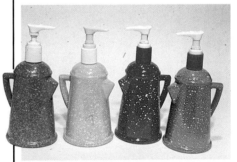

Country Style Coffee Pots
Moisturized 10oz Hand Lotion
1975 *Blue $7.50* **MP $7**
1978 *Yellow $8.50* **MP $6**
1979 *Red $9.50* **MP $6**
1979 *Green $9.50* **MP $6**

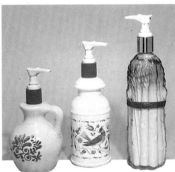

1976 *Country Jug Moisturized Hand Lotion 10oz $8* **MP $5**
1978 *Country Creamery, 10oz Moisturized Hand Lotion $8.50* **MP $5**
1979 *Garden Fresh Moisturized Hand Lotion 10oz $9.50* **MP $5**

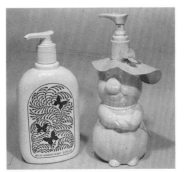

1982 *Silken Soap Dispenser (plastic) 10oz $3.29* **MP 75¢**
1982 *Stylish Lady. Liquid Cleanser or Hand Lotion 8oz $12.50* **MP $5**

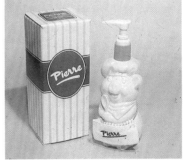

1984 *Pierre Hand Lotion Decanter. Care Deeply Hand Lotion 8oz $12.50* **MP $5**

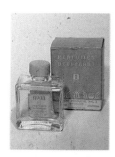
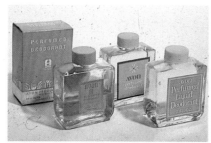
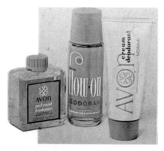
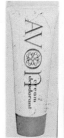
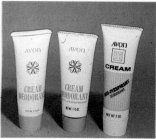

1947-48 only *Perfumed 2oz 59¢* **MP $10** with N.Y.-Montreal label, $14 boxed

1948-54 *Perfumed 2oz 59¢* **MP $6** (Pasadena), $8 boxed
1967-76 *Perfumed 2oz 79¢* **MP $1**
1967-68 *As above 4oz (not shown) $1.25* **MP $4**
1976 *Perfumed 2oz $1.49* **MP $1.50***

1955-67 *Perfumed 2oz 69¢* **MP $2**
1963-66 *Flow-On (glass) 1³/₄oz 89¢* **MP $6**
1960-63 *As above, plastic (not shown)* **MP $4**
1963-66 *Cream 1³/₄oz 79¢* **MP $3**

1960-63 *Cream 1³/₄oz 79¢* **MP $4**

1966 *Cream 1³/₄oz 79¢* **MP 25¢**
1967-70 *Cream 1³/₄oz 79¢* **MP $2**
1970-71 *Cream 1³/₄oz (not shown) 98¢* **MP $4**
1971-76 *Cream 2oz 98¢* **MP 50¢**

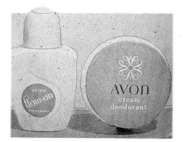
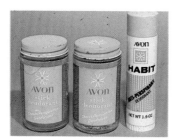
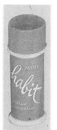
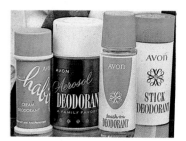

1958-60 *Flow-On 2oz 98¢* **MP $5**
1954-60 *Cream 1oz 49¢* **MP $5**

1956-60 *Stick 1.8oz 79¢* **MP $8**
1960 only *Stick 1.8oz 79¢* **MP $15** (4-A on lid)
1972-76 *Habit 1.5oz $1.50* **MP $1**
1970-72 *As above 1¹/₄oz (not shown) $1.25* **MP $3**

1960-63 *Habit 1¹/₄oz $1* **MP $3**
1963-65 *Habit, Normal 1¹/₄oz $1* **MP $3**
1967-70 *Habit 1¹/₄oz $1.25* **MP $2**
1970 only *Habit 1¹/₄oz $1.25* **MP $4**

1965-67 *Habit 1¹/₄oz $1.25* **MP $3**
1965-66 *Aerosol 3oz $1.25* **MP $4**
1965-66 *Touch-On 1³/₄oz $1.25* **MP $5**
1965-68 *Stick 2³/₄oz $1.25* **MP $3**

DEODORANTS

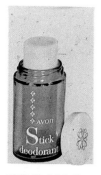
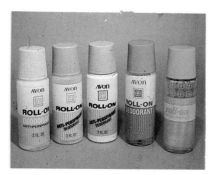
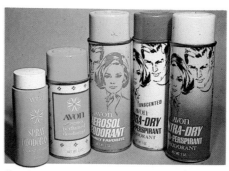
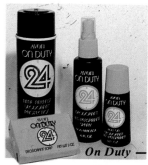

On Duty

1960-63 *Stick 1³/₄oz 89¢* **MP $7**

1969-71 *Roll-On 2oz 98¢* **MP $3**
1972-76 *Roll-On 2oz $1.35* **MP 50¢**
1971-72 *Roll-On 2oz 98¢* **MP $1**
1968-69 *Roll-On 1³/₄oz 98¢* **MP $3**
1966-67 *Roll-On 1³/₄oz 98¢* **MP $4**

1966-67 *Spray 3oz (squeeze bottle) 98¢* **MP $3**
1968-76 *Aerosol Perfumed 4oz $1.25* **MP $1**
1970-76 *Aerosol Family 7oz $1.79* **MP 50¢**
1971-75 *Unscented Ultra-Dry 7oz $1.89* **MP 50¢**
1970-75 *Ultra-Dry 7oz $1.25* **MP 50¢**

1977 *Soap 3oz (special only)* **MP 50¢**
1975 *Aerosol 7oz $2.75* **MP 50¢**
1977 *Spray 4oz $2.29* **MP 50¢**
1976 *Roll-On 2oz $1.49* **MP $1.25***

Dri-N-Delicate —

Feelin' Fresh —
1978-81 *Body Powder 8oz $1.99* **MP 50¢**
1978-81 *Body Splash 8oz $2.29* **MP 50¢**

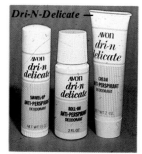
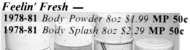
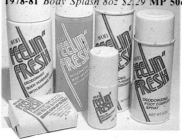
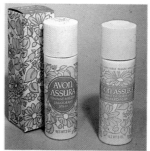
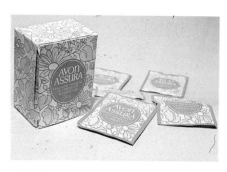

1976 *Swivel-Up Cream 1.5oz $1.69* **MP 50¢**
1976 *Roll-On 2oz $1.49* **MP 25¢**
1976 *Cream 2oz $1.49* **MP 50¢**

1978 *Deodorant Soap 3oz shown in Bonus wrapper, free to customers in introduction campaign* **MP $2**
1978 *Roll-On Deo. 2oz $1.49* **MP 25¢**
1978 *Aerosol Deo. 4oz $2.59* **MP $3***
1978-81 *Foot Comfort Spray 3oz $2.59* **MP 50¢**

1970 *Assura Spray 3oz $1.75* **MP $2**
1972 *Assura Spray Powder 3oz $1.75* **MP 2**

1970-72 *Assura Feminine Hygiene Deodorant Towelettes, 10 per box $1.50* **MP $2 complete**

**Available from Avon at time of publication*

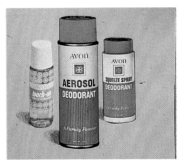

1966 *Touch-On Deodorant 1.75oz* *$1.25* **MP $5**
1968 *Aerosol 7oz $1.75* **MP $1**
1968 *Squeeze Spray 3oz 98¢* **MP $2**

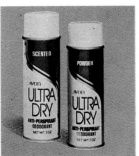

1975 *Ultra Dry Scented 7oz* *$1.98* **MP 50¢**
1975 *Ultra Dry Powder 7oz* *$1.98* **MP 50¢**

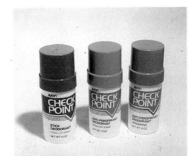

1982 *Checkpoint (left to right) Stick Deodorant 2oz $3.29* **MP $2.49***
Stick Anti-Perspirant, regular scent 2oz $3.29 **MP $2.49***
Stick Anti-Perspirant, unscented 2oz $3.29 **MP $2.49***

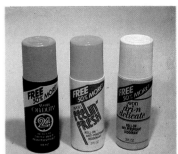

1981 & 1983 *Bonus Size Roll-On Deodorants (left to right)*
On Duty 3oz $1.49 **MP 50¢**
Feelin' Fresh 3oz $1.49 **MP 50¢**
Dri-N-Delicate 3oz $1.49 **MP 50¢**

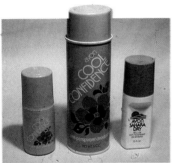

1982 *Cool Confidence Roll-On-Deodorant 2oz $2.19* **MP $1.49***
1982 *Cool Confidence Aerosol Deodorant 4oz $2.99* **MP $2.49***
1983 *Sahara Dry Roll-On Deodorant 1.5oz $2.99* **MP $2***

EARLY AVON DEO- DORANTS

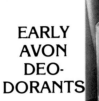

1929-30 *Deodorant 2oz 50¢* **MP $75**

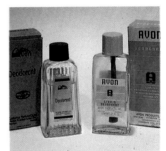

1930-36 *Deodorant 2oz 50¢* **MP $45, $55 boxed**
1944-47 *Liquid Deodorant with Applicator 2oz 59¢* **MP $22, $30 boxed**

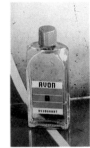

1937-44 *Deodorant 2oz 52¢* **MP $20**

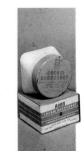

1938-44 *Cream 37¢* **MP $8, $12 Boxed**

(See Men's Deodorants pgs. 236-238)

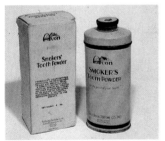

1931-36 *Smoker's Tooth Powder 4oz 50¢* **MP $40, $60 boxed**

DENTAL CARE by AVON

. . . Smoker's Tooth

See additional Tooth Tablets on page 28. Also see additional Smoker's Toothpowders on pages 156 and 236.

odors, especially those of tobacco.

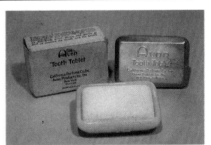

1934 *Tooth Tablet 35¢* **MP $60, $80 boxed**

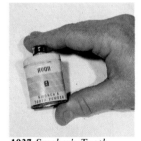

1937 *Smoker's Tooth Powder Sample (Small cap)* **MP $45**

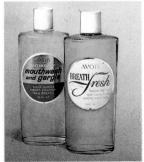

1968 *Antiseptic Mouthwash and Gargle 10oz $1.25* **MP $3**
1968-70 *Breath Fresh 10oz $1.25* **MP $2**

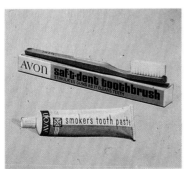

1970 *Saf-D-Dent Toothbrush 98¢* **MP $2 boxed**
1957 *Smoker's Toothpaste 69¢* **MP $3**

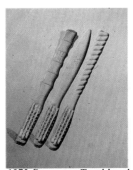

1970 *Decorator Toothbrush Trio Pak $1.75* **MP 25¢ each, $3.50 boxed**

(See also page 28)

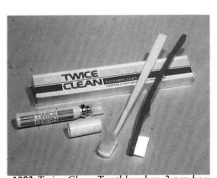

1983 *Twice Clean Toothbrushes, 2 per box, yellow and red, 2 campaigns only $2.99* **MP $3 boxed**
1983 *Twice Fresh Breath Spray, Cool Mint .33oz $2.49* **MP $2***

Available from Avon at time of publication

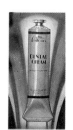 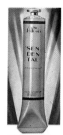 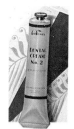 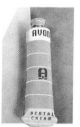 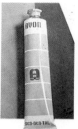 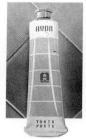 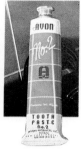 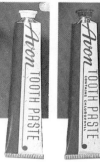

1931-37 *Dental Cream 25¢* **MP $50**

1931-37 *Sen Den Tal 40¢* **MP $50**

1931-37 *Dental Cream No. 2 40¢* **MP $50**

1937-47 *Dental Cream 26¢* **MP $30**

1937-40 *Sen Den Tal 36¢* **MP $35**

1937-49 *Tooth Paste 23¢* **MP $35**

1941-50 *Tooth Paste No. 2, 25¢* **MP $30**

1953-56 *Tooth Paste (white) 49¢* **MP $18**
1953-56 *Tooth Paste (green) with Chlorophyll 49¢* **MP $18**

Dental Cream was a foamy dentifrice, containing no abrasives or strong chemicals.
Sen Den Tal was a mildly abrasive cleanser, especially designed for hard to clean teeth.

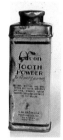 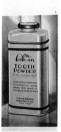 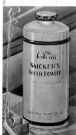

DENTAL CARE BY AVON

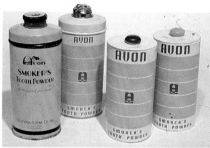 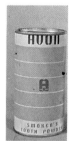 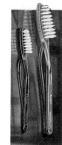

1932-37 *Tooth Powder 35¢* **MP $40**

1930-31 *Tooth Powder 35¢* **MP $45**

1930-31 *Smoker's Tooth Powder 50¢* **MP $45**

Smoker's Tooth Powder cleaned teeth and also destroyed mouth odors, especially those of tobacco.

1931-36 *Smoker's Tooth Powder 50¢* **MP $40**
1938-42 *Smoker's Tooth Powder 51¢* **MP $30**
1944-45 *Smoker's Tooth Powder 51¢* **MP $20**
1942-43 *Smoker's Tooth Powder 51¢* **MP $25**

1943-44 *Smoker's Tooth Powder 51¢* **MP $25**

1932-47 *Tooth Brushes, Amber, Red or Green. Adult 50¢, Youth 35¢* **MP $6 each**

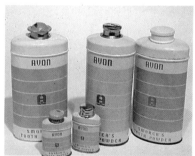 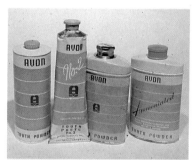 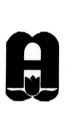 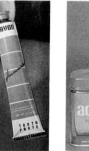 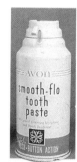

Tooth Powders (left to right) —
1950-54 *Smoker's 57¢* **MP $18**
1936-38 *Smoker's 50¢* **MP $35**
1946-50 *Smoker's 51¢* **MP $20**
1936 *Smoker's Sample (CPC label)* **MP $50**
1937 *Smoker's Sample (lg. cap)* **MP $45**

1943-44 *Tooth Powder 26¢* **MP $25**
1940 only *Tooth Paste No. 2 25¢* **MP $35 (see 1941-50 above)**
1936-49 *Tooth Powder 36¢* **MP $20**
1949-55 *Ammoniated Tooth Powder 49¢* **MP $15**

1949-55 *Ammoniated Tooth Paste 49¢* **MP $20**

1958 *Aqua-Dent 7oz 99¢* **MP $8**

1961 *Smooth-Flo Tooth Paste 5¹/₂oz 89¢* **MP $5**
1958 *As above, with red cap (not shown)* **MP $8**

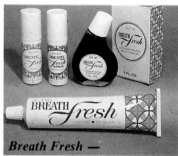 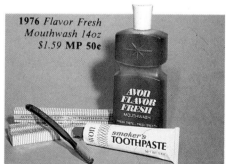 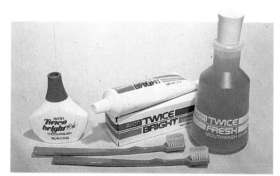

Breath Fresh —

1971 *Spray-Peppermint .5oz $1.50* **MP $1**
1968 *Spray .5oz $1.25* **MP $1**
1970 *Concentrated Mouth Wash 1oz $1.75* **MP $2**
1969 *Tooth Paste 4.75oz 89¢* **MP $2**

1976 *Flavor Fresh Mouthwash 14oz $1.59* **MP 50¢**

1976 *Plaque Control Toothbrush, blue only 98¢* **MP $1.50 boxed**
1978 *Plaque Control Toothbrush in blue, red or green $1.09* **MP $1.50 boxed**
1969 *Smoker's Toothpaste 4.75oz 89¢* **MP $1 (new size, labeling)**

1974-75 *Twice Bright Tooth Polish 2³/₄oz $1.89* **MP $2**
1981 *Twice Bright Toothpaste 5oz $1.89* **MP $1.50***
1981 *Twice Fresh Mouthwash 10oz $2.49* **MP $2***
1981-84 *Twice Clean toothbrushes. Blue and green in 1 box $2.49* **MP $2 boxed**

*Available from Avon at time of publication

Elite and Antiseptic Powders

A body talcum containing a mild deodorant, a baby powder, a foot powder and a powder to relieve skin irritations were benefits provided by Elite. Because of World War II, it was necessary to replace the metal containers with cardboard packaging in 1943. Discontinued in 1955, Elite was followed with its counterpart, Avon Antiseptic Powder.

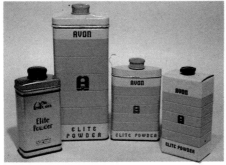
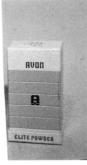
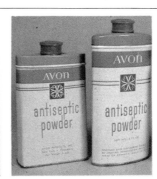
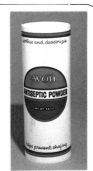

1930-36 *Elite Powder 3oz 35¢* **MP $45**
1930-36 *16oz (not shown) $1* **MP $55**
1936-49 *16oz $1.04* **MP $30**
1936-54 *Elite Powder 37¢* **MP $19**
1944-45 *Elite Powder, cardboard 43¢* **MP $25**
(See also Elite Powders pg. 26)

1943-44 *Elite Powder, cardboard 43¢* **MP $25**

1955-62 *Antiseptic Powder 3oz 59¢* **MP $6**
1962-68 *Antiseptic Powder 2³/₄oz 69¢* **MP $3**

1968-70 *Antiseptic Powder 3.5oz 89¢* **MP $1**

(See also pg. 150)

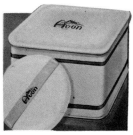

1930-34 *Dusting Powder 8oz $1.35* **MP $50**

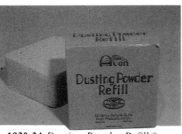

1930-34 *Dusting Powder Refill 8oz $1* **MP $30**

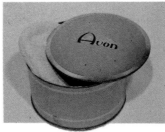

1934-36 *Dusting Powder 13oz $1.20* **MP $40**

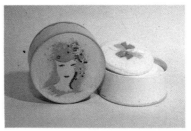

1945 *Beauty Dust from Petal of Beauty Set* **MP $30**

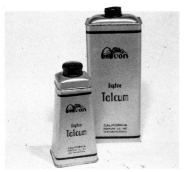

1930 only *Daphne Talcum 35¢* **MP $55**
1931-36 *Daphne Talcum 14¹/₂oz $1* **MP $50**

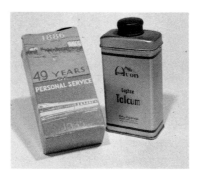

1935 *Daphne Talc in 49th Anniversary Box* **MP $55 in Anniversary box**

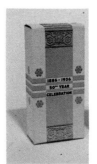

1936 *Daphne Talcum in 50th Anniversary Box (front and back of box shown)* **MP $55 in Anniversary box**

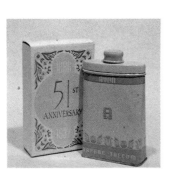

1937 *Daphne Talcum in 51st Anniversary Box* **MP $35 in Anniversary box**

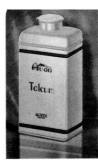

1930 *Talcum 35¢* **MP $45**

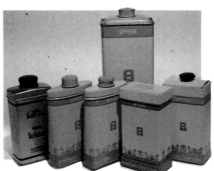

1930-32 *Daphne Talcum 35¢* **MP $45**
1946-50 *Daphne Talcum 39¢* **MP $10**
1936-43 *Daphne Talcum 37¢* **MP $15**
1936-43 *Daphne Talcum 14¹/₂oz $1.04* **MP $45**
1943-44 *Daphne Talcum, cardboard 37¢* **MP $25**
1944-45 *Daphne Talcum, cardboard 37¢* **MP $25**

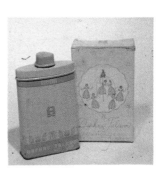

1940 only *Daphne Talc, customer gift with purchase, 10¢* **MP $32 as shown**

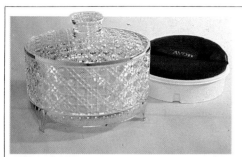

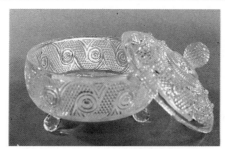

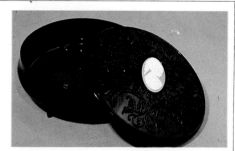

1971 *Crystalique Beauty Dust (plastic) in Hana Gasa, Elusive, Charisma, Regence, Unforgettable, Rapture, Somewhere, Here's My Heart, Topaze, Cotillion, To A Wild Rose and Occur! $8* **MP $7**

1972 *Crystalique Beauty Dust (glass). Same fragrances as 1971 except Hana Gasa and To A Wild Rose, add Moonwind. $8* **MP $11**

1973 *Cameo Beauty Dust Container 5½" diam. Sold empty for $5* **MP $7**

BEAUTY DUST CONTAINERS

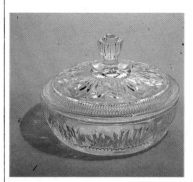

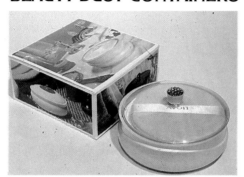

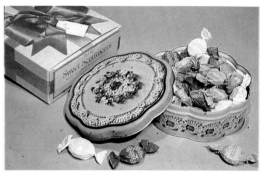

1975 *Beauty Dust Crystalique Container, sold empty $6* **MP $7**

1965 *C-10 Beauty Dust Demonstrator. Box pictures one of 8 containers to fill with choice of Beauty Dust fragrances* **MP $10 box only, $22 complete**

1981 *Sweet Sentiments Valentine Candy in Tin dated "Valentine's Day 1981". Two campaigns only 9oz $7.99* **MP $5 container only**

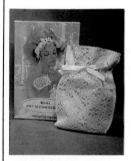

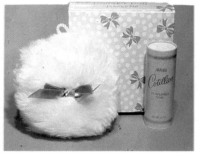

1966 *Pat 'N' Powder Mitt and Beauty Dust in Occur!, Rapture or Unforgettable 2½oz $2.50* **MP $7, $10 boxed**

1980 *Pamper-Puff Powder Mitt with zippered compartment to hold talc. Sold empty $9* **MP $7, $8 boxed**

Powder Mitts

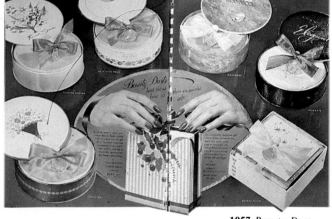

1958 *Beauty Dust 6oz with ribboned ⅝ dram bottle of matching fragrance same as 1957 fragrances (above) $1.95-$2.50* **MP $35, $45 Xmas boxed**

1957 *Beauty Dust 6oz with ribboned ⅝ dram bottle of matching fragrance in Cotillion, Forever Spring, To A Wild Rose, Nearness, Elegante & Bright Night $1.95-$2.50* **MP $35, $45 Xmas boxed**

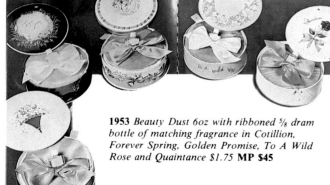

1953 *Beauty Dust 6oz with ribboned ⅝ dram bottle of matching fragrance in Cotillion, Forever Spring, Golden Promise, To A Wild Rose and Quaintance $1.75* **MP $45**

1956 *Beauty Dust 6oz with ribboned ⅝ dram bottle of matching fragrance. Same fragrances as 1957, except Quaintance replaces Elegante $1.95* **MP $40, $50 Xmas boxed**

BEAUTY DUST GIFTS

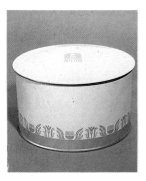
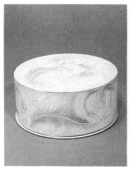
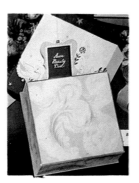
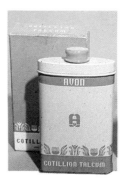
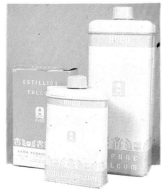

1936-49 *Dusting Powder 13oz $1.20* **MP $35**

1942-48 *Beauty Dust 6oz $1.10* **MP $38**

1943-44 *Beauty Dust in gift box $1.10* **MP $45, $55 boxed**

1937-46 *Cotillion Talcum 2¾oz 35¢* **MP $15, $18 boxed**

1946-50 *Cotillion Talcum 2¾oz 37¢* **MP $10, $13 boxed**
1946-50 *Daphne Talcum 14½oz $1.04* **MP $30**

TALCS AND DUSTING POWDERS

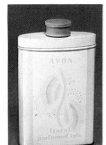
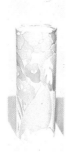
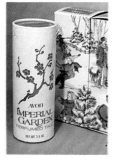
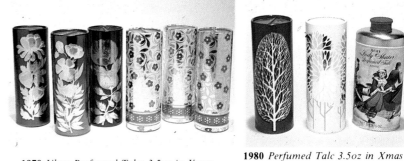
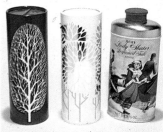

1958-61 *Floral Talc 59¢* **MP $12**

1978 *Talc 3.5oz in Burst of Spring box in 6 Frag. $2* **MP $1**

1974 *Perfumed Talcs 3.5oz in 4 Xmas scene gift boxes. 7 frag. $1.50 and $2* **MP $2.50 each with box**

1979 *Ultra Perfumed Talcs 3.5oz in Xmas Gift wrap, 6 fragrances $3* **MP $2**
1979 *Perfumed Talcs in Xmas Gift wrap, 10 frag. $2.50* **MP $1.50**

1980 *Perfumed Talc 3.5oz in Xmas Gift wrap (red) 6 frag. $3* **MP $1**
1980 *Ultra Perfumed Talc 3.5oz in Xmas wrap (silver) 7 frag. $3.50* **MP $1.50**
1979-80 *Lady Skater Talc in Sweet Honesty and Ariane 3.75oz $5.50* **MP $3**

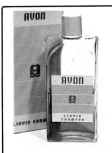
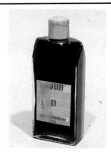
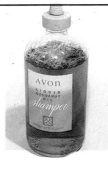
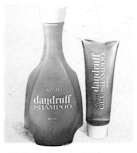
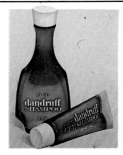
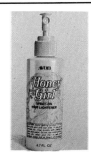

1937 *Liquid Shampoo 6oz 51¢* **MP $20, $25 boxed**

1937 *Pre-Shampoo Oil 2oz 52¢* **MP $25**

1956 *Cocoanut Oil Shampoo 16oz $1.59* **MP $25**

1967-70 *Dandruff Shampoo 8oz $1.50* **MP $4**
1967-70 *Dandruff Gel Shampoo 3oz 98¢* **MP $3**

1970-75 *Dandruff Shampoo 8oz $1.50* **MP $2.50**
1970-75 *Dandruff Gel Shampoo 3oz 98¢* **MP $1.50**

1973 *Honey Girl Spray-On Hair Lightener 4.7oz $2.25* **MP $3**

HAIR CARE

1976 *Natural Sheen Hair Dress and Conditioner 3oz $2* **MP 50¢**

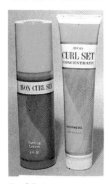
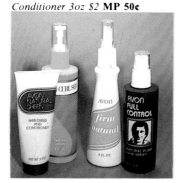
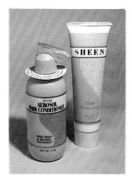
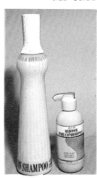
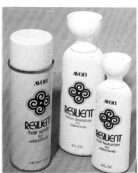

Curl Set —
1968 *Setting Lotion 8oz $1.50* **MP 75¢**
(1964 *As above, but 7oz $1.50* **MP $2)**
1966 *Concentrate 6oz $1.50* **MP 75¢**

1975 *Curl Set Setting Lotion 8oz $1.98* **MP 25¢**
1977 *Firm and Natural Hair Spray 6oz $2.29* **MP 50¢**
1980 *Full Control Natural Pump Hair Spray 6oz $2.29* **MP 50¢**

1971 *Aerosol Hair Conditioner 2oz $3* **MP 75¢ (label change)**
1966 *Sheen Hair Dressing 2oz $1* **MP $2**

1969 *Gentle Lotion Shampoo 8oz $.150* **MP $1.50**
1967-71 *Aerosol Hair Cond. 2oz $3* **MP $2**

1972 Resilient —
Hair Spray 7oz $2 **MP 50¢**
Shampoo 8oz $3 **MP 50¢**
Hair Texturizer 4oz $2.50 **MP 50¢**

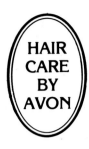

HAIR CARE BY AVON

More than 80 years ago, a lady used Bandoline for graceful, wavy hair.

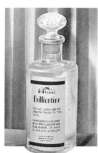

1929-30 *Brilliantine 2oz 50¢* **MP $80**

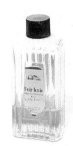

1930-36 *Hair Tonic Eau de Quinine for Oily Hair 6oz 90¢* **MP $50** *16oz $1.75* **MP $65**

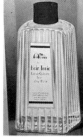

1930-36 *Hair Tonic Eau de Quinine for Dry Hair 6oz 90¢* **MP $50** *16oz $1.75* **MP $65**

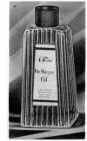

1930-36 *Pre-Shampoo Oil 2oz 75¢* **MP $50**

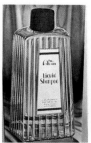

1930-36 *Liquid Shampoo 6oz 75¢* **MP $50,** *16oz $1.50* **MP $65**

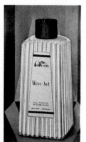

1930-36 *Wave Set 4oz 75¢* **MP $50**

Eau de Quinine, a delicately scented hair tonic, was used to help prevent dandruff, stop falling hair and retard the graying of the hair.

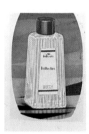

1930-36 *Brilliantine 2oz 50¢* **MP $50**

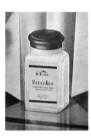

1930-36 *Bandoline Hair Dressing and Wave Lotion 35¢* **MP $50**

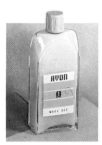

1937-43 *Wave Set 4oz 52¢* **MP $18**

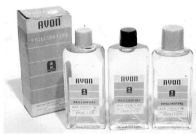

1936-47 *Brilliantine 2oz 52¢* **MP $15** **(Montreal label), $18 boxed**
1944-45 *Brilliantine 2oz 59¢* **MP $18 black lid (Montreal label)**
1943 *Brilliantine 2oz 59¢ (different lid)* **MP $18 (Montreal label)**

If label (right) read **California Perfume Co., Inc., New York-Montreal,** *bottle was issued 1930-1934. If* **Avon Products, Inc., Div.** *is also on label, bottle was issued 1934-1936. (See right)*

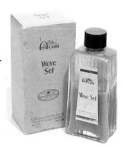

1934-36 *Wave Set 4oz 78¢* **MP $45,** **$55 boxed**

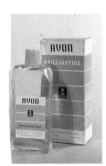

1950-54 *Brilliantine 2oz 59¢* **MP $15,** **$18 boxed with Pasadena Label**

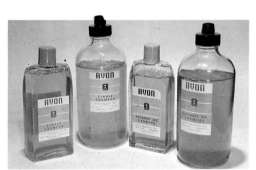

1947-51 *Liquid Shampoo 6oz 51¢* **MP $15,** **$35 Pasadena label without Dist.**
1939-47 *Liquid Shampoo 16oz $1.02* **MP $20,** **$45 with Pasadena label.**
1950-54 *Cocoanut Oil Shampoo (formerly Liquid Shampoo) 6oz 59¢* **MP $18,** *16oz* **MP $30**

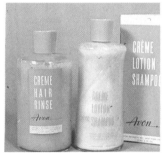

1953-54 *Creme Hair Rinse 6oz 89¢* **MP $20**
1953-54 *Creme Lotion Shampoo 6oz $1* **MP $20,** **$25 boxed**

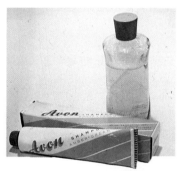

1947-49 *Amber Cream Shampoo 59¢* **MP $22, $30 boxed**
1954-57 *Liquid Cocoanut Oil Shampoo 6oz 79¢* **MP $15,** *16oz $1.59* **MP $25**

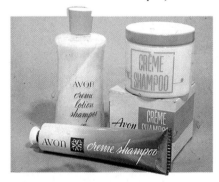

1954-56 *Creme Lotion Shampoo 6oz $1* **MP $18**
1954-60 *Creme Shampoo (tube) 6oz 59¢* **MP $8**
1952-53 *Creme Shampoo (jar) $1* **MP $20,** **$25 boxed**

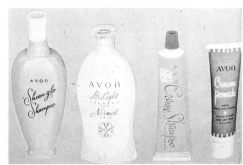

1960-64 *Sheen-Glo Shampoo 6oz $1.19* **MP $6**
1959-62 *Hi-Light Shampoo for Normal (shown), Dry or Oily Hair 6oz $1.19* **MP $5**
1960-62 *Creme Shampoo 2¼oz 69¢* **MP $8**
1961-65 *Cream Pomade 1¾oz 89¢* **MP $4**

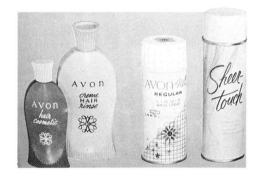

1956-65 *Hair Cosmetic 3oz $1* **MP $3**
1956-64 *Cream Hair Rinse 6oz $1* **MP $3**
1958-64 *AVONnet Regular (shown) or Fine Hair Spray 5oz $1.25* **MP $6**
1961-63 *Sheer-Touch Hair Spray 7oz $1.50* **MP $5**

(See Men's on pages 236-238)

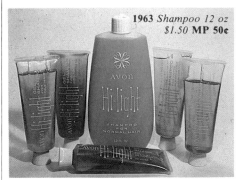

1963 *Shampoo 12 oz*
$1.50 **MP 50¢**

Gel Shampoo. 3oz 79¢
1963 *Oily hair* **MP $1**   **1963** *Dry hair* **MP $1**
1965 *Tinted, bleached, damaged hair* **MP $1**
1963 *Normal hair* **MP $1**
1968 *Dry, bleached or damaged hair* **MP 75¢**

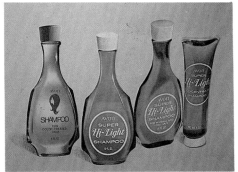

1971-76 *Shampoo for Color-Treated Hair 8oz*
$2 **MP 75¢**
1970-72 *Super Shampoo 12oz $1.79* **MP $1**
1972-75 *Super Shampoo for Normal & Oily Hair*
8oz $1.20 **MP 75¢**
1970-75 *Super Concentrate 5oz $1.50* **MP 75¢**

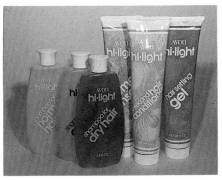

1975-79 *Shampoo for normal, oily and dry*
hair 6.5oz each $1.49 **MP 50¢**
1976 *Creme Rinse 6oz $1.49* **MP 50¢**
1975 *60-second Hair Cond. 6oz $1.49* **MP 50¢**
1975 *Hair Setting Gel $1.49* **MP 50¢**

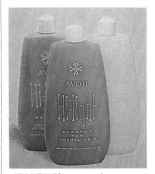

1964-71 *Shampoo for*
bleached or damaged, normal
or oily hair 12oz $1.50
MP 75¢

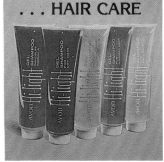

. . . HAIR CARE

1965-67 *Gel Shampoo for dandruff,*
dry, bleached or damaged, normal
or oily hair 9oz $1.75 **MP $1**

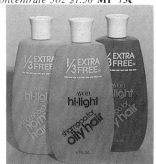

1978 *Shampoo for normal, dry*
or oily hair, extra-size bottle 8.7oz
(1 Campaign only) $1.49 **MP $2**

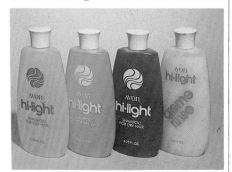

1979-83 *Shampoo for oily, normal and dry*
hair 6¼oz each $1.49 **MP 25¢**
1979 *Creme Rinse 6¼oz $1.49* **MP 50¢**

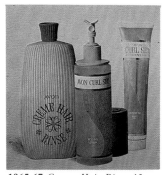

1965-67 *Creme Hair Rinse 12oz*
$1.50 **MP $1**
1964-68 *Curl Set 8oz $1.50* **MP $1**
1966 *Curl Set Concentrate 6oz*
$1.50 **MP $1**

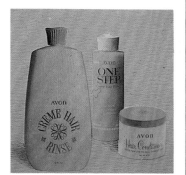

1967 *Creme Hair Rinse 12oz*
$1.50 **MP 75¢**
1968 *One-Step 8oz $1.50* **MP 75¢**
1968 *Hair Conditioner 6oz*
$2.50 **MP 75¢**

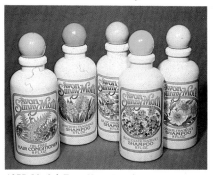

1977-80 *Oil-Free Hair Conditioner* **MP 50¢**
1977-81 *Hyacinth Fragrance Shampoo* **MP 50¢**
1977-80 *Lilac Fragrance Shampoo* **MP 50¢**
1978-80 *Fresh Clover Fragrance Shampoo* **MP 50¢**
1977-81 *Jonquil Fragrance Shampoo* **MP 50¢**

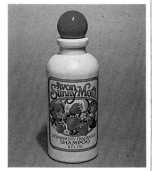

1979-80 *Strawberry*
Fragrance Shampoo
MP 75¢

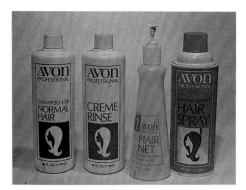

1970's *Professional Hair Products used in*
Avon Beauty Salons, Inc. only. Shampoo 16oz,
Creme Rinse 16oz, Hair Net 8oz and Hair Spray
13oz. Not for retail sale **MP $10 each**

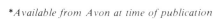

**Available from Avon at time of publication*

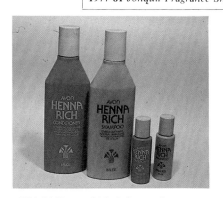

1981-84 *Henna Rich (left to right)*
Conditioner 8oz $3.29 **MP 25¢**
Shampoo 8oz $3.29 **MP 25¢**
Conditioner, trial size 1oz 69¢ **MP 25¢**
Shampoo, trial size 1oz 69¢ **MP 25¢**

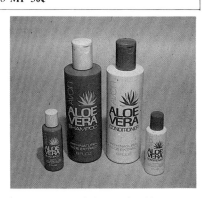

1983 *Aloe Vera (left to right) Shampoo,*
trial size 1oz 39¢ **MP 59¢***
Shampoo 8oz $3.49 **MP $2.50***
Conditioner 8oz $3.49 **MP $2.50***
Conditioner, trial size 1oz 39¢ **MP 59¢***

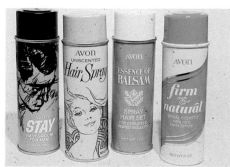
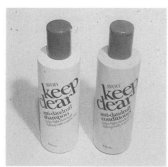
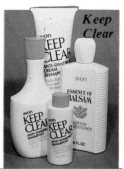
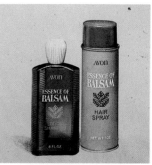

1967-71 *Stay Hair Groom for Men 7oz $1.50* **MP $2**
1968-70 *Unscented Hair Spray 7oz $1.50* **MP $3**
1973-77 *Essence of Balsam Spray Hair Set for Curlers & Heated Rollers 7oz $2.50* **MP $1**
1979-80 *Firm & Natural Herbal Scented Aerosol Hair Spray $2.39* **MP $1.50**

1984 *Keep Clear Anti-Dandruff Shampoo 8oz $3.49* **MP $2***
1984 *Keep Clear Anti-Dandruff Conditioner 8oz $3.49* **MP $2***

. . . HAIR CARE

1978 *Anti-Dandruff Shampoo 7oz $2.29* **MP 50¢**
1979 *Anti-Dandruff Cream Shampoo 7oz $2.49* **MP 50¢**
1977 *Trial Size 2oz 25¢* **MP 50¢**
1973 *Essence of Balsam Conditioner 8oz $3* **MP 50¢**

1973 *Essence of Balsam Shampoo 8oz $3* **MP 50¢**
1974 *Hair Spray 7oz $2.50* **MP $1**

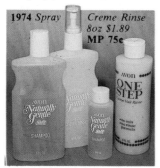
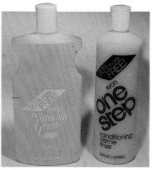
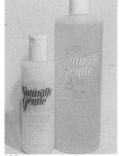
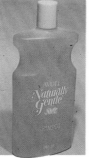
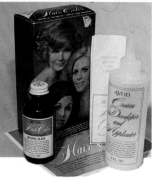

1974 *Spray* **Creme Rinse** *8oz $1.89* **MP 75¢**

Naturally Gentle —
1976 *Shampoo 8oz $1.79* **MP $2**
1976 *Shampoo Trial Size 2oz 25¢ with other purchase* **MP 25¢**
1976 *One Step Creme Hair Rinse 8oz $1.39* **MP 25¢**

1982 *Naturally Gentle Shampoo bonus bottle 24oz (1 Campaign only) $3.99* **MP $1**
1982 *One Step Creme Rinse bonus size 24oz (1 Campaign only) $2.69* **MP $1**

1984 *Naturally Gentle — Essence of Camomile Conditioner 8oz $2.99* **MP $2***
Essence of Camomile Shampoo 16oz $3.99 **MP $3***

1983-84 *Naturally Gentle Shampoo 24oz $5.29* **MP, $1**

1969-70 *Hair Color (Test areas only). Cream Developer, Hair Colorant 2oz each and plastic gloves $2.50* **MP $25 complete**

Protem —

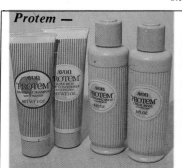
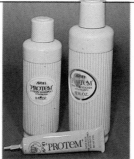
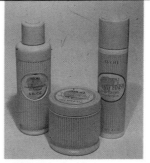
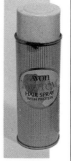
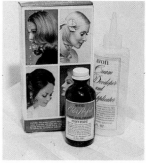

1974 *Dandruff Shampoo 3oz $2.50* **MP 50¢**, *1973 (not shown) $2* **MP $1**
1975 *Super Rich Hair Conditioner 3oz $2.50* **MP 50¢**
1972 *Conditioning Hair Set 6oz $2* **MP 50¢**, *1969 (different lid)* **MP $1**
1975 *Creme Rinse 6oz $3* **MP 50¢**

1971 *Lotion Shampoo 8oz $3* **MP 50¢**
1974 *Hair Conditioner 12oz $5* **MP 50¢**
1975 *Super Rich Hair Conditioner 1oz Trial Size 69¢* **MP 50¢**

1970 *Hair Conditioner 6oz $3* **MP 50¢**
1969 *Creme Shampoo 5oz $2.50* **MP 50¢**
1970 *Instant Finish Hair Gloss 4oz $1.75* **MP 50¢**

1972 *Hair Spray 7oz $2* **MP 50¢**

1971-74 *Color Perfect Hair Color. Cream Developer, Hair Colorant 2oz each and plastic gloves $2.50* **MP $4 complete**

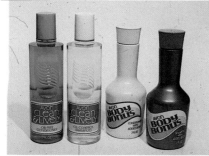
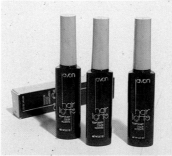
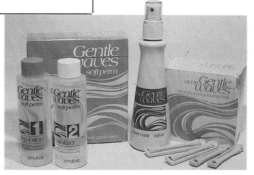

1980-82 *Clean & Lively Oil-Free Conditioner 7oz $2.59* **MP 25¢**
1980-82 *Clean & Lively Oil-Control Shampoo 7oz $2.59* **MP 25¢**
1980-83 *Body Bonus Conditioner 7oz $2.99* **MP 25¢**
1980-83 *Body Bonus Shampoo 7oz $2.99* **MP 25¢**

1981-82 *Hair Lights Color Accents in Moonlight Copper, Sunlight Gold, Starlight Ash ½oz $6* **MP 50¢**

*Available from Avon at time of publication

1982-84 *Gentle Waves Soft Permanent. Waving Lotion and Neutralizer 3.75oz each, Foamer Application Bottle, 100 end papers and instructions $5.79 kit* **MP $3**
1982 *Gentle Waves Hair Mist 6oz $3.49* **MP $3***
1982 *Gentle Wave Curlers, 20 med. & 30 small rods $4.99* **MP $2**

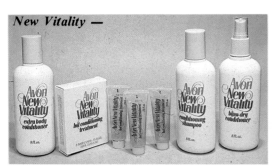

New Vitality —

1978-81 *Extra Body Conditioner 8oz $2.49* **MP 75¢**
1978-82 *Hot Conditioning Treatment. Box of three .75oz tubes $2.49* **MP 50¢**
1978-81 *Conditioning Shampoo 8oz $2.49* **MP 75¢**
1979-81 *Blow-Dry Conditioner 8oz $2.49* **MP 75¢**

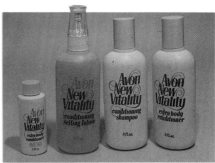

1981-82 *New Vitality —*
Extra Body Conditioner, trial size 1oz 69¢ **MP 75¢**
Conditioning Setting Lotion 8oz $3.29 **MP 75¢**
Conditioning Shampoo 8oz $3.29 **MP 75¢**
Extra Body Conditioner 8oz $3.29 **MP 75¢**

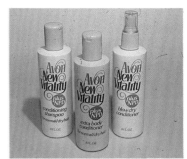

1984 *New Vitality Plus NPD —*
Conditioning Shampoo 8oz $3.49
MP $2.50*
Extra Body Conditioner 8oz $3.49
MP $2.50*
Blow Dry Conditioner 8oz $3.49
MP $2.50*

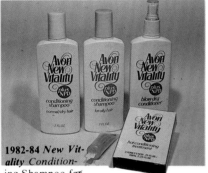

1982-84 *New Vitality* Conditioning Shampoo for
Normal/Dry Hair 7oz $3.29 **MP 50¢**. *Conditioning Shampoo for Oily Hair 7oz $3.29* **MP 50¢**. *Blow Dry Conditioner 7oz $3.29* **MP 50¢**. *Hot Conditioning Treatment, Box of three .75oz tubes $3.29* **MP 50¢**

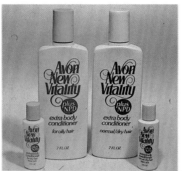

1982-84 *New Vitality Extra Body Conditioner (left to right) — For Oily Hair, trial size 1oz 75¢* **MP 59¢***. *For Oily Hair 7oz $3.29* **MP 50¢**. *For Normal/Dry Hair 7oz $3.29* **MP 50¢**. *For Normal/Dry Hair, trial size 1oz 75¢* **MP 59¢***

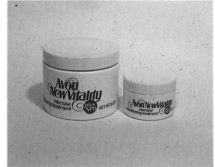

1983 *Intensive Conditioning Treatment 6oz $3.49* **MP $2.50***
1983 *Intensive Conditioning Treatment, trial size 1oz 49¢* **MP 59¢***

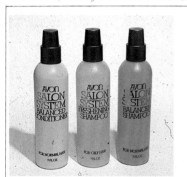

SALON
SYSTEM

1981-83 *Salon System ($4.50 each)*
Balanced Conditioner 7oz **MP 50¢**
Freshening Shampoo 7oz **MP 50¢**
Balanced Shampoo 7oz **MP 50¢**
Freshening Detangler 7oz **MP 50¢**

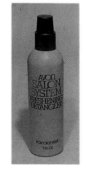

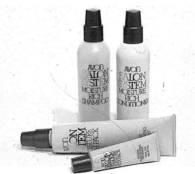

Moisture Rich Shampoo 7oz **MP 50¢**
Moisture Rich Conditioner 7oz **MP 50¢**
Moisture Rich Pack Intense Conditioning Treatment 5oz **MP 50¢**
Trial Size 1oz 69¢ **MP 75¢**

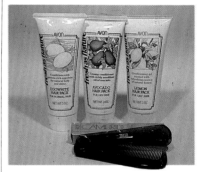

1983 only *Fresh as Nature Hair Beauty Pack in Eggwhite, Avocado or Lemon 3oz $2.49* **MP $1 each**
1982 *Cambridge Collection. Folding Tortoise Comb $3.50* **MP $2.50***

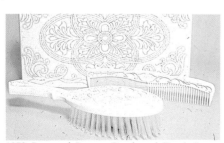

1972 *Past and Present Brush and Comb Set $6* **MP $8**

**BRUSHES
and BRUSH & COMB SETS**

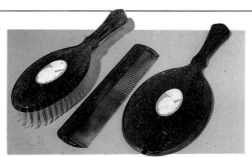

1973 *Cameo Brush and Comb Set. Brush 8" long, comb 7" long $7* **MP $7**
1973 *Cameo Dresser Vanity Mirror, 10" long $5* **MP $7**

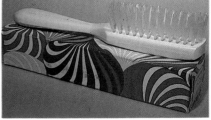

1967 *Professional Style Hairbrush in Ivory or Pink (shown in Xmas box) with purchase of another Hair product $1.50. Value $3* **MP $6, $8 in Xmas box**

*Available from Avon at time of publication

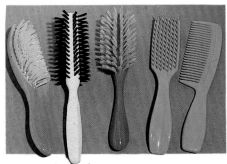

1971 *Flair, 8" long $3* **MP $1**
1975 *Full Round, 8" long $5* **MP $1**
1971 *Natural Bristle, 8" long $9* **MP $3**
1975 *Brush and Comb for Long Wet Hair, both 8" long $4* **MP $2**

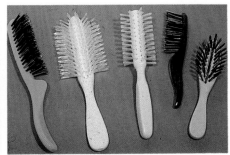

1970 *Styling, 8" $3* **MP $2**
1970 *Half Round, 8" $3* **MP $2**
1977 *Full-Round Brush Petite, 7" $4* **MP $1**
1969 *Mini-Brush, 6" $1.50* **MP $1**
1978 *Flair Mini-Brush 5½" $3.50* **MP $1**

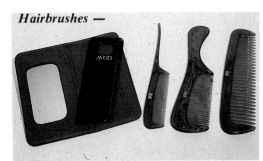

Hairbrushes —

1980 *Pursemates Mirror and Comb. U.S. only $4.99 with a $5 purchase* **MP $9** *retail*
1981 *Cambridge Collection. Rattail Comb, Handled Comb and Wide-Tooth Comb $3 each* **MP $2.50 ea.***
1983 *Cambridge Mini-Handled Comb 6½" $2.50 (not shown)* **MP $1.50**

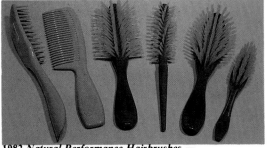

1982 *Natural Performance Hairbrushes —*
Brush and Comb for Long or Wet Hair 8" $5 **MP $3.50**
Half-Round 8" $5 **MP $4***
Blow Dry Curling Brush 8" $5 **MP $2**
Flair 8" $5 **MP $4***
Mini 6" $2.99 **MP $2.50***

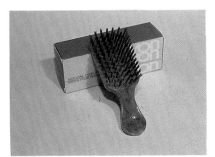

1983 *Natural Performance Men's Club Brush 7" $7* **MP $5***

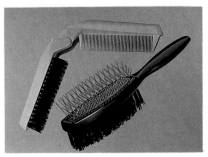

1974 *Folding Comb & Brush $2.75* **MP $2**
1973 *Two-in-One Wig Brush $5.50* **MP $5**

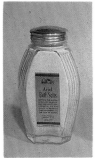

1930-33 *Ariel Bath Salts 63¢* **MP $75**

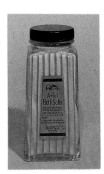

1933-36 *Ariel Bath Salts 10oz 75¢* **MP $60**

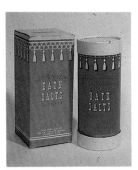

1944-45 *Bath Salts. Jasmine (shown) Vernafleur, Pine and Attention 5oz 69¢* **MP $30**

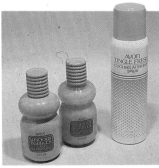

1981 *Luscious Bubbles "Try-It" size Bubble Bath and Foaming Cleanser (2 Campaigns only) 3.5oz $3.50* **MP $1**
1982 *Tingle Fresh 4oz $6.50* **MP 50¢**

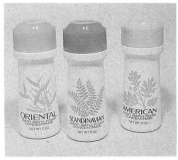

1981-84 *International Bath Foam Collection. Oriental, Scandinavian & American 2oz $6* **MP $1**

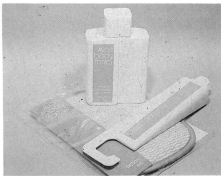
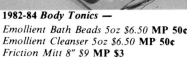

1982-84 *Body Tonics —*
Emollient Bath Beads 5oz $6.50 **MP 50¢**
Emollient Cleanser 5oz $6.50 **MP 50¢**
Friction Mitt 8" $9 **MP $3**

*Available from Avon at time of publication

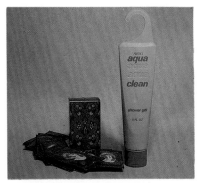

1983 *Victorian Bubble Bath Concentrate. Ten 2oz packets $3* **MP $2 complete**
1983 *Aqua Clean Shower Gel 5oz $5* **MP $2.50***

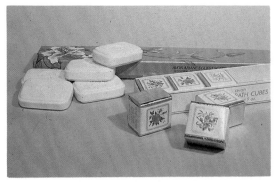

1983 *Five Guest Soaps in Tasha, Soft Musk, Odyssey, Candid, Timeless, Ariane or Foxfire 1oz ea. (2 brochures only) $6* **MP $4**
1984 *Floral Bath Cubes in Roses, Roses, Wild Jasmine, Honeysuckle, Hawaiian White Ginger. Six 1.5oz cubes $6* **MP $5***

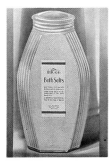 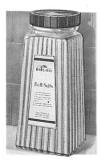 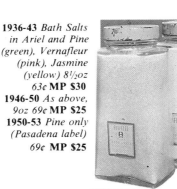 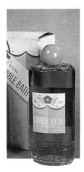 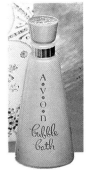

1936-43 *Bath Salts in Ariel and Pine (green), Vernafleur (pink), Jasmine (yellow) 8½oz 63¢* **MP $30**
1946-50 *As above, 9oz 69¢* **MP $25**
1950-53 *Pine only (Pasadena label) 69¢* **MP $25**

1929-33 *Bath Salts 10oz 75¢* **MP $80**

1933-36 *Bath Salts 10oz 75¢* **MP $60**

1944-45 *Bubble Bath 8oz $2.25* **MP $42, $52 boxed**

1951 *Bubble Bath 4oz $1.29* **MP $20, $25 boxed**

1959 *Bubble Bath 8oz $1.69* **MP $4**

BATH OILS, BUBBLES AND SALTS

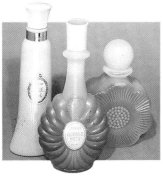 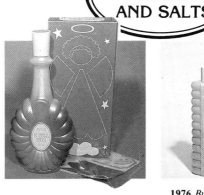 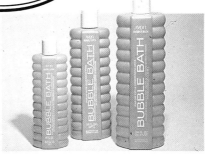 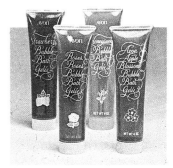

1964 *Bubble Bath 8oz $1.98* **MP $4**
1967 *Bubble Bath 8oz $2* **MP $2**
1975 *Bubble Blossom Bubble Bath 14oz $7* **MP $3**

1968 *Santa's Helper. Bubble Bath 8oz $2* **MP $7 with Xmas box**

1976 *Bubble Bath 8oz and 16oz with ingredients listed on front $3 & $5.50* **MP $2* and $4***
1980 *Bubble Bath 24oz $8* **MP $7***

Bubble Bath Gelee:
1972 *Strawberry 4oz $3* **MP $1**
1975 *Roses, Roses 4oz $3.50* **MP 50¢**
1977 *Apple Blossom 4oz $3.50* **MP 50¢**
1977 *Honeysuckle 4oz $3.50* **MP 50¢**

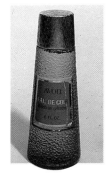 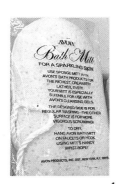 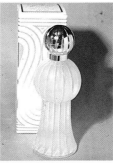 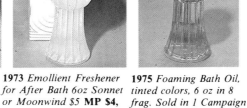 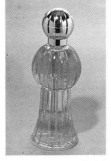 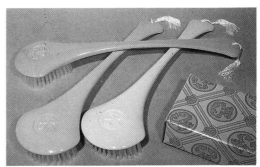

1972 *Eau De Cool 6oz $5* **MP $4.50**

1972 *Avon Bath Mitt $1.50* **MP $3.50**

1973 *Emollient Freshener for After Bath 6oz Sonnet or Moonwind $5* **MP $4, $5 boxed**
1974 *Imperial Garden and Charisma* **MP $4, $5 boxed**

1975 *Foaming Bath Oil, tinted colors, 6 oz in 8 frag. Sold in 1 Campaign only $6* **MP $11 with Bath Oil label, $13 boxed**

Avon Bath Brushes — 15½" long:
1977 *Blue $8.50* **MP $6**
1978 *Yellow and Ivory $8.50* **MP $6**

Trial Sizes —

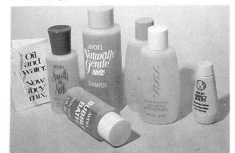 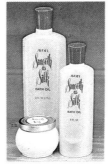 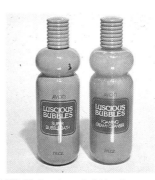 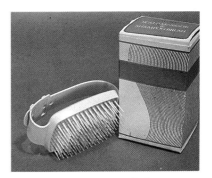

1978 *Smooth as Silk Bath Oil 1oz & "29¢ off" coupon. 29¢ with purchase* **MP 40¢**
1976 *Naturally Gentle Shampoo 2oz 25¢ with purchase* **MP 40¢**
1977 *Skin-So-Soft 1oz 25¢ with purchase* **MP 40¢ (blue cap), $1 (white cap)**
1977 *Bubble Bath 1oz 25¢ with purchase* **MP 25¢**

1978 *Smooth as Silk Bath Oil 8oz $5* **MP $6***
1978 *Smooth as Silk Bath Oil 16oz $8.50* **MP $9***
1980 *Smooth as Silk Skin Softener 5oz $5.50* **MP $4***

1980-83 *Luscious Bubbles Super Bubble Bath 7oz $5* **MP 50¢**
1980-83 *Luscious Bubbles Foaming Creamy Cleanser 7oz $5* **MP 50¢**

1973-75 *Scalp Massage and Shampoo Brush $1.75* **MP $1.75, $2 boxed**

*Available from Avon at time of publication

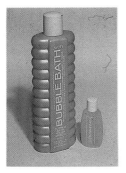

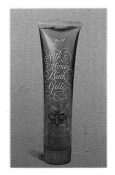

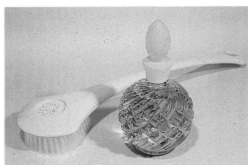

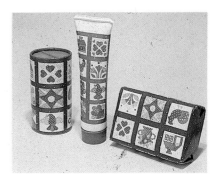

1984 *Fresh Green Bubble Bath 16oz $7* **MP $4***. *24oz $9* **MP $6***
1984 *Fresh Green Bubble Bath, trial size 1oz 49¢* **MP 25¢**

1972 *Silk & Honey Bath Gelee 4oz $3* **MP $1.25**

1981 *Bath Brush, beige 15½" $12.50* **MP $10***
1981 *Soft Swirls Bath Decanter. Skin-So-Soft or Smooth as Silk Bath Oil 8oz $12* **MP $7**

1981 *Winter Tuck-Ins. Powder Sachet 1.25oz $2* **MP 50¢**
Rich Moisture Hand Cream 1oz $2 **MP 50¢**
Soap 3oz $2 **MP $2**

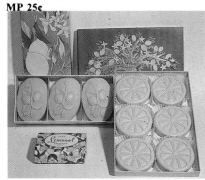

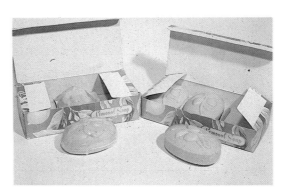

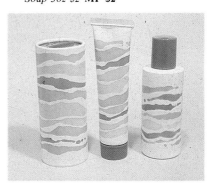

1954-58 *Lemonol Soap. Three cakes $1* **MP $28**
1966 *Lemonol Soap Slices. Six 1½oz cakes $2.25* **MP $26**
1964 *Lemonol Soap 3oz 39¢* **MP $5**

1950-54 *Lemonol Soap. Three cakes 79¢* **MP $35**
1962-63 *Lemonol Soap. Three cakes (flat edge) $1.19* **MP $28**

1981 *Pretty Portables — 69¢ each with $5 purchase. Ultra Talc, choice of 7 fragrances 1.5oz* **MP 50¢**. *Hand Cream, choice Rich Moisture, Vita Moist, Moisture Garden 1oz* **MP 50¢**. *Bubble Bath 2oz* **MP 50¢**

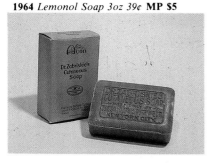

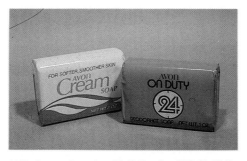

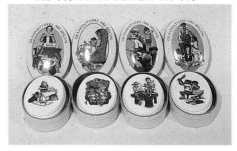

1935-36 only *(with G.H. Seal on box) Dr. Zabriskie's Soap 3oz 26¢* **MP $40 boxed**

1981 *Cream Soap 3oz $1.49/3 cakes* **MP $1.49/3 cakes***
1982 *On Duty Soap 3oz $1.49/3 cakes* **MP $1.49/3 cakes***

1983 *Grandmothers Are Special. 2.5oz decal soap in coordinated tin box. Baking or Reading $7.50* **MP $6**
1983 *Grandfathers Are Special. 2.5oz decal soap in coordinated tin box. Fishing or Mending $7.50* **MP $6**

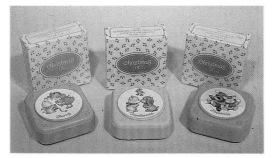

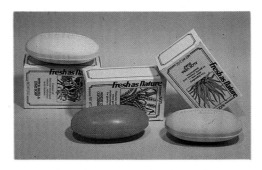

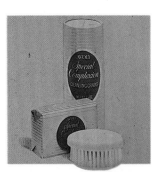

1983 *Christmas Wishes Decal Soaps 2oz each (left to right)*
"Sharing" Bayberry frag. $3 **MP $2 boxed**
"Togetherness" Mistletoe & Holly frag. $3 **MP $2 boxed**
"Happiness' Mint frag. $3 **MP $2 boxed**

1982 *Fresh As Nature Soap in Witch-Hazel & Lyme, Wheat Germ & Glycerine or Aloe Vera 3oz $2.50* **MP $1.50***

*Available from Avon at time of publication

1972 *Special Complexion Cleansing Grains 4.5oz $1.75* **MP $2**
1969 *Special Complexion Bar 3oz 75¢* **MP 3**
1970 *Complexion Beauty Brush 2½" $3* **MP $3**

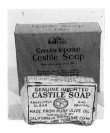
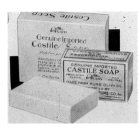
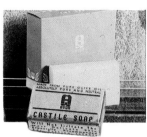
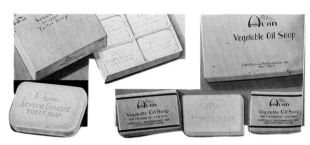

1929-30 *Castile Soap 2 cakes 60¢* **MP $50**

1930-37 *Castile Soap 2 cakes 62¢* **MP $40**

1937-40 *Castile Soap 2 cakes 62¢* **MP $35**
1941-43 *(not shown)* **Genuine Imported** *dropped from wrapper* **MP $40**

1930-36 *Savona Bouquet Toilet Soap. Six 4¹/₂oz cakes 50¢* **MP $100**

1930-36 *Vegetable Oil Soap, 3 cakes 45¢* **MP $80**

INDIVIDUAL and BOXED SOAPS

"Vegetable Oil Soap contains soothing vegetable oils to prevent dry, taut or chapped skin when hard water must be used."

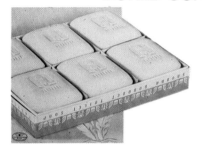
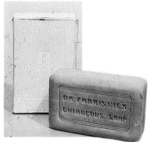
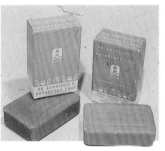
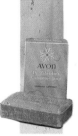
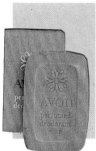

1936-43 *Savona Bouquet Toilet Soap. Box of 6 cakes 51¢* **MP $75**

1942-46 *Dr. Zabriskie's Soap 3oz 33¢* **MP $25 boxed**

1936-42 *Dr. Zabriskie's Soap 3oz 26¢* **MP $35**
1936 only *With CPC label on box* **MP $40 boxed**
1947-54 *Dr. Zabriskie's Soap (Pasadena label) 3oz 43¢* **MP $12 boxed**

1954-62 *Dr. Zabriskie's Soap 3oz in 4-A designed box 43¢* **MP $16**

1963 only *Perfumed Deo. Soap boxed 3oz 39¢* **MP $14**
1964 only *Perf. Deo. Soap, wrapped (not shown) 39¢* **MP $13**

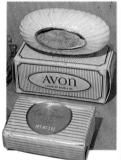
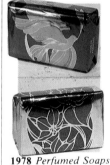
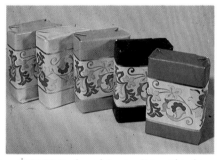
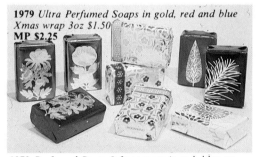

1966 *Complexion Bar 4oz $1.25* **MP $4**
1969 *Special Complexion Bar 3oz 75¢* **MP $3**

1978 *Perfumed Soaps (top) in 8 frag., red, blue or green Xmas pkg. 3oz each $1.25* **MP $3**
1977 *Perfumed Soaps (bottom) in 6 frag., red, blue or green Xmas pkg. 3oz each $1.25* **MP $3**

1974-75 *Perfumed Soaps, Xmas pkg. 3oz each: Field Flowers, Sonnet, Roses, Roses, Moonwind, Bird of Paradise, (Charisma not shown) $1.25* **MP $4**

CHRISTMAS WRAPPED SOAPS

1979 *Ultra Perfumed Soaps in gold, red and blue Xmas wrap 3oz $1.50* **MP $2.25**

1979 *Perfumed Soap, 8 fragrances in red, blue or green foil (center) $1.50* **MP $2.25**
1980 *Perfumed Soap in Moonwind or Charisma in red Xmas wrap $2.25* **MP $2.25**
1980 *Bar Soap for Men in 3 fragrances in brown & white Xmas wrap $1.75* **MP $2.25**
1980 *Ultra Perfumed Soap in silver Xmas wrap 3oz $2.25* **MP $2.25**

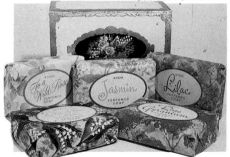
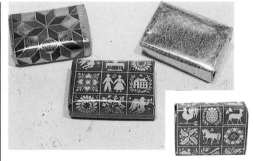
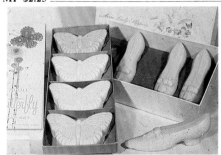

1963 *Soap Treasures with choice of Soaps, 13 frag. available. Only Lilac and Lily of the Valley issued with floral wraps; all others in solid color wraps with white 4-A design band. (Incorrect assortment shown — see p. 168) $1.95* **MP $35**

1982 *(top) Perfumed Soap in 7 Ultra frag. 3oz $2.25* **MP $2**
1981 *Perfumed Soap in 9 Ultra frag. 3oz $2.25* **MP $2**
1982 *Perfumed Soap in Moonwind, Charisma, Sweet Honesty 3oz $2.25* **MP $2**
1982 *Men's Bar Soap in 4 frag. 3oz $2.25* **MP $2**

1966 *Butterfly Soap Set. Four 1¹/₂oz cakes $2* **MP $25**
1965 *Lady Slippers Gift Soap. Four 1¹/₂oz cakes $2.25* **MP $27**

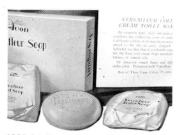

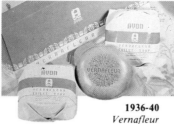

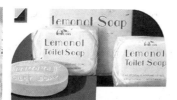

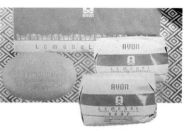

1930-36 *Vernafleur Cold Cream Toilet Soap. Box of 3 cakes 75¢* **MP $80**

1936-40 *Vernafleur Cold Cream Toilet Soap. Box of 3 cakes 77¢* **MP $75**

1930-36 *Lemonol Toilet Soap. Box of 3 cakes 50¢* **MP $80** *Carton of 12 cakes (not shown) $1.75* **MP $130**

1936-40 *Lemonol Toilet Soap. Box of 3 cakes 51¢* **MP $65** *Carton of 12 cakes $1.79* **MP $105**

Vernafleur Toilet Soap, a floral-scented soap containing basic cold cream, was especially suited for skin constantly exposed to the outdoors.

Lemonol Soap was also used as a shampoo to cleanse and lighten blonde and auburn hair instead of a lemon rinse.

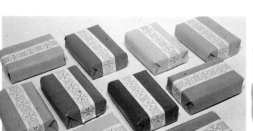

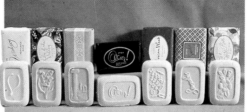

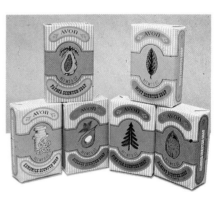

1961-64 *Assortment of Soaps, all 3oz each, 39¢ each* **MP $6 each**
Floral in violet wrap
Lemonol in yellow wrap
Cotillion in pink wrap
Here's My Heart in blue
Rose Geranium and To A Wild Rose in rose wrap
Persian Wood in red wrap
Royal Jasmine in chartreuse
Somewhere in lilac wrap
Royal Pine in green wrap
Topaze in yellow wrap

Assortment of Soaps, all 3oz each:
1964 *Wishing 39¢* **MP $6**
1963 *Lily of the Valley 39¢* **MP $6**
1961 *Topaze 39¢* **MP $5**
1965 *Occur! 49¢* **MP $5**
1964 *Persian Wood 39¢* **MP $5**
1966 *Somewhere 49¢* **MP $5**
1964 *To A Wild Rose 39¢* **MP $6**

1971 *Country Store Scented Soaps 3oz Papaya, Mint, Camomile, Avocado, Pine Tar, Almond 75¢* **MP $2.25**

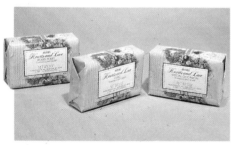

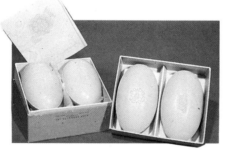

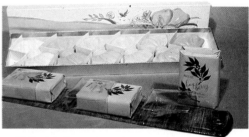

1981 *Hearts and Lace Glycerine Soap in Roses, Roses (pink), Special Occasion (red) and Lilac (lavender) 3oz $2* **MP $2**

1945 *Facial Soap, 2 cakes with "Personal Note" 59¢* **MP $32**
1955 *Facial Soap, 2 cakes 89¢* **MP $21**

1962 *Gift Bows. Six cakes $2.25* **MP $32**
1967 *Bayberry Gift Soaps. Caddy Holder contains three 3oz Bayberry scented soaps $3* **MP $26 complete**

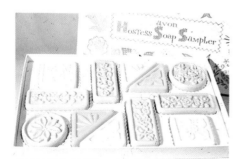

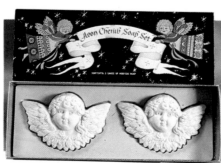

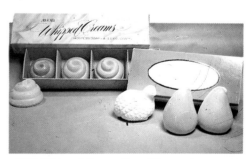

1964 *Hostess Soap Sampler. 12 molded cakes $2.50* **MP $25**

1966 *Cherub Soap Set. Two 3oz cakes $2* **MP $25**

(See Men's p. 240, Children's p. 259)

1968 *Whipped Cream. Four 1½oz each soaps $3* **MP $12**
1968 *Partridge and Two Pear Soaps 2oz each $3* **MP $9**

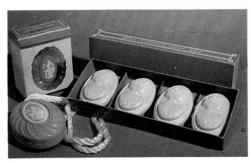

1969 *Cameo Soap with rope 4oz $1.75* **MP $7**
1966 *Cameo Soaps. Four 1½oz cakes $2* **MP $21**

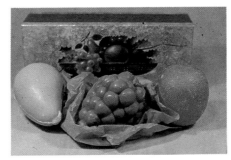

1969 *Fruit Bouquet Perfumed Soaps 2oz each $3* **MP $12**

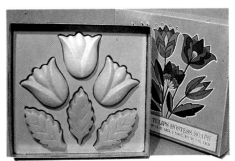

1970 *Spring Tulips. Six cakes boxed $3.50* **MP $13**

... BOXED SOAPS

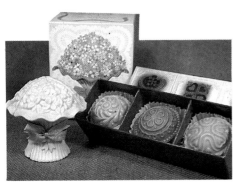

1972 *Hostess Bouquet. Three 2oz cakes $3.50* **MP $8**
1971 *Cupcake Soap Set. Three 2oz cakes $3* **MP $9**

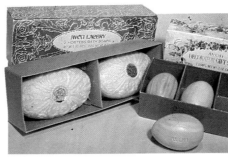

1972 *Lacery Hostess Bath Soaps, 2 cakes 5oz each $4* **MP $8**
1969 *Decorator Gift Soaps. Three 2oz cakes $3* **MP $11**

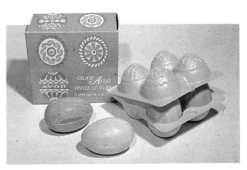

1971 *Grade Avon Hostess Soaps, 4 cakes 2oz each $4.50* **MP $13**

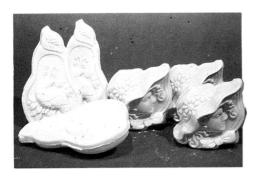

1974 *Partridge 'N Pear Hostess Fragranced Soaps $4* **MP $7**
1974 *Golden Beauties Hostess Soaps. Three 2oz soaps $3* **MP $7**

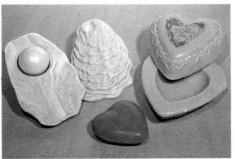

1972 *Hidden Treasure. Bird of Paradise Perfume "pearl" ⅛oz and two Soaps $6* **MP $13**
1978 *A Token of Love. Pink decal Soap holds red heart-shaped Soap 6oz total $6* **MP $7**

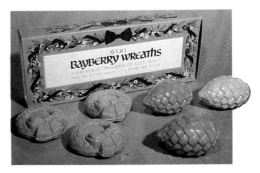

1975 *Bayberry Wreaths. Three 1½oz Bayberry scented Soaps $5* **MP $7**
1970 *Pine Cone Soaps (box not shown). Three Pine scented 2oz Soaps $3* **MP $10**

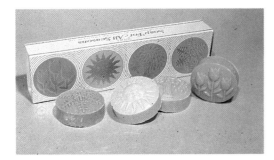

1973 *Soap For All Seasons, 4 cakes 1½oz each $3.50* **MP $8**

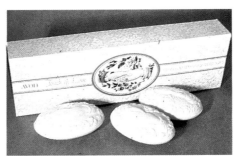

1975 *Touch of Love. Three 2oz Spring Lavender fragranced Soaps $5* **MP $7**

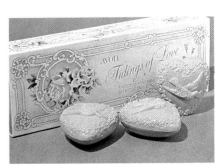

1975 *Tidings of Love. Three 2oz Hostess fragranced Soaps $4* **MP $7**

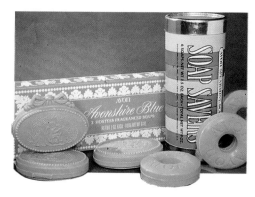

1973 *Avonshire Blue Hostess Soaps. Three 2oz cakes $3* **MP $8**
1973 *Soap Savers. Six spearmint scented 1½oz Soaps $4.50* **MP $8, $1 each soap**

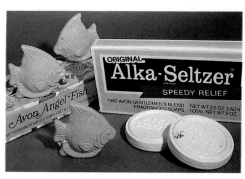

1978 *Angel Fish. Three 2oz Soaps $5.50* **MP $7**
1978 *Alka-Seltzer Soaps. Two 2½oz cakes in Special Occasion fragrance for her and Gentlemen's Blend for him $5* **MP $6**

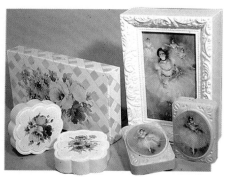

1978 *Country Garden Hostess Soaps. Two 3oz Special Occasion fragranced decal Soaps $6* **MP $7**
1978 *Beauty in Motion Ballet Picture and Soaps. Two 3½oz Special Occasion fragranced decal Soaps. Lid serves as framed ballet picture to hang $10* **MP $10**

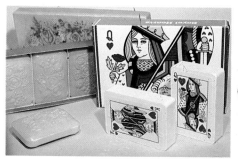

1959 *Hostess Bouquet Soaps. Four guest-size cakes $1.39* **MP $27**
1978 *Royal Hearts Hostess Soaps. Two 3oz Festive fragranced decal Soaps $6* **MP $7**

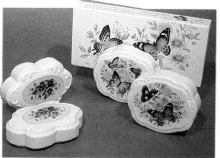

1976 *Bouquet of Pansies. Two 3oz Special Occasion fragranced decal Soaps $5.50* **MP $6**
1977 *Butterflies Hostess Soaps. Two 3oz Special Occasion fragranced decal Soaps $5.50* **MP $6**

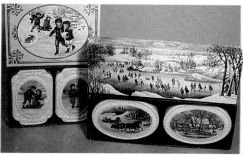

1977 *Winter Frolics. Two 3oz decal Soaps $5.50* **MP $6**
1976 *Winterscape Boxed Soaps, two 3oz Special Occasion fragranced decal Soaps $5.50* **MP $6**

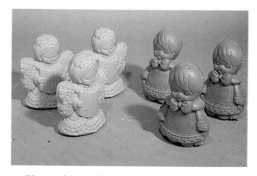

1975 *Angel Lace Hostess fragranced Soaps. Three 2oz cakes $4* **MP $7 boxed**
1976 *Little Choir Boys Hostess Soaps. Three 2oz cakes $5* **MP $6 boxed**

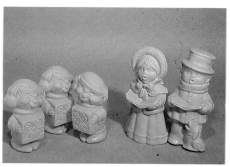

1977 *Merry Elfkins Guest Soaps. Three 2oz Festive fragranced cakes $5.50* **MP $6**
1978 *Christmas Carollers. Two 3oz Special Occasion fragranced Soaps $5.50* **MP $6**

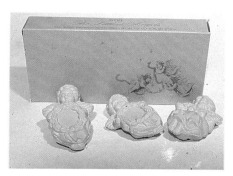

1980 *Littlest Angels Hostess Soaps, 3 cakes 2oz each $5.50* **MP $6**

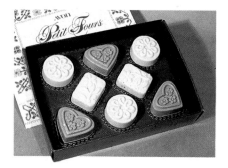

1975 *Petit Fours. Eight 1oz Soaps in 3 shapes $6* **MP $9**

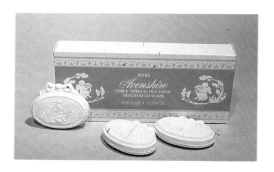

1979 *Avonshire Hostess Soaps. Three 2oz Special Occasion fragranced Soaps $6* **MP $7**

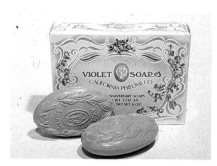

1980 *California Perfume Co. 1980 Anniversary Soaps. Two 3oz Violet scented Soaps $5.50* **MP $6**

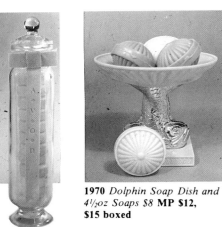

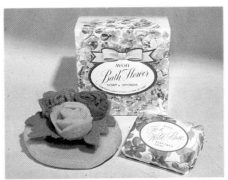

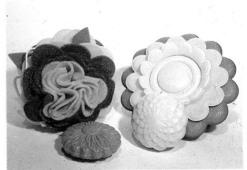

1970 Dolphin Soap Dish and 4½oz Soaps $8 **MP $12, $15 boxed**

1965 Decorator Soap Miniatures. 12 cakes 9¾" high $4.50 **MP $20, $25 boxed**

1965 Bath Flower Set. Flowered sponge and 3oz cake To A Wild Rose Soap $2.50 **MP $17 boxed**

1969 Bath Blossoms. Flower-shaped Sponge with loop to hang up and 3oz Soap $3.50 **MP $10**
1979 Bath Blossoms Sponge serves as soap holder for 3oz Special Occasions Soap $8 **MP $8**

SOAP DISHES AND CONTAINERS

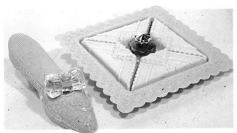

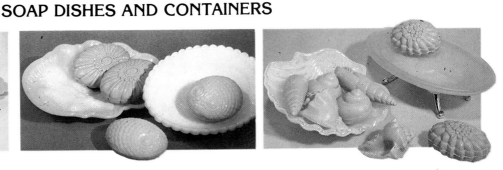

1970 Lady Slipper Soap 5oz with Glass Bow Perfume ⅛oz Charisma or Cotillion $5 **MP $15 Soap and Perfume MP $6 each**
1972 Fragrance and Frills. Perfume ⅛oz and four 1½oz Soaps in Field Flowers or Bird of Paradise $6.75 **MP $10**

1970 Heavenly Soap Dish, milkglass. Two 2oz Soaps $5 **MP $12**
1971 Owl Soap Dish, two 2oz owl Soaps $4.50 **MP $10**

1972 Gift of the Sea. Six 1oz seashell Soaps and dish $6 **MP $11**
1971 Decorator Soap Dish and two 2 oz Soaps $7 **MP $9**

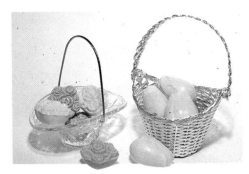

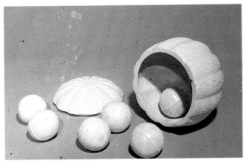

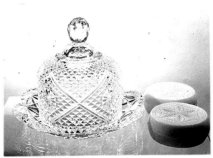

1972 Flower Basket, five 1oz Hostess fragranced Soaps $6 **MP $8**
1978 Treasure Basket. Handwoven aluminum basket and four 1½oz Soaps $13.50 **MP $11**

1973 Melon Ball Guest Soaps. Plastic "melon" with six 1oz melon scented soap balls $4.50 **MP $8 complete, $4 container only**

1973 Butter Dish and three 3oz Hostess scented Soaps $8.50 **MP $14**

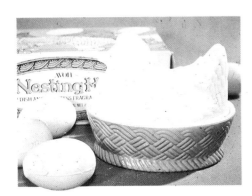

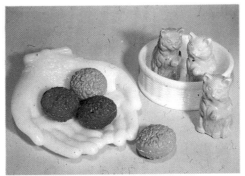

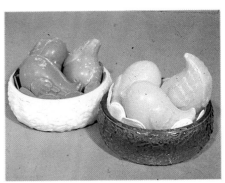

1973 Nesting Hen Soap Dish and four 2oz Soaps $8.50 **MP $12**

1969 Touch of Beauty Soap Dish (made in Mexico) and two dark pink and two light pink Soaps $5 **MP $13**
1973 Sittin' Kittens Soap Dish, three 2oz Hostess scented molded Soaps $5 **MP $6**

1973 Love Nest Soap Dish, three 1oz Soaps $4 **MP $6**
1978 Love Nest Soap Dish (green) three 1½oz Special Occasion scented Soaps $6.50 **MP $6**

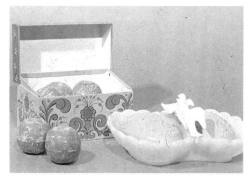

1974 *Recipe Treasures, Metal recipe box holds five 1½oz orange scented balls of Soap* **$6 MP $8**
1974 *Lovebirds Soap Dish and two 4oz Hostess scented Soaps* **$8 MP $10**

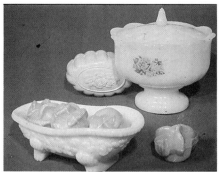

1974 *Beauty Buds Soap Dish, four 1oz Hostess scented Soaps* **$7.50 MP $8**
1974 *Hostess Blossoms Flower Arranger Soap Dish and Hostess Fragrance Soap 4oz Adaptable plastic lid serves as flower holder* **$8 MP $10**

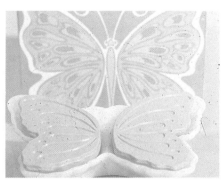

1975 *Wings of Beauty Soap Dish and two 2oz Hostess scented Soaps* **$7.50 MP $9**

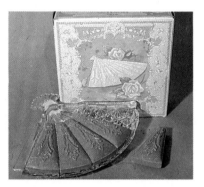

1974 *Hostess Fancy Soap Dish and five 1oz fan-shaped Soaps* **$7.50 MP $9**

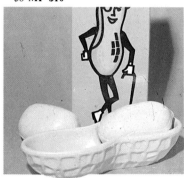

1975 *Nutty Soap. Plastic shell dish with two 3oz peanut-scented Soaps* **$6 MP $6**

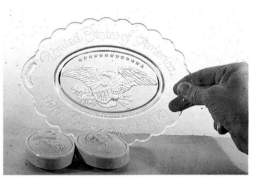

1975 *Bicentennial Plate and two 3oz Special Occasion scented Soaps* **$9 MP $10**

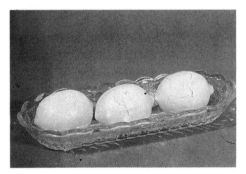

1975 *Sunny Lemon Soap Dish and three 2oz lemon scented Soaps* **$6 MP $7**

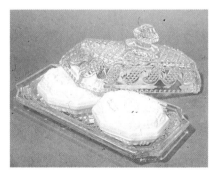

1975 *Crystalucent Covered Butter Dish and two 3oz Soaps* **$11 MP $11**

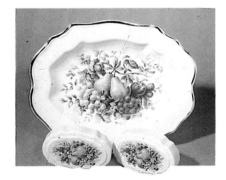

1976 *Nature Bountiful Ceramic Plate, edged in 22k gold and two 5oz Special Occasion scented decal Soaps* **$25 MP $25, $15 plate only**

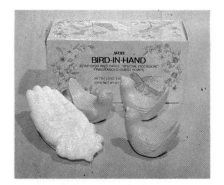

1979 *Bird-In-Hand Soap Dish and three 1.5oz Special Occasion scented Soaps* **$8.50 MP $9 boxed**

(See also Fragrance Lines and Collections, p. 188)

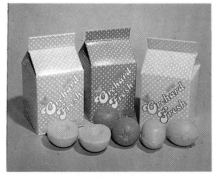

1980 *Orchard Fresh Guest Soaps, six 1oz Peach, Orange or Lemon scented Soaps per carton* **$6 MP $6**

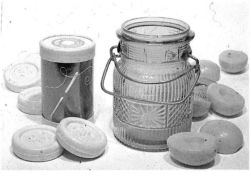

1977 *Button, Button Guest Soaps, five 1oz Special Occasion scented Soaps in cardboard "spool"* **$6 MP $6**

1977 *Country Peaches Soap Jar, six 1oz peach scented Soaps* **$8.50 MP $7**

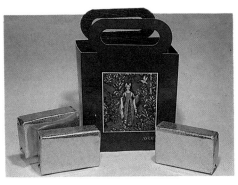

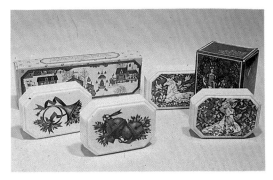

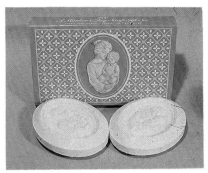

1981 *Holiday Gift Soaps. Choice of 3 Ultra Soaps in tapestry-designed cardboard bag 3oz each (2 Campaigns only) $7* **MP $6**

1982 *Country Christmas Decal Soaps. Two 3oz cakes $6* **MP $5**
1981 *Tapestry Hostess Decal Soaps. Two 3oz cakes $6.50* **MP $6**

1983 *Mother's Joy Hostess Soaps. Two 3oz $5.50* **MP $5**

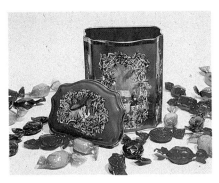

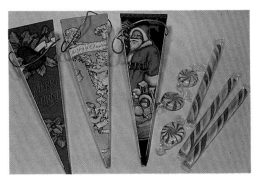

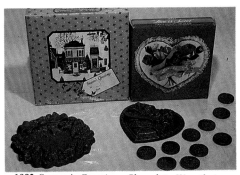

1981 *Holiday Treats. Filled hard candy in "1981" dated tin canister 9oz (2 Campaigns only) $8.99* **MP $4 canister only**

1982 *Country Christmas Ornament with Candy. Cardboard cones with two 4oz bags of peppermint candy sticks and starlights. Hanging cord inc. $8.99 ea. set* **MP $1 each cone only**

1982 *Season's Greetings Chocolate Wreath 4oz (2 Campaigns only) $6.99* **MP $3**
1983 *Love is Sweet Chocolate Heart 4oz (2 Campaigns only) $6.99* **MP $3**
1982 *Love is Sweet Chocolate samples. Ten per pkg. 50¢* **MP 50¢**

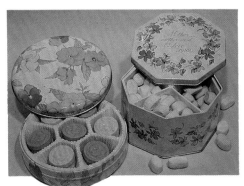

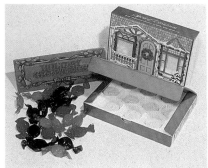

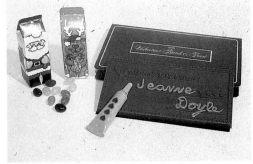

1983 *Pansy Patch Mints in tin canister 4oz (2 Campaigns only) $8.99* **MP $3 canister only**
1982 *Loving Treats Buttermints in collector's tin dated "Mother's Day 1982" 7oz (2 Campaigns only) $9.99* **MP $4 container only**

1983 *Holiday Greetings Christmas Candy in Coffee, Rum and Cinnamon flavors 4oz (2 Campaigns only) $3.99* **MP $4**
1983 *Spirit of Christmas Cream Mint Wreaths 4oz (2 Campaigns only) $4.99* **MP $5**

1983 *Jolly Jelly Beans in cherry, marshmallow & lime flavors in Santa or Rudolph cardboard-ornament box 89¢ each* **MP $1**
1984 *Valentine Bank & Trust Inscribable Chocolate 4oz and 3oz tube of frosting (2 Campaigns only) $6.99* **MP $7**

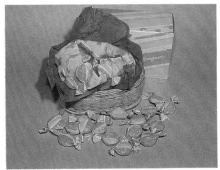

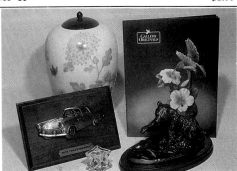

1984 *Mother's Day Candy Bouquet. Lime and grape candy with chocolate centers in wicker basket 7oz (2 Campaigns only) $6.99* **MP $7**

Gallery Originals —

Gallery Originals were tested for Christmastime selling in one Branch only in 1982, the Kansas City Branch. The program passed its test marketing with flying colors and Gallery Originals were sold nationwide for the 1983 Holiday Season. The 1984 Gallery Catalog introduced a selection of Museum Reproductions from four of America's foremost museums.

1983 *Heirloom Beauty Porcelain Ginger Jar 10½" $75* **MP $85**
1983 *Gallery Originals Catalog* **MP 50¢**
1982-83 *Sentimental Journey Car Plaque. 1955 Thunderbird (shown) or 1953 Corvette $18.50 each* **MP $25**
1982-84 *Star Bright Stackable Star Crystal Candleholder $5 each* **MP $7**
1982-83 *Wonders of Wildlife Grizzly Bear Figurine, Bronze-tone cast metal on mahogany base $65* **MP $75**

GALLERY ORIGINALS

Christmas Cards

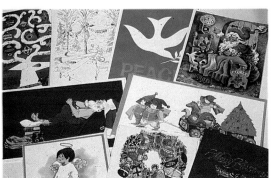

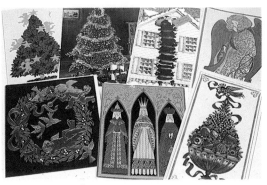

left top —
#4 Ornamental Reindeer $8 **MP $1.50**
#15 Winter Wonderland $8 **MP $1.50**
#11 Dove of Peace $9 **MP $1.75**
#22 Wake Up, Comet $6 **MP $1**
center —
#36 Snoozing Santa $7 **MP $1.25**
#16 Bringing Home Tree $5 **MP 75¢**

right, top —
#12 Christmas Tree Cherubs $10 **MP $2**
#31 Christmas Eve $7 **MP $1.25**
#30 Stack of Good Wishes $6 **MP $1**
#29 The Christmas Angel $8 **MP $1.25**

bottom —
#34 Little Angel $4 **MP $1**
#20 Christmas Wreath $4 **MP $1**
#28 Merry Christmas $5 **MP $1**

1971 Christmas Greeting Cards. *Designed exclusively for Avon, were sold in a Test Market area by a limited number of Representatives in Newark Branch. There were 36 different designs, 25 cards of one design in a box. MP is for 1 card w/env.*

bottom —
#9 Christmas Wreath Cherubs $10 **MP $2**
#13 The Three Kings $7 **MP $1.25**
#35 Christmas Centerpiece $7 **MP $1.25**

Vitamins

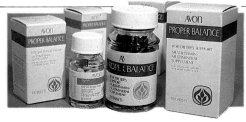

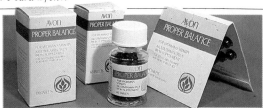

In 1979 Proper Balance Vitamins were offered in test markets, in 8 Divisions, Springdale Branch. Due to results over the last three years, Avon has made the decision not to expand its Vitamin business further at this time.

*The Whole Family Multivitamin Supplement, 60-tablet size $3.49 **MP $3** 100 size $4.99 **MP $4***

*Dieter's Support Multivitamin Multimineral Supplement, 60-tablet size $4.49 **MP $4** 100 size $6.49 **MP $5***

*Woman's Vitality Mutli vitamin/Plus Iron Suppt. 60-tablet $3.99 **MP $3** 100 size $5.99 **MP $5***

*14-day trial size Woman's Vitality Vitamins, 1 per customer during C-14 & 15, 1979 49¢ **MP $2***

Avon Books

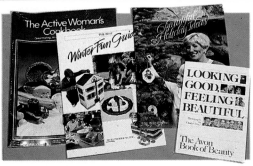

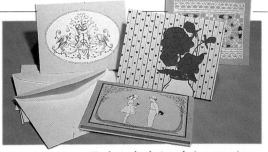

1980 *The Active Woman's Cookbook, U.S. only, with purchase $2.50 **MP $3***
1981 *Winter Fun Guide, U.S. only, one campaign with purchase $2.99 **MP $4***
1980 *Beautiful Holiday Ideas, U.S. only, one campaign with purchase $2.99 **MP $4***
1981 *Looking Good, Feeling Beautiful. Abridged paperback version of hardcover book. Sold with purchase in C-12 only 50¢ **MP $2.50***

1981 *Love Notes. Exclusively designed. 4 notes w/eps. Free with purchase in C-2, U.S. only **MP $1.50** set of 4*

Cologne and Toilet Water Atomizers

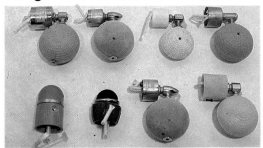

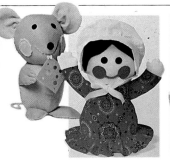

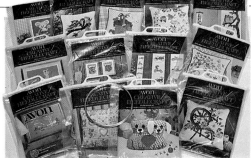

24-karat gold-plated with rubber bulbs—
1955 A. *Fits Golden Promise Cologne and Toilet Water $1 **MP $7***
1950 B. *Toilet Water Atomizer fits Flowertime, Lily of the Valley, Cotillion and To A Wild Rose 89¢ **MP $8***
1955 C *Fits Cotillion and Bright Night Cologne and Cotillion, Forever Spring, Nearness and To A Wild Rose Toilet Water $1 **MP $7***
1954 D. *Young Hearts Cologne Atomizer from Neat and Sweet Set **MP $7***
1950 E. *Fits Perfumed Deodorant only 49¢ **MP $4***
1950 F. *Fits Deodorant for Men only 49¢ **MP $4***
1955 G. *Fits Nearness, Forever Spring, Quaintance, To A Wild Rose Cologne and Quaintance Toilet Water $1 **MP $7***
1942 H. *Fragrant Mist Set Atomizer (wartime issue) **MP $10***

*1973 House Mouse Doll-Making Kit, 11" high $7 **MP $10***
*1973 Calico Kate Doll-Making Kit, 11" high $7 **MP $10***

Needlecraft Kits

Market Prices *are for Kit complete with pattern, needle, yarn and accessories*

top: 1974 Pals on Parade Picture 6x8" $6 **MP 9**
1973 Owl Mates Pillow 14x14" $9 **MP $12**
1974 Bushel of Strawberries Pillow 14x14" $10 **MP $13**
1974 Thirteen Original Colonies Pillow 14x14" $10 **MP $13**
1975 Tree Owls Wall Hanging 40x6" $12 **MP $15**
center: 1973 Myrtle Turtle Picture 8x10" $5 **MP $8**
1975 First Prize at the County Fair, 3 pictures 4x5" $8 **MP $11**
1974 Vintage Cars Wall Hanging 40x6" $12 **MP $15**
1974 Spring Violets Pillow 14x14" $9 **MP $12**
bottom: 1972 Lakescape Picture 18x24" $12 **MP $15**
1974 Floral Sentiments Pillow 14x14" $10 **MP $13**
1974 Love 'n Stuff Pillow-Making Kit $8 **MP $11**
1975 Spinning Wheel & Wild Roses 14x14" $12 **MP $15**

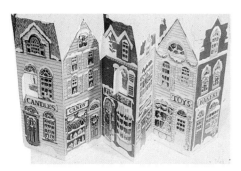

1982 *Christmas Surprise "Scratch and Sniff" Calendar 18"x8" $6.50* **MP $5**

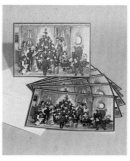

1983 *Holiday Greeting Cards. Victorian designed cards 4¼"x6", pkg. of 6 free with purchase* **MP $2**

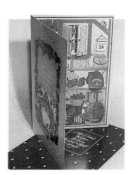

1983 *Mrs. Claus's Kitchen Surprise Calendar with 6 "scratch and sniff" scents $6.50* **MP $5**

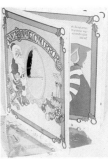

1982 *Santa's Magic Mirror Christmas Record & Picture Book. 12 page picture book contains 33-1/3 record (1 Campaign only) $1.49 with purchase* **MP $5**

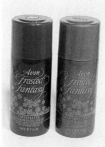

1982 *Frosted Fantasy Windowpane Frost, crystalline white, in Mountain Pine fragrance 4oz $3.29* **MP 50¢**
1983 *Frosted Fantasy in Christmas green, Mountain Pine fragrance 4oz $3.79* **MP 75¢**

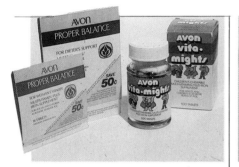

1980 *Women's Vitality Vitamins, 14-day trial size with 50¢ coupon* **MP $3**
1980 *Dieter's Support Vitamins, 14-day trial size with 50¢ coupon* **MP $3**
1980 *Vita-Mights Children's Chewable Multi-Vitamins, 100 tablets* **MP $10**

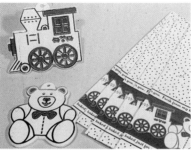

1983 *Holiday Cookie Kit. "Teddy Bear" and "Train" plastic cookie cutters, 5 gift bags and recipe card $7.50* **MP $6**

. . . Vitamins

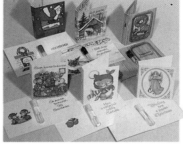

1983 *Holiday Surprise Gift Cards. Each card holds inch of fragrance. Choice of 6 designs and frags. (2 Campaigns only) $2.50 set of three* **MP 50¢ each**

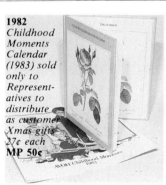

1982 *Childhood Moments Calendar (1983) sold only to Representatives to distribute as customer Xmas gifts 27¢ each* **MP 50¢**
(See also pg. 288)
1982 *Calendar of Roses (1983) diary/date keeper book 7"x9" $2.99 with purchase* **MP $10 retail value**

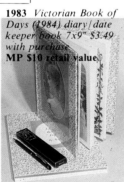

1983 *Victorian Book of Days (1984) diary/date keeper book 7x9" $3.49 with purchase* **MP $10 retail value.**

1983 *Genuine Onyx Accent Pen. Red or black finish ballpoint pen, 5¼" in flannel pouch $28* **MP $22***

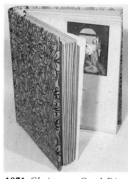

1971 *Christmas Card Display Album. Used by Representatives in Newark Test Market area, contains all 36 designed Christmas Cards* **MP $125** *(See pg. 174)*

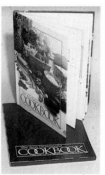

1983 *International Cookbook 7⅞x10¼", 96-pages (1 Campaign only) $3.99 with purchase* **MP $10, $11 boxed**

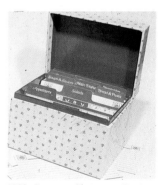

1982 *Country Christmas Recipe Box (cardboard) with 20 Better Homes & Gardens recipe cards, 30 blank cards and 8 tab dividers (1 Campaign only) $2.99 with purchase* **MP $10 retail value**

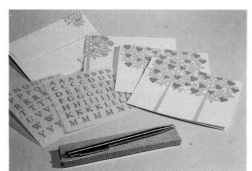

1983 *Initially Yours Note Cards. Package of 4 with eps. and sheet of transfer initials. Free with purchase* **MP $2, retail value**
1981 *Initial Pen, 5⅛" in flannel pouch. Choice of initial $18* **MP $10**

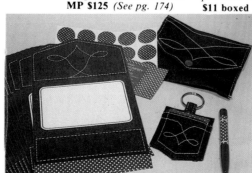

1981 ***Pockets Collection —***
Fragranced Postalettes. 15 sheets notepaper, Sweet Honesty Sachet packet .18oz & decorative seals $6 **MP $3 complete**
Pocket. Tote lined with red & white polka dots 5"x5½" $7 **MP $4**
Key Holder 2"x3" $5 **MP $3**
Colorstick for Lips .05oz $3.50 **MP $1**

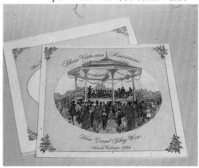

1983 *Those Victorian Americans Calendar (1984) sold only to Representatives to distribute as customer Christmas gift 30¢ each* **MP 50¢**
(See also p. 288)

**Available from Avon at time of publication*

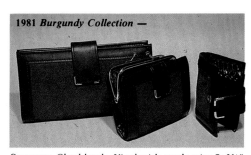

1981 Burgundy Collection —

Secretary Checkbook. Vinyl with suede trim 7x3¾"
$18 **MP $10**
French Purse 4x3¾" $16 **MP $8**
Key Case 3½x3¾" $10 **MP $5**

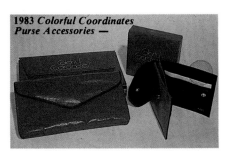

1983 Colorful Coordinates
Purse Accessories —

Slim Clutch with checkbook cover and 6
plastic windows 7⅝x4⅛" in red (shown) or
navy $21 **MP $18***
Slim Billfold 3⅞x3⅝" in red or navy $16
MP $14*

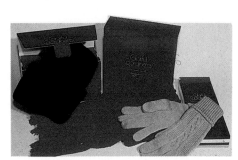

1983 Colorful Coordinates Knit Accessories.
In red (shown), navy, white or beige —
Knit Hat $16 **MP $8**
Gloves $13 **MP $6**
Fringed Scarf $18 **MP $9**

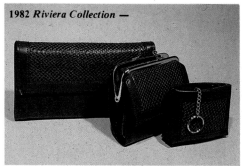

1982 Riviera Collection —

Secretary Checkbook. Vinyl with leather trim 7½x4"
$21 **MP $12**
French Purse 4x3¾" $16 **MP $8**
Coin/Key Case with zipper top 4x3¾" $10 **MP $5**

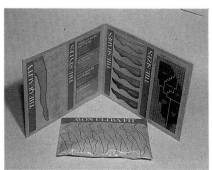

1984 Ultra Fit Pantyhose Color Chart **MP 25¢**
1984 Ultra Fit Pantyhose in Regular $2.79
MP $2.79, *Total Support $6.79* **MP $6.79,**
Control Top $3.79 **MP $3.79** *and Knee Highs*
$3.79 pkg. of 3 **MP $3.79**
(Name later changed to Style & Fit Pantyhose)

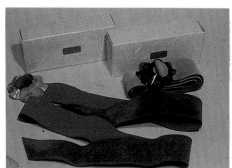

1983 Reversible Suedean Belt in blue/red or tan/
brown. 36" and 40" long, 1½" wide $10 **MP $5 ea.**

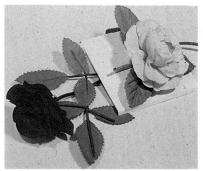

1981 Fabric Rose. Free with Mother's Day
purchase **MP $2**
1983 Perfect Loveliness Corsage with silk-
like flowers 75¢ with purchase **MP $2 retail**
value

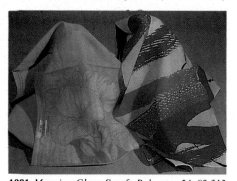

1981 Morning Glory Scarf. Polyester 54x9" $12
MP $10
1982 Autumn Embers Scarf. Polyester 54x9"
$2.99 with purchase **MP $10**

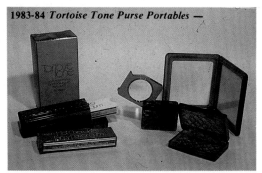

1983-84 Tortoise Tone Purse Portables —

Gum Holder & Fancy Flavor Gum. One pkg. each Hot
Chocolate and Eggnog $6 **MP $2** *holder only*
Magnifying Case, 1¼x1½" $6 **MP $5***
Double Picture Frame, 2½x2¾" $6 **MP $5***
Stamp Holder, 2" long $6 **MP $5***

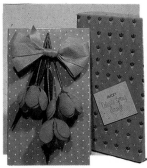

1984 *Delicate Spring Corsage*
75¢ **MP $1** *boxed*

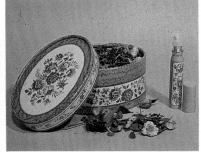

1983 *Natural Blend Potpourri in tin can-*
ister $12 **MP $5** *canister only*
1983 *Natural Blend Potpourri Refresher*
.33oz $4 **MP 50¢**

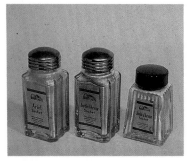

1929-34 *Ariel Powder Sachet 78¢* **MP $60**
1930-34 *Jardin D'Amour Powder*
Sachet $1.04 **MP $75**
1934-37 *Ariel Powder Sachet 78¢*
MP $35

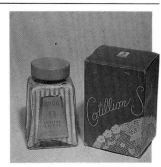

1939 *Gift boxed Cotillion*
Powder Sachet $1.04 **MP $40** *as*
shown

*Available from Avon at time of publication

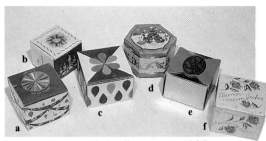

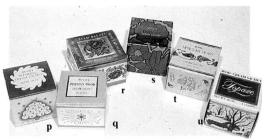

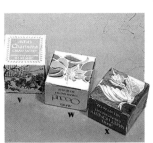

a-1954 *Issued with Cotillion, To A Wild Rose, Forever Spring, Golden Promise & Quaintance* **MP $9**
b-1955 *Issued with above fragrances* **MP $8**
c-1956 *Issued with Cotillion, To A Wild Rose, Forever Spring, Quaintance, Nearness & Bright Night* **MP $8**
d-1957 *Issued with Cotillion, To A Wild Rose, Forever Spring, Nearness, Bright Night & Elegante* **MP $8**
e-1958 *Issued with above fragrances* **MP $8**
f-1958 *72nd Anniversary Box issued with 1957 fragrances* **MP $9**

(below left)
g-1959 *Issued with Cotillion, To A Wild Rose, Nearness, Bright Night, Persian Wood, Here's My Heart* **MP $8**

p-1965 *Issued with To A Wild Rose, Somewhere, Unforgettable, Here's My Heart, Persian Wood, Wishing, Rapture, Occur!, Cotillion, Topaze* **MP $7**
q-1966 *Issued with above fragrances* **MP $7**
r-1968 *Issued with 1965 fragrances* **MP $7**
s-1969 *Issued with 1965 fragrances, add Charisma, Brocade & Regence* **MP $6**
t-1970 *Issued with above fragrances, add Hana Gasa and Elusive* **MP $6**
u-1973 *Issued with above fragrances, delete Wishing, add Bird of Paradise, Sonnet, Roses & Moonwind* **MP $5**

v-1974 *Issued in 16 in-line fragrances and 12 floral fragrances* **MP $4**
w-1977 *Issued in 10 fragrances in red, blue or green boxes* **MP $2**
x-1978 *Issued in 10 fragrances in red, blue or green boxes* **MP $2**

CREAM SACHET GIFT BOXES

h-1959 *73rd Anniversary Box issued with above fragrances* **MP $9**
j-1960 *Issued with Cotillion, To A Wild Rose, Nearness, Bright Night, Persian Wood, Here's My Heart & Topaze* **MP $8**
k-1961 *Issued with Cotillion, To A Wild Rose, Persian Wood, Here's My Heart & Topaze* **MP $8**
m-1962 *Issued with above fragrances, add Somewhere* **MP $8**
n-1964 *Issued with above fragrances* **MP $7**

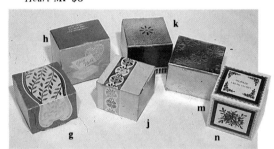

Market Prices *are for Gift Box only.* *(See Fragrance Lines for correct Cream Sachet Jar.)*

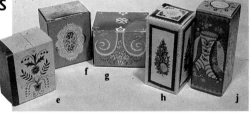

Floral Cream Sachets, .66oz $3 each:

1972 *Violet, Carnation and Gardenia* **MP $1.50**
1974 *Hyacinth and Magnolia* **MP $2.50**
(1975 Lily of the Valley not shown **MP $3)**

Market Prices *are for Gift Box only* *(See Fragrance Lines for correct Powder Sachet Jar. See* **1937** *Gift Box Sachet pg. 52,* **1959** *Gift Box Sachet pg. 67)*

POWDER SACHET GIFT BOXES

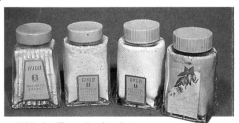

c-1952 *Issued with b-1952 fragrances* **MP $10**
d-1957 *Issued with Cotillion, To A Wild Rose, Quaintance, Nearness, Forever Spring & Bright Night* **MP $8**
e-1958 *Issued with Cotillion, To A Wild Rose, Nearness, Forever Spring, Bright Night & Elegante* **MP $8**
f-1960 *Issued with Cotillion, To A Wild Rose, Persian Wood, Here's My Heart & Topaze* **MP $8**
g-1963 *Issued with above fragrances, add Somewhere* **MP $8**

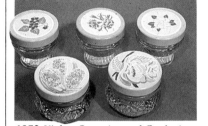

h-1964 *Issued with Cotillion, To A Wild Rose, Persian Wood, Here's My Heart, Somewhere, Topaze & Lavender* **MP $7**
j-1965 *Issued in above fragrances, add Wishing, Rapture & Occur!* **MP $7**

a-1943 *57th Anniversary Box issued with Attention* **MP $15**
b-1952 *Valentine Box issued with Flower Time, Cotillion, Golden Promise & Quaintance* **MP $10**

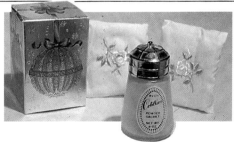

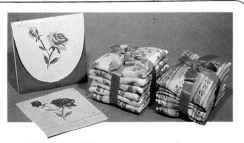

1937 *Cotillion, Jardin d'Amour, Marionette $1.04; Ariel 78¢* **MP $26**
1939-42 *Cotillion, Garden of Love (formerly Jardin d'Amour), Marionette $1.04; Ariel 78¢*
1942 *Above frag. and Attention $1.15* **MP $20 each**
1943 *(ribbed cap) Above frag. $1.15, Ariel 89¢* **MP $8 each**
1946 *Garden of Love $1.19* **MP $20**

1965 *Perfumed Pillowettes, two Powder Sachet Pillows and Powder Sachet, 9 frag. .9oz $3 to $3.75* **MP $22 complete, $14 bottle only**

POWDER SACHETS

1961 *Sachet Pillows, 6 tissue envelopes in package 50¢* **MP $11**
1977 *Lavender Bouquet Sachet Pillows, 6/$7.50* **MP $1 each, $7 boxed**
1978 *French Ribbon Sachet Pillows, 6 fabric sachets with Garlandia frag. $7.50* **MP $6**

Gift Perfumes

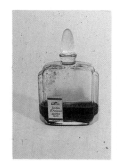

1929 *Jardin d'Amour Perfume 1oz, packaged in bottle with new labeling. Xmas gift to Representatives, never sold to customers.* **MP $200** *(See also pg. 18)*

The captivating fragrance, Jardin d'Amour (pronounced Zhard-dan-damoor) was introduced at Christmas time 1926. Jardin d'Amour means "garden of love" and in 1939 Jardin d'Amour became Garden of Love. The newly named fragrance, available only in Perfume and Powder Sachet, was discontinued in 1949.

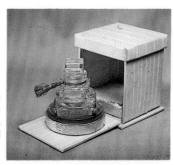

1939 *3 dram Ballad Perfume $3.50* **MP $125, $160 boxed**

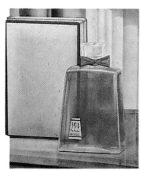

1930 *Perfume "391" 1oz $2.50* **MP $135, $165 boxed** *(1931 Flaconette 1 dram, not shown, $1.25* **MP $75)** *Note: Because of the Excise Tax, imposed in 1932, above prices were increased to $2.60 and $1.30.*

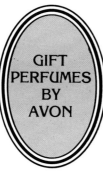

GIFT PERFUMES BY AVON

By reversing the numbers, it appears that "391" perfume introduced the beginning of a new decade, "1930".

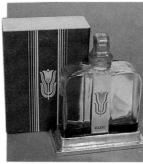

1934-38 *7 dram Bouquet Perfumes. Jardin d'Amour, Bolero, Cotillion $2.60* **MP $100, $130 boxed** **1936** *Add "Lucy Hays" and Topaze* **MP $110** **1938** *Add Courtship and Marionette* **MP $125**

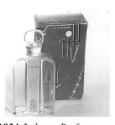

1934 *2 dram Perfume Flaconette in Cotillion, Bolero or Jardin d'Amour (shown with 1936 Xmas box) $1.04* **MP $90, $100 boxed, $135 Xmas boxed** **1936** *Add "Lucy Hays" and Topaze* **MP $100** **1938** *Add Courtship and Marionette* **MP $115**

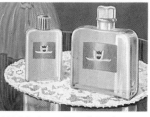

1934 *2 dram Floral Perfume Flaconette, plastic gold lid. Lily of the Valley, Trailing Arbutus, Gardenia, Sweet Pea, 52¢, Rose, Narcissus & Ariel 78¢* **MP $75, $90 boxed** **1934** *7 dram Floral Perfumes. Lily of the Valley, Trailing Arbutus, Gardenia, Sweet Pea $1.56, Rose, Narcissus & Ariel $2.34* **MP $100, $130 boxed**

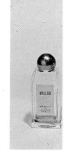

1940-42 *Ballad Perfume Flaconette 1 dram $1.25* **MP $40**

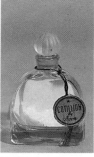

1940 *3 dram Bouquet Perfumes in Cotillion, Courtship, Marionette and Garden of Love $2.25* **MP $100, $125 boxed**

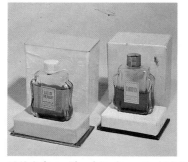

1940 *3 dram Floral Perfumes (gold lid) in Trailing Arbutus, Gardenia, Sweet Pea and Lily of the Valley $1.50* **MP $70, $85 boxed** **1945** *3 dram Floral Perfumes (white lid) with same fragrances as 1940 $1.50* **MP $65, $80 boxed** **1946** *Add Crimson Carnation* **MP $70, $85 boxed**

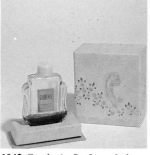

1945 *Gardenia Perfume 3 dram $2.50* **MP $70, $90 boxed** *as shown*

The magic of real flowers is caught in Avon's floral perfumes. Warm, exotic, fresh and sweet as those precious scents.

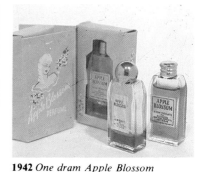

1942 *One dram Apple Blossom Flaconette shown in gift box 75¢* **MP $65 boxed** **1940** *One dram Perfume Flaconette (shown in Apple Blossom, issued in 1941) several frag. 52¢ & 75¢* **MP $40** **1943-44** *One Dram Perfume Flaconette several frag. 59¢ & 85¢* **MP $40** *(1945 Bottle as above, but white plastic lid, not shown* **MP $35)**

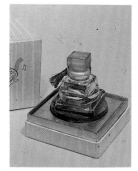

1945 only *Ballad Perfume 3 dram $3.50* **MP $180 in Xmas box**

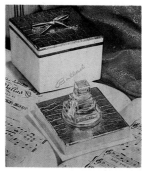

1946 *3 dram Ballad Perfume $3.50* **MP $135, $175 boxed** *(1947 Golden Promise issued in same bottle and box $5* **MP $135, $175 boxed)**

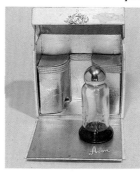

1947 *Perfume 1/2oz $5* **MP $100, $175 boxed**

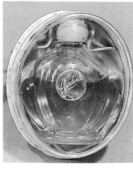

1948 *3 dram Floral Perfume in Gardenia or Lily of the Valley $2.50* **MP $75, $90 boxed**

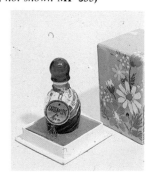

1948 only *Garden of Love Perfume 3 dram $3* **MP $110, $160 boxed**

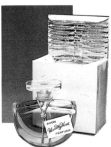

1959 One-ounce Gift Perfume, Cotillion, To A Wild Rose, Bright Night, Nearness $15; Persian Wood and Here's My Heart $17.50 **MP $65, $80 boxed**

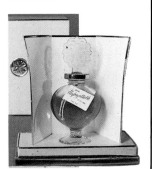

1963 One-ounce Gift Perfume, Crystal imported from France. Glass 4-A embossed stopper. 7 frag. $17.50 to $25 **MP $50, $70 boxed**

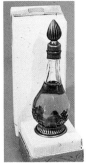

1966 Half-Ounce Perfume in 9 frag. $10 to $12.50 **MP $13, $18 boxed**

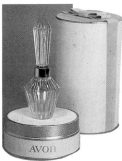

1969 Half-Ounce Perfume in 10 frag. $11 to $15 **MP $11, $17 boxed**

Two dram Perfume Flaconettes —

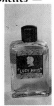 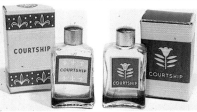 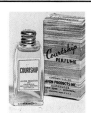 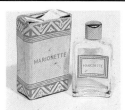

1936 "Lucy Hays" (Mrs. McConnell's maiden name). During March only given as a customer gift, with purchase, in honor of Mrs. McConnell's 51st Wedding Anniversary **MP $50, $85 boxed**

1937 Courtship, gift to Representatives to try before intro and use as a demo **MP $45, $85 boxed**
1937 Courtship, gift in honor of Founder's Campaign (Mr. McConnell) July 6 to 26 only. A Friendship offer of 20¢ with purchase **MP $45, $85 boxed**

1943-44 Courtship Perfume Flaconette 1 dram 85¢ **MP $40, $60 boxed**

1938 Marionette, gift in honor of Founder's Campaign. 20¢ with purchase **MP $40, $80 boxed**

PERFUMES BY THE DRAM

Precious perfume, the richest and purest form of fragrance, in an elegant display of craftsmanship in glass. Each smartly designed bottle merits all the unique packaging devised for it. Who could resist this magnificent collection of Avon masterpieces?

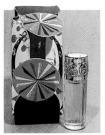 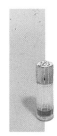 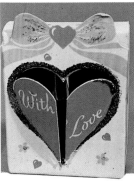 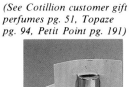 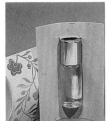

(See Cotillion customer gift perfumes pg. 51, Topaze pg. 94, Petit Point pg. 191)

1953 One dram Perfume bottle shown in Xmas box, 6 frag. $1.75 **MP $12, $25 as shown**

1951 One Dram Perfume in 9 frag. $1.75 **MP $13**

1950 With Love Valentine Perfume, 1 dram, in 9 frag. $1.75 **MP $35 boxed**

1957 One dram Perfume, several frag. in Xmas box $1.75 **MP $15 boxed**

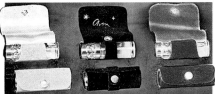 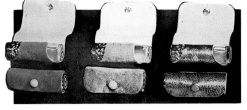

One dram Perfumes in Suedene Wrappers —
1955 Nearness (blue) $2.25 **MP $17**
1955 Bright Night (black) $2.25 **MP $17**
1956 Elegante (burgundy) $2.25 **MP $18**

1956 To A Wild Rose (rose) $2 **MP $17**
1956 Forever Spring (green) $2 **MP $17**
1956 Cotillion (simulated gold kid) $2 **MP $18**

Luscious was the first one-dram perfume issued in a wrap-around case. (See page 73). Long after Luscious was discontinued, all one-dram perfumes were offered in satin lined wraps with iridescent, pearl-like closures.

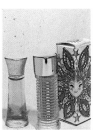 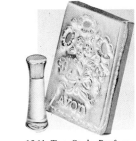 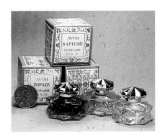

1959-62 Top Style One Dram Perfume in 8 frag. $2 to $2.50 **MP $10**
1962-66 One Dram Perfume in 10 frag. $2.50 to $3.25 **MP $9, $10 boxed**
1966-67 One Dram Perfume in 9 frag. $2.50 to $3.25 **MP $12**
1974-76 One Dram Perfume in 6 frag. $3.75 to $4.25 **MP $5**

1961 Top Style Perfume Xmas boxed $2 to $2.50 **MP $16 Xmas boxed**

1969-74 One Dram Perfume in 15 frag. $2.75 to $3.75 **MP $3**

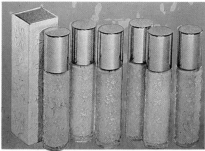

1963 *Perfume Creme Rollette. Somewhere, Topaze, Cotillion $2; Here's My Heart, Persian Wood, To A Wild Rose .33oz $1.75* **MP $6 each, $8 boxed**

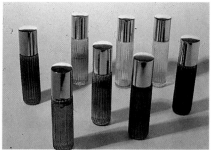

1965 *Perfumed Rollettes in 9 frag. Clear formula, tinted glass .33oz $1.75, $2 and $2.50* **MP $9**

1969 *Perfume Rollette in 8 frag. .33oz $2 & $2.50* **MP 50¢** *(left)*

1973 *Scentiment Perfume Rollette in 3 frag. .33oz $5* **MP $7** *(left)*

PERFUME ROLLETTES

SPRAY ESSENCE

An Avon creation of special fragrance oils with lasting powers similar to perfume. The "perfume" women can afford to wear every day.

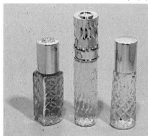

1975 *Perfume Rollette in Moonwind, Charisma & Sonnet .33oz $4.50 ea.* **MP $1**
1975 *Perfume Rollette in 8 frag. .33oz $3 ea.* **MP 50¢**

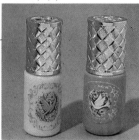

1974 *Scentiment Purse Spray Essence in 3 frag. ¼oz $5* **MP $7** *(right)*

1962 *Crystal Glory Spray Essence in 6 frag. 1oz $4.50 to $5* **MP $17** *(refills, not shown, $2.50 to $3* **MP $7)** *(left)*

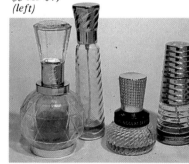

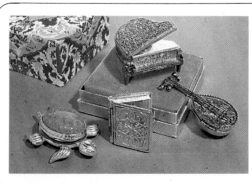

1957 *Essence de Fleurs in 6 frag. 1oz $3* **MP $9, $14 boxed**
1959 *Spray Essence in 6 frag. 1oz $3 to $3.25* **MP $5, $10 boxed**

1966-67 *Spray Essence in 9 frag. 1¼oz $3.50 to $4* **MP $10**
1967 *Spray Essence in 8 frag. Color coded labels $3.50 to $4* **MP $4**
1969 *Spray Essence in Charisma, Brocade & Regence 1¼oz $4.50* **MP $5**
1979 *Spray Essence in 10 frag. ¼oz $3.50* **MP $3**

Perfume Jewelry a la Glace

Table Top Jewelry a la glace. Each refillable gold-toned miniature contains .02oz of Perfume Glace in Moonwind, Elusive, Charisma, Brocade, Regence or Bird of Paradise. Oval refills $1.35 & $2

1971 *Baby Grand $10* **MP $15, $19 boxed**
1971 *Tortoise $9* **MP $10, $14 boxed**
1971 *Memory Book $7* **MP $9, $12 boxed**
1971 *Mandolin $9* **MP $13, $17 boxed**

(See pg. 254 for Glace Jewelry)

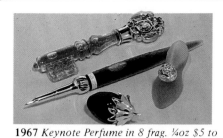

1967 *Keynote Perfume in 8 frag. ¼oz $5 to $6.50* **MP $15, $18 boxed**
1971 *Scent With Love Perfume in 5 frag. ¼oz $6 to $7.50* **MP $10, $13 boxed**
1974 *Strawberry Fair in Sonnet or Moonwind 1/8oz $5 & $6* **MP $7, $9 boxed**
1973 *Precious Slipper Perfume in 3 frag. ¼oz $5 & $6* **MP $7, $9 boxed**

PERFUME PETITE FIGURALS

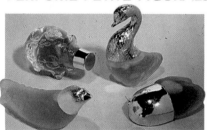

1972 *Perfume Petite (Piglet) in 4 frag. ¼oz $6* **MP $7, $8 boxed**
1974 *Precious Swans Perfume in 3 frag. 1/8oz $6* **MP $7, $9 boxed**
1969 *Love Bird Perfume in 7 frag. ¼oz $6.25 to $7.50* **MP $10, $12 boxed**
1975 *Ladybug Perfume in 3 frag. 1/8oz $6* **MP $5, $6 boxed**

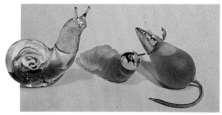

1968 *Perfume Petite (Snail) in 6 frag. ¼oz $6.25 to $7.50* **MP $11, $13 boxed**
1972 *Small Wonder Perfume 1/8oz in 3 frag. $5* **MP $9, $11 boxed**
1970 *Perfume Petite Mouse in 7 frag. ¼oz $6.25 to $7.50* **MP $13, $17 boxed**

1978 *Dapper Snowman Cologne in Sweet Honesty or Moonwind 1oz $5* **MP $3, $4 boxed**

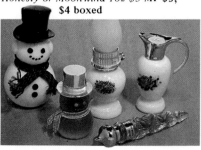

1973 *Snowman Petite Perfume in 3 frag. ¼oz $6* **MP $7, $8 boxed**
1974 *Evening Glow Perfume in 3 frag. .33oz $7* **MP $7, $8 boxed**
1974 *Parisian Garden Perfume in 3 frag. .33oz $7.50* **MP $7, $8 boxed**
1967 *Perfume Flaconette (Icicle) in 9 frag. 1 dram $2.50 to $3.75* **MP $7, $9 boxed**

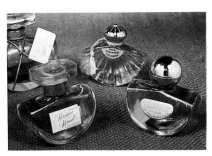

1959 *Gift Magic Cologne. Rocker bottle with flat cap* ¹/₂oz $1 **MP $10**
1962 *Gift Fancy Cologne. Sea shell bottle with gold cord* ¹/₂oz $1 **MP $8**
1967 *Half-ounce Cologne. Rocker bottle with round gold cap.* 12 frag. $1.25 **MP $5**

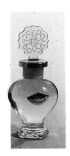

1964 *Half-ounce Cologne in 9 frag.* $1.25 **MP $5, $6 boxed**

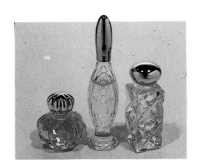

1969 *Minuette Cologne in 10 frag.* ¹/₂oz $1.50 **MP $3**
1970 *Minuette Cologne in 13 frag.* ¹/₂oz $1.50 **MP $2**
1972 *Fragrance Facets Cologne in 11 frag.* ¹/₂oz $1.75 **MP $2**

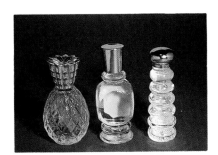

1972 *Pineapple Petite Cologne in 5 frag.* 1oz $3.50 **MP $3**
1975 *Ultra Cologne, Timeless or Unspoken* 1oz $4 **MP $3**
1978 *Cologne Rondelle in 10 frag.* ¹/₂oz $2.50 **MP 75¢**

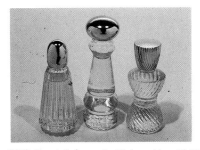

1973 *Demi-Cologne in 12 frag.* ¹/₂oz $1.75 **MP $2**
1975 *Demi-Cologne in choice of 9 frag.* ¹/₂oz $2 **MP $1.50**
1976 *Cologne Petite. Choice of 8 frag.* ¹/₂oz $2 **MP $1.25**

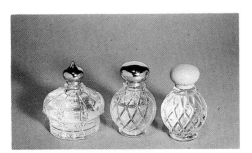

1972 *Cologne Royale in 6 frag.* 1oz $3.50 **MP $4**
1974 *Fragrance Gem Cologne in 11 frag.* ¹/₂oz $2 **MP $2**
1977 *Floral Half-Ounce Cologne in a choice of 6 floral frag.* $2 **MP $1.25**

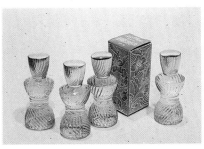

1979 *Anniversary Cologne Petite in Regence, Persian Wood, Rapture and Brocade* ¹/₂oz $2.50 **MP $2, $3 boxed**

COLOGNE MINIATURES

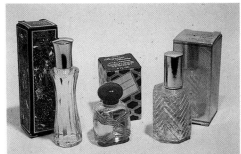

1979 *Cologne Classique in 11 fragrances* .5oz $2.50 **MP $1**
1980 *Precious Hearts Cologne in 6 fragrances* .5oz $3.50 **MP $1, $2 boxed**
1980 *Cologne-Go-Round in Field Flowers, Hawaiian White Ginger, Honeysuckle or Roses, Roses* .5oz $3.50 **MP $1, $2 boxed**

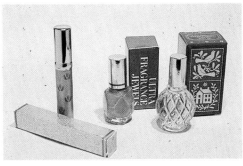

1980 *Crystal Drop Cologne in 8 fragrances* .5oz $3 **MP $1**
1981 *Lovechimes Cologne in Roses, Roses, Charisma, Moonwind or Sweet Honesty* .5oz $3.50 **MP $1, $2 boxed**

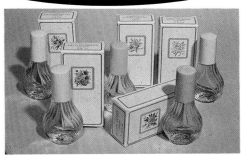

1981 *Floral Colognes in Field Flowers, Hawaiian White Ginger, Roses, Roses, Honeysuckle, Wild Jasmine* .5oz $3 **MP $2***

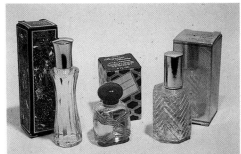

1981 *Fluted Petite in 7 fragrances* .5oz $3.50 **MP $1, $1.25 boxed**
1982 *Fragrance Notables in 6 fragrances* .5oz $4 **MP 75¢, $1 boxed**
1981 *Ultra Shimmer in 4 fragrances* .75oz $5.50 **MP $1.25, $1.50 boxed**

***Available from Avon at time of publication**

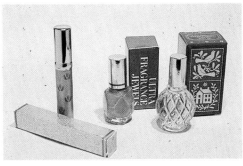

1981 *Ultra Cologne Mini-Spray in 6 fragrances* .33oz $6.50 **MP $1, $1.25 boxed**
1982 *Ultra Fragrance Jewels in 6 fragrances* .33oz $5 **MP 75¢, $1 boxed**
1982 *Vintage Fragrance Cologne in Cotillion, Regence, Here's My Heart, Brocade, Persian Wood & Rapture* .5oz (2 Campaigns only) $3 **MP $1, $1.25 boxed**

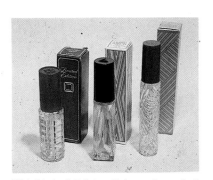

1981 *Limited Edition Cologne Spray in 7 fragrances* .5oz (2 Campaigns only) $4.50 **MP $1.25, $1.50 boxed**
1982 *Ultra Collection Cologne Spray in 6 fragrances* .5oz (2 Campaigns only) $4 **MP $1, $1.25 boxed**
1983 *Ultra Flacon Cologne Spray in 7 fragrances* .5oz $6 **MP $1, $1.25 boxed**

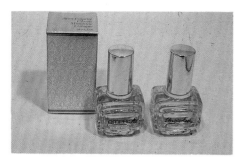

1981 Classic Miniature Cologne in 8 Ultra fragrances .33oz $4 MP $1, $1.25 boxed

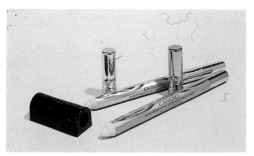

1981 A Stroke of Fragrance Pencil. Foxfire, Tasha, Candid and Timeless in golden case. Odyssey and Ariane in silvery case. .08oz $6 MP $1
1981 A Stroke of Fragrance Pencil Sharpener $1.49 MP $1

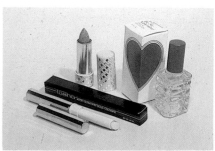

1983 Ultratwist. Solid cologne in 8 Ultra fragrances .05oz $6 MP $6*
1983 Ultra Fragrance Shimmer. Solid Cologne in 7 fragrances .13oz $5 MP $1

1984 Be My Valentine Mini-Cologne for Her in 7 fragrances .5oz (2 Campaigns only) $3.50 MP $1 boxed

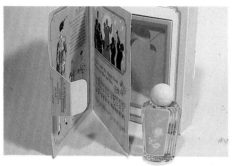

1983 Fragrance Classic. Apple Blossom .5oz in Apple Blossom Time "Storybook" $8.50 MP $7*

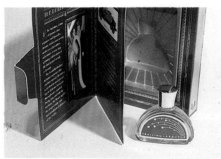

1983 Fragrance Classic. Trailing Arbutus .5oz in The Roaring Twenties "Storybook" $8.50 MP $7*

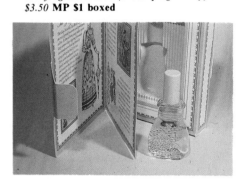

1983 Fragrance Classic. White Lilac .5oz in Gay Nineties "Storybook" $8.50 MP $7*

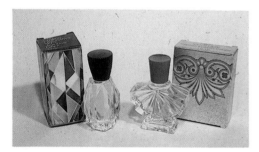

1983 Classic Fragrance Notes Cologne in 9 fragrances .5oz $3.50 MP $2*
1983 Fragrance Keepsake Cologne in Cotillion, Regence, Here's My Heart, Brocade, Persian Wood, Rapture and Somewhere .5oz (2 Campaigns only) $4 MP $1.50, $1.75 boxed

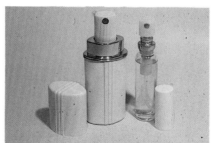

1984 Ultra Cologne Purse Atomizer in 8 fragrances .33oz $7 MP $5
1984 Ultra Cologne Purse Atomizer refill in 8 fragrances .33oz $5 MP $4*

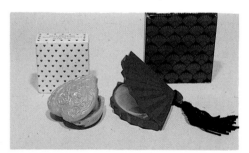

1982 Delicate Heart Perfume Compact in Candid, Tasha and Ariane .10oz $5.50 MP $1, $1.25 boxed
1982 Oriental Fan Perfume Glace Compact in Candid or Timeless .15oz $5.50 MP $1, $1.25 boxed (See also p. 187 & 191)

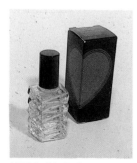

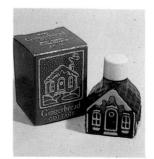

1984 Be My Valentine Mini-Cologne for Him in Wild Country, Rugger, Black Suede and Musk .5oz (2 Campaigns only) $3.50 MP $1 boxed

1983 Gingerbread Cottage Cologne in Charisma or Sweet Honesty .5oz $4.50 MP $1.25, $1.50 boxed

*Available from Avon at time of publication

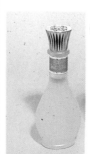

Cologne Silk

— the creamy translucent cologne that smooths on like silk. . . .

1966-68 Cologne Silk. Occur!, Unforgettable (shown), Rapture 3oz $4 MP $4
1967-68 Here's My Heart, To A Wild Rose $3.50: Somewhere, Topaze & Cotillion $3.75 MP $5 ea.
1968 only Brocade & Regence $4.50 MP $6.50 ea.

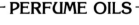
PERFUME OILS

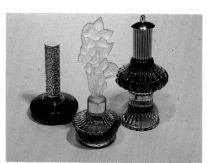

1969-73 Perfume Oil in 9 fragrances 1/2oz $5 to $7.50 MP $5 Hana Gasa & Moonwind MP $6
1971-72 Fragrance Splendor Perfume Oil in 5 fragrances 1/2oz $6 MP $8
1974-76 Perfume Concentre in 5 fragrances 1oz $6 to $7.50 MP $4

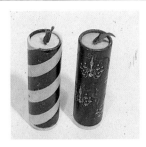

1952 *Cologne Stick in Xmas Wrap $1.25* **MP $27**
1955 *Cologne Stick in Xmas Wrap $1.25* **MP $25**

COLOGNE STICKS

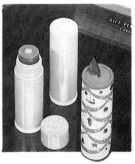

1952-56 *Cologne Stick in Golden Promise, Quaintance, Cotillion, Forever Spring and To A Wild Rose $1.25* **MP $16 each**
1953-54 *Cologne Stick in Xmas Wrap $1.25* **MP $25**

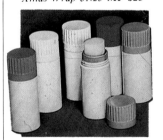

1956-59 *Cologne Stick in Cotillion, To A Wild Rose, Quaintance, Forever Spring $1.25 each; Nearness, Bright Night, Elegante $1.50; Quaintance & Elegante* **MP $10, all others MP $8**

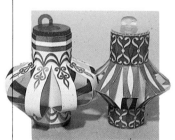

1957 *Cologne Stick in Paper Lantern: Nearness, Bright Night $1.50; Cotillion, To A Wild Rose, Forever Spring and Quaintance $1.25* **Quaintance MP $17, $15 all others**
1956 *(See above for fragrances and regular selling price)* **Quaintance MP $17, all others $15**

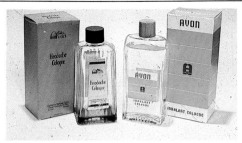

Headache Cologne

1931-36 *Headache Cologne 4oz 75¢* **MP $50, $65 boxed**
1936-40 *Inhalant Cologne 4oz 52¢* **MP $40, $48 boxed**

Headache Colognes, re-named **Inhalant,** *and then called* **Refreshing Cologne,** *were never intended as fragrances. These toiletry Colognes were sprinkled on a handkerchief and then inhaled, providing a soothing treatment for tired nerves, car sickness, fatigue, headache and insomnia. Also refreshing in hot or close atmosphere.*

COLOGNES and COLOGNE MISTS

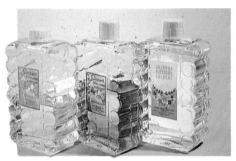

Orchard Blossoms Cologne —
1942 *Cologne 6oz (short neck bottle and cap) from Petal of Beauty Set* **MP $75**
1944-45 *Cologne 6oz $1* **MP $80**
1945 *Cologne 6oz (different label) sold in Petal of Beauty Set only* **MP $75**

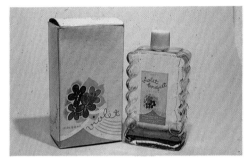

1946-49 *Violet Bouquet Cologne 6oz $1* **MP $80, $105 boxed**

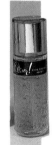

1962 *Occur! Cologne Mist (black label) 2oz $2.50* **MP $7**

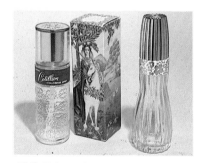

1963 *Cologne Mist 2oz in Cotillion, Somewhere, Topaze, Persian Wood, To A Wild Rose & Here's My Heart $2.25 & $2.50* **MP $6**
1968 *Cologne Mist 2oz in 8 frag. $2.50 & $3* **MP $3**

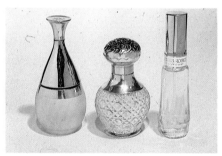

1969 *Cologne Mist in Charisma, Brocade, Regence & (1970 Elusive) 2oz $4.25 each* **MP $4**
1971 *Cologne Mist 2oz in 6 frag. $4.25* **MP $2**
1975 *Cologne Mist 1oz in 6 frag. $3.50* **MP $4**

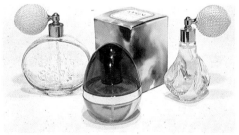

1973 *Cologne Elegante Atomizer in Imperial Garden, Patchwork, Moonwind & Sonnet 3oz $7.50* **MP $8**
1975 *Topalene Cologne Spray Roses, Roses, Moonwind or Patchwork 2¹/₂oz $6.50* **MP $4**
1980 *Ultra Mist Atomizer Cologne in Tasha, Timeless, Ariane, Candid 1.5oz $13* **MP $6**

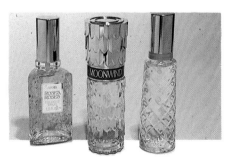

1976 *Cologne Spray in 6 frag. 1.8oz $5* **MP $1**
1977 *Cologne Spray w/neck label in Topaze, Moonwind, Charisma 1.8oz $6.50* **MP $1**
(1974 *Above bottle w/o neck label, Cologne Mist in 10 frag. 2oz $5* **MP $1**)
1975 *Cologne Mist in 10 frag. 2oz $5* **MP $1.50**
(1977 *Above bottle with Cologne Spray in 6 frag. 1.8oz $5* **MP $1**)

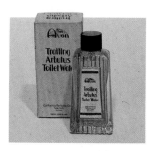

1930-34 *Trailing Arbutus Toilet Water 2oz 75¢* **MP $60, $70 boxed**

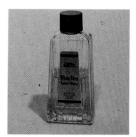

1930-34 *White Rose Toilet Water 2oz 75¢* **MP $60, $70 boxed**

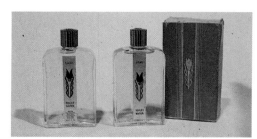

1936-39 *Lilac Toilet Water 2oz 78¢* **MP $45** **1936 only** *Lilac Toilet Water (formerly Lilac Vegetal) 2oz 78¢* **MP $75, $90 boxed**

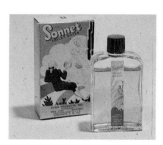

1940 *Sonnet Toilet Water 2oz in "yellow dress" introductory bottle $1.19* **MP $40, $55 boxed**

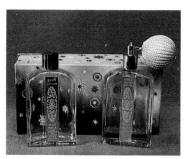

1940-47 *Toilet Water 2oz in Jasmine, Trailing Arbutus, Apple Blossom, Lily of The Valley, Lilac ea. 89¢ and Marionette, Cotillion and Sonnet ea. $1.19* **MP $30, $40 boxed; 1942** *Attention* **MP $30; 1946** *Crimson Carnation,* **1947** *Wishing ea. $1.19* **MP $35, $45 boxed**

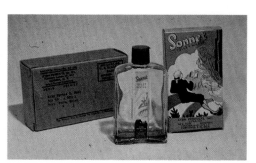

1941 *Sonnet Toilet Water 2oz in "green dress." Representative's demo shown with shipping carton* **MP $55 boxed, $85 as shown**

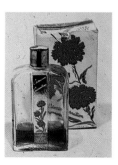

1946 *Crimson Carnation 2oz $1.19* **MP $45, $60 boxed**

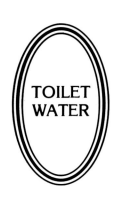

TOILET WATER

ANNIVERSARY KEEPSAKES

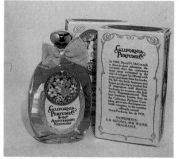

1975 *California Perfume Co. Anniversary Keepsake. Charisma or Sweet Honesty Cologne. (Limited edition bottle — "1975" embossed on back) 1.7oz $6* **MP $7, $9 boxed** *(See also Manager's Award, p. 309)*

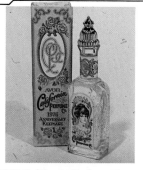

1976 *California Perfume Co. Anniversary Keepsake. 1.7oz Moonwind or Cotillion Cologne. (Limited edition bottle — embossed with "1976") $6* **MP $6, $8 boxed**

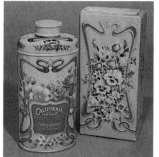

1977 *California Perfume Co. 1977 Anniversary Keepsake (embossed on bottom — "Avon 1977") 3¾oz Trailing Arbutus or Roses, Roses Talc $4* **MP $4, $5 boxed** *(Reps only edition embossed "Anniversary Celebration Talc 1977"* **MP $7**)

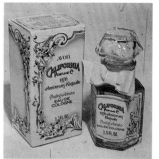

1978 *California Perfume Co. Anniversary Keepsake (embossed on bottom — "Avon 1978") 1.5oz Eau de Cologne in Somewhere, Trailing Abutus & Sweet Honesty $6.50* **MP $5, $6 boxed**

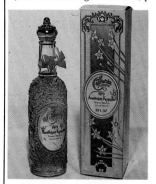

1979 *California Perfume Co. Anniversary Keepsake Eau de Toilette in Trailing Abutus. (Limited edition "Avon 1979" embossed on bottom) 8oz $12* **MP $10, $12 boxed**

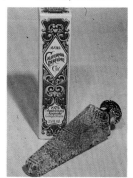

1979 *California Perfume Co. Anniversary Keepsake Cologne Flacon in Trailing Arbutus or Sweet Honesty. (Limited edition "1979" embossed on lid) ¾oz $6.50* **MP $5, $6 boxed**

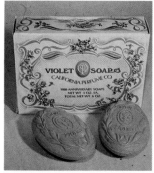

1980 *California Perfume Co. Anniversary Keepsake Violet Soap. Two 3oz violet-scented cakes $5.50* **MP $7**

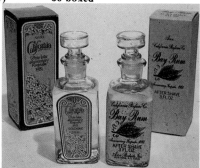

1981 *California Perfume Co. Keepsake Cologne in White Lilac and After Shave in Bay Rum (Dated "1981") All glass bottle is a 1908 replica. 3oz $9.50* **MP $5 boxed**

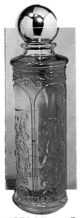

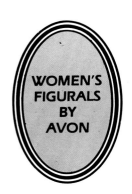

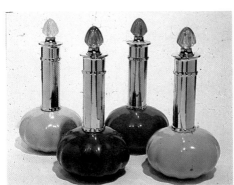

1974 *Winter Garden Cologne Decanter in Topaze, Occur! and Here's My Heart 6oz $6* **MP $5**

1968 *Gift Cologne 4oz in Cotillion, To A Wild Rose, Somewhere, Topaze & Here's My Heart $4* **MP $5**
1975 *Cologne Crystalique Decanter. Moonwind, Sonnet or Imperial Garden 4oz $8* **MP $8**

1972 *Decorator Cologne Mist in Field Flowers (green), Charisma (red), Bird of Paradise (lt. blue) $7 & $8.50* **MP $12,** *Moonwind (dk. blue)* **MP $15**

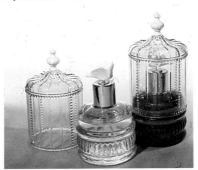

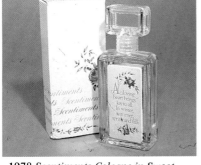

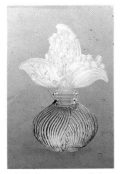

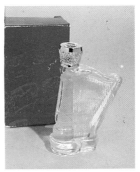

1974 *Song of Love Cologne Mist in Bird of Paradise, Charisma or Sweet Honesty 2oz $6* **MP $5**
1976 *Song of Love Cologne Mist 2oz Here's My Heart or Moonwind $7* **MP $5**

1978 *Scentiments Cologne in Sweet Honesty and Here's My Heart 2oz with Mother's Day Greeting Card on front of bottle $6* **MP $5, $6 boxed**

1979 *Springsong Cologne in Lily of The Valley or Sweet Honesty 1½oz $8* **MP $4**

1978 *Heavenly Music Cologne in Charisma or Topaze 1oz $4.50* **MP $2, $3 boxed**

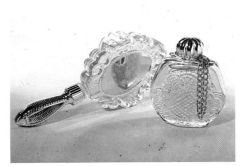

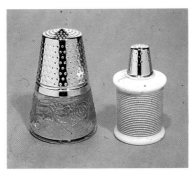

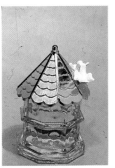

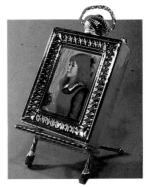

1970 *Looking Glass Cologne in 13 frag. 1½oz $3.50* **MP $8**
1971 *Purse Petite Cologne in 5 frag. 1½oz $4* **MP $7**

1972 *Golden Thimble Cologne in 4 frag. 2oz $4* **MP $5**
1975 *Sewing Notions Cologne in Sweet Honesty, To A Wild Rose or Cotillion 1oz $4* **MP $4**

1974 *Dovecote Cologne in 4 frag. 4oz $6* **MP $6**

1970 *Picture Frame Cologne in 4 frag. Easel, 6"h. 4oz $10* **MP $12**

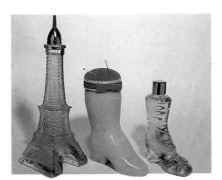

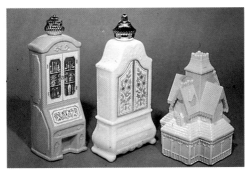

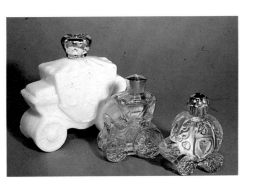

1970 *Eiffel Tower Cologne in 6 frag. 3oz $5* **MP $7, $8 boxed**
1972 *Fashion Boot Pin Cushion Cologne in 4 frag. 5½"h. 4oz $6 to $7* **MP $7**
1975 *High-Buttoned Shoe Cologne 2oz Unforgettable or Occur! $4.50* **MP $4**

1972 *Armoire Decanter. Foaming Bath Oil in 4 frag. 5oz $5* **MP $7**
1972 *Secretaire Decanter. Foaming Bath Oil in 5 frag. 5oz $6 to $7.50* **MP $7**
1972 *Victorian Manor Cologne in 4 frag. 5oz $6* **MP $8**

1972 *Royal Coach Foaming Bath Oil in 4 frag. 5oz $6 to $7* **MP $6**
1973 *Courting Carriage Cologne in Moonwind or Flowertalk 1oz $3.50* **MP $4**
1976 *Magic Pumpkin Coach 1oz Cologne in Bird of Paradise or Occur! $4.50* **MP $3**

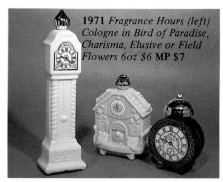

1971 Fragrance Hours (left) Cologne in Bird of Paradise, Charisma, Elusive or Field Flowers 6oz $6 MP $7

1972 Enchanted Hours Cologne in Charisma, Unforgettable, Somewhere or Roses, Roses 5oz $6 MP $6
1973 Beautiful Awakening Cologne in Roses, Roses, Elusive or Topaze 3oz $6 MP $5

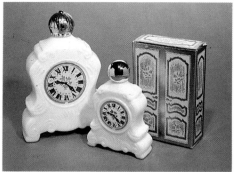

1970 Leisure Hours Bath Oil Decanter Foaming Bath Oil in 6 frag. 5oz MP $5
1974 Leisure Hours Miniature Cologne in Field Flowers, Bird of Paradise or Charisma 1½oz $4 MP $4, $5 boxed

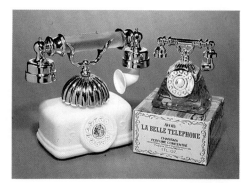

1971 French Telephone 6oz Foaming Bath Oil and ¼oz Perfume in 4 frag. $20 to $22 MP $27
1974 LaBelle Telephone Perfume Concentre in Sonnet, Moonwind or Charisma 1oz $9 MP $7, $8 boxed

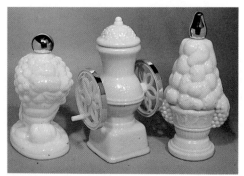

1971 Cornucopia SSS Bath Oil 6oz $6 MP $6
1972 Country Store Coffee Mill Cologne in 4 frag. 5oz $7 to $8 MP $8
1972 Compote Cologne in 4 frag. 5oz $6 to $7 MP $7

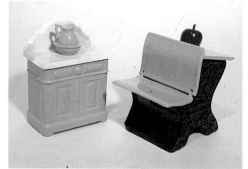

1973 Victorian Washstand Foaming Bath Oil in 3 frag. 4oz $6 MP $6
1973 Remember When School Desk Cologne in 4 frag. $6 MP $8

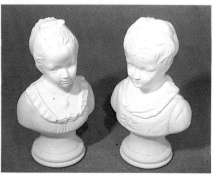

18th Century Classic figurines. Cologne or Foaming Bath Oil in Moonwind or Sonnet 4oz – *1974 Young Girl $7.50 MP $9*
1974 Young Boy $7.50 MP $9

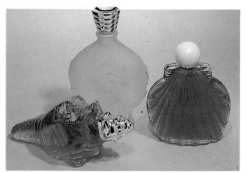

1971 Sea Treasure Foaming Bath Oil in 4 frag. 5oz $6 MP $8
1973 Love Song Decanter 6oz SSS Bath Oil $6 MP $7
1974 Sea Legend Decanter of flint glass. Moonwind or Sonnet Foaming Bath Oil or Roses, Roses Bath Foam 6oz $6 MP $6

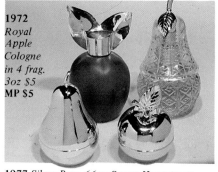

1972 Royal Apple Cologne in 4 frag. 3oz $5 MP $5

1977 Silver Pear .66oz Sweet Honesty or Charisma Cream Sachet $6 MP $4
1974 Pear Lumiere Cologne Mist in Roses, Roses, Bird of Paradise or Charisma 2oz $6 MP $4.50
1976 Enchanted Apple .66oz Charisma or Sonnet Cream Sachet $5.50 MP $5

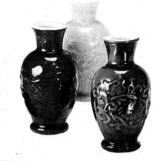

1981 Spring Bouquet Fragranced Vase, glass coated with Jade Blossom scent 6½" high $12 MP $10

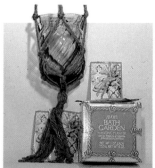

1977 Bath Garden. Hanging Planter and 6 Packets of Mineral Springs Bath Crystals 1oz each $12 MP $11 **complete, $6 Planter only**

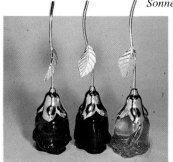

1974 Courting Rose Cologne in 3 frag. 1½oz $6 MP $6.50
1974 Same as left, Red Glass MP $12
1977 Courting Rose Cologne 1½oz Moonwind or Roses, Roses Cologne $6 MP $5

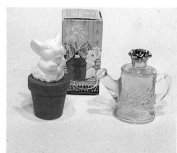

1980 Flower Mouse Cologne in Zany or Cotillion .75oz $6 MP $2
1979 Flower Fancy Cologne in Roses, Roses and Field Flowers 1.25oz $5 MP $3

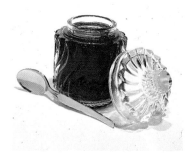

1980 Crystal Clear Hostess Decanter with Stainless Steel Spoon, Strawberry Bubble Bath Gelee 5.5oz $14 MP $8

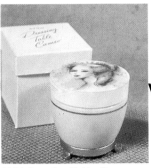

1961 *Dressing Table Cameo Cream Sachet in 6 frag. 1½oz $2.75 to $3.25* **MP $11, $13 boxed**

FOR THE VANITY

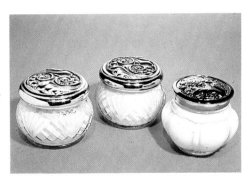

1973 *Rich Moisture Cream (silver lid) 5oz $5* **MP $5**
1973 *Skin-So-Soft Skin Softener (gold lid) 5oz $5* **MP $5**
1975 *Vanity Jar. Rich Moisture Cream or SSS Skin Softener 5oz $6* **MP $4**

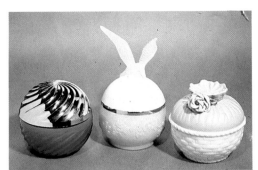

1973 *Sapphire Swirl. Perfumed Skin Softener in Bird of Paradise or Charisma 5oz $5.50* **MP $6**
1974 *Flight to Beauty in Vita Moist, Rich Moisture or Skin-So-Soft Cream 5oz $6* **MP $7**
1974 *Victorian Sewing Basket. Perfumed Skin Softener in Roses, Roses, Bird of Paradise or Charisma 5oz $6* **MP $7**

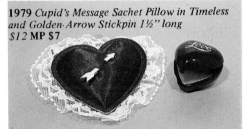

1979 *Cupid's Message Sachet Pillow in Timeless and Golden·Arrow Stickpin 1½" long $12* **MP $7**

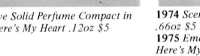

1979 *Scent with Love Solid Perfume Compact in Sweet Honesty or Here's My Heart .12oz $5* **MP $2**

1977 *Oriental Peony Vase Cologne in Moonwind or Sweet Honesty 1½oz $6* **MP $6** *(left)*
1978 *Golden Bamboo Vase Cologne Decanter in Sweet Honesty or Moonwind 1oz $6* **MP $6**

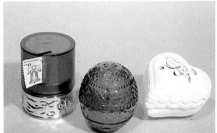

1974 *Scent with Love Cream Sachet in 3 frag. .66oz $5* **MP $5**
1975 *Emeraldesque Cream Sachet in Occur!, Here's My Heart or Sweet Honesty 1oz $4.50* **MP $4**
1976 *Heartscent Cream Sachet in Charisma, Occur! or Roses, Roses .66oz $5.50* **MP $4**

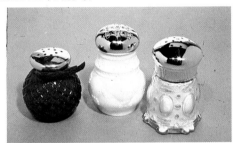

1969 *Powder Sachet (Cranberry) in Charisma, Unforgettable, Cotillion or To A Wild Rose 1½oz $4.50* **MP $10**
1972 *Powder Sachet in 4 frag. 1¼oz $4 to $5* **MP $5**
1973 *Turn-of-Century Powder Sachet Shaker in Charisma or Roses, Roses ¼oz $4.50* **MP $6**

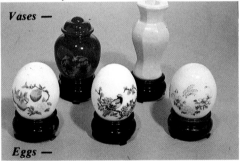

Vases —

Eggs —

1974 *Peach Orchard. Perfume Concentre in Imperial Garden, Moonwind or Sonnet 1oz $7.50* **MP $10**
1975 *Chinese Pheasant. Cologne in Imperial Garden, Charisma or Bird of Paradise 1oz $6.50* **MP $9**
1975 *Delicate Blossoms. Cologne in Patchwork, Sonnet or Charisma 1oz $7.50* **MP $7**

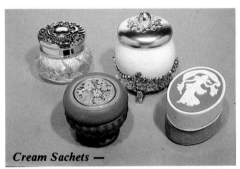

Cream Sachets —

1973 *Vanity Jar in Field Flowers, Charisma or Topaze 1oz $4* **MP $4**
1975 *Gather A Garden in 4 frag. .66oz $5* **MP $3**
1974 *Baroque Cream Sachet in 3 frag. 2oz $7.50* **MP $6**
1975 *Cameo Decanter in 4 frag. .66oz $5* **MP $5**

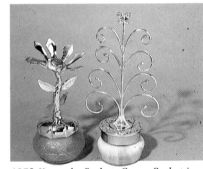

1970 *Keepsake Sachet. Cream Sachet in 5 frag. .66oz $4.50* **MP $6**
1971 *Keepsake Cream Sachet in 5 frag. .66oz $4 to $5* **MP $6**

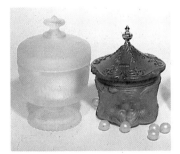

1972 *Period Piece Decanter. Skin Softener in 4 frag. 5oz $7 to $8* **MP $7**
1974 *Venetian Blue Emollient Bath Pearls. Frosted jar with 75 "pearls" in Moonwind, Sonnet or Imperial Garden $7.50* **MP $8**

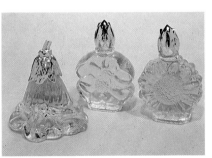

1969 *Petti-Fleur. Elusive, Charisma, Brocade or Regence Cologne 1oz $2.50* **MP $8**
1978 *Dogwood Demi-Decanter Cologne in Moonwind, Apple Blossom ¾oz $4* **MP $2**
1978 *Autumn Aster Demi-Decanter Cologne in Topaze or Sun Blossoms ¾oz $4* **MP $2**

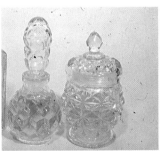

1975 *Crystalier Decanter Cologne in Field Flowers, Roses, Roses or Bird of Paradise 2oz $5* **MP $5**
1973 *Crystal Facets Cologne Gelee in Roses, Roses or Field Flowers 3oz $5* **MP $6**

STUFFED ANIMALS of AVON

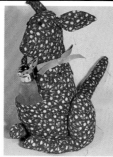
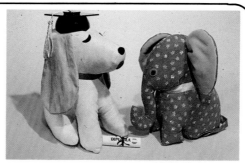

1978 *Kangaroo Two Stuffed Calico Animal and Cologne in Topaze or Sweet Honesty ¾oz $12.50* **MP $11**

1980 *Autograph Hound Stuffed Animal with mortarboard and tassel. Diploma contains .15oz Care Deeply Lip Balm $13.50* **MP $10**
1979 *Ella Elephant Stuffed Animal scented with Garlandia Sachet $9.50* **MP $9.50**

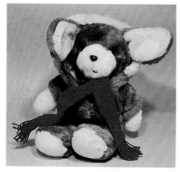
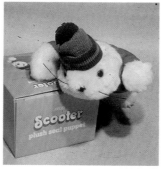
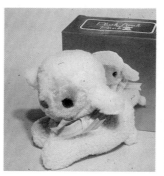

1982 *Plush Puppy with zip-up hooded jacket, T-shirt and scarf $18* **MP $17**

1983 *Scooter Plush Seal Puppet 13" long $20* **MP $18***

1984 *Plush Lamb Bank 6" high $18.50* **MP $16***

Avonshire Blue

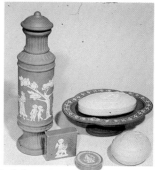

1979 *SSS Decanter ("May 1979") 6oz $13.50* **MP $9**
1979 *Cologne ("May 1979") 6oz in Somewhere or Charisma $13.50* **MP $9**

1971 *Cologne in 4 frag. 6oz $6* **MP $8**
1972 *Soap Dish and oval Soap 5oz $4.50* **MP $8** *(Note: Rare round soaps, demos only* **MP $26**)
1975 *Glace Compact. Moonwind, Elusive, Charisma .10oz $5* **MP $5**

The **Bristol Blue Collection** by Avon presented the very first Avon decanter made of beautifully translucent blue opaline glass. The entire Bristol Blue Collection was inspired by the elegant Bristol Blue opaline glassware made in 18th century Bristol, England, and prized by collectors all over the world.

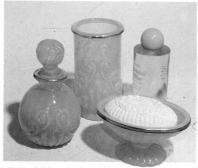

Bristol Blue Collection —
(Imperial Garden, Sonnet or Moonwind)
1974 *Cologne Decanter 5oz $9* **MP $10**
1974 *SSS Bath Oil 5oz $9* **MP $10**
1974 *Soap Dish and Soap 5oz $7* **MP $10**

COLLECTIONS by AVON

American Fashion (see pg. 200)	*Holiday Hostess (see pg. 210)*
American Heirloom	*Hudson Manor*
Anniversary Keepsakes (see pg. 184)	*Mount Vernon*
Avonshire	*Nature's Best (see pg. 206)*
Benjamin J. Bearington (see pg. 206)	*Pennsylvania Dutch*
Bristol Blue	*Petit Point*
Burgundy (see pg. 176)	*Pockets (see pg. 175)*
Burst of Spring	*Private World*
Buttercup	*Riviera (see pg. 176)*
Butterfly Fantasy	*Spring Dynasty*
Cape Cod	*Summer Fantasy*
Castleford	*Tapestry (see also pg. 173)*
Colorful Coordinates (see pg. 176)	*Tender Blossoms*
Country Cupboard	*Tortoise Tone (see pg. 176)*
Country Garden	*Ultra Crystal*
Country Kitchen	*Ultra Vanity*
Crystal	*Victorian (see also pg. 175)*
Delft Blue	*Victoriana*
Emerald Accent	*Whisper of Flowers*
English Provincial	
Flower Fair	
Flowerfrost	
Fostoria (see also pg. 207)	

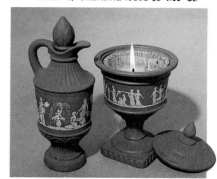

1973 *Avonshire Blue Decanter with Foaming Bath Oil or Skin-So-Soft 6oz $7* **MP $10**
1973 *Perfumed Candle Holder. 9 frag. $9* **MP $12**

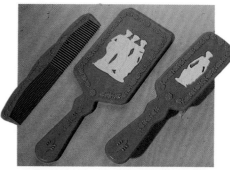

1974 *Vanity Mirror. Plastic with embossed cameo design. 9½" long $6* **MP $8**
1974 *Brush and Comb Set $7* **MP $8**

*Available from Avon at time of publication

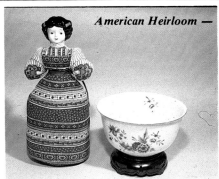

American Heirloom —

1981 *Porcelain Head Doll with Lavender Sachet 10½" high $20* **MP $16.50***
1981 *Porcelain Bowl and plastic stand $25* **MP $20***
1981 *Bowl with "Independence Day 1981" on bottom $25* **MP $25**

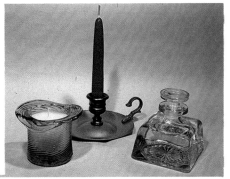

1981 *Pitkin Hat Candle Holder with Fresh Aroma Smoker's Candle $10* **MP $8***
1981 *Chamber Candlestick with 6" Fragranced Taper Candle $16* **MP $12 complete**
1981 *Ship's Decanter. Sweet Honesty Body Splash or Wild Country After Shave 6oz $11,* **MP $5**

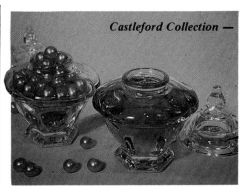

Castleford Collection —

1974 *Emollient Bath Pearls holds 60 "pearls" in Moonwind, Sonnet or Imperial Garden 5"h. $10* **MP $10**
1974 *Cologne Gelee in Apple Blossom, Raining Violets or Roses, Roses 4oz $10* **MP $10**

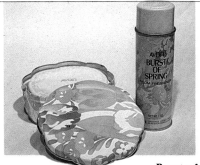

Burst of Spring —

1978 *Beauty Dust Container. Made of tin, sold empty. $6.50* **MP $5**
1978 *Room Freshener 7oz $1.49* **MP 75c**

1978 *Design-wrapped Soap 3oz $1.25* **MP $1.25**
1978 *Scarf sold for $2.50 with $8.50 purchase C-7, value $9* **MP $9**

Available from Avon at time of publication

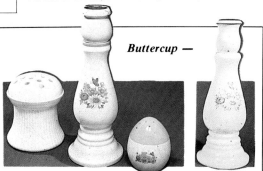

Buttercup —

1974 *Flower Holder perfumed Skin Softener in Moonwind, Sonnet or Imperial Garden 5oz $5* **MP $5**
1974 *Candlestick Cologne in 3 frag. 6oz $7* **MP $9**
1974 *Salt Shaker Cream Sachet, 3 frag. 1½oz $5* **MP $4**
1974 *Candlestick Cologne, later issue with different closure* **MP $7**

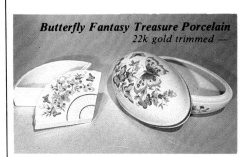

Butterfly Fantasy Treasure Porcelain
22k gold trimmed —

1980 *Fan ("1980") $15* **MP $14**
1978 *Egg ("1974") only 110,000 produced. $14.50* **MP $30**
1978 *Egg with "R" (re-issue) on bottom $24.50* **MP $22**

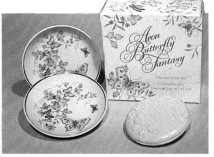

1979 *Two 4" diam. Dishes and Special Occasion Scented Hostess Soap 3oz $16* **MP $16**

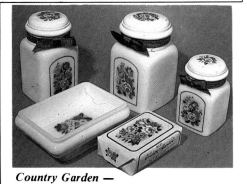

Country Garden —
(in Charisma, Elusive or Bird of Paradise)
1971 *Bath oil 6oz $5.50* **MP $6**
1971 *Beauty Dust 5oz $6* **MP $6**
1971 *Powder Sachet 1¼oz $4.50* **MP $6**
1971 *Soap Dish and Soap $4.50* **MP $7**

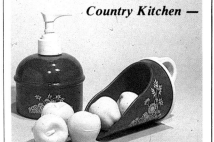

Country Kitchen —

1974 *Hand Lotion 10oz $7* **MP $6**
1974 *Soap Dish plastic "scoop" and 5 apple scented 1oz Soaps $7.50* **MP $8**

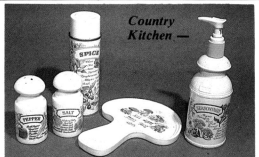

Country Kitchen —

1980 *Ceramic Salt & Pepper Shakers 4" high $12 the set* **MP $10**
1980 *Spice Room Scent 7oz $1.99* **MP $2***
1980 *Ceramic Trivet $12* **MP $10**
1980 *Hand Lotion with Pump Dispenser 10oz $9.50* **MP $9**

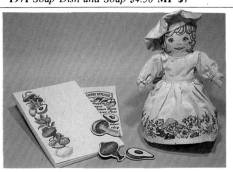

1981 *Magnets and Fragranced Note Pad. 50-page note pad, Country Spice Sachet packet and Avocado, Onion and Mushroom-shaped magnets $7.50* **MP $4 complete**
1982 *Spice Angle 7½" high scented with Spice Garden fragrance $15* **MP $10**

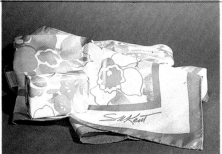

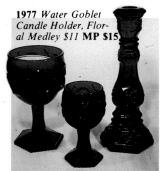

1977 *Water Goblet Candle Holder, Floral Medley $11* **MP $15**

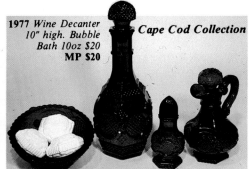

1977 *Wine Decanter 10" high. Bubble Bath 10oz $20* **MP $20**

Cape Cod Collection

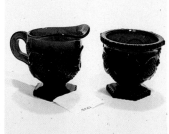

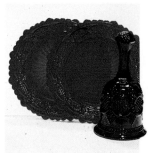

1982 *Sold empty $15* **MP $15***
1976 *Wine Goblet Candlette, Bayberry $8* **MP $9**
1982 *Sold empty $10* **MP $9***
1975 *Candlestick Cologne 3 frag. 5oz $11* **MP $10**

1978 *Dessert Bowl and three 2oz Guest Soaps $11* **MP $10**
1982 *Sold empty $12* **MP $9***
1978 *Salt Shaker Cologne 1½oz $6* **MP $7**
1984 *Sold empty $16.50 set* **MP $13***
1975 *Cruet Decanter with SSS 5oz $11* **MP $10**

1981 *Cream Pitcher Candle Holder $12* **MP $9**
1982 *Sold empty $12* **MP $9***
1981 *Sugar Bowl with 3 Timeless Sachet tablets $12* **MP $9**
1982 *Sold empty $12* **MP $9***

1980 *Dessert Plates, two 7½" diam. $14* **MP $12***
1979 *Hostess Bell, dated "1979" 6½" high with clear glass clapper $15* **MP $15**

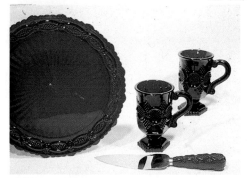

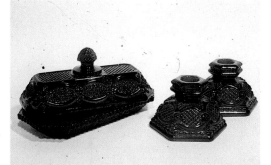

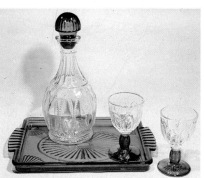

1982 *Dinner Plate 11" diam. $16* **MP $17***
1982 *Pedestal Mugs, two 6oz $17.50* **MP $16***
1981 *Dessert Server 8" long $12.50* **MP $10***

1983 *Covered Butter Dish 7" long $18.50* **MP $15***
1983 *Candle Holder $18.50 set* **MP $15***

Emerald Accent —
1982 *Serving Tray 11½"x7¾" $17.50* **MP $15**
1982 *Decanter 10" high $17.50* **MP $15**
1982 *Cordial Glasses. Set of two, each 4½" high $15* **MP $13**

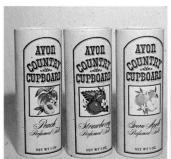

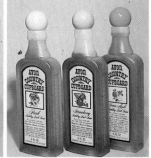

Country Cupboard —
1975 *Talc 5oz in Peach & Strawberry $2.50* **MP 50¢ each**
1977 *Talc 5oz Green Apple $2.50* **MP 50¢**

1975 *Bubbling Bathfoam 6oz in Peach & Strawberry $4.50* **MP 50¢ each**
1977 *Bubbling Bath foam 6oz Green Apple $4.50* **MP 50¢**

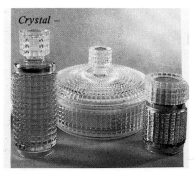

Crystal —

Crystal —
1966 *Cologne in 8 frag. 4oz $3.50 to $5* **MP $6**
1966 *Beauty Dust in 8 frag. 6oz $4.50 to $6* **MP $18**
1970 *Powder Sachet in 4 frag. 1¼oz $4* **MP $6**

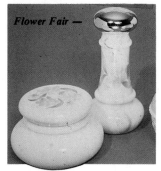

Flower Fair —

1974 *Skin Softener Decanter in Skin-So-Soft 5oz $6* **MP $5**
1974 *Cologne Decanter in Roses, Roses, Sonnet or Moonwind 3oz $7.50* **MP $7**

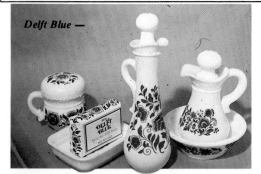

Delft Blue —

1972 *SSS Skin Softener 5oz $5* **MP $6**
1972 *Soap Dish and SSS Soap 3oz $4.50* **MP $7**
1973 *Delft Blue Foaming Bath Oil in Sonnet, Moonwind and Patchwork 5oz $7* **MP $7.50**
1972 *Pitcher and Bowl, SSS Bath Oil 5oz $8.50* **MP $12**

**Available from Avon at time of publication*

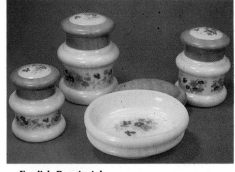

English Provincial —
(in Bird of Paradise or Charisma)
1972 *Powder Sachet 1¼oz $4.75* **MP $6**
1972 *Foaming Bath Oil 8oz $6* **MP $6**
1972 *Soap Dish and 5oz Soap $4.50* **MP $7**
1973 *Cologne 5oz $6* **MP $6**

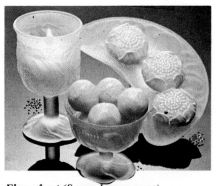

Flowerfrost (Sunny Lemon scent) —
1979 *Goblet and Candlette $14* **MP $13**
1979 *Sherbet Glass and six 1oz Soaps $15* **MP $14**
1980 *Crescent Plate and three 2oz scented Guest Soaps $15* **MP $14**

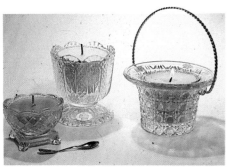

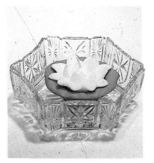

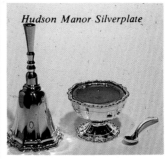

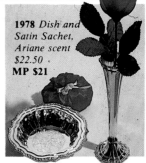

Hudson Manor Silverplate

1978 Dish and Satin Sachet, Ariane scent $22.50 MP $21

1969 *Fostoria Salt Cellar and silver Spoon, Bayberry Candle, non-refillable $6* **MP $9**
1973 *Fostoria Perfumed Candle Holder in 9 frag. $10* **MP $10**
1975 *Fostoria Candlelight Basket in 9 frag. $11.50* **MP $10**

1979 *Fostoria Crystal Pool Floating Candle $15.50* **MP $13**

1978 *Hostess Bell 5½" high $22.50* **MP $21**
1978 *Saltcellar and Spoon with Ariane scented Red Candle 2" high, Spoon 3" long $22.50* **MP $21**

1978 *Bud Vase and Scented Rose. 14" fabric Flower with 2 Tablets Roses, Roses scent. Vase 8" $22.50* **MP $21**

... COLLECTIONS BY AVON

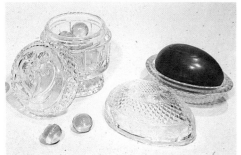

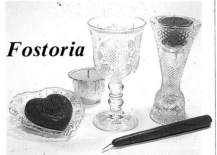

Fostoria

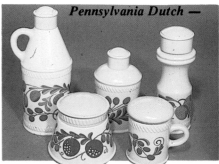

Pennsylvania Dutch —

1974 *Fostoria Compote holds 12 SSS Bath Oil Capsules $10* **MP $11.50**
1977 *Fostoria Egg Soap Dish and 6oz Spring Lilacs scented Soap $15* **MP $10** *("Mother's Day 1977" embossed issue, 2 campaigns only* **MP $15**)

1977 *Heart and Diamond Soap Dish and 5oz Special Occasion scented Soap $9* **MP $9**
1978 *Heart & Diamond Fostoria Loving Cup Candle Holder, Floral Medley $15* **MP $11**
1979 *Heart and Diamond Candlestick with Candlette and Taper $15* **MP $13**

(Patchwork, Sonnet or Moonwind)
1973 *Hand and Body Cream Lotion 10oz $6* **MP $6** *(N/A in Moonwind)*
1973 *Foaming Bath Oil 6oz $6* **MP $6**
1973 *Cologne Decanter 4oz $6* **MP $6**
1973 *Perfumed Skin Softener 5oz $5* **MP $6**
1973 *Powder Sachet Shaker 1¼oz $6* **MP $6**

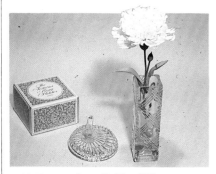

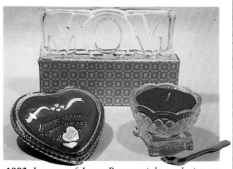

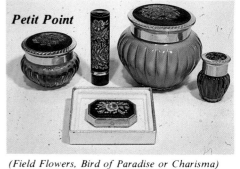

Petit Point

1980 *Fostoria Ring Holder, 3½" wide x 2½" high $10* **MP $9**
1980 *Fostoria Crystal Bud Vase dated "Avon 1980", with pink fabric carnation and fragrance pellet $15.50* **MP $13**

1983 *Images of Love Paperweight and picture frame with removable printed message $12* **MP $10***
1983 *Mom's Pride and Joy picture frame with stencil $14* **MP $12***
1981 *Fostoria Condiment Dish with Fragrance Candle and spoon $13* **MP $9**

(Field Flowers, Bird of Paradise or Charisma)
1974 *Cream Sachet 2"h, 1oz $5* **MP $5**
1970 *Petit Pink Lipstick $2* **MP $4**
1974 *Perf. Skin Softener 3"h, 5oz $5* **MP $5**
1974 *Perfume 2"h, ¼oz $7.50* **MP $7**
1967 *Glace Compact $4.50* **MP $11**

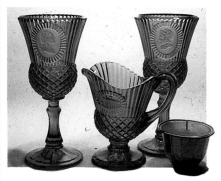

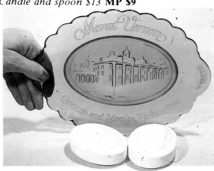

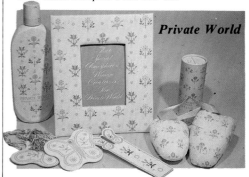

Private World

1976 *George and Martha Washington Candle Holders by Fostoria. Floral Medley fragrance. Each $12.50* **MP $10, $13 Martha**
1977 *Mount Vernon Sauce Pitcher, Fostoria Candle Holder, Floral Medley $15.50* **MP $13**

1979 *Mount Vernon Plate and two 3oz Special Occasion scented Soaps $13* **MP $13**

*Available from Avon at time of publication

1982 *Lingerie Wash 8oz $4* **MP 50¢**
1982 *Picture Frame 6"x7" $12.50* **MP $10***
1982 *Powder Sachet 1.5oz $4* **MP 50¢**
1982 *Butterfly Fragrancers w/cord $7.50* **MP $1**
1982 *Bookmark, free with purchase* **MP 50¢**
1982 *Soft Sachet, with hanging ribbon $10* **MP $2**

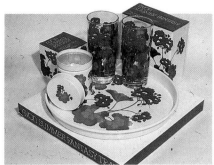

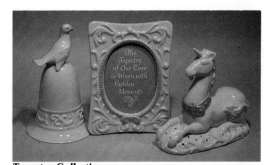

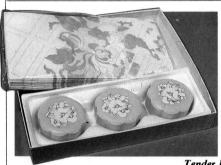

1982 *Spring Dynasty Fragranced Vase. Willow scent 7" high $13.50 ea.* **MP $8**

Summer Fantasy —
1983 *Indoor/Outdoor Candle. Floral Touches scent $12.50* **MP $6 tin container only**
1983 *Glasses. Set of two, 15oz ea. $12.50* **MP $9**
1983 *Tray 12" diam. $11* **MP $9**

Tapestry Collection —
1981 *Porcelain Bell 5" high $18* **MP $15***
1981 *Porcelain Picture Frame 5" high $15* **MP $13**
1981 *Porcelain Unicorn Pomander with Fragranced Wax Chips, Garlandia scent $19* **MP $16**

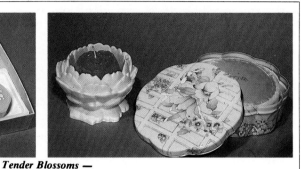

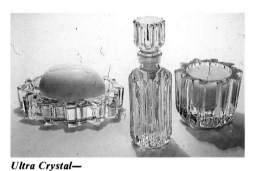

Tender Blossoms —
1977 *Guest Towels and Soaps. 12 Paper Towels and three 2oz Special Occasion fragranced Soaps $6.50* **MP $8**

1977 *Beauty Dust Container. Made of tin, sold empty. $6.50* **MP $6**
1977 *Tender Blossoms Fragrance Candle, Floral Medley scent, non-refillable $6.50* **MP $6**

Ultra Crystal—
1981 *Soap Dish and 4oz Soap in Foxfire, Ariane, Tasha or Timeless $12* **MP $11**
1981 *Cologne Decanter in choice of above fragrances 2oz $12* **MP $10**
1981 *Fragrance Candleholder and Candlette in above fragrances $12* **MP $11**

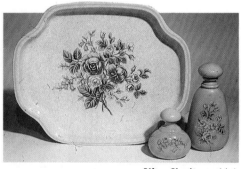

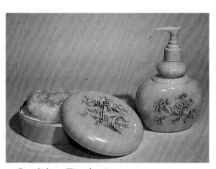

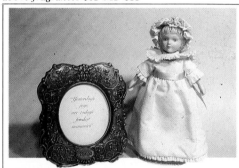

Ultra Vanity — (Ariane, Candid or Timeless)
1980 *Vanity Tray, 12"x10" metal $10* **MP $10**
1980 *Cologne in above fragrances 2oz $9* **MP $8**
1980 *Luxury Bathfoam in above fragrances 6.75oz $8* **MP $6**

1980 *Beauty Dust with Puff in above fragrances 6oz $3.50* **MP $10**
1980 *Soft Body Satin with Pump Dispenser in above fragrances 10oz $12.50* **MP $9**

Victorian Collection —
1983 *Personalized Picture Frame. Metal frame emb. with any 3 initials $25* **MP $15**
1983 *Collector Doll with metal stand. Porcelain head, arms and legs, 8" high $35* **MP $35**
(See Porcelain Music Box pg. 207)

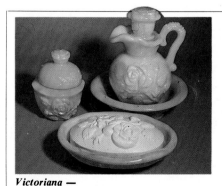

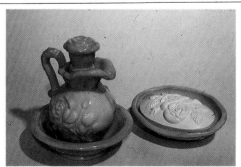

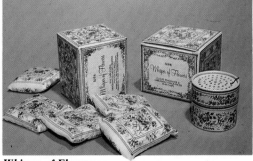

Victoriana —
1972 *Powder Sachet in 2 frag. 1½oz $6* **MP $9**
1971 *Pitcher and Bowl, SSS Bath Oil 6oz $7.50* **MP $13**
1972 *As above with Foaming Bath Oil in 2 frag. $7.50 and $8.50* **MP $13**
1972 *Soap Dish/Soap, 2 frag. $4.50* **MP $8**

1978 *Pitcher and Bowl. Limited edition, embossed "May 1978". Bubble Bath 6oz $13.50* **MP $13**
1978 *Soap Dish and 5oz Special Occasion scented Soap. Dated May 1978 $8.50* **MP $10**

Whisper of Flowers —
1980 *Sachet Pillows in Garlandia fragrance. Set of 5 $9.50* **MP $8**
1980 *Closet Pomander with Garlandia fragranced wax chips $5.50* **MP $5.50 complete, $3 container only**

**Available from Avon at time of publication*

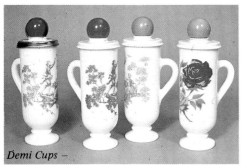
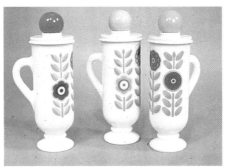
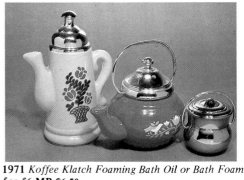

Demi Cups –
1968 *Foaming Bath Oil 3oz $3.50* **MP $8**
1969 *Charisma Foaming Bath Oil 3oz $3.50* **MP $8**
1969 *Regence Foaming Bath Oil 3oz $3.50* **MP $8**
1969 *To A Wild Rose Foaming Bath Oil 3oz $3.50* **MP $9**

1971 *Dutch Treat Demi Cups 3 frag. Cream Lotion 3oz $3.50* **MP $8**

KITCHEN FIGURALS

(See also pages 189-192)

1971 *Koffee Klatch Foaming Bath Oil or Bath Foam 5oz $6* **MP $6.50**
1973 *Little Dutch Kettle Foaming Bath Oil in 2 frag. or Lemon Bathfoam 5oz $6* **MP $6.50**
1976 *Hearthside Decanter .66oz Sweet Honesty or Occur! Cream Sachet $5* **MP $5.50**

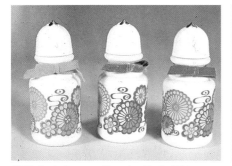
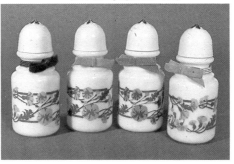
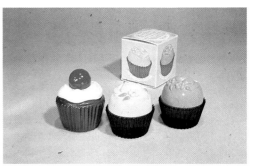

1968 *Bath Seasons Foaming Bath Oil in Honeysuckle, Lilac & Hawaiian White Ginger 3oz $2.50* **MP $8**

1967 *Bath Seasons Foaming Bath Oil in Lily of The Valley, Honeysuckle, Lilac & Jasmine 3oz $2.50* **MP $10**

1974 *Sweet Treat Cologne, Pink and Pretty 1oz $3.35* **MP $5**
1979 *Bon-Bon Cologne in Sweet Honesty (pink) or Cotillion (yellow) .75oz $6* **MP $2.50**

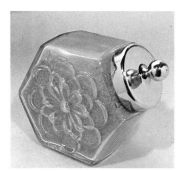
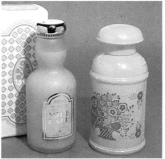
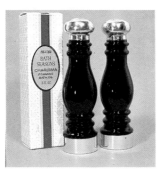
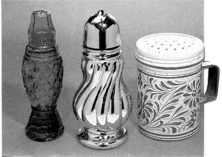

1973 *Country Store Mineral Springs Bath Crystals 12oz $7.50* **MP $7.50**

1974 *Liquid Milk Bath in Moonwind, Sonnet or Imperial Garden 6oz $6* **MP $7**
1973 *Creamery Decanter with Hand and Body Lotion in Roses, Roses or Field Flowers 8oz $6* **MP $7**

1969 *Bath Seasons Foaming Bath Oil in Charisma or Brocade 3oz $3.50* **MP $7 each, $8 boxed**

1976 *Crystalpoint Salt Shaker Cologne in Sonnet or Cotillion 1½oz $4* **MP $4**
1977 *Silver Swirls Salt Shaker Cologne in Sweet Honesty or Topaze 3oz $7.50* **MP $6**
1977 *Country Talc Shaker (metal) Sweet Honesty or Charisma 3oz $7.50* **MP $5**

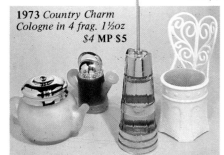
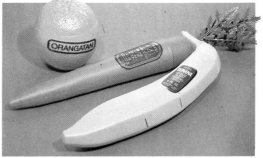
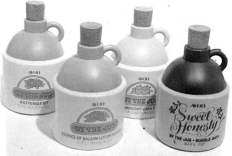

1973 *Country Charm Cologne in 4 frag. 1½oz $4* **MP $5**
1974 *Teatime Powder Sachet in Moonwind, Roses, Roses or Sonnet 1¼oz $6* **MP $6**
1972 *Dream Garden Perfume Oil in 5 frag. ½oz $6* **MP $12**
1972 *Sweet Shoppe Pin Cushion Cream Sachet in 6 frag. 1oz $5 to $6* **MP $9**

1976 *Orangatan. 6oz Bronze Glory Tanning Lotion $4* **MP $2**
1978 *Karrot Tan. 9" plastic carrot holds 4oz Bronze Glory Tanning Lotion $7.50* **MP $3**
1974 *Sunana Bronze Glory Tanning Lotion 6oz $3.50* **MP $3**

By the Jug –
1974 *Astringent 10oz $4* **MP $4**
1974 *Essence of Balsam Lotion Shampoo 10oz $4* **MP $4**
1974 *Strawberry Bath Foam 10oz $4* **MP $4**
1976 *Sweet Honesty Bubble Bath 10oz $5* **MP $3**

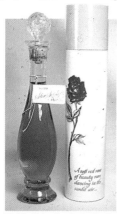
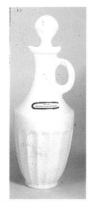
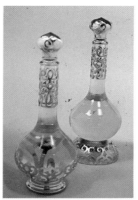
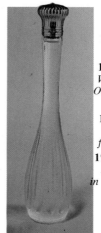
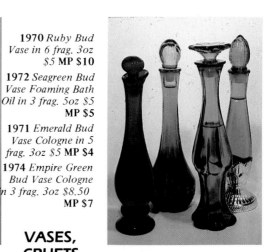

1962 *Skin-So-Soft Bath Oil 10¼"h. $3.50* **MP $14 with card/label, $18 boxed**

1963 *Bath Urn opal glass. Perf. Bath Oil 6 frag. $3.50/$3.75* **MP $15 with label**

1968 *Riviera Cologne in Brocade or Regence 4oz $6* **MP $9** *(Shown also with reversed base)*

1964 *Deluxe Bath Decanter, Skin-So-Soft 6oz $3.50* **MP $12 with neck tag** *(not shown)*

1970 *Ruby Bud Vase in 6 frag. 3oz $5* **MP $10**

1972 *Seagreen Bud Vase Foaming Bath Oil in 3 frag. 5oz $5* **MP $5**

1971 *Emerald Bud Vase Cologne in 5 frag. 3oz $5* **MP $4**

1974 *Empire Green Bud Vase Cologne in 3 frag. 3oz $8.50* **MP $7**

VASES, CRUETS and URNS

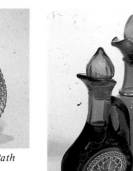
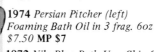
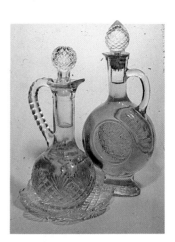

1974 *Regency Skin-So-Soft Bath Oil 6oz $6.50* **MP $6**
1975 *Golden Flamingo Foaming Bath Oil in Bird of Paradise, Charisma or Field Flowers 6oz $7.50* **MP $5**

1974 *Persian Pitcher (left) Foaming Bath Oil in 3 frag. 6oz $7.50* **MP $7**

1972 *Nile Blue Bath Urn, Skin-So-Soft Bath Oil 6oz $7.50* **MP $8**

1974 *Nile Green Bath Urn Foaming Bath Oil in Field Flowers, Bird of Paradise or Charisma $7.50* **MP $8**

1973 *Cruet Cologne Set, 4 frag. 8oz $15* **MP $16**

1966 *Skin-So-Soft Decanter (Cruet) 10oz $5* **MP $10**

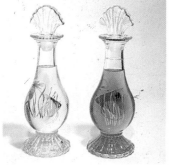
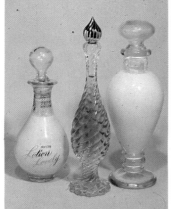
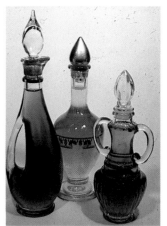

1978 *Sea Fantasy Bud Vase, SSS 6oz $10.50* **MP $7**
1979 *Sea Fantasy Bud Vase (reissue) Light Bouquet SSS, Smooth As Silk Bath Oil or Bubble Bath 6oz $11* **MP $7**

1964 *Lotion Lovely Body Lotion in 7 frag. 8oz $3 to $4* **MP $8**

1967 *Cologne Classic in 8 frag. 4oz $3.50 to $5* **MP $6**

1972 *Classic Beauty Decanter Hand & Body Lotion in 2 frag. 10oz $5* **MP $6**

1967 *Bath Urn, Skin-So-Soft 8oz $5* **MP $9**

1965 *Skin-So-Soft Urn 10oz $5* **MP $9**

1974 *Athena Bath Urn (right) Foaming Bath Oil in 3 frag. 6oz $8.50* **MP $7**

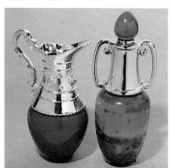
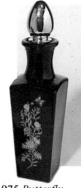
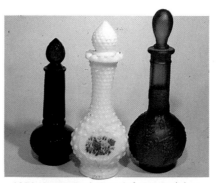
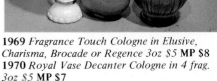
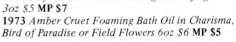

1973 *Venetian Pitcher Cologne Mist in 4 frag. 3oz $8* **MP $7**
1974 *Marblesque Cologne Mist in Imperial Garden, Moonwind or Sonnet 3oz $8.50* **MP $6**

1975 *Butterfly Garden Vase Cologne in Roses, Roses, Bird of Paradise or Topaze 6oz $8* **MP $8**

1973 *Garnet Bud Vase Cologne in 4 frag. 3oz $6* **MP $5**
1973 *Hobnail Bud Vase Cologne in 2 frag. 4¾oz $7* **MP $7**
1973 *Grape Bud Vase. Skin-So-Soft Bath Oil 6oz $6.50* **MP $6**

1969 *Fragrance Touch Cologne in Elusive, Charisma, Brocade or Regence 3oz $5* **MP $8**
1970 *Royal Vase Decanter Cologne in 4 frag. 3oz $5* **MP $7**
1973 *Amber Cruet Foaming Bath Oil in Charisma, Bird of Paradise or Field Flowers 6oz $6* **MP $5**

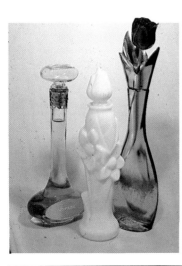

1968 *Bud Vase (left) Cologne in 8 frag. 4oz $4 to $5* MP $8

1973 *Floral Bud Vase. Foam of Roses Bathfoam or Field Flowers Foaming Bath Oil 5oz $6* MP $6

1971 *Cologne Elegante in 5 frag. 4oz $8.50 to $10* MP $15

1972 *Victorian Lady Foaming Bath Oil in 4 frag. 5oz $6* MP $7

1969 *Classic Decanter SSS Bath Oil 6oz $6* MP $10

1971 *Sea Maiden Skin-So-Soft Bath Oil 6oz $6* MP $8

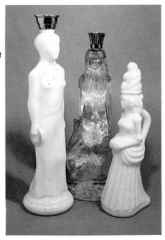

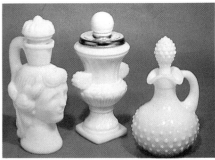

1972 *Grecian Pitcher Skin-So-Soft Bath Oil 5oz $6* MP $7
1971 *Bath Urn Foaming Bath Oil or Bath Foam 5oz $5* MP $8
1972 *Hobnail Decanter Foaming Bath Oil or Bathfoam in 4 frag. 5oz $7 to $8* MP $7

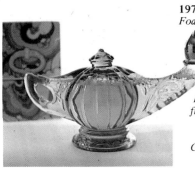

1971 *Aladdin's Lamp Foaming Bath Oil in 5 frag. 6oz $7.50* MP $12

1971 *Parlor Lamp Cologne 3oz & Perfumed Talc ¼oz in 5 frag. $7.50 to $9* MP $10

1970 *Courting Lamp Cologne in 5 frag. 5oz $7* MP $12

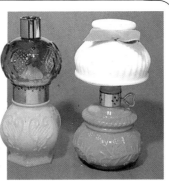

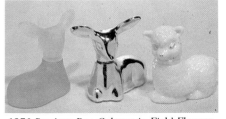

1976 *Precious Doe Cologne in Field Flowers or Sweet Honesty ½oz $4* MP $3
1978 *Silver Fawn Cologne in Sweet Honesty or Charisma ½oz $4* MP $3
1977 *Little Lamb Cologne in Sweet Honesty or Topaze ¾oz $5* MP $3

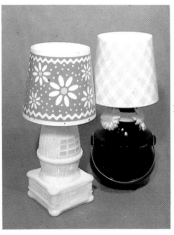

1976 *Country Charm Cologne in Field Flowers or Sonnet 4.8oz $10* MP $7

1973 *Hearth Lamp Cologne in 3 frag. 8oz $8.50* MP $8

1973 *Tiffany Lamp Cologne in 4 frag. 5oz $8 to $9* MP $10

1974 *Ming Blue Lamp Foaming Bath Oil in 3 frag. 5oz $7.50* MP $6

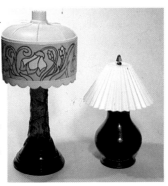

A GLASS MENAGERIE

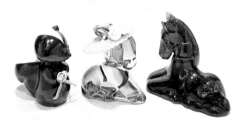

1978 *Sniffy Cologne Decanter in Sweet Honesty or Topaze 1¼oz $7* MP $5
1978 *Little Burro Cologne, straw-like hat and flower. Charisma or Sweet Honesty 1oz $6* MP $5
1979 *Gentle Foal Cologne in Charisma or Sun Blossoms 1.5oz $7* MP $3

LAMPS BY AVON

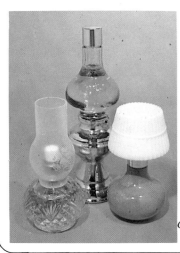

1973 *Chimney Lamp (left) Cologne Mist in 3 frag. 2oz $6.50* MP $6

1976 *Library Lamp Cologne in Charisma or Topaze 4oz $9* MP $6 *(center)*

1975 *Charmlight Decanter Cream Sachet and 2oz Cologne in Imperial Garden, Moonwind or Sonnet $8* MP $6

1976 *Mansion Lamp Cologne in Bird of Paradise or Moonwind 6oz $11* MP $9

1973 *Hurricane Lamp Cologne in 4 frag. 6oz $9.50* MP $10

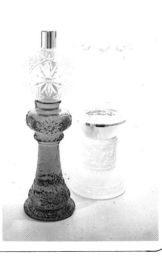

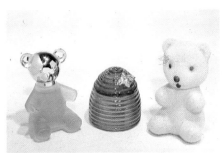

1976 *Teddy Bear. ¾oz Topaze or Sweet Honesty Cologne $4.50* MP $3
1978 *Honey Bee Cologne in Moonwind or Honeysuckle 1¼oz $6* MP $3
1977 *Fuzzy Bear Cologne in Sweet Honesty or Occur! $6.50* MP $5

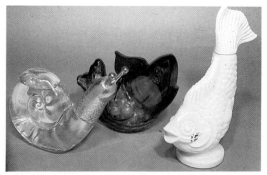

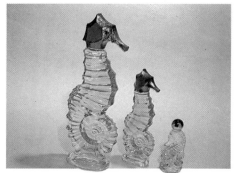

1968 *Dolphin, Skin-So-Soft Bath Oil $5* **MP $9**
1973 *Dolphin Miniature Cologne in Charisma or Field Flowers 1½oz $4* **MP $4**

1973 *Bath Treasure (Snail) Skin-So-Soft Decanter 6oz $7.50* **MP $8**
1974 *Song of the Sea, 80 bath "pearls" in 3 frag. $8.50* **MP $8.50**
1973 *Sea Spirit Foaming Bath Oil, 3 frag. 5oz $6* **MP $6**

1970 *Sea Horse Decanter, Skin-So-Soft Bath Oil 6oz $6* **MP $8**
1973 *Sea Horse Miniature Cologne in Unforgettable or Here's My Heart 1½oz $4* **MP $4**
1980 *Seahorse Miniature Cologne in Charisma, Sweet Honesty, Moonwind and Occur! .5oz $3.50* **MP $1.50**

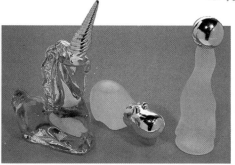

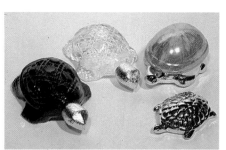

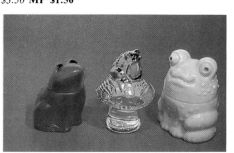

1974 *Unicorn Cologne Decanter in 4 frag. 2oz $5* **MP $4**
1977 *Baby Hippo Cologne in Sweet Honesty or Topaze 1oz $5* **MP $3**
1976 *Lovable Seal Cologne in Here's My Heart or Cotillion 1oz $4* **MP $2**

1971 *Treasure Turtle Cologne in 14 frag. 1oz $3.50* **MP $4**
1977 *Treasure Turtle Cologne (clear) in Sweet Honesty or Charisma 1oz $4.50* **MP $3**
1975 *Precious Turtle Cream Sachet in Roses, Roses or Patchwork .66oz $5.50* **MP $4**
1978 *Golden Turtle Solid Perfume Compact in Sweet Honesty or Candid .07oz $7* **MP $4**

1977 *Emerald Prince Cologne in Sweet Honesty or Moonwind 1oz $5* **MP $4**
1976 *Fairytale Frog Cologne. Sweet Honesty or Sonnet 1oz $4.50* **MP $2**
1973 *Enchanted Frog Cream Sachet Decanter in Sonnet or Moonwind 1½oz $5* **MP $4**

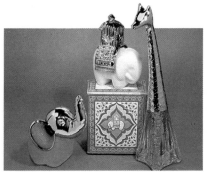

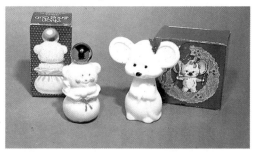

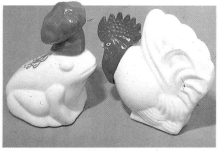

1974 *Good Luck Elephant Cologne in Sonnet, Imperial Garden or Patchwork 1½oz $5* **MP $4**
1977 *Royal Elephant Cologne in Topaze, Charisma 1½oz $6* **MP $4**
1975 *Graceful Giraffe Cologne in Topaze or To A Wild Rose 1½oz $5.50* **MP $3**

1979 *Snug Cub Cologne in Sweet Honesty or Occur! 1oz $6* **MP $3**
1979 *Merry Mouse Cologne in Cotillion or Zany .75oz $6* **MP $3**

1975 *Handy Frog Decanter with Moisturized Hand Lotion 8oz $7.50* **MP $7**
1973 *Country Kitchen Hand Lotion 6oz $6* **MP $8**

. . . A GLASS MENAGERIE . . .

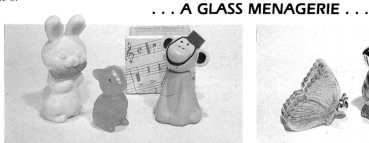

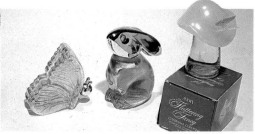

1974 *Swiss Mouse Cologne in Roses, Roses, Field Flowers or Bird of Paradise 3oz $6* **MP $5**
1977 *Tree Mouse Cream Sachet in Charisma or Sweet Honesty .66oz $6* **MP $3**

1979 *Fuzzy Bunny Cologne in Sweet Honesty or Honeysuckle 1oz $7.50* **MP $4**
1979 *Charming Chipmunk Cologne in Sweet Honesty or Field Flowers .5oz $5.50* **MP $2**
1979 *Monkey Shines Cologne in Sonnet or Moonwind 1oz $7.50* **MP $4**

1972 *Butterfly Cologne in 5 frag. 1½oz $4* **MP $5**
1974 *Snow Bunny Cologne in 4 frag. 3oz $6* **MP $5**
1980 *Fluttering Fancy Cologne in Charisma or Sweet Honesty 1oz $7.50* **MP $5**

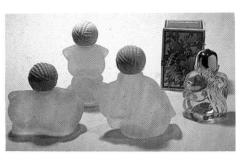

1981 *Frisky Friends Cologne. Pink cap: Hawaiian White Ginger, Yellow: Roses, Roses, Blue: Honeysuckle 1oz $6.50 ea.* **MP $3**
1982 *Autumn Scurry Cologne in 3 frag. 5oz $4* **MP $1**

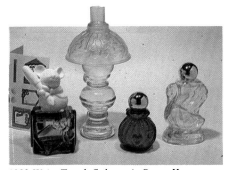

1982 *Write Touch Cologne in Sweet Honesty or Charisma 1oz $7.50* **MP $3**
1981 *Nostalgic Glow Cologne in 3 frag. 1oz $7.50* **MP $4**
1983 *Heartstrings Cologne in 3 frag. .5oz $4.50* **MP $1**
1981 *Winged Princess Cologne in 3 frag. .5oz $4.50* **MP $1**

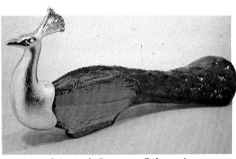

1973 *Regal Peacock Decanter Cologne in Moonwind, Patchwork or Sonnet 4oz $7* **MP $9**

BIRDS
of
AVON

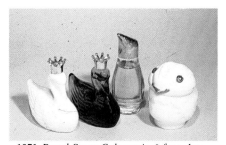

1971 *Royal Swan Cologne in 6 frag. 1oz $3.50* **MP $6**
1974 *Royal Swan Cologne in 4 frag. 1oz $3.50* **MP $8**
1975 *Pert Penguin Cologne in Cotillion or Field Flowers 1oz $4* **MP $2**
1973 *Snow Bird Cream Sachet Decanter in 3 frag. 1½oz $5* **MP $3**

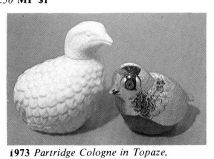

1973 *Partridge Cologne in Topaze, Unforgettable, Occur! and Somewhere 5oz $6.50* **MP $7**
1974 *Robin Red-Breast Cologne in Roses, Roses, Bird of Paradise and Charisma 2oz $5* **MP $5**

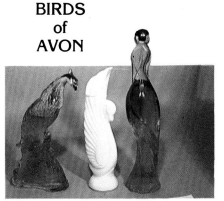

1970 *Bird of Paradise Cologne Decanter 8"h, 5oz $6* **MP $8**
1972 *Swan Lake Cologne in 4 frag. 3oz $5 to $6* **MP $6**
1971 *Flamingo Decanter Cologne in 4 frag. 5oz $5.50* **MP $8**

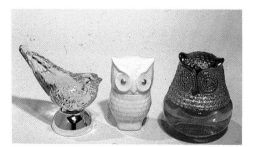

1971 *Song Bird Cologne in 5 frag. 1½oz $4* **MP $5**
1972 *Precious Owl Cream Sachet in 4 frag. 1½oz $4 to $5* **MP $5**
1974 *Owl Fancy Cologne Gelee, Raining Violets or Roses, Roses 4oz $6* **MP $6**

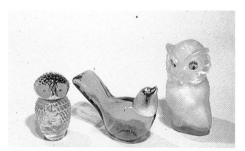

1974 *Baby Owl Cologne. 1oz Occur! or Sweet Honesty $4* **MP $2**
1975 *Bird of Happiness Cologne in 4 frag. 1½oz $5* **MP $4**
1976 *Snow Owl, 1¼oz Moonwind or Sonnet Powder Sachet $7* **MP $4**

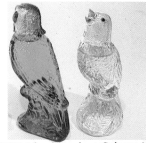

1977 *Island Parakeet Cologne in Charisma or Moonwind 1½oz $6* **MP $4**
1979 *Golden Notes Cologne in Moonwind or Charisma 1¾oz $6* **MP $3**

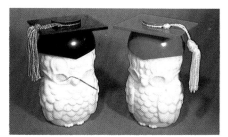

1975 *Dr. Hoot Cologne 4oz Sweet Honesty or Wild Country $7.50* **MP $5**
1977 *Dr. Hoot Cologne (blue hat) 4oz Sweet Honesty or Wild Country $7.50* **MP $7**

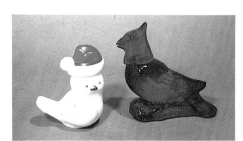

1979 *Precious Chickadee Cologne in Here's My Heart and Sun Blossoms 1oz $6* **MP $3**
1979 *Red Cardinal Cologne in Bird of Paradise or Charisma 2oz $6.50* **MP $3**

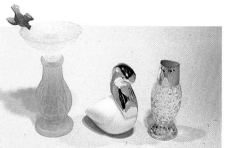

1977 *Song of Spring. 1oz Sweet Honesty or Topaze Cologne $6* **MP $4**
1978 *Love Bird Cologne in Charisma or Moonwind 1½oz $6* **MP $3**
1980 *Owl Miniature Cologne in Ariane, Timeless, Candid and Tasha .6oz $4* **MP $1**

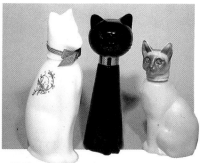

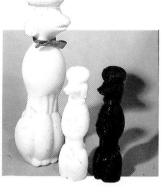

**A
KENNEL
OF
CATS
AND
DOGS**

*1971 Ming Cat Cologne in 4 frag. $6.50 to
$8* **MP $10**
*1975 Tabatha Spray Cologne in Imperial Garden
Bird of Paradise, Cotillion 3oz $7.50* **MP $7**
*1978 Royal Siamese Cologne in Cotillion or
Moonwind 4.5oz $8.50* **MP $7**

*1973 Suzette Foaming Bath Oil
Decanter in 5 frag. 5oz $6* **MP $5**
*1972 Bon Bon Cologne in 5 frag.
1oz $3.50* **MP $4**
*1973 Bon Bon (black) Cologne in
4 frag. 1oz $3.50* **MP $5**

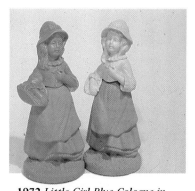

*1972 Little Girl Blue Cologne in
Brocade, Unforgettable, Cotillion and
Somewhere 3oz $6* **MP $9**
*1974 Pretty Girl Pink Cologne in
Unforgettable, Somewhere, Occur! and
Topaze 3oz $6* **MP $12**

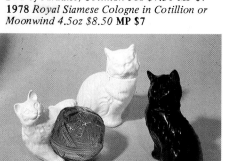

*1973 Kitten Petite Cologne in Moonwind or
Sonnet 1½oz $4* **MP $4**
*1972 Kitten Little Cologne in 5 frag. 1½oz
$4* **MP $4**
*1975 Kitten Little (black) Cologne in Bird
of Paradise, Roses, Roses or Sweet Honesty
1½oz $3.50* **MP $4**

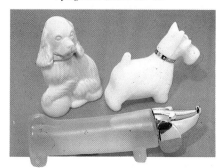

*1974 Lady Spaniel Cologne in Moonwind,
Sonnet or Patchwork 1½oz $4.50* **MP $5**
*1973 Queen of Scots Cologne in 5 frag.
1oz $4* **MP $4**
*1973 Dachshund Cologne in 4 frag. 1½oz
$4* **MP $4**

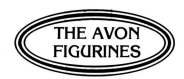

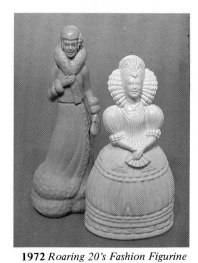

*1972 Roaring 20's Fashion Figurine
Cologne in Unforgettable, Topaze,
Somewhere and Cotillion 3oz $6*
MP $11
*1972 Elizabethan Fashion Figurine
Cologne 4oz in Charisma, Field
Flowers, Bird of Paradise $6 and
Moonwind $7* **MP $12**

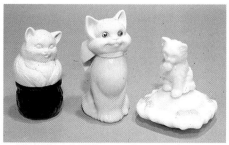

*1974 Kitten's Hideaway Cream Sachet in
Field Flowers, Bird of Paradise or Charisma
1oz $5* **MP $5**
*1975 Blue Eyes Cologne in Topaze or Sweet
Honesty 1½oz $6* **MP $4**
*1976 Sitting Pretty Cologne in Charisma or
Topaze 1½oz $6* **MP $4**

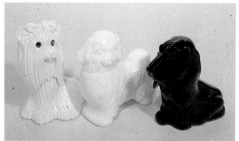

*1976 Princess of Yorkshire Cologne in Topaze or
Sweet Honesty 1oz $6* **MP $3**
*1974 Royal Pekingese Cologne in Topaze,
Unforgettable and Somewhere 1½oz $4* **MP $3**
*1978 Baby Bassett Cologne in Sweet Honesty or
Topaze 1¼oz $5* **MP $3**

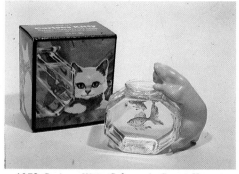

*1979 Curious Kitty Cologne in Sweet Honesty or
Here's My Heart 2.5oz $7.50* **MP $4, $5 boxed**

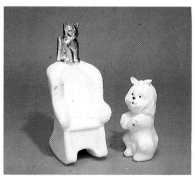

*1971 Sitting Pretty Cologne in 5 frag.
4oz $6* **MP $7**
*1979 Sweet Tooth Terrier Cologne in
Cotillion or Topaze 1oz $6* **MP $3**

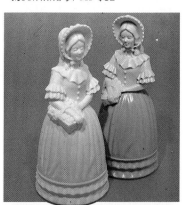

*1971 Victorian Fashion Figurine (left)
Cologne in Field Flowers, Elusive, Bird of
Paradise or Brocade 4oz $6* **MP $13**
*1973 Victorian Fashion Figurine
Cologne in Field Flowers, Charisma,
Bird of Paradise 4oz $6* **MP $40**

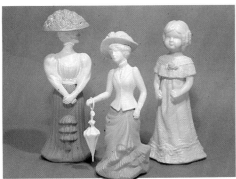

1974 *Gay Nineties Fashion Figurine in Topaze, Unforgettable or Somewhere 3oz $6* **MP $11**
1979 *On The Avenue Figurine Cologne in Unforgettable or Topaze 2oz $9* **MP $8**
1979 *Adorable Abigail Cologne in Regence or Sweet Honesty 4.5oz $13* **MP $10**

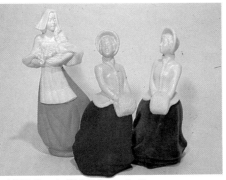

1973 *Dutch Girl Cologne in Topaze, Unforgettable or Somewhere 3oz $6* **MP $9.50**
1977 *Skater's Waltz Cologne in Charisma or Moonwind 4oz $8.50* **MP $7**
1979 *Skater's Waltz Cologne (blue) in Charisma or Cotillion 4oz $10* **MP $7**

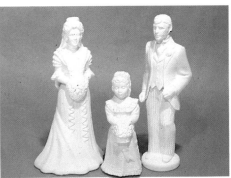

1976 *Bridal Moments Cologne in Sweet Honesty or Unforgettable 5oz $9* **MP $8**
1979 *Wedding Flower Maiden Cologne in Sweet Honesty or Unforgettable 1.75oz $7* **MP $6**
1978 *Proud Groom Cologne in Unforgettable or Sweet Honesty 2oz $9* **MP $8**

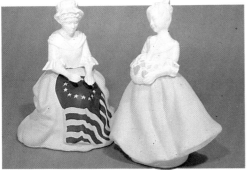

1976 *Betsy Ross Cologne in Sonnet or Topaze 4oz $6.99 dated July 4, 1976* **MP $11 Available 2 campaigns only.** *In milk glass* **MP $25**
1974 *Flower Maiden Cologne in Somewhere, Topaze and Cotillion 4oz $6* **MP $8**

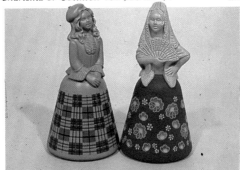
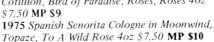

1975 *Scottish Lass in Sweet Honesty, Cotillion, Bird of Paradise, Roses, Roses 4oz $7.50* **MP $9**
1975 *Spanish Senorita Cologne in Moonwind, Topaze, To A Wild Rose 4oz $7.50* **MP $10**

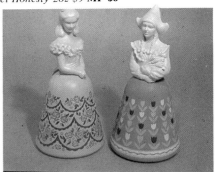

1976 *American Belle in Sonnet or Cotillion Cologne 4oz $7.50* **MP $6**
1977 *Dutch Maid Cologne in Sonnet or Moonwind 4oz $7.50* **MP $6.50**

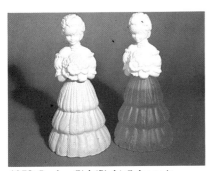

1978 *Garden Girl (Pink) Cologne in Charisma or Sweet Honesty Cologne 4oz $7* **MP $5**
1975 *Garden Girl Cologne in Sweet Honesty, Somewhere, Cotillion, To A Wild Rose 4oz $7* **MP $6**

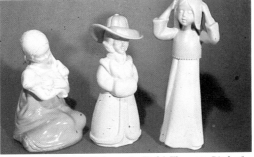

1973 *Dear Friends Cologne in Field Flowers, Bird of Paradise, Roses, Roses 4oz $6* **MP $12**
1973 *Little Kate Cologne in Charisma, Bird of Paradise or Unforgettable 3oz $5* **MP $9**
1974 *Sweet Dreams Cologne in Sweet Honesty or Pink & Pretty 3oz $6* **MP $15**

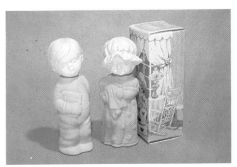

1979 *Sweet Dreams Cologne in Somewhere or Zany 1.25oz $7.50* **MP $5.50**
1980 *Little Dream Girl Cologne in Sweet Honesty or Occur! 1.25oz $7.50* **MP $5.50**

. . . THE AVON FIGURINES

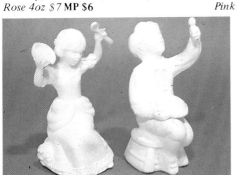

1978 *Little Miss Muffet Cologne in Topaze or Sweet Honesty 2oz $7* **MP $6**
1979 *Little Jack Horner Cologne in Topaze or Roses, Roses 1.5oz $7.50* **MP $6***

* Available from Avon at time of publication

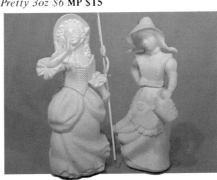

1976 *Little Bo-Peep Cologne in Sweet Honesty or Unforgettable 2oz $7* **MP $6**
1977 *Mary, Mary Cologne in Sweet Honesty or Topaze 2oz $7* **MP $6**

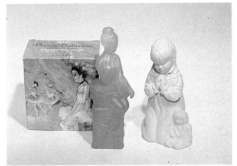

1981 *Prima Ballerina Cologne in Sweet Honesty or Zany 1oz $7.50* **MP $6.50**
1981 *First Prayer Cologne in Charisma, Topaze or Occur! 1.5oz $8.50* **MP $7**

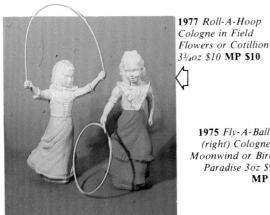

1977 *Roll-A-Hoop Cologne in Field Flowers or Cotillion 3³/₄oz $10* **MP $10**

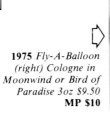

1975 *Fly-A-Balloon (right) Cologne in Moonwind or Bird of Paradise 3oz $9.50* **MP $10**

1976 *Catch-A-Fish Cologne in Field Flowers or Sonnet 3oz $9.50* **MP $6.50**

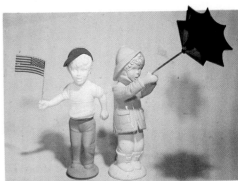

1980 *Marching Proud Cologne in Sweet Honesty or Topaze 2oz $14.50* **MP $12*** **(Last Figurine in the Motion series)**
1979 *Tug-A-'Brella Cologne in Moonwind or Cotillion 2.5oz $12.50* **MP $10**

1975 *Skip-A-Rope Cologne in Sweet Honesty, Bird of Paradise or Roses, Roses 4oz $9.50* **MP $10**

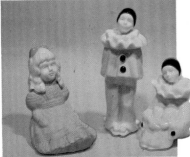

1982 *Pierrot Cologne in Occur! (center) or Sweet Honesty 1.75oz $12.50* **MP $9**

1982 *Pierrette Cologne in Occur! or Sweet Honesty (right) 1.75oz $12.50* **MP $9**

1982 *Precious Priscilla Cologne in Moonwind or Sweet Honesty (left) 3oz $12.50* **MP $10***

American Fashion Thimble Collection. Miniature hand-painted porcelain replicas. Each 2" high.
1982 *Victorian 1890 Edition $13* **MP $10***
1982 *Gibson 1900 Edition $13* **MP $10***
1983 *Cavalier 1923 Edition $13* **MP $10***
1983 *Flapper 1927 Edition $13* **MP $10***
1983 *Art Deco 1928 Edition $13* **MP $10***
1983 *Floral Fantasy 1938 Edition $13* **MP $10***
1984 *Big Band Era 1942 Edition $13* **MP $10***
1984 *Christian Dior's "New Look" Edition $13* **MP $10***

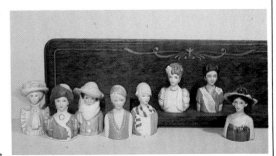

1983 *Thimble Display Rack 12¹/₂" long $16.50* **MP $13***

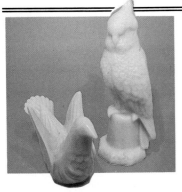

1974 *Delicate Dove, Sun Forest or Summer Breeze scent $6* **MP $7**
1972 *Cockatoo, Floral Medley scent $6* **MP $8**

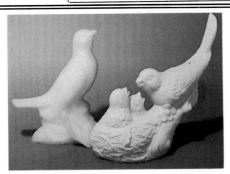

1974 *Sign of Spring, Fernerie scent $6* **MP $7**
1978 *The Nestlings, Garlandia scent $8* **MP $6**

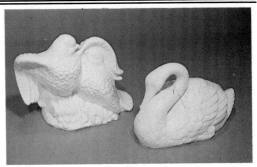

1979 *Two Turtledoves, Potpourri scent $11* **MP $10**
1980 *Tender Love, Potpourri scent $12* **MP $11**

DECORATIVE POMANDERS

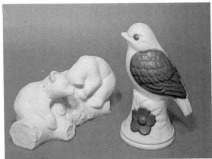

1979 *Honey Bears, Floral Medley scent $9* **MP $8**
1975 *Meadow Bird, Fernerie scent $7.50* **MP $8**

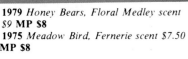

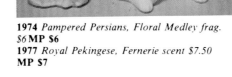

1974 *Pampered Persians, Floral Medley frag. $6* **MP $6**
1977 *Royal Pekingese, Fernerie scent $7.50* **MP $7**

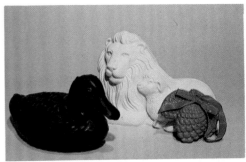

1974 *Duck Decoy, Wild Country or Deep Woods scent $8* **MP $9**
1980 *Peaceful Partners, Fragrant Seasons scent $13* **MP $10**
1980 *Pine Cone Cluster Hanging Pomander, Mountain Pine scent $5.50* **MP $4**

*Available from Avon at time of publication

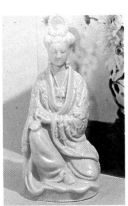
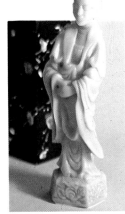
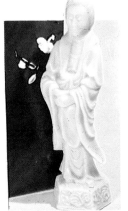
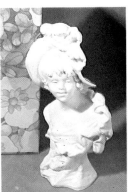
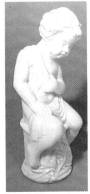
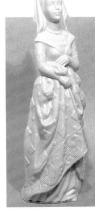

1975 *Coral Empress, Fragrant Seasons scent $6* **MP $8**

1972 *Oriental Figurine, Potpourri scent $6* **MP $10**

1973 *Oriental Figurine, Potpourri scent 10''high $6* **MP $9**

1976 *Parisian Mode, Garlandia scent $7.50* **MP $6**

1975 *Florentine Cherub, Fragrant Seasons scent $7.50* **MP $7**

1977 *Florentine Lady, Fragrant Seasons scent $8* **MP $6**

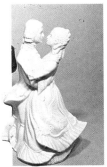
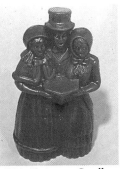
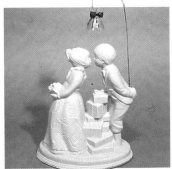
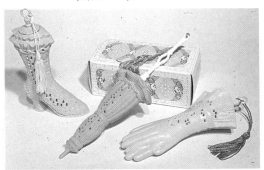

1978 *Viennese Waltz, Potpourri scent $9* **MP $7**

1974 *Christmas Carollers, Festival Garlands scent $7.50* **MP $8**

1979 *Under the Mistletoe, Potpourri scent $12.50* **MP $11**

1978 *Frilly Boot Closet Pomander, Potpourri wax chips $6* **MP $3**
1976 *Parasol Closet Pomander, Potpourri $5* **MP $3**
1979 *Lacy Gloves Closet Pomander, Garlandia scent $6* **MP $3**

. . . DECORATIVE POMANDERS

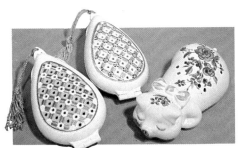
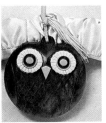
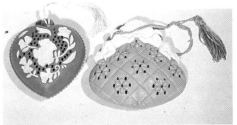
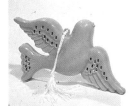

1967 *Lavender Closet Pomander, refillable $5* **MP $7**
1970 *Potpourri Closet Pomander, refillable $5* **MP $7**
1978 *Pampered Piglet Ceramic Pomander, Meadow Morn $10* **MP $9**

1974 *Wise Eyes Closet Pomander, Fernerie scent $4* **MP $6**

1973 *Heartscent Closet Pomander, Potpourri scent $4* **MP $6**
1977 *Sweet Cherubs Closet Pomander, Potpourri scent $5* **MP $4**

1979 *Fresh Flight Pomander, Potpourri scent $6* **MP $5**

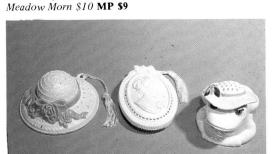
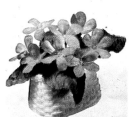
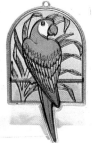
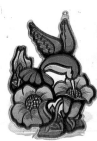
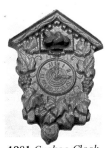

1975 *Picture Hat Pomander, Potpourri scent $5* **MP $5**
1980 *Cameo Closet Pomander, Potpourri scent $6* **MP $5**
1980 *Flirtatious Frog Ceramic Pomander, Fernerie scent $11* **MP $10**

1981 *Basket of Violets Pomander in white opal glass holds fabric violets, Violet scented chips $13* **MP $10**

1981-84 *Tropical Splendor Hanging Window Pomander $12* **MP $9**

1980 *Fragrant Flight Window Pomander, Flowerburst scent $12* **MP $10**

(See "Whisper of Flowers" page 192)

1981 *Cuckoo Clock Hanging Wall Pomander, Spiced Apple scented chips $12* **MP $9**

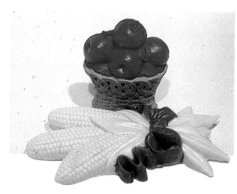

1978 *Bountiful Harvest, Spiced Apple scent $9.50* **MP $9**

1979 *Autumn Harvest Hanging Pomander, Garlandia scent $10.50* **MP $9**

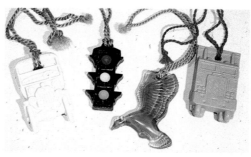

1979 *Model T Car Pomander, Country Morning scent $3.50* **MP $2**
1980 *Traffic Stopper Car Pomander, Country Morning scent $4* **MP $3**
1980 *Wild Game Car Pomander, Meadow Morn scent $5.50* **MP $4**
1981 *Keep On Truckin' Car Pomander, Fernerie scent $5* **MP $3**

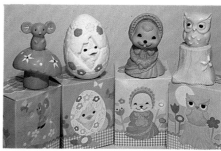

1981 *Heralds of Spring Mini-Pomanders Potpourri scent. Mouse, Chick, Chipmunk and Owl each 3" high $6* **MP $4**

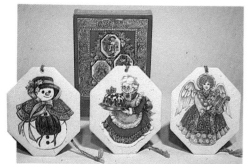

1980 *Fragrant Tree Trimmings. Set of 3 Mountain Pine scented fabric ornaments with a different design on each side. Cords included $9 a set* **MP $9**

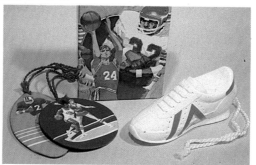

1981 *Go For It! Football and Basketball fabric scented Pomanders $8 set* **MP $6**
1981 *Sneakin' Round Pomander, Country Morning scent wax chips and blue decals $7* **MP $5**

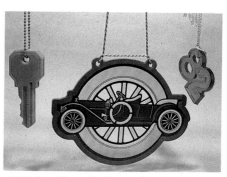

1981 *Sure Start Car Pomander, Meadow Morn scent $5.50* **MP $3**
1981 *Vintage Motorcar Pomander, Country Morning scent $14* **MP $10**
1982 *1982 Graduate Pomander, Herbal Mist scent (2 Campaigns only) $5.50* **MP $5**

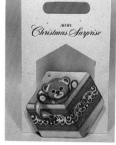

1982 *Christmas Surprise Fragranced Ornament, Holiday Spice scent $5* **MP $3**

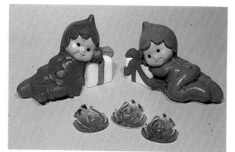

1982 *Santa's Helpers Pomander, Festive Garlands scent. Boy (left) or Girl $8 each* **MP $7 each**
1981 *Hidden Scents Sachet Nuggets, Meadow Morn scent $6.50* **MP $4**

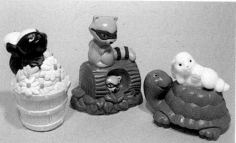

1982 *Woodland Charmers Mini Pomanders. Skunk in flower basket, Raccoons with log or Rabbit with tortoise, Fernerie scent $8.50 each* **MP $6 each**

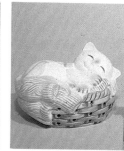

1983 *Cat-Napper Ceramic Pomander, Meadow Morn scented wax chips $16.50* **MP $13**

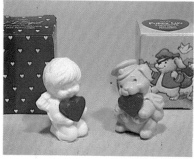

1982 *L'il Cupid Pomette, Potpourri scent (2 Campaigns only) $5* **MP $3**
1983 *Puppy Luv Pomette, Garlandia scent $5* **MP $2**

(See also p. 210 & 211)

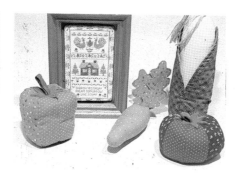

1983 *Calico Garden Fabric Pomander, Fernerie scent. Pepper, Carrot, Corn or Tomato $9 each* **MP $7**
1982 *An American Tradition Pomander, plastic 5"x7" wall frame $12* **MP $10**

*Available from Avon at time of publication

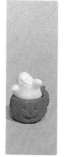

1983 *Littlest 'Boo' Pomette, Halloween Treat scent (2 Campaigns only) $4.50* **MP $3**

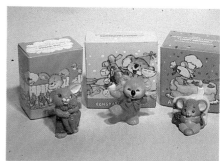

1984 *Merry Messenger Pomette in greeting carton, Special Occasion scent. "Thank You" with Bunny, "Congratulations" with Koala and "Happy Birthday" with Mouse $6.50 each* **MP $5* each**

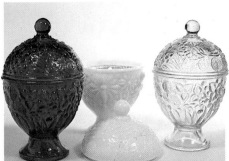

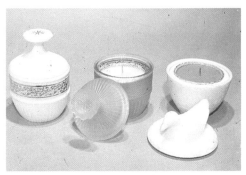

Perfumed Pedestal Candle Containers
  1965 *Red $4* **MP $17**
  1964 *White $3.50* **MP $15**
  1965 *Amber $4* **MP $17**

CANDLES by AVON

1967 *First Christmas Candle, Frankincense and Myrrh, non-refillable $5* **MP $14**
1969 *Perfumed Candle and pedestal-snuffer lid in 9 frag. $7.50 and $8* **MP $10**
1974 *Golden Pine Cone Fragrance Candlette, Bayberry fragrance $6* **MP $6.50**

1966 *Perfumed Candle (white) in 9 frag. $4.25 to $5* **MP $15**
1967 *Perfumed Candle (frosted) in 8 frag. each in a different colored aluminum cup that shows through the glass $4.50* **MP $16**
1970 *Nesting Dove in 7 frag $7.50* **MP $10**

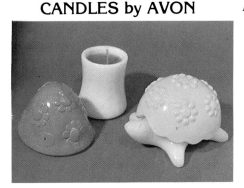

1972 *Mushroom Candle, Garden Spice (non-refillable) $5* **MP $8**
1972 *Turtle Candle, Garden Spice (non-refillable) $5* **MP $8**

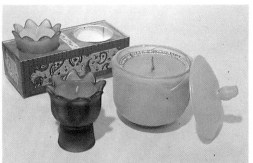

1971 *Floral Medley Perfumed Candles 1.3oz (non-refillable) $5.50* **MP $10**
1972 *Glow of Roses Perfumed Candle and Container $7* **MP $9**

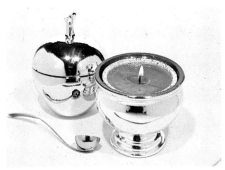

1968 *Golden Apple in 9 frag. $5.75 to $6.50* **MP $15**
1969 *Wassail Bowl Candle Holder with silver ladle $8* **MP $13**

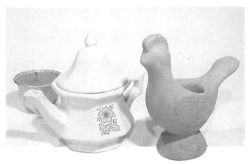

1972 *China Teapot, genuine china, 2 cup size with Perfumed Candle (available one campaign only) $12.50* **MP $20**
1976 *Terra Cotta Bird Fragrance Candlette Holder $8* **MP $7.50**

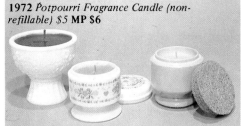

1972 *Potpourri Fragrance Candle (non-refillable) $5* **MP $6**

1973 *Hearts and Flowers Candle, Floral Medley scent $5* **MP $5**
1974 *Kitchen Crock Candlette, Meadow Morn fragrance $5* **MP $6.50**

1979 *Bunny Ceramic Planter Perfumed Candle Holder in Floral Medley or Spice Garden $18* **MP $15**

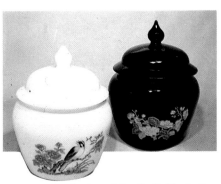

1971 *Dynasty Perfumed Candle Holder in 7 frag. $7.50* **MP $12**
1974 *Lotus Blossoms Perfumed Candle and Holder in 9 frag. $10* **MP $12**

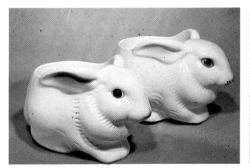

1977 *Bunny Ceramic Planter Candle Holder in 5 frag., hand-painted and "Handcrafted in Brazil" on bottom. Did not appear in brochure, sold only during C-15-77 at $10.99* **MP $13**
1978 *Bunny Planter-Candle Holder made in U.S. in Roses, Roses or Floral Medley $15* **MP $13**

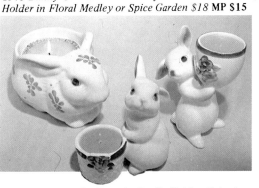

1980 *Bunny Bright Ceramic Candle Holder, Spiced Apple fragrance Candlette $14* **MP $12**
1981 *Sunny Bunny Ceramic Candle Holder, dated Avon 1981. Floral Medley fragrance Candlette $16.50* **MP $14**

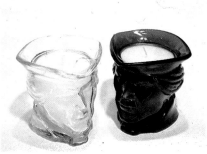

1979 *Revolutionary Soldier Fresh Aroma Smoker's Candle, non-refillable $8* **MP $10**
1979 *As above, issued in amber glass $9* **MP $9**

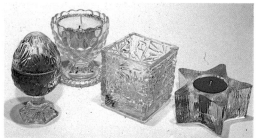

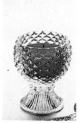

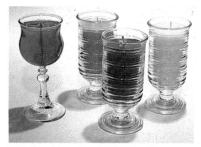

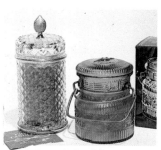

1979 *Crystalglow Clearfire Transparent Candle, Softscent fragranced Amethyst candle $13.50* **MP $10**
1974 *Ovalique Perfumed Candle Holder in 9 frag. $10* **MP $8**
1978 *Winter Lights Candlette, Moonwind fragrance $10* **MP $9**
1980 *Starbright Candle with Bayberry (red) or Floral Medley (white) scent $11* **MP $8**

1975 *Facets of Light Candlette, Bayberry scent $6* **MP $6**

1980 *Sparkling Swirl Clearfire Transparent Candle, Softscent fragrance $14.50* **MP $12**
1980 *Sherbet Dessert Candle, Spiced Apple scent (pink), Strawberry scent (red), Lemon scent (yellow) $10* **MP $9**

1969 *Crystal Candelier, Frankincense and Myrrh scented candle chips and wick 6½"h $7* **MP $12 complete**
1979 *Country Spice Candle, Spiced Apple scent $10.50* **MP $8**

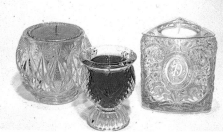

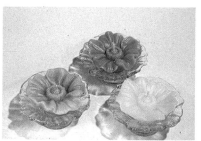

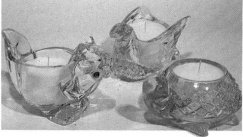

1972 *Crystal Glow Candle Holder $10* **MP $12**
1979 *Clearfire Transparent Candle, Softscent fragrance $12* **MP $8***
1980 *Personally Yours Candle, Meadow Morn scent, issued with 26 gold foil alphabet letters $14* **MP $11**

1980 *Floral Light Candle, Floral Medley scent in choice of yellow, lavender or green candle $9* **MP $7**

. . . CANDLES BY AVON

1978 *Bright Chipmunk Candelette, Spice Garden fragrance $9.50* **MP $7**
1977 *Dove in Flight Candlette, Meadow Morn $9.50* **MP $7**
1978 *Sparkling Turtle, Meadow Morn $9.50* **MP $6**

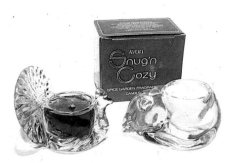

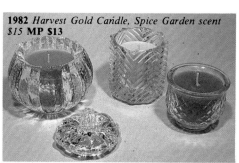

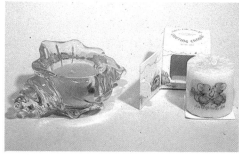

1979 *Shimmering Peacock Clearfire Candle, Softscent fragrance $12.50* **MP $11**
1981 *Snug 'N Cozy Fragrance Candle, Spice Garden scent $12* **MP $11**

*Available from Avon at time of publication

1982 *Harvest Gold Candle, Spice Garden scent $15* **MP $13**
1982 *Ultra Shimmer Perfumed Candle, Tasha Foxfire, Timeless or Odyssey scent $11* **MP $8***
1982 *Spice Cupboard Candle, Spice Ginger (shown) Frosty Mint, Chocolate, Vanilla or Apple scent $6.50* **MP $5**

1983 *Coral Glow Fragranced Candle, Tropical Breeze scent $15* **MP $12**
1983 *Rain or Shine Greeting Candle in "Greeting Card" carton, Spice Garden scented candle $6.50* **MP $5 complete**

CANDLESTICKS BY AVON

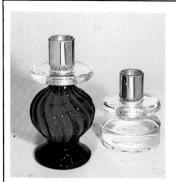

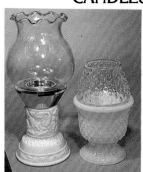

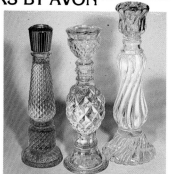

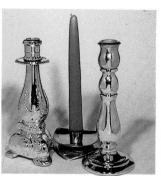

1970 *Candlestick Cologne in 5 frag. 4oz $6* **MP $11**
1974 *Cologne and Candlelight in Imperial Garden, Roses, Roses or Charisma 2oz $5* **MP $5**

1973 *Hurricane Lamp Cologne in 4 frag., candle not included $9.50* **MP $10**
1973 *Hobnail Patio Candle Holder in 8 frag. $9* **MP $10**

1970 *Crystallite Candlestick Cologne in 6 frag. 4oz $5.50* **MP $6**
1973 *Regency Candlestick Cologne in 4 frag. 4oz $8* **MP $8**
1976 *Opalique Candlestick Cologne in 2 frag. 5oz $12* **MP $8**

1972 *Candlestick Cologne in 4 frag. $7 & $8.50* **MP $8**
1970 *Danish Modern Set. Scented Taper 9"h, $4.50* **MP $8.50**
1966 *Candlestick Cologne in 3 fragrances 3oz $3.75* **MP $13**

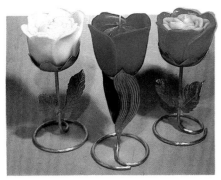

1973 *Sunshine Rose Fragrance Candle, Rose scent* $8.50 **MP $9.50**
1973 *Flaming Tulip Candle, Floral Medley scent* $8.50 **MP $9.50**
1971 *Floral Fragrance Candle, Floral Medley fragrance* $8.50 **MP $11**

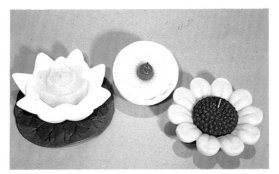

1972 *Water Lily Fragrance Candle, non-refillable,* $5 **MP $6**
1974 *Greatfruit Fragrance Candle, Grapefruit scented* $5 **MP $5**
1975 *Black-Eyed Susan Candle, Wild Flowers fragrance, non-refillable* $6 **MP $5**

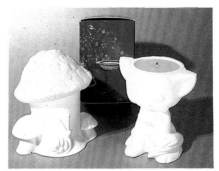

1975 *Enchanted Mushroom, Meadow Morn scent, non-refillable* $6 **MP $7**
1975 *Catnip Fragrance Candle, Floral Medley scent, non-refillable* $5 **MP $8**

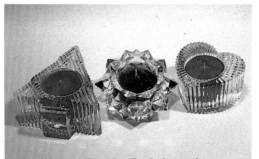

1981 *Glistening Tree Candle, Softscent frag-rance in Ruby (shown) or Emerald* $12 **MP $10**
1981 *Gem Glow Clearfire Transparent Candle in Emerald, Amber or Ruby, Softscent fragrance* $13 **MP $10**
1982 *Love Light Clearfire Transparent Candle, Softscent fragrance* $13 **MP $10**

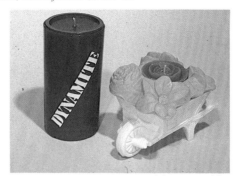

1975 *Dynamite Fragrance Candelette, reusable as pencil holder* $6.50 **MP $6**
1979 *Garden Bounty, Meadow Morn scent* $9.50 **MP $8**

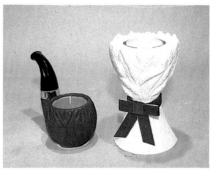

1979 *Fresh Aroma Smoker's Candle, non-refillable* $9 **MP $8**
1980 *Harvest Time Candle in glass holder, Spice Garden scent* $12 **MP $11**

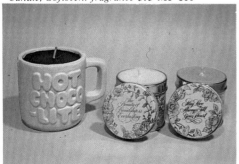

1981 *Hot Choco-Lite Candle, Chocolate scent* $9 **MP $7**
1982 *Scentiments Candle, Floral Medley scent in "Friendship" canister or "Love" canister* $8.50 *each* **MP $7 each**

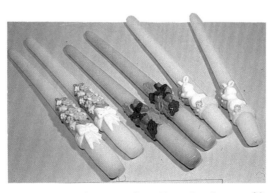

1982 *Fragranced Decorated 10" Taper Candles, set of 2 Flower Fancy, Floral Medley scent* $9 **MP $8**
Shades of Autumn, Spice Garden scent $10 **MP $9**
Easter Surprise, Garlandia scent $13 **MP $10**

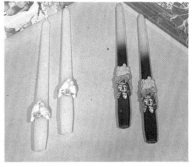

1983 *Love Birds Fragranced Tapers with removable dated ceramic love bird huggers* $18.50 *set of 2* **MP $15***
1983 *Autumn Harvest Sculptured Tapers 10"* $10 *set of 2* **MP $9**

. . . CANDLES BY AVON

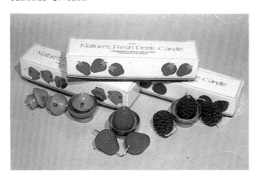

1984 *Nature's Fresh Petite Candles, Mushroom, Strawberry or Pine Cone. Carton of 3 with metal holder* $8.50 *each set* **MP $7**

**Available from Avon at time of publication*

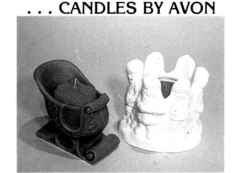

1975 *Sleigh Light Candle, Bayberry scent, non-refillable* $7 **MP $6**
1980 *Glow of Christmas Candle in glass holder, Floral Medley scent* $12 **MP $11**

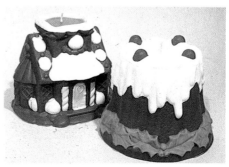

1977 *Gingerbread House Candle, Frankincense and Myrrh scented, non-refillable* $7 **MP $7**
1978 *Plum Pudding Candle, Frankincense and Myrrh scented, non-refillable* $9 **MP $8**

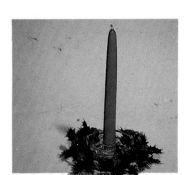

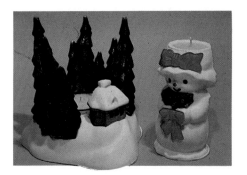

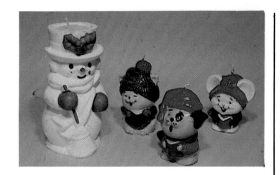

1980 *Holiday Candle Dish with Wreath and 8" Taper Candle. Red in Floral Medley scent. Off-white in Spice Garden and Green in Bayberry* **$11 MP $11**

1979 *Winter Wonderland Candle in glass holder, Bayberry scent $19* **MP $17**
1979 *Mrs. Snowlight Candle, Bayberry scented, non-refillable $9* **MP $8**

1981 *Mr. Snowlight Candle, Bayberry scented $9* **MP $8**
1981 *Carolling Trio Candles. Crooning Cat, Howling Hound or Melodic Mouse $7.50 each* **MP $5 each**

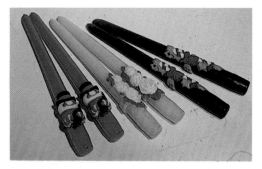

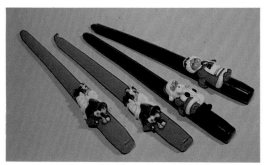

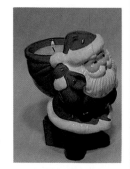

1980 *Fragranced Decorated 10" Taper Candles, Set of two, Bayberry scented $7* **MP $8** *Dapper Snowman in Red, Winter Rose in Off-white, Candy Cane and Holly in Green*

1981 *Christmas Chimes 10" Taper Candles, Bayberry Scent $9* **MP $8**
1981 *Mr. & Mrs. Christmas 10" Taper Candles, Bayberry scent $9* **MP $8**

1982 *Ho-Ho Glow Ceramic Candle Holder, Bayberry scent $18* **MP $16**

. . . CANDLES BY AVON

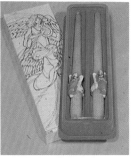

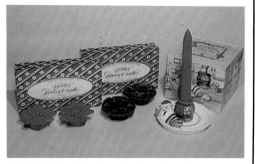

1982 *Stocking Surprise 10" Taper Candles, Bayberry scent (2 Campaigns only) $10* **MP $10**
1981 *Holiday Hostess 10" Taper Candles, Bayberry scent $9* **MP $8**

1983 *Heavenly Angel Ceramic Huggers and 10" Tapers, Bayberry scent $18.50* **MP $15**

1983 *Holiday Floating Candles, Fragrant Seasons scent. Poinsettia or Holly and Berry Wreaths. Set of 2 $6.50* **MP $6**
1983 *Snuggly Mouse Ceramic Candle Holder with 6" Festive Fragrance taper candle $18.50* **MP $15**

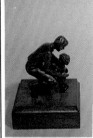

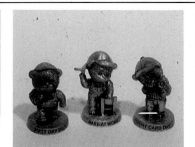

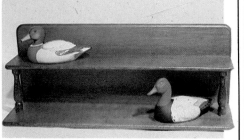

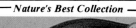

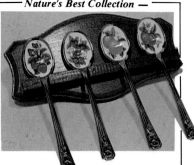

1984 *A Father's Arms Figurine. Dated metal figurine on solid wood base $24;* **MP $22**

Benjamin J. Bearington Pewter Figurines — *$16.50 each*
1983 *"First Day Back"* **MP $16**
1983 *"Hard at Work"* **MP $16**
1984 *"Report Card Day"* **MP $16**

Collector Duck Series — *Each cast metal duck carries the Avon Collectibles Logo.*
1983 *Mallard $16.50* **MP $13***
1984 *Canvasback $16.50* **MP $13***
1983 *Display Rack, solid mahogany 12½" $18.50* **MP $15***

Inlaid porcelain spoon 5", $12 each.
1981 *Wooden Display Rack 7" long $10* **MP $10**
1981 *Strawberry decal spoon* **MP $12**
1982 *Raspberry* **MP $12**
1982 *Orange* **MP $12**
1982 *Plum* **MP $12**

*Available from Avon at time of publication

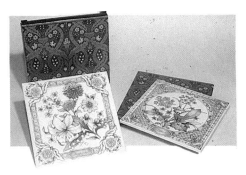

1983 *Floral Expression Collector Tiles, Happiness (left) and Love 6"x6" $12.50 each* **MP $10 each**

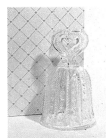

1984 *Fostoria Treasured Moments Bell 4¼" high $18.50* **MP $15***

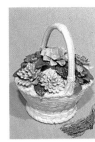

1980 *Porcelain Floral Bouquet. Hand-painted Bisque, dated 1980 on bottom $19* **MP $18***

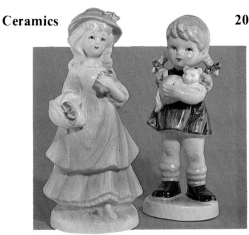

1973 *Jennifer Ceramic Figurine $9.99* **MP $45**
1973 *My Pet Ceramic Figurine $9.99* **MP $40**

CERAMICS

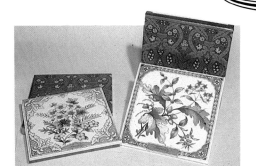

1983 *Floral Expression Collector Tiles. Friendship (left) and Hospitality 6"x6" $12.50 each* **MP $10 each**

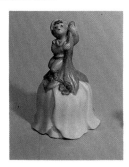

1983 *"Good Luck" Bell. Hand-painted porcelain $18.50* **MP $15**

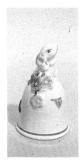

1984 *Bunny Bell. Hand-painted, dated "1984" $15* **MP $13***

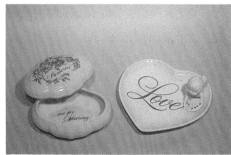

1983 *Avon Memories Porcelain Music Box. Trimmed in 14k gold, plays "Try To Remember" melody $35* **MP $30***
1984 *Cupid's Message Porcelain Dish 5" wide $15* **MP $13***

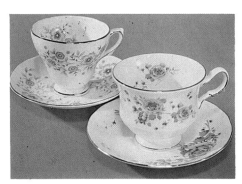

1974 *Blue Blossoms Cup/Saucer $11.50* **MP $16**
1974 *Pink Roses Cup/Saucer $11.50* **MP $16** *(Both made in England with 22k gold trim.)*

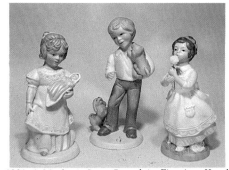

1981 *A Mother's Love Porcelain Figurine. Hand-painted, dated "1981" $23* **MP $20**
1981 *Best Friends Porcelain Figurine. Hand-painted, dated "1981" $23* **MP $20**
1982 *Wishful Thoughts Porcelain Figurine. with fabric dandelion $25* **MP $23**

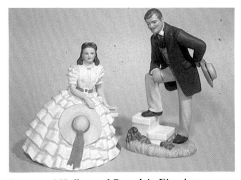

Images of Hollywood Porcelain Figurines —
1983 *Vivien Leigh as Scarlet O'Hara 4½" high $36* **MP $33***
1984 *Clark Gable as Rhett Butler 5¾" high $36* **MP $33***

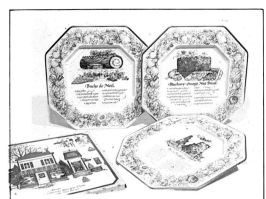

1982 *Hospitality Sweets Recipe Plates. 7" octogonal metal plate with recipe ingredients on front. Recipe card inc. with each. Plum Pudding Buche de Noel or Blueberry-Orange Nut Bread $7.50 each* **MP $6 each**

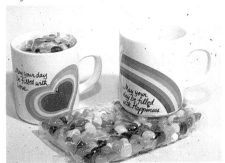

1984 *Love Mug and Happiness Mug. Each ceramic mug dated "Easter 1984" holds 8oz package of jelly beans (2 Campaigns only) $9.99* **MP $6 mug only**

**Available from Avon at time of publication*

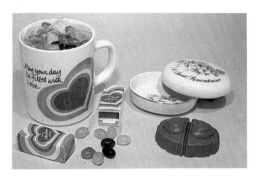

1983 *Love Mug with Jelly Beans 8oz (2 Campaigns only) $9.99* **MP $6 mug only**
1982 *A Sweet Remembrance. Porcelain box trimmed in 22k gold, dated "Valentine's Day 1982", holds 1.75oz Swiss chocolate (2 Campaigns only) $17.50* **MP $14 box only**

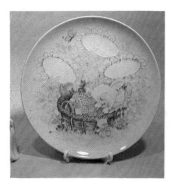

1983 *Sweet Dreams Keepsake Plate 7⅝" diam. $18.50* **MP $16**

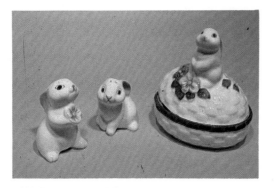

1983 *Bunny Mates Salt and Pepper Shakers $15.50 set* **MP $13**
1982 *Bunny Luv Trinket Box, made in Brazil. Dated "1982" $17.50* **MP $15**

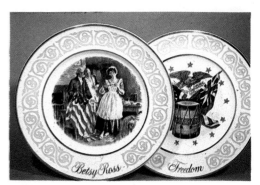

1973 *Betsy Ross Plate 9" diam. $15* **MP $25**
1974 *Freedom Plate 9" diam. $15* **MP $25**
Both Plates produced by Enoch Wedgewood (Tunstall) Ltd., England

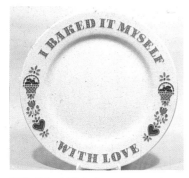

1982 *Baked With Love Plate 9" diam. Dated "1982" $22* **MP $18**

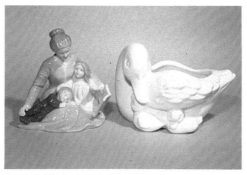

1984 *A Mother's Touch Figurine. Dated "Mother's Day 1984" $48* **MP $43**
1984 *Mother's Love Ceramic Planter with Oxalis plant and pkg. of growing medium (3 Campaigns only) $14.99* **MP $14 planter only**

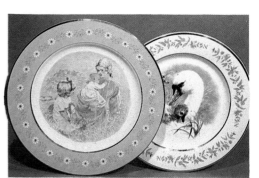

1974 *Tenderness Plate 9" diam. Created exclusively for Avon by Alvarez of Spain $15* **MP $22** *(Representative's Commemorative edition with inscription on back* **MP $27**)
1975 *Gentle Moments Plate 9" diam. Made in England by Wedgewood $17* **MP $22**

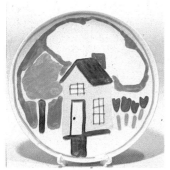

1982 *Children's Personal Touch Plate 7⅝" diam. with room to personalize $16* **MP $14**

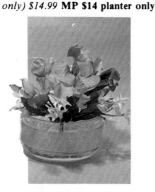

1982 *Crystalline Bowl with Fragranced Flowers and Odyssey fragrance tablet $22* **MP $15**

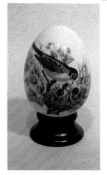

1984 *Four Seasons Porcelain Egg and wooden stand, "Spring" $18.50* **MP $15***

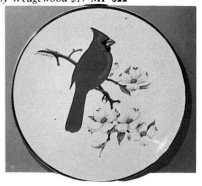

1974 *Cardinal Plate 10" diam. Cardinal decal designed and painted by Don Eckelberry $18* **MP $30**

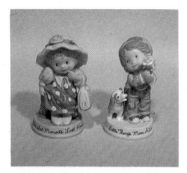

1983 *"Cherished Moments" 1981 Mother's Day Figurine $20* **MP $18**
1983 *"Little Things" 1982 Mother's Day Figurine $20* **MP $18**

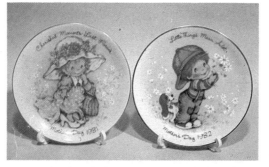

1981 *"Cherished Moments" 1981 Mother's Day Plate 5" with display easel $12* **MP $14**
1982 *"Little Things" 1982 Mother's Day Plate 5" with easel $14* **MP $14**

Available from Avon at time of publication

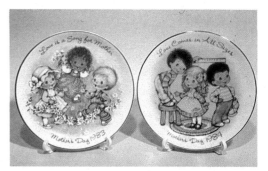

1983 *"Love Is a Song" 1983 Mother's Day Plate 5" with easel $15* **MP $14**
1984 *"Love Comes in All Sizes" 1984 Mother's Day Plate 5" with easel $15* **MP $14**

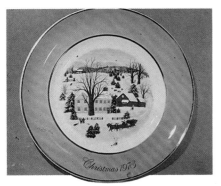

1973 *Christmas Plate "Christmas on the Farm", 9" diam. Produced by Wedgwood $15* **MP $85**

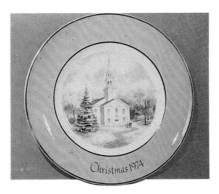

1974 *Christmas Plate "Country Church", 9" diam. Produced by Wedgwood $16* **MP $50**

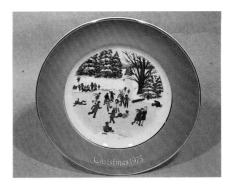

1975 *Christmas Plate "Skaters on the Pond", 9" diam. Produced by Wedgwood $18* **MP $32**

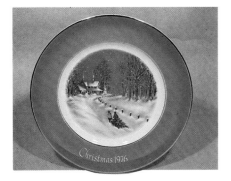

1976 *Christmas Plate "Bringing Home The Tree", 9" diam. Produced by Wedgwood $18* **MP $32**

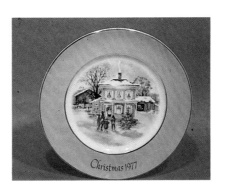

1977 *Christmas Plate "Carollers in The Snow", 9" diam. Produced by Wedgwood $19.50* **MP $30**

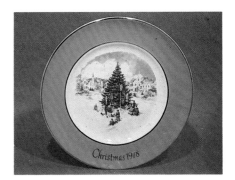

1978 *Christmas Plate "Trimming The Tree", 9" diam. Produced by Wedgwood $21.50* **MP $30**

CHRISTMAS PLATES & FIGURINES

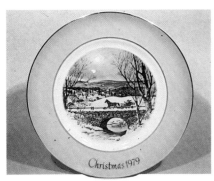

1979 *Christmas Plate "Dashing Through the Snow", 9" diam. Produced by Wedgwood $24* **MP $26**

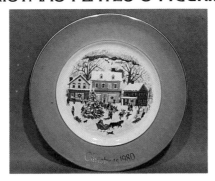

1980 *Christmas Plate "Country Christmas", 9" diam. Produced by Wedgwood and last in this design series $25* **MP $26**

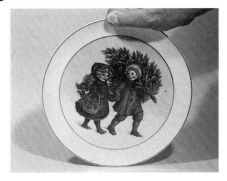

1981 *Christmas Plate without lettering on the front* **MP $75**

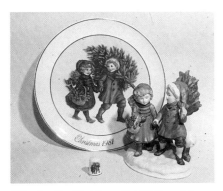

"Sharing the Christmas Spirit" Porcelain —
1981 *Christmas Plate 9" diam. Dated and trimmed in 22k gold $26* **MP $30**
1981 *Christmas Figurine $60* **MP $64**
1982 *Thimble, dated "1981" $12* **MP $12**

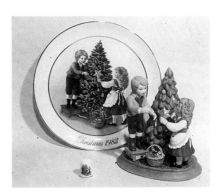

"Keeping the Christmas Tradition" Porcelain —
1982 *Christmas Plate 9" diam. Dated and trimmed in 22k gold $30* **MP $30**
1982 *Christmas Figurine $65* **MP $65**
1982 *Thimble "1982" $12* **MP $12**

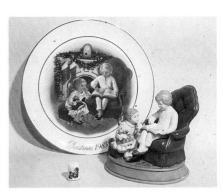

"Enjoying the Night Before Christmas" Porcelain —
1983 *Christmas Plate 9" diam. Dated and trimmed in 22k gold $30* **MP $30**
1983 *Christmas Figurine $65* **MP $65**
1983 *Thimble "1983" $12* **MP $12**

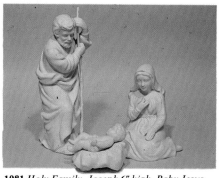

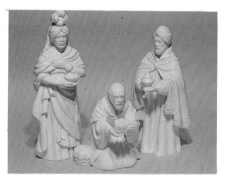

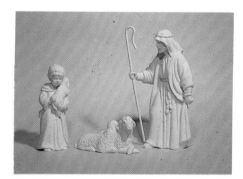

1981 *Holy Family. Joseph 6" high, Baby Jesus in Manger 2½" long and Mary 4" high $45 set* **MP $42.50 set***

1982 *The Magi. Balthasar 6½" high, Melchior 4¼" high and Kaspar 7½" high $23 each* **MP $23.50***

1983 *Shepherd Boy 4¾" high* $24 **MP $19.50***
1983 *Sheep 4" long $18* **MP $13.50***
1983 *Shepherd 6½" high $28* **MP $22.50***

Nativity Collectibles: Porcelain bisque figurines are handcrafted, dated and have initials of the artist, Michael Whitaker Arike.

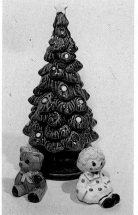

CHRISTMAS FIGURALS

1979 *Merry Christmas Tree Hostess Set. Ceramic Pomander Centerpiece and Rag Doll and Teddy Bear Shakers. Only one or two sets were sold to Representatives $29* **MP $30**

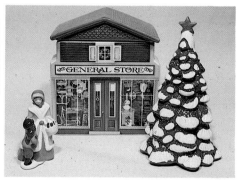

1982 *McConnell's Corner. Handcrafted and hand-painted collection.*
Town Shoppers 3" high $15 **MP $15**
General Store 5¾" high $32 **MP $32**
Town Tree 6" high $17 **MP $17**

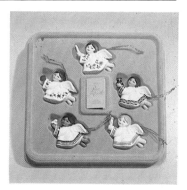

1983 *"Peace on Earth" Angels Ornament collection. Hand-painted porcelain ornaments, each 2½" wide $42* **MP $38**

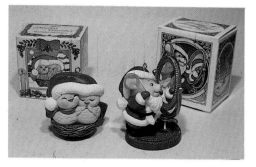

1982 *Nestled Together Keepsake Ornament, plastic, Dated "1982" $9* **MP $7**
1982 *Melvin P. Merrymouse Ornament, plastic. Dated "1982" $12* **MP $10**

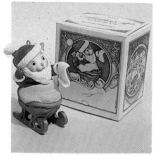

1983 *Melvin P. Merrymouse Ornament, plastic. Dated "1983" $12.50* **MP $10**

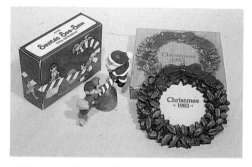

1983 *Santa's Seesaw Tree Ornament, plastic $12.50* **MP $10**
1983 *Captured Moments Frame Ornament, plastic and dated $8* **MP $6**

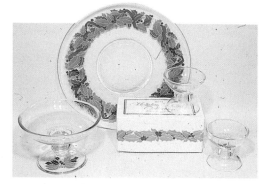

1981 *Holiday Hostess Compote 4" high $14* **MP $12**
1981 *Holiday Hostess Platter 11" diam. $18* **MP $16**
1981 *Holiday Hostess Candlesticks 3" high $12 pair* **MP $10 pair**

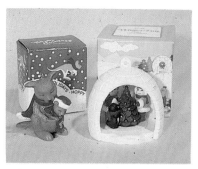

1983 *Hoppy Holidays Ornament, plastic $8* **MP $6**
1983 *Winter Fun Tree Ornament, plastic $12* **MP $10**

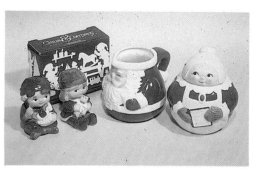

1983 *Claus & Company Porcelain Collection —*
Santa's Helpers Salt & Pepper Shakers. Boy and Girl $16 set **MP $13**
Santa Claus Creamer $16 **MP $13**
Mrs. Claus Sugar Bowl $16 **MP $13**

(See also p. 173 and 202 and Christmas candles pgs. 205-206)

*Available from Avon at time of publication

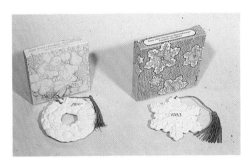

1980 *Christmas Ceramic Wreath with golden metallic cord, dated 1980 in 14k gold $10* **MP $11**
1983 *Christmas Ceramic Snowflake with golden metallic cord, dated 1983 in 14k gold $12* **MP $12**

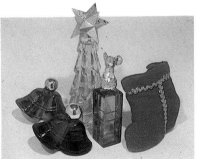

1974-75 *Christmas Bells Cologne in 4 frag. 1oz $4.50* **MP $4.50**
1979-80 *Christmas Bells Cologne (red glass) in 2 frag. 1oz $5* **MP $3**
1972 *Crystaltree Cologne in Moonwind or Sonnet 3oz $7.50* **MP $5**
1978 *Peek-A-Mouse Cologne in Sweet Honesty or Unforgettable 1oz in red cloth stocking $7* **MP $6 complete**

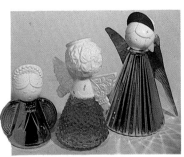

1968 *Golden Angel Foaming Bath Oil in 4 frag. 4oz $3.50* **MP $11 with wings**
1976 *Golden Angel Cologne in Sweet Honesty or Occur! 1oz $5* **MP $4**
1974 *Heavenly Angel Cologne in Unforgettable, Sweet Honesty or Occur! 2oz $5* **MP $6**

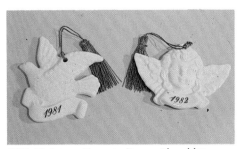

1981 *Christmas Ceramic Dove with golden metallic cord, dated 1981 in 14k gold $10* **MP $10**
1982 *Christmas Ceramic Angel with golden metallic cord, dated 1982 in 14k gold $12* **MP $12**

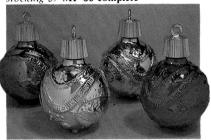

1967 *Christmas Ornament Bubble Bath 4oz green, silver, gold and red. $1.75 each* **MP $10**

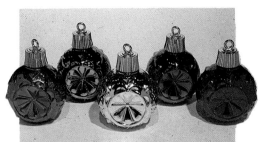

1968 *Christmas Sparkler Bubble Bath 4oz in blue, green, gold, red,each $2.50* **MP $9, Purple MP $35**

CHRISTMAS FIGURALS

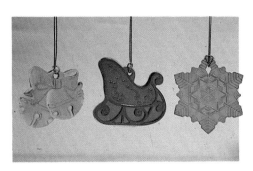

1982 *Seasonal Scents Pomander Ornaments, Mountain Pine scent. Jingle Bells, Country Sleigh and Shimmering Snowflake $5 each* **MP $4 ea.**

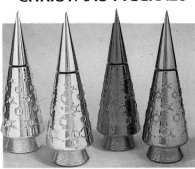

1968 *Christmas Tree Bubble Bath 4oz Silver, gold, red and green, each $2.50* **MP $9**

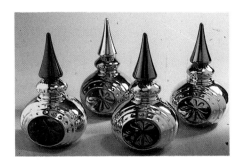

1969 *Christmas Cologne in 4 fragrances — red: Unforgettable, gold: Topaze, blue: Occur!, green: Somewhere 3oz each $3.50* **MP $8**

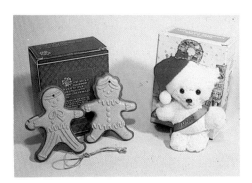

1981 *Gingerbread Joys Fragranced Wax Ornaments, Spiced Apple scent $7.50 set* **MP $7**
1982 *Baby's 1982 Keepsake Ornament. Stuffed Teddy Bear with ribbon dated 1982 $8* **MP $8**

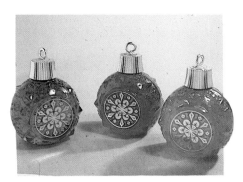

1970 *Christmas Ornament (plastic) Bubble Bath 5oz each $2.50* **MP $6**

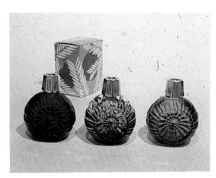

1979 *Festive Facets Cologne in Charisma (red), Sweet Honesty (green) and Here's My Heart (blue), 1oz $4.50* **MP $3**

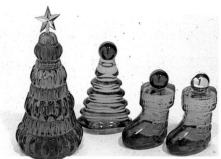

1974 *Yuletree Cologne in Sonnet, Moonwind or Field Flowers 3oz $6* **MP $4**
1975 *Touch of Christmas Cologne in Unforgettable or Imperial Garden Cologne 1oz $4* **MP $3**
1976 *Christmas Surprise Cologne in Sweet Honesty, Moonwind, Charisma or Topaze 1oz $4* **MP $2 Red cap, $3 Silver cap**

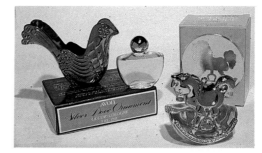

1976 *Silver Dove Ornament dated "Christmas 1976" holds ½oz bottle of Bird of Paradise or Occur! Cologne $7* **MP $8**
1979 *Rocking Horse Tree Ornament in Sweet Honesty or Moonwind Cologne .75oz $6.50* **MP $5**

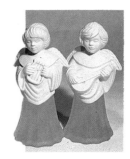

1978 *Angel Song (Lyre) Cologne in Here's My Heart or Charisma 1oz $5* **MP $3**
1979 *Angel Song (Mandolin) Cologne in Unforgettable or Moonwind $5.50* **MP $3.50**

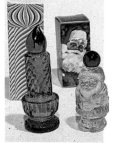
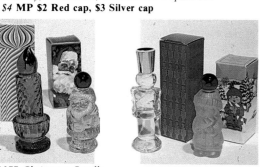
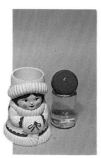
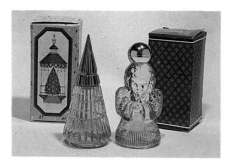

1977 *Christmas Candle (left) Cologne in 4 frag. 1oz $4* **MP $2**
1978 *Jolly Santa Cologne in Topaze or Here's My Heart 1oz $1.49 with purchase* **MP $1**

1980 *Christmas Soldier Cologne in 4 fragrances .75oz $3.50* **MP $2**
1980 *Song of Christmas Cologne in 3 fragrances .75oz $5.50* **MP $2**

1981 *Christmas Charmer Candlestick Holder Cologne in Zany or Charisma .33oz $9* **MP $7**

1982 *Crystallique Tree Cologne in Foxfire, Odyssey or Timeless .5oz $5* **MP $3**
1981 *Heavenly Angel Cologne in Ariane, Candid or Timeless .5oz $4.50* **MP $2**

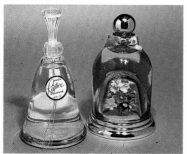

1965 *Fragrance Belle Cologne in 8 frag. 4oz $3.50 to $5* **MP $20 with tag**
1973 *Bell Jar Cologne in 4 frag. 5oz $6* **MP $8**

BELLS by AVON

1975 *Crystalsong Cologne in Sonnet $7.50 or Timeless 4oz $8.50* **MP $7**
1976 *Hospitality Bell Cologne in Moonwind, or Roses, Roses 3¾oz $8* **MP $7 ("Avon '76")**
1977 *Rosepoint Bell Cologne in Charisma or Roses, Roses 4oz $8.50* **MP $7 ("Avon '77" embossed on base)**

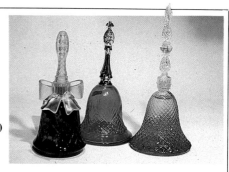

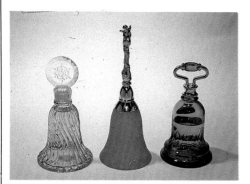

1980 *Crystal Snowflake Christmas Bell Cologne in 4 fragrances 3.75oz $10* **MP $9**
1979 *Cherub Hostess Bell Cologne in Bird of Paradise or Topaze 3.75oz ("1979") $9* **MP $8**
1978 *Emerald Bell Cologne in Sweet Honesty, Roses, Roses 3¾oz $8.50* **MP $7 ("Avon-'78")**

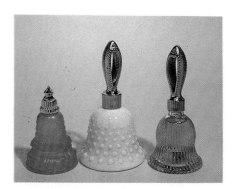

1978 *Joyous Bell Cologne in Charisma or Topaze 1oz $5* **MP $3**
1973 *Hobnail Bell Cologne in 5 frag. 2oz $5* **MP $5**
1968 *Fragrance Bell Cologne in 9 frag. 1oz $2* **MP $7**
(See also pages 211 & 213)

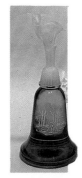

1981 *Moonlight Glow Annual Bell Cologne in Moonwind or Topaze. Last in the series of Christmas Bells, dated 1981 3oz $11* **MP $11**

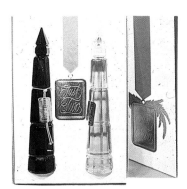

1965 *Just Two. Tribute After Shave Lotion, black, and Rapture Cologne, clear 3oz each $5.50* **MP $85, $32 black, $36 clear**

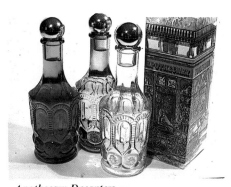

Apothecary Decanters —
1972 *Breath Fresh Mouthwash 8oz $3.50* **MP $4**
1973 *Spicy After Shave 8oz $4* **MP $4**
1973 *Lemon Velvet Moisturizing Friction Lotion 8oz $4* **MP $4**

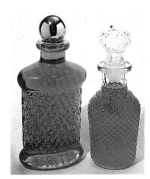

1974 *Breath Fresh Mouthwash 8oz $4* **MP $3**
1976 *Flavor Fresh Mouthwash 6oz $4* **MP $2**

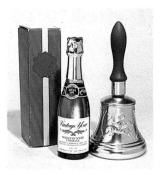

1978 *Vintage Year in Wild Country or Sweet Honesty Cologne 2oz $6* **MP $5**
1979 *Paul Revere Bell in Clint After Shave or Sweet Honesty Body Splash 4oz $9* **MP $9**

FIGURALS FOR MEN OR WOMEN

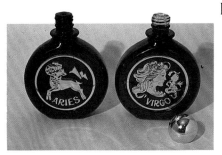

1975 *Star Signs Decanter in Wild Country After Shave or Sweet Honesty Cologne 4oz and embossed personalized Star Sign decal $7* **MP $5 black glass** *(left)* **MP $10 painted glass** *(right)*

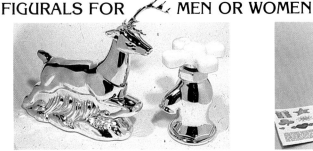

1976 *Wilderness Classic in Deep Woods After Shave or Sweet Honesty Cologne 6oz $10* **MP $9**
1977 *Just a Twist in Deep Woods After Shave or Sweet Honesty Cologne 2oz $5* **MP $3**

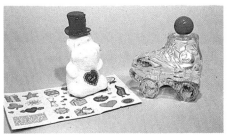

1980 *Huggable Hippo and sheet of decals in Light Musk After Shave or Zany Cologne 1.75oz $6* **MP $4**
1980 *Rollin' Great in Lover Boy or Zany Cologne 2oz $6* **MP $3**

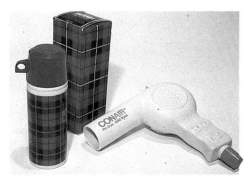

1978 *Plaid Thermos Brand Decanter in Wild Country After Shave or Sweet Honesty Body Splash 3oz $6* **MP $4**
1978 *Conair 1200 Blow Dryer with Naturally Gentle Shampoo 6oz $6* **MP $4**

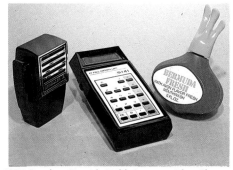

1977 *Breaker 19 with Wild Country After Shave or Sweet Honesty Cologne 2oz $5* **MP $3**
1978 *It All Adds Up! in Deep Woods After Shave or Sweet Honesty Body Splash 4oz $8.50* **MP $6**
1978 *Bermuda Fresh Mouthwash, plastic onion holds 6oz $4.50* **MP $2**

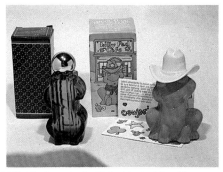

1981 *Big Spender in Light Musk After Shave or Sweet Honesty Cologne 1oz $5.50* **MP $3**
1982 *Huggable Hop-A-Long in Light Musk After Shave or Sweet Honesty Cologne and decals 1oz $6.50* **MP $4**

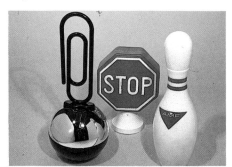

1978 *Get The Message in Clint After Shave or Sweet Honesty Cologne 3oz $9.50* **MP $7**
1975 *Stop! Decanter in Wild Country After Shave or Sweet Honesty Bath Freshener 4oz $5.50* **MP $3**
1978 *Strike! Decanter in Wild Country A/Shave or Sweet Honesty Cologne 4oz $5.50* **MP $3**

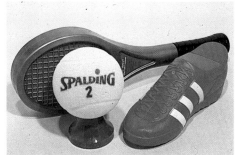

1975 *Tennis Anyone? in Spicy After Shave or Sweet Honesty After Bath Freshener 5oz $5* **MP $3**
1977 *Mixed Doubles in Spicy After Shave or Sweet Honesty Body Splash 3oz $6* **MP $4**
1978 *On The Run in Wild Country After Shave or Sweet Honesty Body Splash 6oz $6* **MP $4**

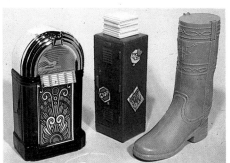

1977 *Juke Box with Wild Country After Shave or Sweet Honesty Cologne 4.5oz $6.50* **MP $4**
1977 *Locker Time with Wild Country After Shave or Sweet Honesty Body Splash 6oz $5.50* **MP $3**
1979 *Dingo Boot with Wild Country After Shave or Sweet Honesty Body Splash 6oz $5.50* **MP $4**

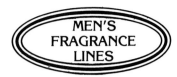

MEN'S FRAGRANCE LINES

Dorothy Bernard's
FRAGRANCE DATING GUIDE
For Men and Boys

1929 *Bay Rum (formerly Aromatic Bay Rum and California Bay Rum)*

1931 *After Shaving Lotion (renamed Original 1965)*

1959 *After Shower 'Vigorate*

1961 *Deluxe Spice (later Spicy)*

1963 *Tribute*

1964 *Blue Blazer (for Young Men) "4-A"*

1965 *Leather Original*

1966 *Island Lime Sports Rally (for Boys)*

1967 *Wild Country*

1968 *Windjammer*

1969 *Bravo Excalibur*

1970 *Oland*

1971 *Tai Winds*

1972 *Deep Woods Sure Winner (for Boys-Tai Winds fragrance)*

1973 *Blend 7*

1975 *Everest*

1976 *Clint*

1978 *Trazarra*

1979 *Weekend Avon Naturals: Brisk Spice Cool Sage Crisp Lime Light Musk*

1980 *Black Suede Lover Boy Rookie (for Boys)*

1981 *Rugger*

1982 *CJ*

1983 *Cordovan Musk for Men*

1984 *Cool Seas Feraud Pour Homme*

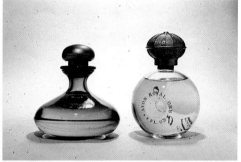

1964 *Captain's Choice, After Shave Lotion in 3 frag. or After Shower Cologne 8oz each $2.50 & $2.75* **MP $16. 1965** *Spicy Pre-Electric Shave* **MP $17**
1965 *Royal Orb in Spicy or Original After Shave Lotion 8oz $3.50* **MP $25**

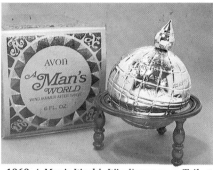

1969 *A Man's World. Windjammer or Tribute After Shave Lotion 6oz $5* **MP $8 with stand, boxed**

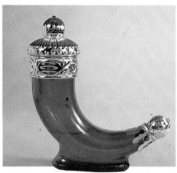

1966 *Viking Horn in Spicy, Original or Blue Blazer After Shave 7oz $7* **MP $22**

MEN'S FIGURALS

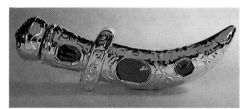

1968 *Scimitar in Windjammer or Tribute After Shave 6oz $6* **MP $20**

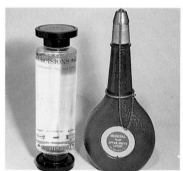

1965 *Decisions, Spicy After Shave Lotion 8oz $2.50* **MP $27**
1966 *Alpine Flask in Spicy, Blue Blazer or Original After Shave 8oz $4* **MP $56**

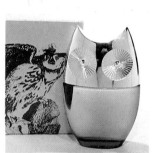

1969 *Wise Choice in Leather or Excalibur After Shave Lotion 4oz $4* **MP $5**

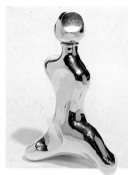

1969 *Futura in Excalibur or Wild Country Cologne 5oz $7* **MP $26**

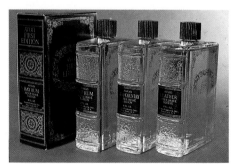

1967 *First Edition in Bay Rum, Wild Country or Leather After Shave 6oz $3.50* **MP $8 each, $10 boxed**

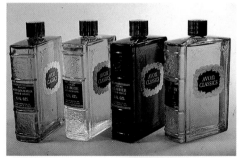

***Classics** (After Shave Lotion) —*
1969 *Windjammer 6oz $3.50* **MP $9**
1969 *Tribute 6oz $3.50* **MP $8**
1969 *Leather 6oz $3.50* **MP $9**
1969 *Wild Country 6oz $3.50* **MP $8**

(See page 45 for CPC Fragrance Dating Guide, page 46 for Women's and Girl's Fragrance Line Dating)

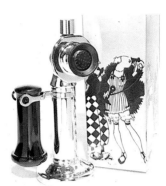

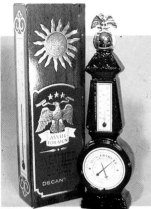

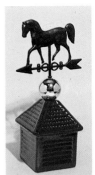

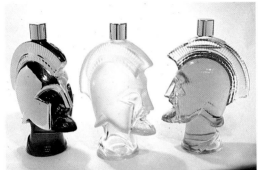

1969 *Avon Calling. Wild Country or Leather Cologne in phone 6oz. Talc in receiver 1¼oz $8* **MP $12, $16 boxed**

1969 *Weather-Or-Not in Leather, Tribute or Wild Country After Shave 5oz $5* **MP $6**

1977 *Weather Vane in Wild Country or Deep Woods After Shave 4oz $6.50* **MP $4**

Warrior (in Tribute fragrance only):
1967 *After Shave Lotion 6oz $4.50* **MP $18**
1968 *Cologne, frosted 6oz $4* **MP $7**
1971 *Cologne, clear 6oz $4* **MP $6**

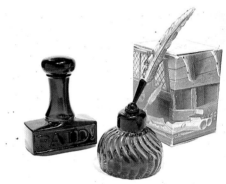

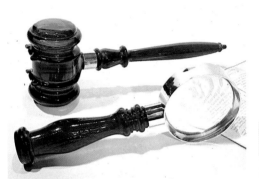

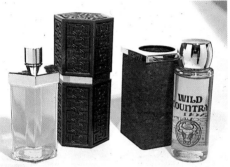

1970 *Stamp Decanter in Spicy or Windjammer After Shave Lotion 4oz $4* **MP $6**
1969 *Inkwell Decanter, Windjammer or Spicy After Shave Lotion 6oz $6* **MP $9, $11 boxed**

1967 *Gavel in Spicy, Original or Island Lime After Shave $4* **MP $17**
1979 *Super Sleuth Magnifier in Wild Country or Everest After Shave 2oz $9.50* **MP $8**

1968 *After Shave Caddy in Leather or Island Lime 6oz $7* **MP $20**
1977 *Desk Caddy in Clint or Wild Country Cologne 4oz $10* **MP $8**

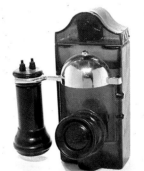

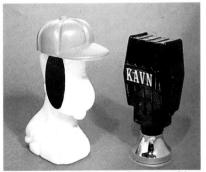

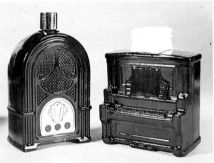

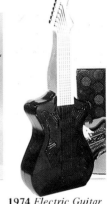

1973 *Avon Calling 1905 in Spicy or Wild Country After Shave 7oz and Talc ¾oz $10* **MP $10**

1969 *Snoopy Surprise Package. Excalibur or Wild Country After Shave or Sports Rally Lotion 5oz $4* **MP $7**
1975 *On the Air in Spicy, Wild Country or Deep Woods After Shave Lotion 3oz $5* **MP $4**

1972 *Remember When Radio in Wild Country or Spicy After Shave or Hair Lotion 5oz $4* **MP $5**
1972 *Piano Decanter in Tai Winds or Tribute After Shave 4oz $4* **MP $5**

1974 *Electric Guitar in Wild Country After Shave or Sure Winner Lotion 6oz $5* **MP $5, $6 boxed**

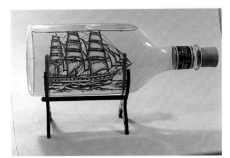

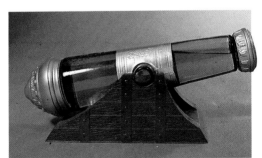

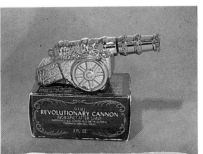

1970 *Captain's Pride in Windjammer or Oland After Shave 6oz $5* **MP $7 with stand**

1966 *Defender (Cannon) in Leather, Island Lime or Tribute After Shave 6oz $5* **MP $21**

1975 *Revolutionary Cannon in Spicy or Blend 7 After Shave 2oz $5.50* **MP $4, $5 boxed**

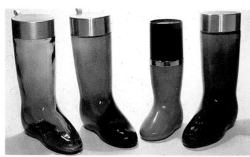
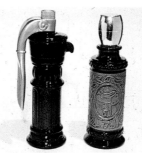
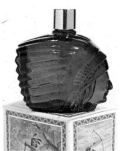
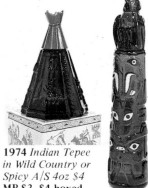

Leather —
1965 *All-Purpose Lotion for Men, silver cap 8oz $5* **MP $12**
1966 *All-Purpose Cologne, gold cap 8oz $5* **MP $6**
1966 *Spray Cologne 3oz $4* **MP $5**
1971 *Cologne, no strap 8oz $5* **MP $5**

1968 *Pump Decanter in Wild Country, Windjammer or Leather After Shave 6oz $5* **MP $7**
1980 *Boots 'N Saddle After Shave in Wild Country or Weekend 7oz $11* **MP $9**

1972 *Indian Chieftain in Spicy After Shave or Hair Lotion 4oz $3.50* **MP $4, $5 boxed**

1974 *Indian Tepee in Wild Country or Spicy A/S 4oz $4* **MP $3, $4 boxed**
1975 *Totem Pole in Wild Country, Deep Woods or Spicy After Shave 6oz $6.50* **MP $6**

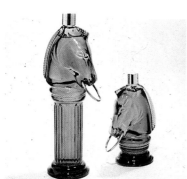
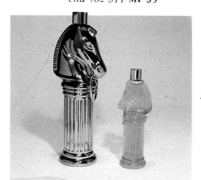

AVON AMERICANA

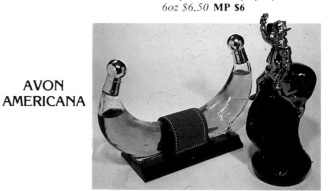

Pony Post After Shave Lotion —
1966 *(Green) Leather, Island Lime or Tribute 8oz $4* **MP $10**
1968 *(Green) Choice of 3 frag. or Pre-Electric Shave 4oz $3.50* **MP $5**

1972 *(Gold) Tai Winds or Leather 5oz $5* **MP $7**
1973 *Miniature in Spicy or Oland 1½oz $4* **MP $3**

1967 *Western Choice. 1 each Wild Country and Leather After Shave 3oz each $6* **MP $22**
1971 *Bucking Bronco, Oland or Excalibur After Shave Lotion 6oz $6* **MP $8**

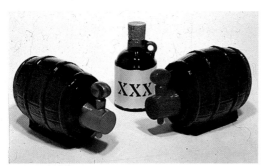
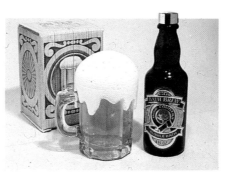
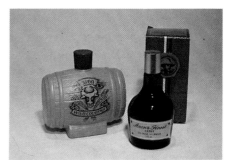

1974 *After Shave on Tap (gold) in Wild Country or Oland 5oz $4* **MP $5**
1978 *Little Brown Jug in Deep Woods or Tai Winds After Shave 2oz $4.50* **MP $3**
1976 *After Shave on Tap in Wild Country or Spicy 5oz $4* **MP $4**

1979 *On Tap Mug After Shave in Wild Country or Deep Woods 4oz $8* **MP $7**
1979 *Bath Brew. Wild Country Bubble Bath 4oz $5* **MP $4**

1980 *By The Barrel with Wild Country Shampoo or Bubble Bath 8oz $6* **MP $3**
1980 *Avon's Finest Cologne in Trazarra or Clint $6* **MP $4**

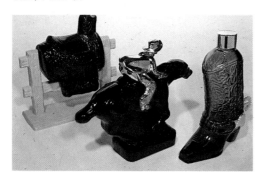
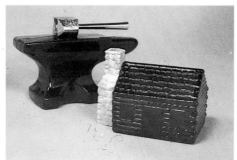
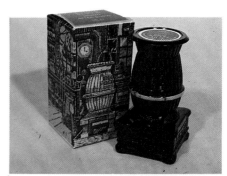

1971 *Western Saddle in Wild Country or Leather After Shave 5oz $7.50* **MP $7**
1971 *Pony Express. Leather or Wild Country After Shave 5oz $6* **MP $7** *(one of the "Transportation" group of figurals)*
1973 *Western Boot in Wild Country or Leather After Shave 5oz $5* **MP $5**

1972 *Blacksmith's Anvil in Deep Woods or Leather After Shave 4oz $5* **MP $6**
1973 *Homestead Decanter in Electric Pre-Shave or Wild Country After Shave 4oz $4* **MP $4**

1970 *Pot Belly Stove. Bravo or Excalibur After Shave 5oz $4* **MP $5, $7 boxed**

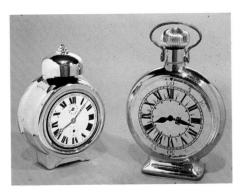
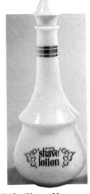
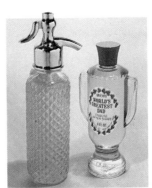
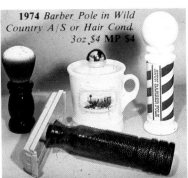

1974 *Barber Pole in Wild Country A/S or Hair Cond. 3oz $4* **MP $4**

1978 *No Cause for Alarm in Tai Winds or Deep Woods After Shave 4oz $9* **MP $8**
1968 *Daylight Shaving Time in Spicy, Leather or Wild Country After Shave 6oz $5* **MP $8**

1963 *Close Harmony A/S in 3 frag. or After Shower Lotion 8oz $2.25* **MP $25**

1973 *Bottled by Avon. Oland or Windjammer A/S 5oz $4* **MP $5**
1971 *World's Greatest Dad, Electric Pre-Shave Spicy or Tribute A/S 4oz $3.50* **MP $5**

1976 *Barber Shop Brush (left) Cologne in Tai Winds or Wild Country 1½oz $4* **MP $3**
1973 *Super Shaver in Bracing Lotion or Spicy A/S 4oz $4* **MP $4**
1974 *Ironhorse Shaving Mug in Blend 7, Deep Woods or Leather A/S $7.50* **MP $8**

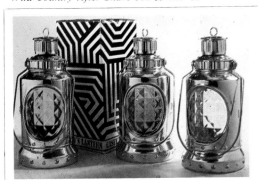

1966 *Casey's Lantern in Island Lime, Leather or Tribute After Shave 10oz $6 each.* Red **MP $48, $55 boxed.** *Green and Amber* **MP $58, $65 boxed**

LANTERNS

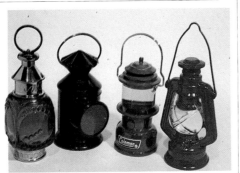

1974 *Whale Oil Lantern in Wild Country, Tai Winds or Oland After Shave 5oz $7* **MP $7**
1975 *Captain's Lantern 1864 in Wild Country or Oland After Shave 7oz $7.50* **MP $6**
1977 *Coleman Lantern in Wild Country or Deep Woods Cologne 5oz $8.50* **MP $6**

1979 *Country Lantern in Deep Woods or Wild Country After Shave 4oz $8* **MP $5**

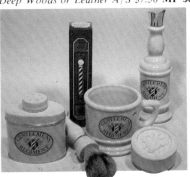

1982 *Gentlemen's Regiment Collection —*
Talc in Black Suede or Wild Country 3.5oz $7 **MP $3.50**
Shaving Brush 6" $11 **MP $9**
Shaving Mug & Soap 3oz $17 **MP $14**
After Shave Decanter in Black Suede or Wild Country 4.5oz $12.50 **MP $10**

MEN'S MINI-COLLECTIONS

It was the mid-sixties that marked the beginning of Avon's series of mini-collections, but how many collectors could realize back then the significance a Pipe Dream Decanter, a Stein, Twenty Paces or a Casey's Lantern would play in their yet-to-be discovered hobby?

If he's a car buff . . . and what American man isn't . . . he'll delight in the Avon cars, the most successful decanter series ever! Nature lovers will love the series of Wild Animals and Sea Creatures, Avon's sculptured denizens of the deep.

If he's a chess player, Avon provides the Chess Mates. If he's into transportation, there's a wide array of popular vehicles. Some for travel, some for work and some just for fun!

And those unique decanters with a bit of nostalgia for the exciting days of the Old West . . . Avon found it an inspiration for the American series of men's decanters.

No matter what the hobby, there's a series to capture the fancy of any man in Avon's treasure of mini-collections.

Americana	Nature
Automotive	Patriotic
Cars	Pipes
Chessmen	Sports
Guns	Steins & Mugs
Lanterns	Transportation

1982 *Dad's Pride and Joy. Fostoria picture frame/ paperweight 6½" long with stencil $12* **MP $10**

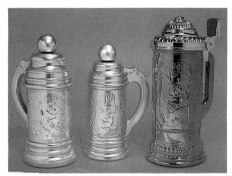

1965 *Stein in 4 frag. A/S 8oz $3.50 to $4* **MP $13**
1968 *Stein in Spicy, Windjammer or Tribute After Shave 6oz $4.50* **MP $11**
1972 *Hunter's Stein in Deep Woods or Wild Country After Shave 8oz $10* **MP $14**

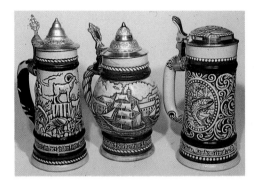

1976 *Collector's Stein of Stoneware. Holds plastic bottle of Cologne in 8oz Everest or Wild Country $30* **MP $40**
1977 *Tall Ships Ceramic Stein. Holds plastic bottle of Cologne in Wild Country or Clint 8oz $30* **MP $40**
1978 *Sporting Stein. Holds plastic bottle of Cologne in Trazarra or Wild Country 8oz $30* **MP $40**

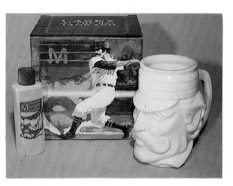

1980 *Casey At The Bat Tankard. Glass tankard holds plastic bottle of Weekend or Wild Country After Shave 4oz $17.50* **MP $15, $11 mug only**

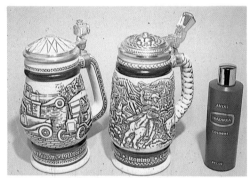

1979 *Car Classics Ceramic Stein. Holds plastic bottle of Trazarra Cologne 8oz $37.50* **MP $40**
1980 *Western Round-Up Ceramic Stein. Holds plastic bottle of Wild Country or Trazarra Cologne 8oz $45* **MP $45**

STEINS and MUGS

A series of Collector Ceramic Steins, with metal flip-top lids, was introduced in 1976. Handcrafted in Brazil, each is numbered and dated. A series of lidless miniature steins began in 1982. Each hand-painted replica is numbered and dated.

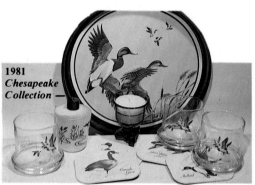

1981 Chesapeake Collection —

Glass with After Shave. Holds plastic bottle of Weekend or Wild Country 7oz $11 **MP $5**
Tray 12" diam. $9 **MP $9**
Jigger Candle. Fresh Aroma scent $13 **MP $10***
Drinking Glasses. Set of two 8oz $10 **MP $8**
Coasters. Set of four felt-backed metal $10 **MP $8**

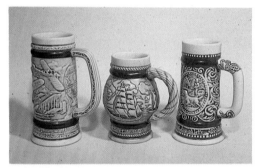

Miniature Steins —
1982 *Flying Classics 5½" high. Replica of 1981 Collectors Stein $15* **MP $15**
1982 *Tall Ships 4½" Replica of 1979 stein $15* **MP $13***
1983 *Sporting 5" Replica of 1978 stein $15* **MP $13***

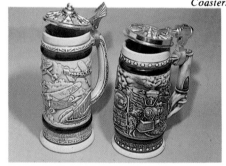

1981 *Flying Classics Ceramic Stein 9½" high $45* **MP $45**
1982 *Age of the Iron Horse 8½" high $45* **MP $40***

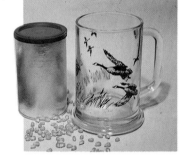

1982 *The Perfect Combo. Glass mug dated 1982 holds Gourmet Popcorn 10oz (2 Campaigns only) $9.99* **MP $10, $7 mug only**

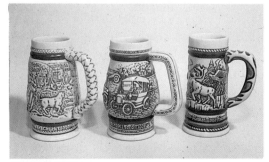

Miniature Steins —
1983 *Western Round-Up 5" high. Replica of 1980 stein $15* **MP $15**
1982 *Vintage Cars. 5" Replica of 1979 Car Classics stein $15* **MP $15**
1983 *Endangered Species. 5" Replica of 1976 stein $15* **MP $15**

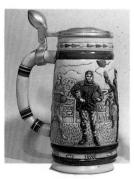

1983 *Great American Football Stein 9" high $45* **MP $40***

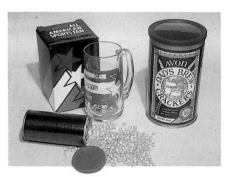

1983 *All American Sports Fan Mug with Popcorn 11oz (2 Campaigns only) $9.99* **MP $10, $7 mug only**
1983 *Dad's Brew Crackers in fiberboard canister 8oz (2 Campaigns only) $6.99* **MP $3**

*Available from Avon at time of publication

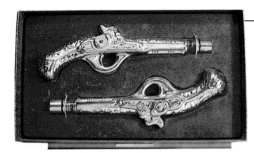

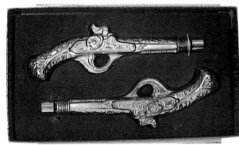

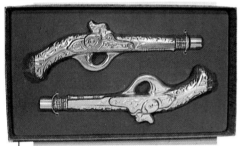

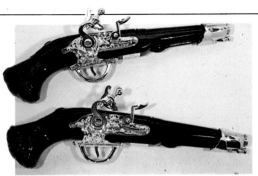

1973 *Dueling Pistol 1760 in Deep Woods or Tai Winds After Shave 4oz $10* **MP $11**
1974 *Dueling Pistol II (black glass) in Wild Country or Tai Winds After Shave 4oz $10* **MP $10**

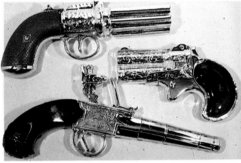

1976 *Pepperbox Pistol 1950. Everest or Tai Winds Cologne 3oz $12* **MP $10**
1977 *Derringer in Deep Woods or Wild Country Cologne 2oz $8* **MP $6**
1978 *Thomas Jefferson Handgun in Everest or Deep Woods Cologne 2¼oz $12.50* **MP $9**

1967 *Twenty Paces Set. Wild Country or Leather All Purpose Cologne and After Shave 3oz each $11.95, box lined in red* **MP $50,** *in black* **MP $125,** *in blue* **MP $160**

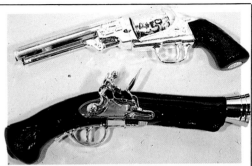

1975 *Colt Revolver 1851. Wild Country or Deep Woods After Shave 3oz $12* **MP $10**
1976 *Blunderbuss Pistol 1780. After Shave in Everest or Wild Country 5½oz $12* **MP $10**

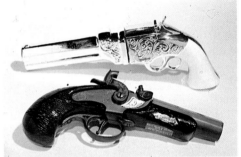

1979 *Volcanic Repeating Pistol in Wild Country or Brisk Spice Cologne 2oz $14* **MP $11**
1980 *Philadelphia Derringer in Light Musk or Brisk Spice After Shave 3oz $12* **MP $9**

GUNSHOP

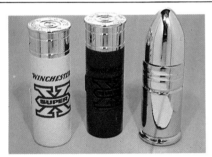

1976 *Good Shot! Deep Woods (yellow) or Wild Country (red) After Shave 2oz $4 each* **MP $3**
1977 *Wild West. Everest or Wild Country After Shave 1½oz $5* **MP $3**

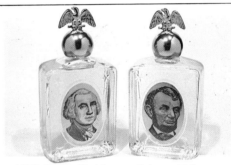

1970 *George Washington. Spicy or Tribute After Shave 4oz $3.50* **MP $4**
1971 *Abraham Lincoln. Leather or Wild Country After Shave 4oz $3.50* **MP $4**

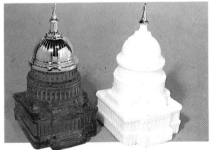

1970 *Capitol Decanter. Leather or Tribute After Shave 5oz $5* **MP $6**
1976 *Capitol Decanter. Wild Country or Spicy After Shave 4½oz $7* **MP $5**

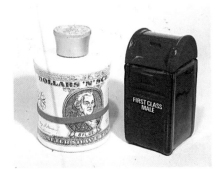

1966 *Dollars 'N' Scents. Spicy After Shave Lotion 8oz $2.50* **MP $27**
1970 *First Class Male. Wild Country or Bravo After Shave or Liquid Hair Lotion 4oz each $3* **MP $6**

PATRIOTIC REPLICAS

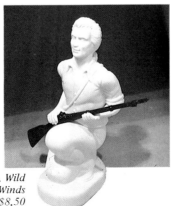

1975 *Minuteman. Wild Country or Tai Winds After Shave 4oz $8.50* **MP $7**

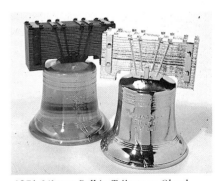

1971 *Liberty Bell in Tribute or Oland After Shave or Cologne 5oz $5 & $6* **MP $6**
1976 *Liberty Bell. Oland or Deep Woods After Shave 5oz $7* **MP $5**

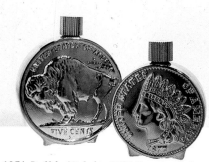

1971 *Buffalo Nickel in Wild Country, Spicy After Shave or Hair Lotion 5oz $5* **MP $9**
1970 *Indian Head Penny. Excalibur, Tribute or Bravo After Shave 4oz $4* **MP $9**

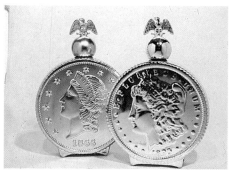

1971 *$20 Gold Piece in Windjammer After Shave or Electric Pre-Shave 6oz $5* **MP $9**
1970 *Liberty Dollar. Oland or Tribute After Shave 6oz $5* **MP $9**

1979 *President Lincoln, dated 1979, in Deep Woods or Everest After Shave 6oz $13* **MP $11**

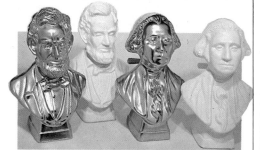

1973 *President Lincoln in Tai Winds or Wild Country After Shave 6oz $6* **MP $8**
1979 *President Washington, dated 1979, in Wild Country or Tai Winds After Shave 6oz $13* **MP $11**
1974 *President Washington in Tai Winds or Deep Woods After Shave 6oz $8* **MP $8**

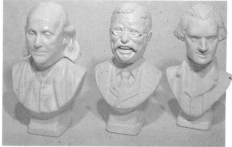

1974 *Benjamin Franklin in Wild Country or Tai Winds After Shave 6oz $8* **MP $8**
1975 *Theodore Roosevelt in Wild Country or Tai Winds After Shave 5oz $9* **MP $8**
1977 *Thomas Jefferson in Wild Country or Everest After Shave 5oz $10* **MP $7**

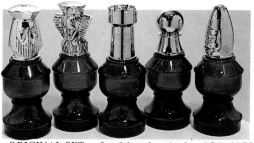

ORIGINAL SET – *3oz $4 each, raised to $5 in 1975. Unless noted,* **MP $5 each, $5.50 boxed**
1971 only *Smart Move (above, left) in Tribute or Oland* Cologne **MP $10, $13 boxed**
1974-78 *in Wild Country A/S or Hair Cond.*
1972-73 *King in Tai Winds or Oland* **MP $7, $10 boxed** (**MP $8 with Tai Winds, $11 boxed**)
1974-78 *King in Wild Country or Oland (Add $3 for 1974 box)*
1973-74 *Queen in Oland or Tai Winds After Shave* **MP $7, $10 boxed**
1974-78 *Queen in Wild Country or Deep Woods (add $3 for 1974 box)*
1973-74 *Rook in Oland or Spicy A/S* **MP $7** with Oland label, **$10 boxed. Spicy boxed MP $1**
1974-78 *Rook in Spicy or Wild Country (add $3 for 1974 box)*
1974-78 *Pawn in Wild Country or Electric Pre-Shave (add $3 for 1974 box)*
1974-76 *Bishop in Wild Country, Blend 7 After Shave or Hair Lotion* **MP $6 with Hair Lotion label, $7 boxed**
1977-78 *Bishop in Wild Country or Blend 7 A/S*

OPPOSING SET –
(Chess Pieces II) 3oz $5 each, **MP $5, $5.50 boxed**
1975-78 *King II in Spicy A/S or Hair Lotion*
1975 *Smart Move II in Wild Country After Shave, Hair Lotion or Hair Conditioner*
1975 *Bishop II in Spicy A/S or Hair Lotion*
1975 *Rook II in Wild Country A/S or Hair Lotion*
1975 *Queen II in Spicy A/S or Hair Cond.*
1975 *Pawn II in Spicy A/S or Hair Cond.*

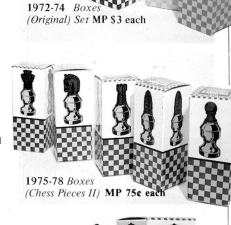

1972-74 *Boxes (Original) Set* **MP $3 each**

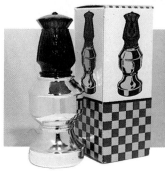

1975-78 *Boxes (Chess Pieces II)* **MP 75¢ each**

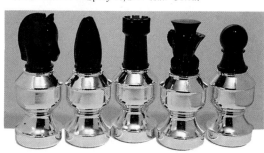

THE CHESSMEN from AVON

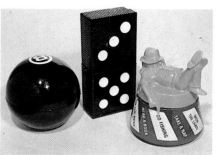

1973 *Eight Ball in Spicy After Shave, Electric Pre-Shave or Hair Lotion 3oz $4* **MP $4**
1978 *Domino After Shave Decanter in Tai Winds or Everest 1½oz $5* **MP $5**
1978 *Weekend Decision Maker in Tai Winds or Wild Country After Shave 3oz $9* **MP $7**

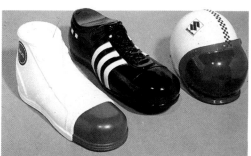

1974 *Just for Kicks in Spicy After Shave or Sure Winner Lotion 7oz $4.50* **MP $5**
1974 *Super Shoe. Sure Winner Bracing Lotion or Hair Trainer 6oz $4* **MP $4**
1976 *Motocross Helmet 6oz Wild Country After Shave or Protein Hair Lotion with Decals $5.50* **MP $4**

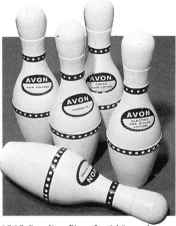

1960 Bowling Pins. 5 of 10, each a different 4oz Men's product $1.19 each **MP $17**

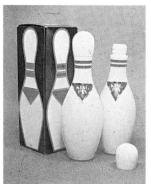

1969 King Pin. Wild Country or Bravo After Shave Lotion 4oz $3 **MP $4**

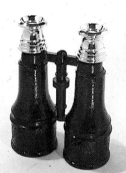

1973 Marine Binoculars in Tai Winds or Tribute After Shave & Cologne 4oz each $10 **MP $8**

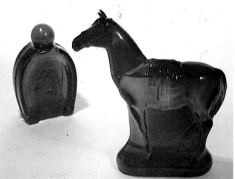

1974 Triple Crown in Spicy After Shave or Hair Conditioner 4oz $4 **MP $3**
1975 Sport of Kings, 5oz Wild Country, Spicy or Leather After Shave $7.50 **MP $6**

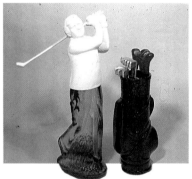

1975 Perfect Drive. Spicy After Shave or Hair/Scalp Conditioner 4oz $7.50 **MP $9**
1969 The Swinger. Bravo or Wild Country After Shave Lotion 5oz $5 **MP $8**

WORLD OF SPORTS

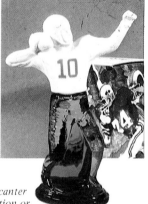

1973 Pass Play Decanter in Sure Winner Lotion or Wild Country After Shave 5oz $5.75 **MP $8**

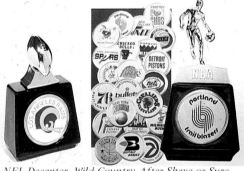

Opening Play — (Sports Rally Bracing Lotion, Wild Country or Spicy After Shave) —
1968 Gold without stripe 6oz $4 **MP $17**
1968 Clear glass **MP $100**
1969 Shiny gold without stripe **MP $30**
1968 Gold with stripe $4 **MP $14**

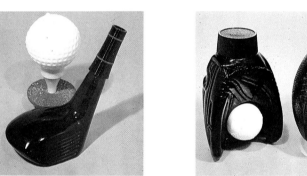

1973 Tee-Off Decanter in Spicy After Shave, Electric Pre-Shave or Hair Lotion 3oz $4 **MP $5**
1973 Long Drive Decanter in Deep Woods After Shave or Electric Pre-Shave 4oz $5 **MP $5**

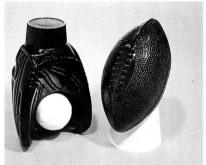

1971 Fielder's Choice Hair Trainer, After Shave or Bracing Lotion 5oz $4 **MP $5**
1970 First Down Decanter Wild Country After Shave or Sports Rally Bracing Lotion 5oz $4 **MP $6**

1976 NFL Decanter. Wild Country After Shave or Sure Winner Bracing Lotion 6oz choice of 28 embossed metal insignia emblems $8 **MP $6**
1977 NBA Decanter in Wild Country After Shave or Sure Winner Lotion 6oz $9.50 **MP $7** Choice of 22 embossed emblems **MP 75¢ each**

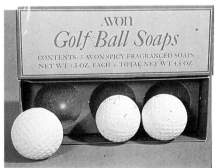

1974 Golf Ball Soaps, Spicy scented, three 1½oz each $3.50 **MP $7**

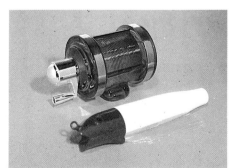

1970 The Angler. Windjammer or Wild Country After Shave 5oz $5 **MP $6**
1977 Sure Catch. Spicy or Wild Country After Shave 1oz $5 **MP $3**

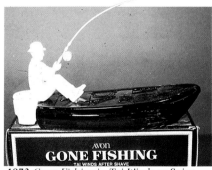

1973 Gone Fishing in Tai Winds or Spicy After Shave 5oz $7 **MP $7, $8** boxed (Also one of the "Transportation" figurals)

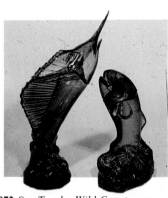
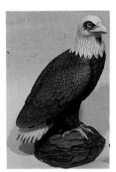
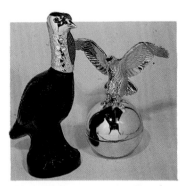
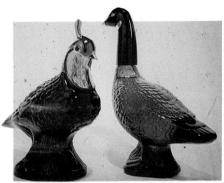

1972 *Sea Trophy Wild Country or Windjammer After Shave Lotion 5½oz $6* **MP $8**
1973 *Rainbow Trout in Deep Woods or Tai Winds After Shave 5oz $6* **MP $7**

1982 *Pride of America. Porcelain Eagle dated "1982" 7¾" $35* **MP $35**

1974 *Wild Turkey in Deep Woods or Wild Country After Shave 6oz $7.50* **MP $7**
1976 *Bold Eagle After Shave in Tai Winds or Wild Country 3oz $11* **MP $9**

1973 *Quail in Blend 7, Deep Woods or Wild Country After Shave 5½oz $7* **MP $8**
1973 *Canada Goose in Deep Woods or Wild Country After Shave or Cologne 5oz $7 & $8* **MP $7**

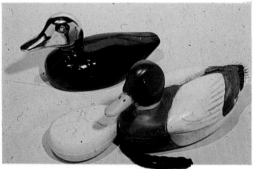
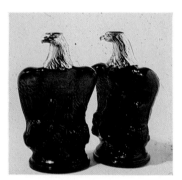
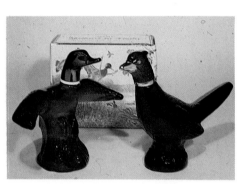

1967 *Mallard in Blue Blazer, Tribute or Spicy After Shave 6oz $5* **MP $13**
1978 *Wild Mallard Ceramic Organizer and Clint Soap 4oz $25* **MP $25***. Those ind. numbered and dated May 1978 sold for 2 Campaigns only* **MP $28**

American Eagle After Shave in Oland or Windjammer 5oz $5
1971 *(amber)* **MP $7**
1973 *(black)* **MP $5**

Avon NATURE SERIES

1974 *Mallard-in-Flight in Wild Country or Tai Winds After Shave or Cologne 5oz $8 & $9* **MP $8**
1972 *Pheasant Decanter in Oland or Leather After Shave 5oz $7* **MP $10**
1977 *Pheasant in Deep Woods or Wild Country After Shave 5oz $9* **MP $7**

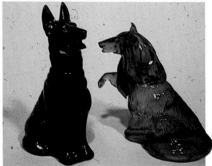
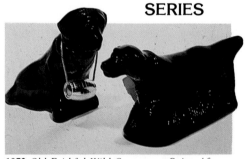
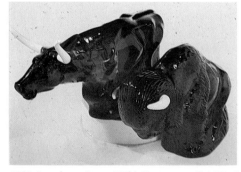

1975 *Noble Prince Wild Country After Shave or Electric Pre-Shave Lotion 4oz $6.50* **MP $6**
1977 *Faithful Laddie in Wild Country or Deep Woods After Shave 4oz $7* **MP $5**

1972 *Old Faithful Wild Country or Spicy After Shave Lotion 5oz $6* **MP $10**
1973 *"At Point" in Deep Woods or Tribute After Shave 5oz $5* **MP $6**

1975 *Longhorn Steer. Wild Country or Tai Winds After Shave 5oz $9* **MP $9**
1975 *American Buffalo Wild Country or Deep Woods After Shave 5oz $7.50* **MP $8**

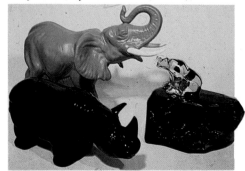
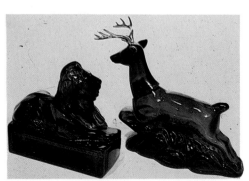
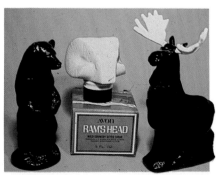

1972 *Big Game Rhino, Spicy or Tai Winds After Shave 4oz $5* **MP $8**
1977 *Majestic Elephant in Wild Country or Deep Woods After Shave 5½oz $11* **MP $8**
1976 *Artic King Everest After Shave 5oz $7* **MP $5**

1973 *Classic Lion in Wild Country, Tribute or Deep Woods After Shave 8oz $7.50* **MP $8**
1973 *Ten Point Buck in Wild Country or Leather After Shave 6oz $8.25* **MP $9**

1977 *Kodiak Bear 6oz Wild Country or Deep Woods After Shave $8* **MP $6**
1975 *Ram's Head Decanter in Blend 7 or Wild Country After Shave 5oz $6.50* **MP $6**
1974 *Alaskan Moose in Wild Country or Deep Woods After Shave 8oz $8* **MP $9**

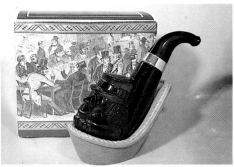

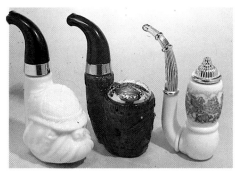

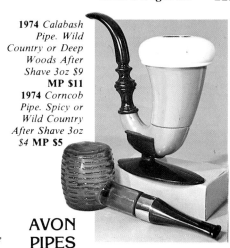

1967 Pipe Dream in Spicy, Tribute or Leather After Shave 6oz $5 **MP $20, $25 boxed**

1972 Bulldog Pipe in Wild Country or Oland After Shave $5 or Cologne $6 **MP $8**
1974 American Eagle Pipe in Tai Winds or Wild Country Cologne $7.50 **MP $8**
1973 Dutch Pipe in Tai Winds or Tribute Cologne 2oz $8 **MP $10**

1974 Calabash Pipe. Wild Country or Deep Woods After Shave 3oz $9 **MP $11**
1974 Corncob Pipe. Spicy or Wild Country After Shave 3oz $4 **MP $5**

AVON PIPES

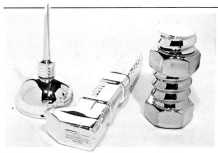

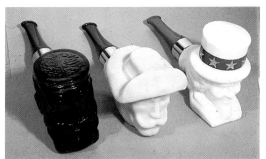

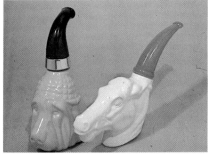

1971 Pipe Full. After Shave Lotion in 4 frag. amber glass 2oz $3.50 **MP $7, $8 boxed**
1972 Pipe Full (green) in Tai Winds or Spicy After Shave 2oz $3.50 **MP $5**

1973 Collector's Pipe in Windjammer or Deep Woods After Shave 3oz $4 **MP $6**
1975 Pony Express Rider Pipe 3oz Wild Country or Tai Winds Cologne $6.50 **MP $7**
1975 Uncle Sam Pipe 3oz Wild Country or Deep Woods After Shave $6.50 **MP $7**

1976 Bloodhound Pipe. 5oz Wild Country or Deep Woods After Shave $7 **MP $7**
1976 Wild Mustang Pipe, 3oz Wild Country of Deep Woods Cologne $7 **MP $7**

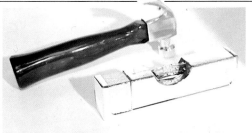

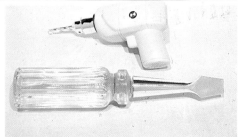

1978 Smooth Going After Shave in Deep Woods or Everest 1½oz $5 **MP $4** *(left)*
1977 Firm Grip After Shave in Wild Country or Everest 1½oz $5 **MP $4**
1976 Big Bolt After Shave in Deep Woods or Wild Country 2oz $4 **MP $3**

1978 On The Mark After Shave in Wild Country or Everest 2½oz $7.50 **MP $6**
1978 On The Level After Shave in Deep Woods or Everest 3oz $6 **MP $5**

1979 Power Drill in Wild Country After Shave or Pre-Electric Shave 5oz $7.50 **MP $5.50**
1976 One Good Turn After Shave in Deep Woods or Everest 3oz $6 **MP $5**

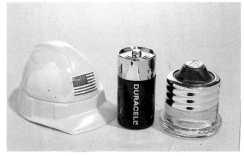

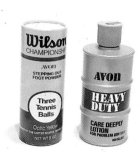

1977 Hard Hat After Shave in Deep Woods or Everest 4oz $6.50 **MP $4**
1976 Super Charge. Spicy or Everest After Shave 1½oz $4 **MP $4**
1977 Right Connection in Oland or Wild Country After Shave 1½oz $4 **MP $3**

1978 Quaker State Heavy Duty Powdered Hand Cleanser 12oz $4.50 **MP $3**
1979 Dutch Boy Heavy Duty Powdered Hand Cleanser 12oz $5 **MP $3**
1980 Turtle Wax Heavy Duty Powdered Hand Cleanser 10oz $6.50 **MP $3**

1980 Wilson Championship Stepping Out Foot Powder 5oz $3.50 **MP $2**
1980 Heavy Duty Care Deeply Lotion 10oz $6.50 **MP $3**

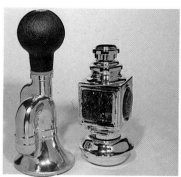

1970 *It's a Blast in Oland or Windjammer After Shave 5oz $7* **MP $11**
1973 *Auto Lantern in Deep Woods or Oland After Shave 5oz and 1¼oz Talc $14* **MP $15**

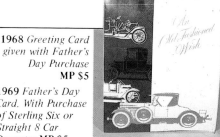

1968 *Greeting Card given with Father's Day Purchase* **MP $5**
1969 *Father's Day Card. With Purchase of Sterling Six or Straight 8 Car Decanter* **MP $5**

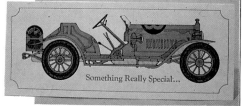

Something Really Special...

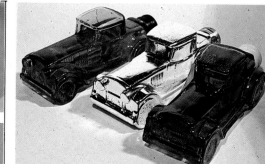

1968 *Sterling Six. Tribute, Spicy or Leather After Shave 7oz Smooth top $4* **MP $35** *Ribbed top (not shown) $4* **MP $8**
1978 *Sterling Six (Silver) "May 1978" in Tai Winds or Deep Woods After Shave 7oz $13* **MP $12**
1973 *Sterling Six II. Wild Country or Tai Winds After Shave 7oz $5* **MP $6**

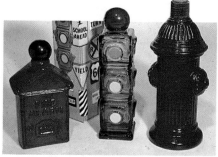

1974 *Fire Alarm Box in Spicy After Shave, Electric Pre-Shave or Hair Lotion 4oz $4* **MP $4**
1974 *Stop 'n Go. Wild Country or Spicy After Shave 4oz $5* **MP $6, $7 boxed**
1975 *No Parking. Wild Country After Shave or Electric Pre-Shave 6oz $6* **MP $4**

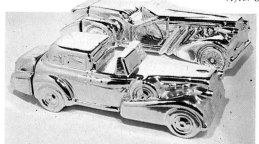

1969 *Solid Gold Cadillac. Excalibur, Wild Country or Leather After Shave 6oz $5* **MP $10**
1970 *Silver Duesenberg Oland or Wild Country After Shave 6oz $6* **MP $10**

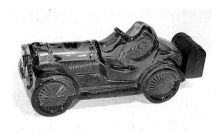

1969 *Straight Eight. Windjammer, Wild Country or Island Lime After Shave 5oz $3.50* **MP $8**

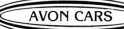

AVON CARS

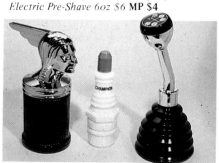

1976 *Chief Pontiac in Tai Winds or Deep Woods After Shave 4oz $8* **MP $8**
1975 *Spark Plug. After Shave in 3 frag. 1½oz $3* **MP $2**
1978 *Super Shift in Sure Winner Lotion or Everest Cologne 4oz $9* **MP $6**

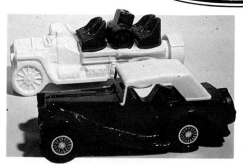

1974 *Thomas Flyer 1908. Oland or Wild Country After Shave 6oz $7.50* **MP $7**
1974 *1936 M.G. Tai Winds, Wild Country or Blend 7 After Shave 5oz $7* **MP $8**

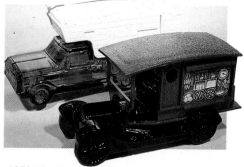

1972 *The Camper. Deep Woods or Oland After Shave 4oz and Talc 5oz $9* **MP $10**
1973 *Country Vendor. Wild Country or Spicy After Shave 5oz $7* **MP $10**

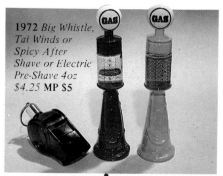

1972 *Big Whistle, Tai Winds or Spicy After Shave or Electric Pre-Shave 4oz $4.25* **MP $5**
1976 *Remember When Gas Pump (red) After Shave in Deep Woods or Wild Country 4oz $7* **MP $8**
1979 *Remember When Gas Pump After Shave in Cool Sage or Light Musk 4oz $9* **MP $7**

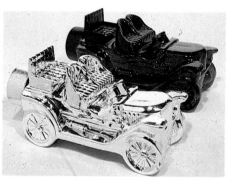

1978 *Stanley Steamer (Silver) "May 1978" in Tai Winds or Deep Woods After Shave 5oz $13* **MP $12**
1971 *Stanley Steamer. Windjammer or Wild Country After Shave or Cologne 5oz $5 and $6* **MP $8**

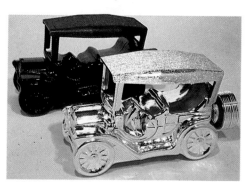

1969 *Touring T. Excalibur or Tribute After Shave 6oz $6* **MP $10**
1978 *Touring T (Silver) "May 1978" in Deep Woods or Everest After Shave 6oz $13* **MP $12**

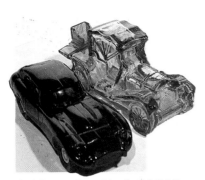
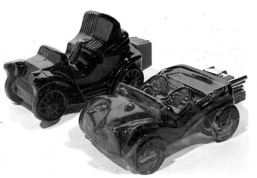
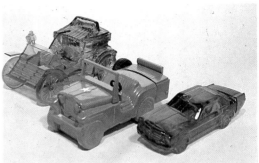

1973 Jaguar. Deep Woods or Wild Country After Shave 5oz $6 **MP $7**
1970 Packard Roadster. Oland or Leather Cologne 6oz $6 **MP $9**

1970 Electric Charger. Leather, Wild Country or Spicy After Shave 5oz $4 **MP $7**
1971 Dune Buggy Spicy After Shave, Sports Rally Lotion or Hair Lotion 5oz $5 **MP $7**

1973 Haynes-Apperson 1902. Blend 7 or Tai Winds After Shave 4½oz $6 **MP $7**
1974 Army Jeep. Wild Country or Spicy After Shave 4oz $6 **MP $7**
1976 '64 Mustang. 2oz Spicy or Tai Winds After Shave $5 **MP $4**

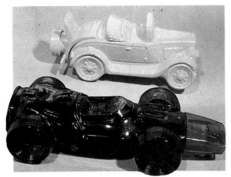
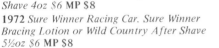
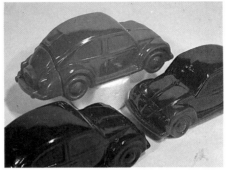
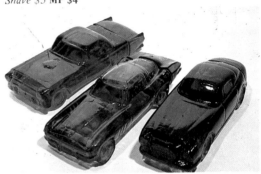

1972 Model "A". Wild Country or Leather After Shave 4oz $6 **MP $8**
1972 Sure Winner Racing Car. Sure Winner Bracing Lotion or Wild Country After Shave 5½oz $6 **MP $8**

1973 Blue Volkswagen. Oland or Windjammer After Shave 4oz $4 **MP $6**
1970 Black Volkswagen. Elec. Pre-Shave Wild Country or Spicy After Shave 4oz $4 **MP $6**
1972 Red Volkswagen. Sports Rally, Oland or Wild Country After Shave 4oz $4 **MP $10**

1974 Thunderbird '55. Wild Country or Deep Woods After Shave 2oz $4 **MP $5**
1975 Corvette Stingray '65. Spicy, Deep Woods or Wild Country After Shave 2oz $4 **MP $7**
1975 Ferrari '53. Wild Country After Shave or Protein Hair Lotion 2oz $4 **MP $7**

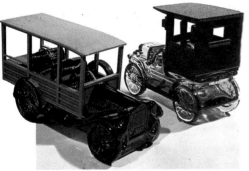
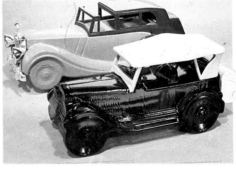
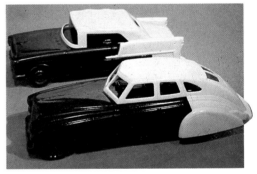

1971 Station Wagon. Tai Winds or Wild Country After Shave 6oz $6 **MP $8**
1972 1906 Reo Depot Wagon. Oland or Tai Winds After Shave 5oz $6 **MP $8**

1972 Rolls-Royce. Deep Woods or Tai Winds After Shave 6oz $8 **MP $9**
1972 Maxwell '23. Deep Woods or Tribute After Shave or Cologne 6oz $6 & $7 **MP $8**

1975 '55 Chevy. Wild Country After Shave or Electric Pre-Shave Lotion 5oz $8.50 **MP $10**
1975 Pierce Arrow '33. Wild Country or Deep Woods After Shave 5oz $7.50 **MP $8**

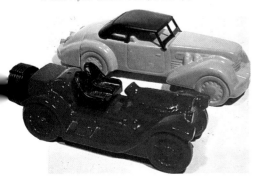
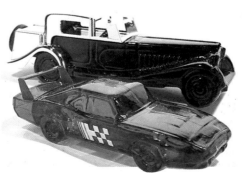
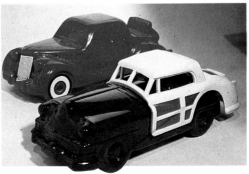

1974 Cord '37. Tai Winds or Wild Country After Shave 7oz $8 **MP $9**
1974 Stutz Bearcat 1914. Oland or Blend 7 After Shave 6oz $7 **MP $8**

1974 Bugatti '27. Wild Country or Deep Woods After Shave or Cologne 6½oz $8 and $9 **MP $10**
1974 Stock Car Racer. Wild Country After Shave or Electric Pre-Shave Lotion 5oz $7 **MP $7**

1976 '36 Ford After Shave in Tai Winds or Oland 5oz $8 **MP $8**
1976 '48 Chrysler Town and Country. Everest or Wild Country After Shave 4½oz $9 **MP $9**

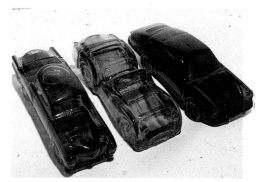

1975 *'51 Studebaker Wild Country or Spicy After Shave 2oz $5* **MP $7**
1975 *Triumph TR3 '56, Wild Country or Spicy After Shave 2oz $5* **MP $7**
1976 *'68 Porsche Spicy or Wild Country After Shave 2oz $5* **MP $6**

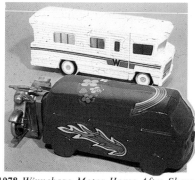

1978 *Winnebago Motor Home After Shave in Wild Country or Deep Woods 5oz $10.50* **MP $11**
1975 *Volkswagen Bus with 4 peel-off decals. Tai Winds After Shave or Sure Winner Bracing Lotion 5oz $6.50* **MP $8**

TRANSPORTATION

From the very early models of the Covered Wagon and the Stage-coach to the latest racers and Big Rigs, these classy "world of transportation" copies are pure joy to Avon collectors.

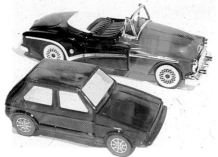

1979 *'53 Buick Skylark in Clint or Everest After Shave 4oz $14* **MP $12**
1980 *Volkswagen Rabbit in Light Musk Cologne or Sure Winner Lotion $9.50* **MP $7**

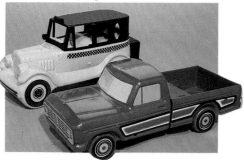

1977 *1926 Checker Cab. 5oz Wild Country or Everest After Shave $8* **MP $8**
1978 *Ford Ranger Pickup. After Shave in Wild Country or Deep Woods 5oz $10.50* **MP $9.50**

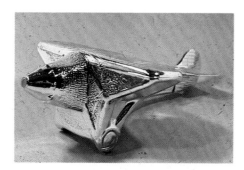

1970 *Spirit of St. Louis. Windjammer or Excalibur After Shave 6oz $8.50* **MP $16**

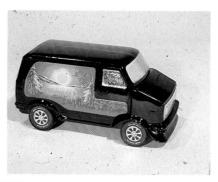

1979 *Vantastic After Shave in Everest or Wild Country and Decals 5oz $9.50* **MP $8**

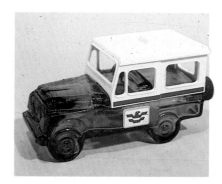

1977 *Extra Special Male After Shave in Deep Woods or Everest 3oz $6.50* **MP $7**

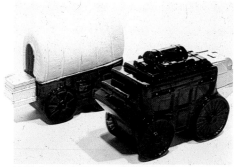

1970 *Covered Wagon. Wild Country or Spicy After Shave 6oz $5* **MP $9**
1970 *Stagecoach Decanter. Wild Country or Oland After Shave 5oz $5* **MP $9**
1977 *Re-issue with "R" embossed on bottom Wild Country or Tai Winds 5oz $6* **MP $5**

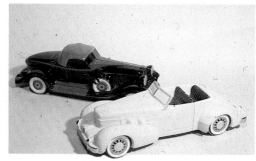

1983 *1932 Auburn Boattail Speedster. Handcrafted ceramic with platinum trim, dated, 8½" long $35* **MP $35**
1984 *1937 Cord. Handpainted ceramic, dated, 9" long (last of Ceramic Antique Cars) $36* **MP $36**

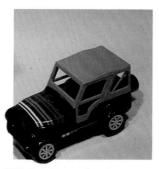

1981 *Jeep Renegade in Trazarra Cologne or Sure Winner Bracing Lotion 3oz $11.50* **MP $8**

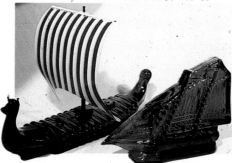

1977 *Viking Discoverer After Shave in Wild Country or Everest 4oz $12.50* **MP $12**
1972 *American Schooner in Oland or Spicy After Shave 4½oz $6* **MP $8**

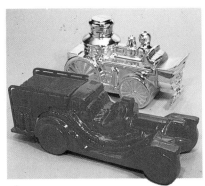

1971 *First Volunteer in Oland or Tai Winds Cologne 6oz $8.50* **MP $11**
1975 *Fire Fighter 1910 in Wild Country or Tai Winds After Shave 6oz $8* **MP $9**

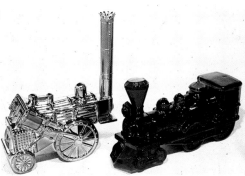

1974 *Golden Rocket 0-0-2 in Tai Winds or Wild Country After Shave 6oz $8* **MP $10**
1971 *The General 4-4-0 in Tai Winds or Wild Country After Shave 5½oz $7.50* **MP $11**

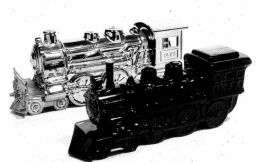

1973 *Atlantic 4-4-2 in Deep Woods or Leather After Shave or Cologne 5oz $9 and $10* **MP $12**
1976 *Cannonball Express 4-6-0 in Deep Woods or Wild Country Cologne or After Shave 3¼oz $9 and $8* **MP $9**

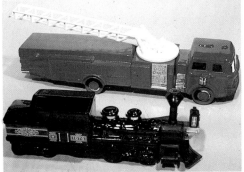

1978 *Red Sentinel Fire Truck After Shave 3.5oz and Talc 6oz in Wild Country or Deep Woods $14.50* **MP $14**
1978 *1876 Centennial Express After Shave in Wild Country or Everest 5oz $10.50* **MP $10**

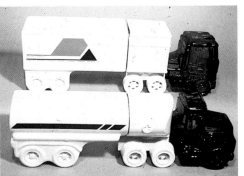

1977 *Highway King After Shave 4oz & Talc 6.5oz in Wild Country or Everest $12.50* **MP $11**
1975 *Big Rig. 3½oz After Shave and 6oz Talc in Wild Country or Deep Woods $12.50* **MP $12**

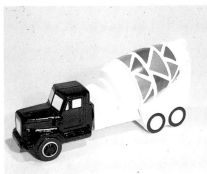

1979 *Cement Mixer After Shave 3oz and Talc 6oz in Wild Country or Everest. With decorative decals $15* **MP $14**

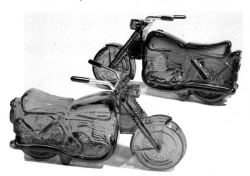

1974 *Super Cycle (blue) After Shave in Wild Country or Spicy 4oz $6* **MP $7**
1971 *Super Cycle in Island Lime or Wild Country After Shave or Sports Rally Bracing Lotion 4oz $6* **MP $8**

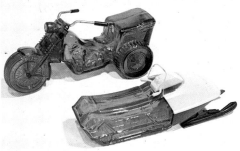

1973 *Road Runner in Wild Country After Shave or Sure Winner Lotion 5½oz $7* **MP $7**
1973 *Snowmobile in Oland or Windjammer After Shave 4oz $7* **MP $8**

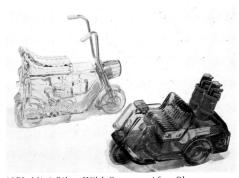

1972 *Mini-Bike. Wild Country After Shave or Sure Winner Bracing Lotion or Avon Protein Hair Lotion 4oz $6* **MP $7**
1972 *The Avon Open in Wild Country or Windjammer After Shave 5oz $6* **MP $10**

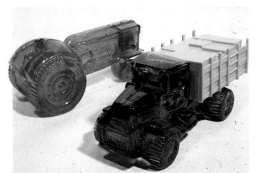

1973 *The Harvester in Wild Country After Shave or Hair Lotion 5½oz $6* **MP $7**
1973 *Big Mack in Windjammer or Oland After Shave 6oz $6* **MP $9**

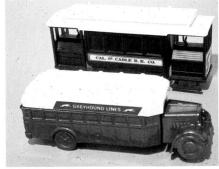

1974 *Cable Car in Wild Country or Leather After Shave 6oz $8* **MP $9**
1976 *'31 Greyhound. 5oz Spicy or Everest After Shave $9* **MP $8**

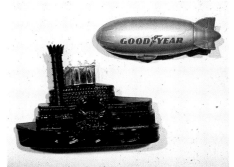

1978 *Goodyear Blimp After Shave in Wild Country or Everest 2oz $7.50* **MP $7**
1971 *Side Wheeler. Wild Country or Spicy After Shave Lotion 5oz $6* **MP $7**

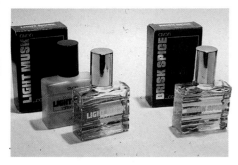

1979 *Light Musk After Shave (plastic) 3oz $3*
MP 50¢
1979 *Light Musk Cologne 2oz $4* **MP $1 boxed**
1979 *Brisk Spice Cologne 2oz $4* **MP $1 boxed**

AVON NATURALS

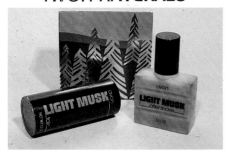

1979 *Fragrance Gift Set, 1.5oz Talc and 3oz
After Shave in Brisk Spice, Cool Sage or Light
Musk $5* **MP $5**
1979 *Above Set with Talc and 2oz Cologne $6*
MP $6

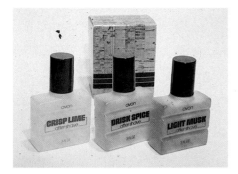

1980 *Avon Naturals After Shave Sampler Set.
Three 3oz After Shave in Brisk Spice, Cool Sage
and Light Musk $10.50* **MP $10**

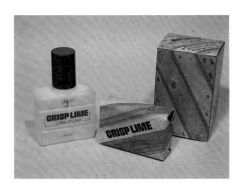

1981 *Avon Naturals After Shave and Soap
Set. 3oz each in Crisp Lime, Light Musk or
Brisk Spice $6* **MP $4 boxed, Soap only MP $3**

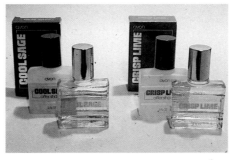

1979 *Cool Sage After Shave (plastic) 3oz $3*
MP 50¢
1979 *Cool Sage Cologne 2oz $4* **MP $1 boxed**
1979 *Crisp Lime After Shave (plastic) 3oz $3*
MP 50¢
1979 *Crisp Lime Cologne 2oz $4* **MP $1 boxed**

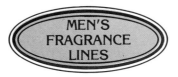

MEN'S
FRAGRANCE
LINES

*A variety of fragrances, each with
its own unique design and color*

(See Fragrance Dating Guide pg. 214)

BRAVO

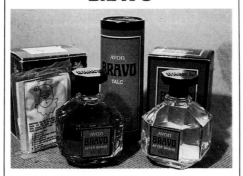

1969 *Santa's Helper After Shave 4oz with
Santa decals to decorate box $1.98* **MP $11**
1969 *Talc 3½oz $1.25* **MP $3**
1969 *After Shave 4oz $2* **MP $4**

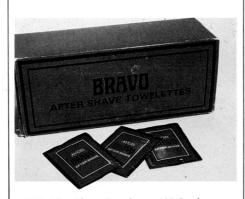

1969 *After Shave Towelettes. 100 Student
Samples* **MP 15¢ each, $20 full box**

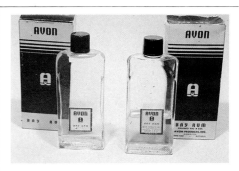

1936-39 *Bay Rum After Shave 4oz 52¢* **MP $40,
$50 boxed**
1939 *Bay Rum After Shave 4oz 52¢* **MP $35,
$45 boxed**

Bay Rum

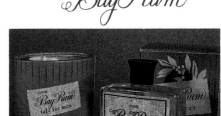

1964 *Bay Rum Gift Set. After Shave Lotion
and Talc 4oz each $2.50* **MP $42**
1964 *Talc only $1.25* **MP $16**
1964 *After Shave Lotion only $1.25* **MP $16**

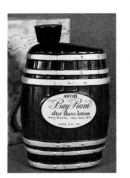 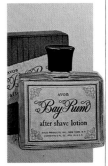

1965 *Bay Rum Keg.
After Shave Lotion 8oz
$2.50* **MP $23**

1964 *Bay Rum After
Shave 4oz $1.25*
MP $16, $20 boxed

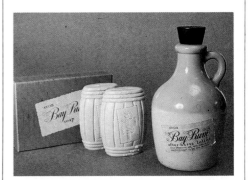

1964 *Bay Rum Boxed Soaps, two 3oz cakes
$1.25* **MP $33**
1962 *Bay Rum Jug After Shave Lotion 8oz
$2.50* **MP $20**

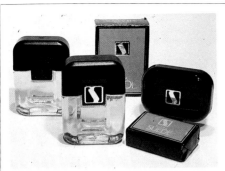

1980 *After Shave 4oz $7* **MP $7***
1980 *Cologne 4oz $9.50* **MP $9***
1980 *Gift Soap with Case 3oz (Sold only for 2 campaigns) $6.50* **MP $7, $5.25 Case only**

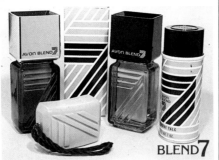

BLEND**7**

1973 *Cologne 5oz $5* **MP $4**
1973 *Shower Soap 5oz $2.50* **MP $10**
1973 *Emollient After Shave 5oz $5* **MP $4**
1974 *Spray Talc 7oz $3* **MP $2**

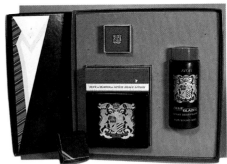

1965 *Blue Blazer Deluxe Set. After Shave Lotion 6oz, Deodorant 1³⁄₄oz and Tie Tac $5.50* **MP $75, Tie Tac MP $18**

BLACK SUEDE

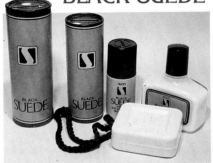

1982 *Bonus Size Talc 5¹⁄₄oz (1 Campaign only) $3.50* **MP $2**
1981 *Talc 3.5oz $3.50* **MP $2.50***
1982 *Roll-On Deodorant 2oz $2.19* **MP $1.69***
1981 *After Shave Soother 4oz $6* **MP $1**
1982 *Shower Soap-On-a-Rope 5oz $6* **MP $4***

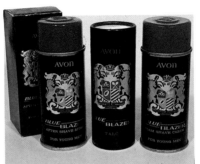

1964 *After Shave Spray 5¹⁄₂oz $1.95* **MP $13, $16 boxed**
1964 *Talc 3¹⁄₂oz $1.25 ("For Young Men" omitted)* **MP $15**
1964 *Foam Shave Cream 6oz $1.25* **MP $13**

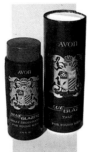

1967 *Spray Deodorant (2³⁄₄oz on front, short issue) $1.25* **MP $15**
1964 *Talc 3¹⁄₂oz $1.25* **MP $10**

BLUE BLAZER

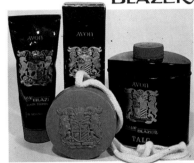

1964 *Shower Soap-On-a-Rope 5oz $1.50* **MP $18**
1964 *Hair Dress 4oz $1.25* **MP $12, $15 boxed**
1964 *European Talc* **MP $15**

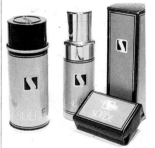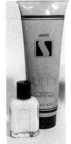

1981 *Spray Talc 4oz $5* **MP $3**
1980 *Cologne Spray 3oz $9.50* **MP $7***
1981 *Bar Soap 3oz $2.25* **MP $1.25***

1983 *Mini After Shave Soother .5oz $3* **MP 50¢**
1984 *After Shave Conditioner 4oz $6.50* **MP $4***

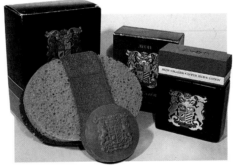

1966 *Soap and Sponge 3oz $2.50* **MP $22, $25 boxed**
1964 *After Shave Lotion 6oz $1.95* **MP $22, $26 boxed**

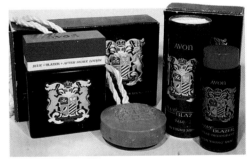

1964 *Blue Blazer Set No. 1. After Shave 6oz and Shower Soap 5oz $3.45* **MP $55**
1964 *Set No. II. Talc 3¹⁄₂oz and Spray Deodorant 2³⁄₄oz $2.50* **MP $32**

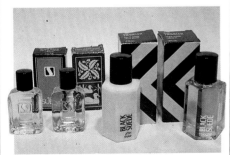

1981 *Gift Edition Cologne .5oz $3.50* **MP $2***
1982 *Gift Edition Cologne .5oz $3.50* **MP $1 Xmas boxed**
1981 *Traveler After Shave 2oz $4* **MP 50¢ boxed**
1981 *Traveler Cologne 2oz $5* **MP 75¢ boxed**

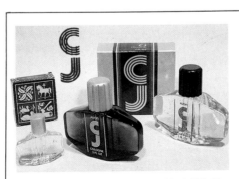

1982 *Gift Edition Cologne .5oz $3.50* **MP $1 Xmas boxed**
1982 *Cologne 3oz $8.50* **MP $2 boxed**
1982 *After Shave 3oz $6.50* **MP $1.50 boxed**

*Available from Avon at time of publication

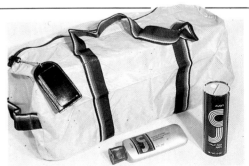

1982 *CJ Tote Bag $5.99 with purchase* **MP $15 value**
1983 *Invigorating Shampoo and Body Cleanser 4oz $5* **MP $1**
1982 *Talc 3.5oz $3.50* **MP 50¢**

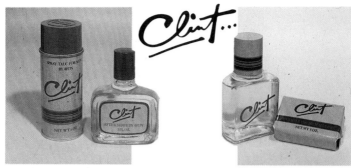
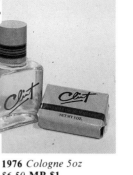

1976 Shower Soap 5oz $4.50 MP $5
1977 Spray Talc 7oz (short issue) $4
MP $3
1977 Talc 3½oz $2.50 MP 50¢

1979 Spray Talc 4oz $4.50
MP $2
1976-81 After Shave 5oz $5
MP $1

1976 Cologne 5oz
$6.50 MP $1
1976 Bar Soap 3oz
$1.25 MP $3

1977 Gift Set. Cologne and Shower
Soap 5oz each $12.50 MP $15

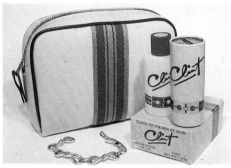
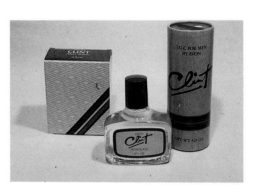
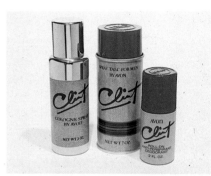

1976 Travel Kit. Canvas with vinyl interior 8x5"
$14 MP $16
1976 Wrist Chain $12 MP $11
1977 Travel Set for Men. After Shave 3oz and
Talc 1½oz $5 MP $5, $2 each

1981-84 After Shave 4oz $6 MP $1, $1.25 boxed
1982 Bonus Size Talc 5¼oz (1 Campaign only)
$3.50 MP $2

1980 Spray Cologne 3oz $8.50 MP $2
1977 Spray Talc 7oz (short issue) $4 MP $3
1979 Roll-On Deodorant 2oz $1.69 MP 50¢

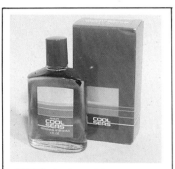
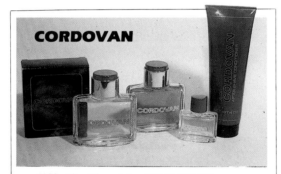
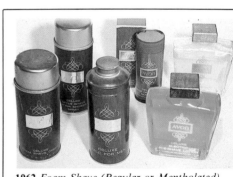

1984 Refreshing After Shave 4oz
$5 MP $3*

COOL SEAS

CORDOVAN

1983 After Shave 2.5oz $10.50 MP $8*
1983 Cologne 2.5oz $13.50 MP $9.50*
1983 Mini Cologne .5oz $3.50 MP $2*
1984 After Shave Conditioner 4oz $6.50 MP $4*

1962 Foam Shave (Regular or Mentholated)
6oz $1.35 MP $11
1962 After Shower Spray-A/S 5½oz $1.98 MP $11
1962 Talc for Men 4oz $1.35 MP $10
1961 Stick Deodorant 2¾oz $1.35 MP $12
1962 After Shave Lotion 6oz $1.79 MP $27
1962 Electric Pre-Shave Lotion 6oz $1.79 MP $27

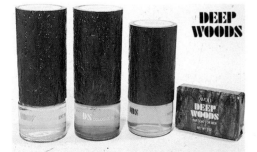
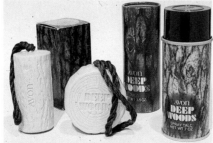
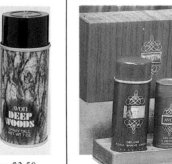

DEEP WOODS

1973 Emollient After Shave 5oz $5 MP $4
1972 Cologne 5oz $5 MP $3
1973 Cologne Spray 3oz $5 MP $4
1976 Bar Soap 3oz $1.25 MP $3

*Available from Avon at time of publication

1972 Shower Soap-On-a-Rope 5oz $2.50
MP $8
1975 Shower Soap-On-a-Rope 5oz $4.50
MP $7
1977 Talc 3.5oz $2.50 MP 75¢
1972 Spray Talc 7oz $3 MP $1

Deluxe

In 1961 "Deluxe"
was the name of
newly designed
packaging that
contained Spicy
fragrance. In
1962 "Deluxe"
became the name
of a new mens'
fragrance line.

1962 Deluxe Set for Men. Choice
of Foam Shave Cream, Stick
Deodorant and After Shave-After
Shower Spray $4.98 MP $45

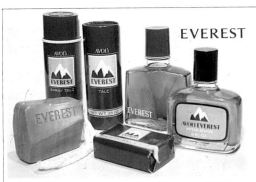

EVEREST

1975 *Shower Soap-On-a-Rope 5oz $4.50* **MP $5**
1976 *Bar Soap 3oz $1.25* **MP $3**
1975 *Spray Talc 7oz $4* **MP $1**
1977 *Talc 3.5oz $2.50* **MP 75¢**
1975 *Cologne 5oz $6.50* **MP $2**
1975 *After Shave 5oz $5* **MP $2**

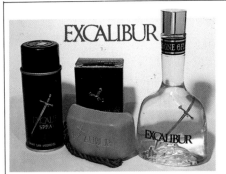

EXCALIBUR

1970 *Spray talc 7oz $3* **MP $3**
1970 *Soap-On-A-Rope 5oz $2.50* **MP $9, $12 boxed**
1969 *Cologne 6oz $5* **MP $7**

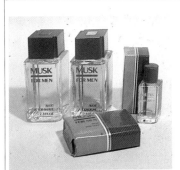

1983 *After Shave 2.8oz $7* **MP $6***
1983 *Cologne 2.8oz $9* **MP $7***
1984 *Mini Cologne .5oz $3.50* **MP $2***
1984 *Bar Soap 3oz $2.50* **MP $1.25***

MUSK

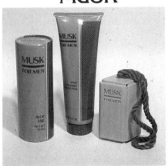

1983 *Talc 3.5oz $3.50* **MP $2.50**
1984 *After Shave Conditioner 4oz $6.50* **MP $4***
1983 *Shower Soap-On-a-Rope 5oz $6* **MP $4***

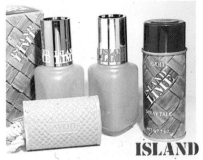

ISLAND LIME

1973-74 *After Shave 6oz $4* **MP $8 boxed**
1974 *After Shave (green lettering) 6oz $4* **MP $7**
1972 *Spray Talc 7oz $3* **MP $1**
1966 *Soap-On-a-Rope 6oz $2* **MP $25**

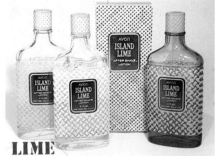

1967 *Clear Glass, light yellow weave 6oz $3* **MP $13, $16 boxed**
1966 *Clear Glass, dark yellow weave 6oz $3* **MP $16, $19 boxed**
1969 only *Green Glass 6oz $4* **MP $26, $28 boxed**

1969-73 *After Shave 6oz $4* **MP $3**

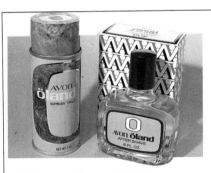

1970 *Spray Talc 7oz $3* **MP $1**
1975 *After Shave 5oz $5* **MP $2**

öland

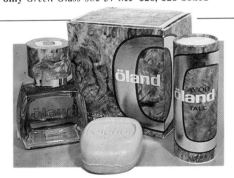

1970 *Gift Set. Cologne 6oz, Talc 3½oz and Soap 5oz $8* **MP $20**

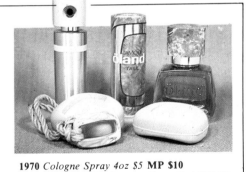

1970 *Cologne Spray 4oz $5* **MP $10**
1970 *Talc 3½oz Shaker top (from Set)* **MP $5**
1970 *Cologne 6oz $5* **MP $3**
1970 *Shower Soap-On-a-Rope 5oz $2.50* **MP $9**
1970 *Soap 5oz (from Set only)* **MP $5**

AVON ORIGINAL

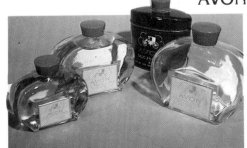

1956 *After Shave Lotion 2oz (Sets only)* **MP $8**
1949 *After Shave Lotion 4oz 49¢* **MP $10**
1949 *Talc for Men 2.6oz 43¢* **MP $8**
1949 *Cologne for Men 6oz $1.50* **MP $18** *(2oz 69¢ MP $10; 4oz in Sets only MP $15 Not Shown: Deodorant 2oz MP $8, 4oz in Sets only MP $10)*

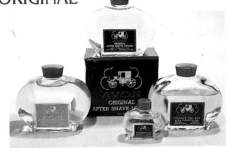

1949 *After Shave Lotion 4oz 49¢* **MP $10**
1965 *Original After Shave (no Avon on label or box) 4oz 98¢* **MP $8, $10 boxed**
1954 *Cologne 4oz (issued in Personal Note Set)* **MP $18**
1949 *After Shave Sample ½oz* **MP $10, Cologne Sample (not shown) MP $15**

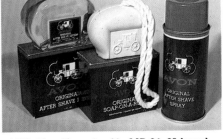

1965 *After Shave 4oz 98¢* **MP $6, $8 boxed**
1966 *Soap-On-a-Rope 5oz $1.75* **MP $18, $22 boxed**
1965 *After Shave Spray 5½oz $1.50* **MP $10**

*Available from Avon at time of publication

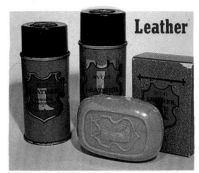

Leather

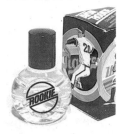

LOVER BOY ROOKIE

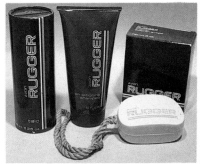

1966 *Aerosol Deodorant 4oz $1.50* **MP $6**
1969 *Spray Talc 7oz $3* **MP $3**
1966 *Bath Soap 5oz $1.75* **MP $18**
(See Cologne, Boots page 216)

1980 *Lover Boy After Shave 3oz $5* **MP $1**
1980 *Lover Boy Cologne 3oz $6* **MP $1**

1980 *Rookie Cologne 2.5oz $3.50* **MP $2** *boxed*

1982 *Bonus Size Talc 5¼oz (1 Campaign only) $3.50* **MP $2**
1982-83 *Conditioning Shampoo 5oz $4.50* **MP $1**
1982 *Shower Soap-On-a-Rope 5oz $6* **MP $4***

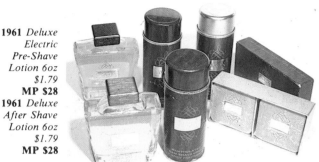

1961 *Deluxe After Shower Powder 4oz $1.35* **MP $15**

1961 *Deluxe Electric Pre-Shave Lotion 6oz $1.79* **MP $28**
1961 *Deluxe After Shave Lotion 6oz $1.79* **MP $28**

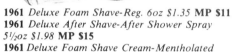

1961 *Deluxe Foam Shave-Reg. 6oz $1.35* **MP $11**
1961 *Deluxe After Shave-After Shower Spray 5½oz $1.98* **MP $15**
1961 *Deluxe Foam Shave Cream-Mentholated 6oz $1.79* **MP $11**
1961 *Deluxe Oatmeal Soap for Men, two 4oz cakes $1.35* **MP $30**

. . . . . . *Deluxe Men's Gifts in 1961 contained a Spicy fragrance. The same packaging in 1962 was used for "Deluxe", a Forest-Fresh fragrance. (See page 230)*

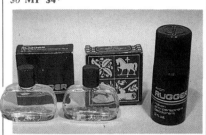

1981 *Gift Edition Cologne .5oz $3.50* **MP $2***
1982 *Gift Edition Cologne .5oz $3.50* **MP $1** *Xmas boxed*
1982 *Roll-On Deodorant 2oz $2.19* **MP $1.69***

AVON **Spicy**

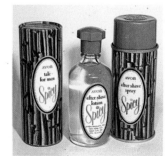

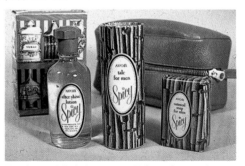

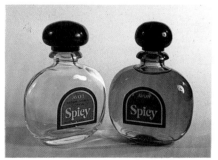

1965 *Talc 3½oz 89¢* **MP $6**
1965 *After Shave 4oz 98¢* **MP $8**
1965 *After Shave Spray 5½oz $1.50* **MP $6**

1966 *Spice O'Life Set. 3½oz Talc and 4oz After Shave Lotion $1.96* **MP $25**
1965 *Overnighter Set. 4oz After Shave Lotion, 3½oz Talc and 3oz Soap, all in Spicy $7.50* **MP $45; Soap MP $7**

1967 *After Shave Lotion, clear 4oz $1.25* **MP $4**
1967 *After Shave Lotion, amber 4oz $1.25* **MP $6**

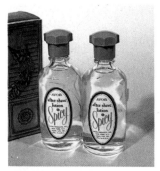

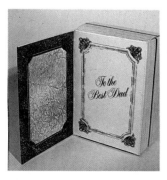

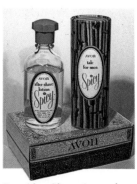

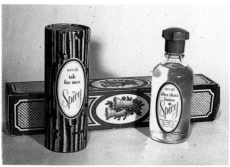

1965 *Christmas Wreath. Two 4oz After Shave $1.95* **MP $25**

1965 *First Edition Father's Day Gift Set. After Shave 4oz and Talc 3½oz $1.87* **MP $32** *(Left, inside cover of box)*

1965 *Holiday Spice. Talc and After Shave Lotion $1.85* **MP $25**

Available from Avon at time of publication

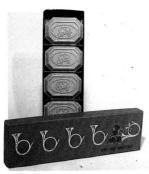

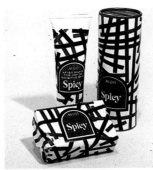

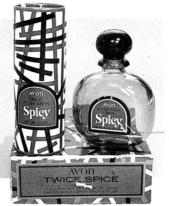

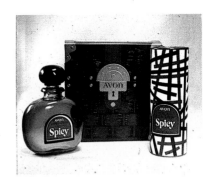

1965 *Soap Miniatures 1½oz each $2* **MP $25**

. . . AVON **Spicy**

1967 *Oatmeal Soap 3oz 98¢* **MP $6**
1967 *After Shave for Dry/Sensitive Skin 2oz 98¢* **MP $4**
1967 *Talc 3½oz 98¢* **MP $1**

1967 *Twice Spice Set. 3½oz Talc and 4oz After Shave Lotion $2.23* **MP $16**

1968 *Spicy Treasure Set. After Shave Lotion 4oz and 3½oz Talc $2.23* **MP $15**

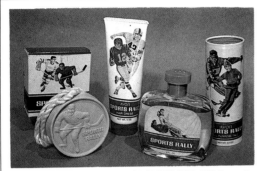

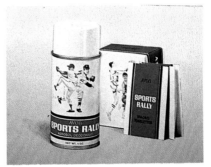

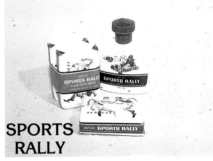

1966 *Deodorant Soap 4oz $1.50* **MP $15, $19 boxed**
1966 *Hair Dress 4oz $1* **MP $8**
1966 *Bracing Lotion 4oz $1.50* **MP $11**
1966 *Talc 3½oz $1* **MP $6**

1966 *Aerosol Deodorant 4oz $1.25* **MP $7**
1966 *Bracing Lotion Towelettes 12 per box $1.25* **MP $10 each box**

SPORTS RALLY

1966 *Sports Rally Clear Skin Soap 3oz each $1 pair* **MP $12**
1966 *Sports Rally Clear Skin Lotion, plastic 4oz $1.25* **MP $5**

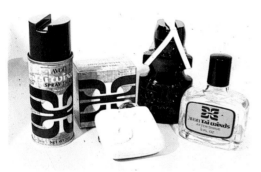

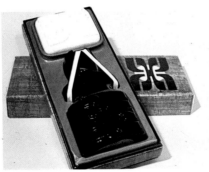

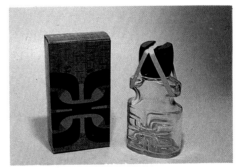

1971 *Spray Talc 7oz $3* **MP $1**
1971 *Soap with rope 5oz $2.50* **MP $6**
1971 *Cologne 5oz $5* **MP $7**
1975 *After Shave 5oz $5* **MP $2**

Tai winds

1971 *Gift Set. Cologne and Soap $8* **MP $16**

1971-75 *After Shave Lotion 5oz $3.50* **MP $3, $5 boxed**

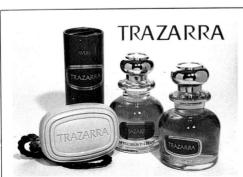

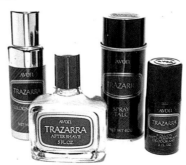

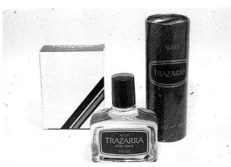

TRAZARRA

1978 *Shower Soap 5oz $5.50* **MP $5**
1978 *Talc 3½oz $2.50* **MP 50¢**
1978 *After Shave Lotion 4oz $6* **MP $1**
1978 *Cologne 4oz $8.50* **MP $4**

1980 *Cologne Spray 3oz $8.50* **MP $3**
1980 *After Shave 5oz $6* **MP $3**
1979-81 *Spray Talc 4oz $4.50* **MP $1**
1979 *Roll-On-Deodorant 2oz $1.69* **MP 50¢**

1981 *After Shave Lotion 4oz $6* **MP $1.25 boxed**
1982 *Bonus Size Talc 5¼oz (1 Campaign only) $3.50* **MP $2**

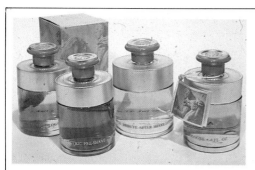

1964 Cologne with neck tag 4oz $2.50 **MP $14,
$17 boxed**
1963 Electric Pre-Shave 4oz $1.75 **MP $10,
$13 boxed**
1963-67 After Shave 6oz $2.50 **MP $10**
1967-68 All Purpose Cologne with neck tag 4oz $3
MP $16, $19 boxed

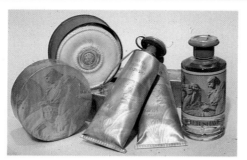

1963 Soap, boxed, 1 round bar 4oz $1.75 **MP $26**
1963 Cream Hair Dress 4oz tube $1.75 **MP $9,
$13 boxed**
1964 Shampoo 4oz tube $1.75 **MP $9, $13 boxed**
1967 After Shave 4oz $2.25 **MP $6**

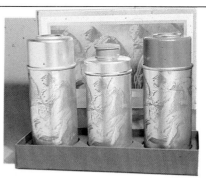

1963 Tribute Gift Set No. 1. 5½oz After
Shave-After Shower Spray, 4oz Talc and
choice of 6oz Regular or Mentholated Foam
Shaving Cream $6.50 **MP $40**

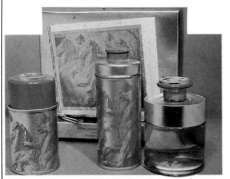

1963 Tribute Gift Set No. 2. Gift card
attached. 6oz After Shave Lotion, 4oz Talc
and 3oz Aerosol Deodorant $6.50 **MP $40**

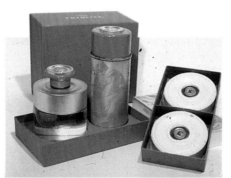

1964 Tribute Shave Set. 6oz After Shave
and 6oz Regular or Mentholated Foam
Shaving Cream $4.25 **MP $30**
1966 Boxed Soap, 2 round bars 3oz each
$1.75 **MP $23** (See Tribute "Warriors" pg. 215)

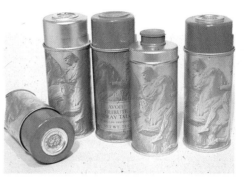

1963-67 Aerosol Deodorant 3oz $1.75 **MP $8**
1963-67 After Shave-After Shower Spray 5½oz
$2.50 **MP $8**
1969 Spray Talc 7oz $3 **MP $7**
1963 Talc 4oz $1.75 **MP $5**
1963 Foam Shave Cream, Regular or Mentholated
6oz $1.75 **MP $8**

TRIBUTE

*Tribute . . . distinctively,
outspokenly masculine
packaging, each container
captures the classic
beauty and splendor of
ancient Greece.*

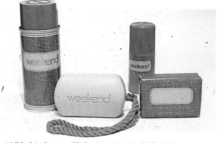

1979-81 Spray Talc 4oz $4.50 **MP $2**
1979 Shower Soap 5oz $5 **MP $5**
1979 Roll-On Deodorant 2oz $1.69 **MP 50¢**
1979 Bar Soap 3oz $1.50 **MP $3**

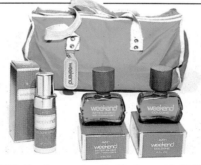

1979 Get-Away nylon Duffle Bag, with $8.50
purchase, $4.99 **MP $15**
1980 Cologne Spray 3oz $8.50 **MP $3**
1979-80 After Shave 4oz $6 **MP $3** (short issue)
1980-81 After Shave (not shown) 5oz $6 **MP $5**
1979 Cologne 4oz $8.50 **MP $4**

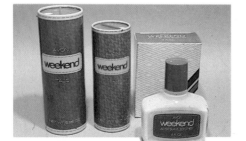

1982 Bonus Size Talc 5¼oz (1 Campaign only)
$3.50 **MP $2**
1981 Talc 3.5oz $3.50 **MP 50¢**
1981 After Shave Soother 4oz $6 **MP $1**

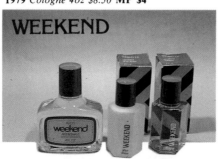

WEEKEND

1981 After Shave Lotion 4oz $6 **MP $1**
1981 Traveler After Shave 2oz $4 **MP 50¢ boxed**
1981 Traveler Cologne 2oz $5 **MP 75¢ boxed**

WINDJAMMER

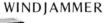
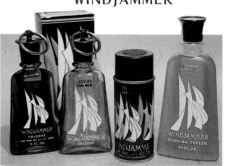

1969 Cologne, paper label 5oz $4 **MP $6**
1968 Cologne, painted label 5oz $4 **MP $11**
1968 Spray Talc 7oz $2.50 **MP $3**
1969 Rubdown Cooler (plastic) 10oz $3 **MP $3**

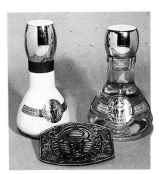
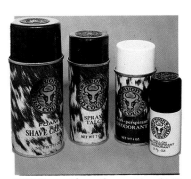
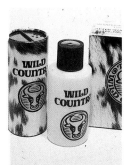
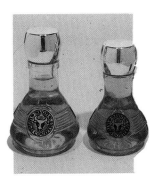
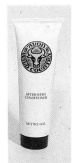

1968 Cologne Spray 2½oz $4 **MP $6**
1968-76 Cologne 6oz $4 **MP $3**
1976 Belt Buckle with any Wild Country purchase $1.99 **MP $4**

1970 Foam Shave Cream 11oz $1.75 **MP $1**
1969 Aerosol Spray Talc 7oz $3 **MP $1**
1975 Aerosol Deo. 4oz $1.79 **MP $1**
1978 Roll-On-Deo. 2oz $1.59 **MP $1.69***

1977 Travel Set. Talc 1.5oz and After Shave 3oz $5 **MP $6 $2 each container**

1976-81 Cologne 6oz $6.50 **MP $2**
1981 Cologne 4oz $10 **MP $8***

1984 After Shave Conditioner 4oz $6.50 **MP $4***

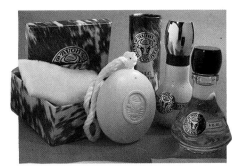
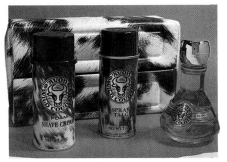
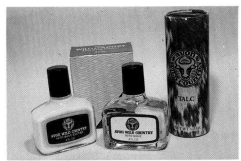

1967 Body Powder 6oz $4 **MP $15**
1967 Shower Soap-On-a-Rope 6oz $2 **MP $6**
1971 Talc 3½oz $1.50 **MP $2.50***
1968 Cologne Spray 2½oz $4 **MP $6**
1971 After Shave Lotion 4oz $3 **MP $1.50**

1970 Saddle Kit. Foam Shave Cream 6oz, Spray Talc 7oz and Cologne 6oz $16 **MP $16, $11 kit only**

1981 After Shave Soother 4oz $6 **MP $1**
1981 After Shave Lotion 4oz $6 **MP $6***
1982 Bonus Size Talc 5¼oz (1 Campaign only) $3.50 **MP $2**

WILD COUNTRY

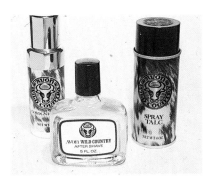
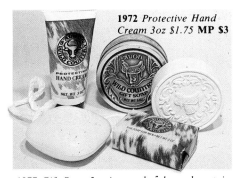
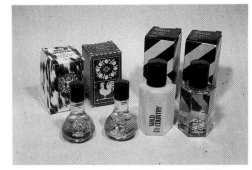

1980 Spray Cologne 3oz $8.50 **MP $3**
1975 After Shave 5oz $5 **MP $3**
1979-81 Spray Talc 4oz $4.50 **MP $1**

1972 Protective Hand Cream 3oz $1.75 **MP $3**
1977 Gift Soap 5oz in metal embossed container $4 **MP $6**
1975 Soap-On-a-Rope 5oz $4 **MP $4***
1976 Bar Soap 3oz $1.25 **MP $1.25***

1981 Gift Edition Cologne .5oz $3.50 **MP $2***
1982 Gift Edition Cologne .5oz $3.50 **MP $1 Xmas boxed**
1981 Traveler After Shave 2oz $4 **MP 50¢ boxed**
1981 Traveler Cologne 2oz $5 **MP 75¢ boxed**

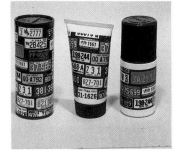

1982 On The Road Again —(2 Campaigns only) Wild Country Talc 1.5oz $2 **MP 75¢**
Wild Country Shave Cream 1oz $2 **MP 75¢**
Wild Country Roll-On Deodorant 2oz $2 **MP 75¢**

MEN'S TOILETRIES

For the discriminating man . . . . . . a wide choice of toiletries, many within a unique packaging theme.

*Available from Avon at time of publication

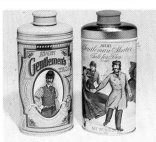

1979 Gentlemen's Talc, Tin holds Wild Country, Clint or Trazarra Talc 3.75oz $5 **MP $2**
1979 Gentleman Skater Talc, Tin holds Clint or Trazarra Talc 3.75oz $5.50 **MP $2**

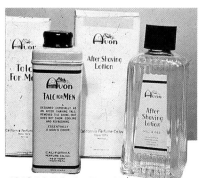

1930-36 *Talc for Men 35¢* **MP $45,**
$55 boxed
1930-36 *After Shaving Lotion 4oz 35¢*
MP $50, $60 boxed

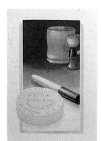

1930 *Styptic Pencil*
10¢ **MP $10**
1930-36 *Shaving Soap*
MP $75 boxed

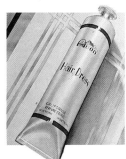

1930-35 *Hair Dress, tube*
50¢ **MP $28**

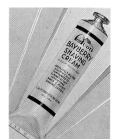

1930-35 *Bayberry*
Shaving Cream 35¢
MP $28

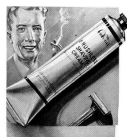

1934-35 *Brushless*
Shaving Cream 50¢
MP $28

MEN'S TOILETRIES

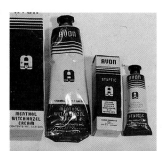

1936-44 *Menthol Witch Hazel*
Cream, tube 37¢ **MP $15,**
$20 boxed
1944-49 *Styptic Cream 17¢*
MP $20, $27 boxed

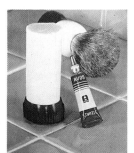

1937-48 *Shaving Stick in*
bakelite holder 36¢ **MP $20**
1937-43 *Styptic Cream 15¢*
MP $25

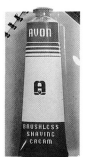

1936-49 *Brushless*
Shaving Cream 41¢
MP $15

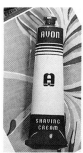

1936-49 *Shaving*
Cream 36¢ **MP $15**

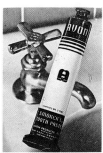

1941 *Smoker's Tooth*
Paste 39¢ **MP $15**

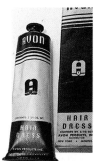

1936-49 *Hair Dress*
37¢ **MP $15, $20**
boxed

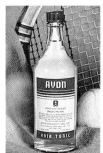

1938-39 *Hair Tonic*
6oz 52¢ **MP $45,**
$55 boxed

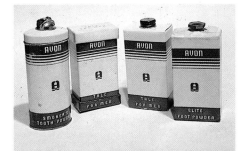

1938-43 *Smoker's Tooth Powder, issued only in*
Men's Sets **MP $15**
1943 only *Talc for Men 43¢* **MP $45**
1945 only *Talc for Men 43¢* **MP $45**
1944-45 *Elite Powder (with hexagon cap) 43¢*
MP $45

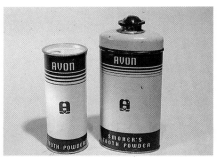

1944-45 *Tooth Powder 57¢* **MP $22**
1946 *Smoker's Tooth Powder, issued*
in Men's Sets **MP $16**

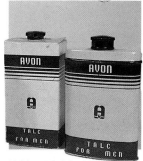

1944 only *Talc for Men,*
cardboard with hexagon lid
2-5/8oz 43¢ **MP $45**
1936-42, then 1946-49 *Talc for*
Men 37¢ & 39¢ **MP $18**

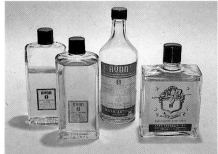

1942-49 *After Shaving Lotion 4oz 43¢* **MP $25**
1936-41 *After Shaving Lotion 4oz 37¢* **MP $35**
1939-40 *Hair Lotion 6oz (shown) 52¢* **MP $40**
(1941-49 *Hair Lotion as above with Good*
Housekeeping Seal on front label **MP $35**
1939-43 *Hair Lotion 16oz $1.35* **MP $50)**
1946-49 *Cologne for Men 6oz $1.50* **MP $80**

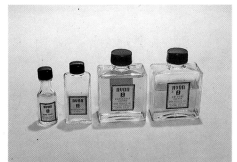

1939 *Hair Tonic Sample ¼oz* **MP $50**
1937 *After Shaving Lotion Sample ½oz* **MP $40**
1947-49 *Deodorant for Men 2oz 59¢* **MP $22**
1948 *Cologne for Men 2oz (issued in Men's Sets)*
MP $30

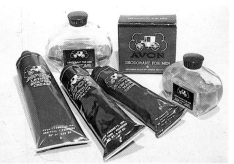

1949-59 *Lather Shaving Cream 3-7/8oz 49¢* **MP $12**
1949-59 *Brushless Shaving Cream 4-1/8oz 49¢*
MP $12
1949-57 *Cream Hair Dress 2¼oz 49¢* **MP $12**
1954-57 *Deodorant for Men 4oz (Sets only)* **MP $10**
1949-58 *Deodorant for Men 2oz 63¢* **MP $9,**
$11 boxed

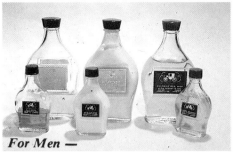

For Men —
1949-58 *Liquid Hair Lotion 4oz 59¢* MP $15
1949-58 *Cream Hair Lotion 4oz 59¢* MP $15
1953 *Cologne for Men 4oz (Before and After Set only)* MP $25
1950's *Liquid and Cream Hair Lotion Samples 1oz each* MP $25
1953 *Liquid Shampoo 1oz (Parade Dress Set only)* MP $25

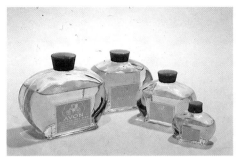

For Men —
1949-58 *Cologne 6oz $1.50* MP $15
1949-57 *Cologne 4oz (Sets only)* MP $15
1952-58 *Cologne 2oz 69¢* MP $12
1950's *Cologne ½oz Sample* MP $25

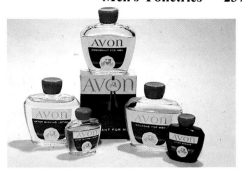

For Men —
1958-62 *After Shaving Lotion 4oz 79¢* MP $8
1958-62 *After Shaving Sample ½oz* MP $12
1958-62 *Deodorant 2oz 69¢* MP $9, $10 boxed
1958 *Cologne 2oz (Happy Hours Set only)* MP $15
1959 *After Shower Sample ½oz* MP $15

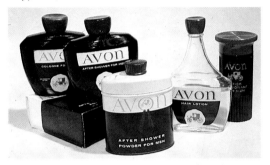

1958-59 *Cologne for Men 4oz $1.25* MP $15, $19 boxed
1959-62 *After Shower for Men 4oz $1.25* MP $12, $15 boxed
1959-62 *After Shower Powder for Men 3oz 89¢* MP $8
(1958-59 only *Talc for Men, not shown, same can as above 69¢* MP $15)
1958-62 *Liquid Hair Lotion 4oz 89¢* MP $10
1959-61 *Stick Deodorant for Men 2½oz $1* MP $12

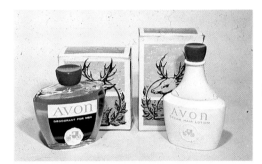

1958 *Deodorant for Men 2oz in Christmas Box 69¢* MP $15
1958 *Cream Lotion 4oz in Christmas Box 89¢* MP $14

1960-61 *Deodorant for Men 2oz (issued in First Prize & Gold Medallion Sets)* MP $12, $20 boxed

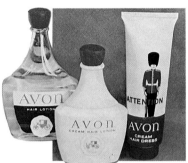

1958 *Liquid Hair Lotion 4oz 89¢* MP $10
1958-62 *Cream Hair Lotion 4oz 89¢* MP $8
1959 *Attention Hair Dress 4oz 89¢* MP $10

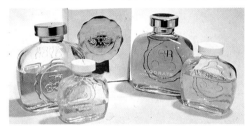

1960-62 *Spice After Shaving Lotion 8oz $1.89* MP $18, $25 boxed
1960-61 *After Shower for Men 2oz (issued in First Prize & Gold Medallion Sets)* MP $12, $20 boxed
1961-62 *'Vigorate After Shaving Lotion 8oz $2.50* MP $20, $28 boxed
1961-62 *Spice After Shaving Lotion 4oz $1.25* MP $10, $15 boxed

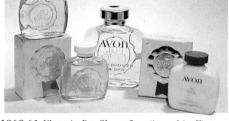

1960-61 *Electric Pre-Shave 2oz (issued in First Prize & Gold Medallion Sets)* MP $12, $20 boxed
1961-62 *After Shower for Men 8oz $2.50* MP $20, $28 boxed
1960-61 *Cream Hair Lotion 2oz (issued in First Prize & Gold Medallion Sets)* MP $10, $18 boxed

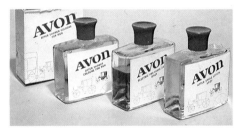

1962-65 *After Shower Cologne for Men 4oz $1* MP $8, $10 boxed
1962-65 *Electric Pre-Shave–Spicy 4oz 89¢* MP $8, $10 boxed
1962-65 *After Shave Lotion–Spicy 4oz 89¢* MP $8, $10 boxed

1962-65 *Brushless Shave Cream–Spicy 4oz 89¢* MP $6

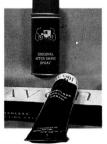

1965-66 *Original After Shave Spray 5½oz $1.50* MP $11
1959-62 *Brushless (shown) or Lather Shaving Cream 5oz 79¢* MP $10, $14 boxed

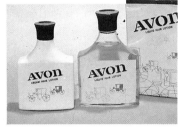

1962-65 *Cream Hair Lotion 4oz 89¢* MP $6
1962-65 *Liquid Hair Lotion 4oz 89¢* MP $7, $9 boxed

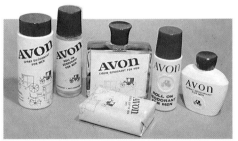

For Men —
1962-65 *Spray Deodorant 2¾oz 89¢* MP $4
1963-65 *Roll-On Deodorant 1¾oz 89¢* MP $5
1962-65 *Liquid Deodorant 2oz 79¢* MP $4
1960-63 *Roll-On Deodorant (plastic) 1¾oz 89¢* MP $4
1959 *Spray Deodorant 2¾oz 89¢* MP $6
1963-65 *Oatmeal Soap 3oz 39¢* MP $12

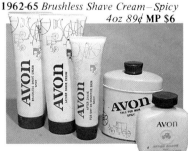

1962-65 *Lather Shave Cream –Spicy 4oz 89¢* MP $6
1962-65 *After Shave for Dry or Sensitive Skin–Spicy 2oz 89¢* MP $7
1962-65 *Talc for Men–Spicy 3oz 89¢* MP $12
1960-61 *After Shave for Dry or Sensitive Skin 2oz 89¢* MP $10

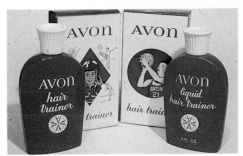

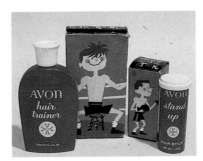

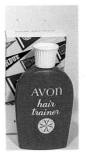

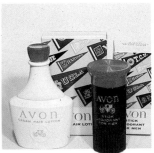

1958 Hair Trainer 4oz 89¢ **MP $3, $11 in Xmas box**
1959 Hair Trainer 4oz 89¢ **MP $3, $11 in Xmas box**

1960-61 Hair Trainer 4oz 89¢ **MP $3, $10 in Gift box**
1958-63 Stand Up Hair Stick 79¢ **MP $5**
1960-61 Above in Gift box shown **MP $10**

1959 Hair Trainer 4oz 89¢ **MP $3, $10 in Xmas box**

1959 Cream Hair Lotion 4oz in Christmas Box 89¢ **MP $14**
1959 Stick Deodorant for Men 2½oz $1 **MP $12, $19 in Xmas box**

. . . . MEN'S TOILETRIES

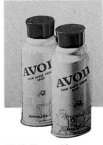

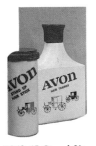

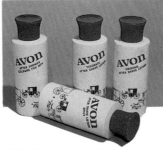

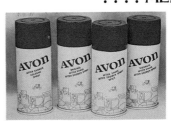

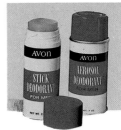

1962 Foam Shave Cream, Mentholated 6oz 89¢ **MP $5**
1962 Foam Shave Cream, Regular 6oz 89¢ **MP $5**

1963-65 Stand Up Hair Stick 1½oz 89¢ **MP $6**
1962-65 Hair Trainer 4oz 89¢ **MP $10**

1963-65 Plastic bottles 2oz issued only in 1963 Jolly Holly Day, 1964 Christmas Trio and 1965 King for a Day in choice of 9 daily-use products **MP $4 each**

1963-65 After Shower Cologne Spray 5.5oz $1.75 **MP $4**
1963-65 Original After Shave-After Shower Spray 5.5oz $1.50 **MP $4**
1962-65 After Shave-After Shower Spray 5.5oz $1.50 **MP $4**
1963-65 'Vigorate After Shave-After Shower Spray 5.5oz $1.75 **MP $4**

1968 Stick Deodorant for Men 2.25oz $1.25 **MP $4**
1968 Aerosol Deodorant for Men 4oz $1.25 **MP $4**

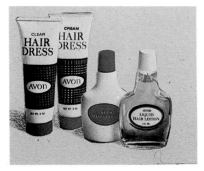

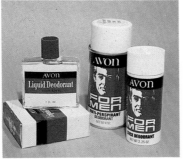

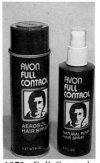

1966-72 Clear Hair Dress 4oz 98¢ **MP $2**
1966-72 Cream Hair Dress 4oz 98¢ **MP $2**
1966-70 Cream Hair Lotion 4oz 98¢ **MP $3**
1966-71 Clear Hair Lotion 4oz 98¢ **MP $3**

1966 Liquid Deodorant for Men 2oz 79¢ **MP $3**
1970 Spray Deodorant for Men 4oz $1.25 **MP $3**
1971 Stick Deodorant for Men 2¼oz $1.25 **MP $3**

Protein Hair Products —
1972 Hair Spray 7oz $1.75 **MP $1.50**
1972 Hair Lotion 6oz $1.75 **MP $1.50**
1973 Hair Managing Control $1.75 **MP $1.50**
1972 Cream Hair Dress 4oz $1.59 **MP $1.50**

1979 Full Control Aerosol Hair Spray 6oz $2.39 **MP $2** (short issue)
1980-83 Full Control Pump Hair Spray 6oz $2.99 **MP 50¢**

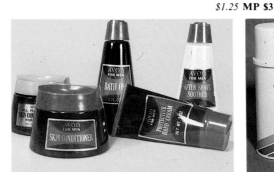

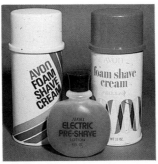

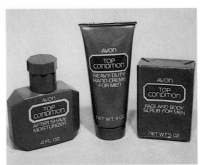

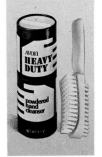

1966 All-Purpose Skin Conditioner 5oz $2.50 **MP $7**
1969 Skin Conditioner 5oz $2.50 **MP $4**
1968 Bath Oil 4oz $2.50 **MP $6**
1969 Hand Cream tube 3oz $1.50 **MP $2**
1968 After Shave Soother 4oz $2.50 **MP $4**

1978-82 Foam Shave Cream 11oz $1.79 **MP 50¢**
1976 Electric Pre-Shave Lotion 4oz $1.49 **MP 50¢**
1971 Foam Shave Cream 11oz $1.50 **MP 75¢**

1982-84 **Top Condition for Men —** After Shave Moisturizer 4oz $5 **MP $1**
Heavy Duty Hand Creme 3oz $3.50 **MP 75¢**
Face and Body Scrub 5oz $3.50 **MP $1**

1973 Heavy Duty Powdered Hand Cleanser 10oz $1.25 **MP 75¢**
1973 Hand & Nail Brush $2.50 **MP $4**

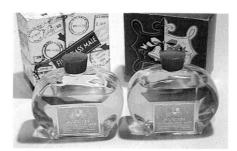

1953-56 *First Class Male gift box holds Cologne for Men 6oz $1.50* **MP $26 boxed**
1957 *Royal Order gift box holds Cologne for Men 6oz $1.50* **MP $26 boxed**

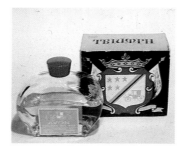

1956 *Triumph gift box holds Cologne for Men 6oz $1.50* **MP $26 boxed**

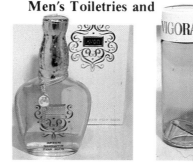

1959 *After Shower for Men 8oz $2.50* **MP $62 with neck cord, $70 boxed**

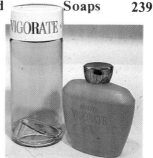

1959 *'Vigorate Lotion 8oz $2.50* **MP $50, $75 boxed**
1960 *'Vigorate Lotion 4oz $1.25* **MP $13**

A GENTLEMAN'S CHOICE

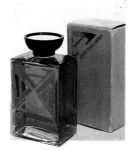

1964 *"4-A" After Shave Lotion 6oz $2* **MP $20, $25 boxed**

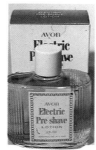

1966 *Electric Pre-Shave Lotion 4oz 89¢* **MP $2**

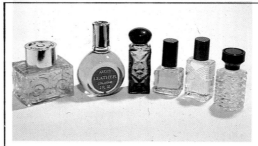

1969 *Gentlemen's Choice in 5 frag. 2oz $1.75* **MP $4**
1970 *Gift Cologne in 4 frag. 2oz $3* **MP $3**
1977 *Cologne Miniature in 3 frag. ½oz $2* **MP $2**
1978 *Cologne Miniature in 4 frag. ½oz $2.50* **MP $2**
1979 *Cologne Accent for Men in 7 fragrances .5oz $2.50* **MP $2**
1980 *Gift Cologne for Men in 8 frag. .5oz $3* **MP $1**

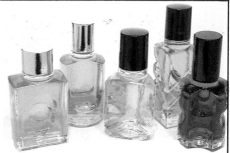

1974 *Gift Cologne in 4 frag. 2oz $2.50* **MP $3**
1975 *Gift Cologne in 4 frag. 2oz $3* **MP $3**
1976 *Gift Cologne in 5 frag. 2oz $3* **MP $2**
1977 *Gift Cologne in 4 frag. 2oz $3* **MP $2**
1978 *Gift Cologne in 4 frag. 2oz $3* **MP $2**

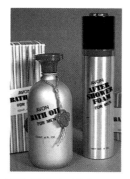

1965-67 *Bath Oil for Men 4oz $2.50* **MP $20**
1965-67 *After Shower Foam for Men 4oz $2.50* **MP $15**

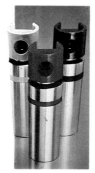

1970 *Cologne Spray for Men 4oz in Oland, Wild Country and Leather $5* **MP $6**

MEN'S GIFT COLOGNES

"Small Colognes with big collecting appeal"

(See also Men's Fragrance Lines pgs. 229-235)

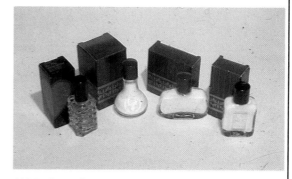

1984 *Be My Valentine Mini Cologne for Him in Wild Country, Rugger, Black Suede or Musk .5oz (2 Campaigns only) $3.50* **MP $1 boxed**
1983 *Mini After Shave Soothers in Wild Country, Rugger or Black Suede .5oz $3 each* **MP 50¢, 75¢ boxed**

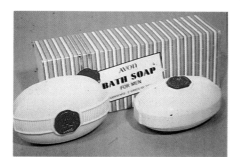

1966-67 *Bath Soap for Men, two 5oz cakes $2.50* **MP $27**

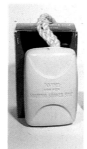

1972 *Men's Shampoo/Shower Soap-On-A-Rope 5oz $2.50* **MP $9**

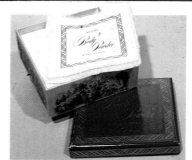

1967 *Body Powder for Men 6oz $4* **MP $13**

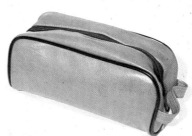

1980 *Travel Case, all vinyl, fully lined. Sold in U.S. only with $7.50 purchase in C-23. $5.99* **MP $11 value**

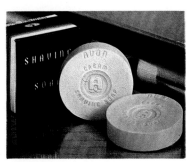

1936 *Shaving Soap, two cakes 31¢*
MP $70 boxed

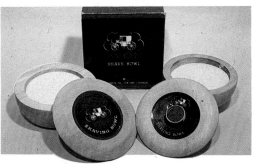

1949-53 *Shaving Bowl $1* **MP $50, $60 boxed**
1953-56 *Shaving Bowl $1.25* **MP $45, $55 boxed**

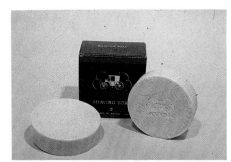

1949-57 *Shaving Soap, two cakes 59¢* **MP $50**
boxed

SOAPS FOR MEN

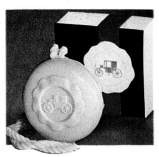

1960-62 *Shower Soap-On-A-Rope 6oz $1.35* **MP $36**

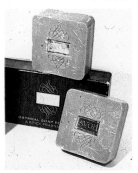

1961-63 *Oatmeal Soap for Men. Two 4oz cakes $1.35* **MP $30**

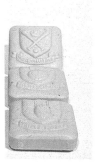

1964 *Most Valuable. Three 3oz Soaps $1.35* **MP $30 boxed**

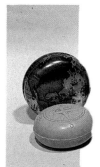

1982 *Ancient Mariner Box with Soap 5oz $10* **MP $9, $4 tin only**

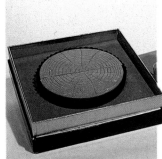

1966-67 *Lonesome Pine Soap. Two 2oz cakes $2* **MP $25**

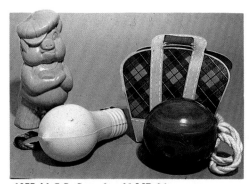

1977 *M.C.P. Soap 8oz $5* **MP $6**
1967 *Light of My Life. Light Bulb shaped Soap-On-a-Rope 5oz $1.50* **MP $20**
1960 *Bowl 'em Over, Avonlite Bowling Ball shaped soap on a cord 6.4oz $1.19* **MP $45 with box, $30 Soap only**

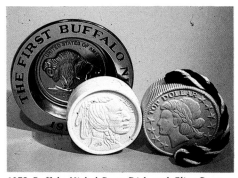

1978 *Buffalo Nickel Soap Dish and Clint Soap 4oz $10.50* **MP $10**
1966 *Top Dollar Spicy scented Soap-On-a-Rope $1.75* **MP $23, $35 boxed**

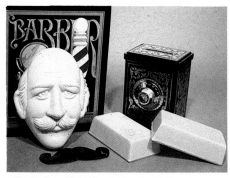

1978 *Barber Shop Duet. 5oz Wild Country molded Soap and Mustache Comb $5* **MP $6 boxed**
1978 *Safe Combination Change Bank with two 3oz Tai Winds scented soap in the shape of gold bars. Embossed metal bank made in England $9.50* **MP $9**

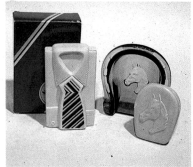

1978 *Suitably Gifted Soap with necktie decal. Deep Woods fragrance 6oz $6.50* **MP $7**
1979 *Lucky Horseshoe Soap Dish and Soap 3.5oz $9.50* **MP $10**

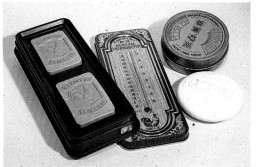

1979 *Farmer's Almanac Thermometer and two 3oz Gentleman's Blend scented soaps. A 1980 Farmer's Almanac with purchase $10.50* **MP $10**
1980 *Perpetual Calendar Container and 5oz Classic Blend scented soap. Metal container made in England $10* **MP $10**

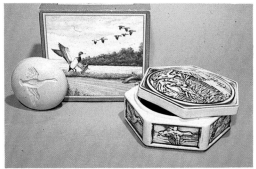

1980 *Birds of Flight Ceramic Box with Trazzara scented soap 5oz. Box made in Brazil $25* **MP $25, $15 box only**

(See Golf Ball Soaps pg. 221)

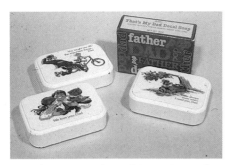

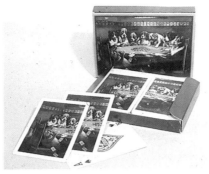

1983 *That's My Dad Decal Soaps, 3oz each. Choice of "We love you, Dad," "You taught me all the important things, Dad" or "You're always there when I need you, Dad" $3 each* **MP $2***

1984 *Dad's Lucky Deal Decal Soap and Card Set. Playing cards 2½"x3½" and soap 3oz $9* **MP $7***
(See also Men's Fragrance Lines pgs. 228-235 and Men's Sets pgs. 244-253.)

MEN'S SETS BY AVON

Avon sets for Men came on the collecting scene during the 30's with only a few wartime sets issued from 1942 thru 1945. The 50's proved to be a popular decade for Men's Sets, and the 60's, too provided numbers of fine collectibles in this important category. Fewer sets in the 70's and 80's indicate heightened value for the sets that remain in private collections.

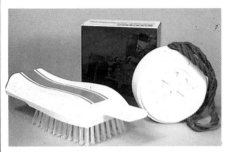

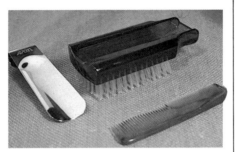

1972 *Sure Winner Brush and Comb $3.50* **MP $7**
1972 *Sure Winner Soap-On-a-Rope $2.25* **MP $13, $16 boxed**

1972 *Trio Valet. Brush, Comb & Shoehorn $5* **MP $9**

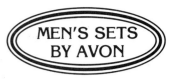

1930 *Hair Treatment Set for Men. Liquid Shampoo 6oz, Pre-Shampoo Oil 2oz, Hair Tonic (for dry or oily hair) 6oz and Hair Dress $2.75* **MP $210**

BRUSHES and BRUSH SETS

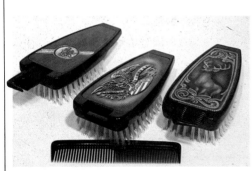

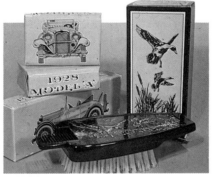

1969 *Brush and Comb Valet $5* **MP $10**
1975 *Brush and Comb Valet $6.50* **MP $8**
1978 *Brush and Comb Valet $9* **MP $8**

1974 *Model "A" Soap Set in Tai Winds or Wild Country 3oz each $3* **MP $10**
1974 *Outdoorsman Brush and Comb Valet $5* **MP $8, $9 boxed**

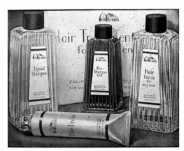

1930-32 *Humidor Shaving Set. Bay Rum 4oz, Lilac Vegetal 2oz, Styptic Pencil, Menthol Witch Hazel Cream, Bayberry Shaving Cream, Talc for Men $2.60* **MP $235**

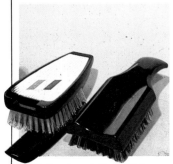

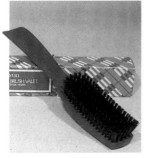

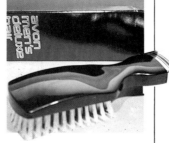

1970 *Brush and Comb Valet $4* **MP $9**
1970 *Club Brush $4* **MP $7**

1974 *Clothes Brush Valet with Shoehorn $7.50* **MP $8, $10 boxed**

1978 *Men's Deluxe Hair Brush $9* **MP $8**

(See also pg. 253)

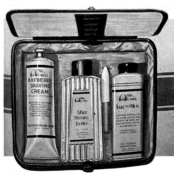

1931 *Men's Traveling Kit, 7¼x6½x2" contains Bayberry Shaving Cream, After Shave Lotion 4oz, Styptic Pencil and Talc $1.95* **MP $160**

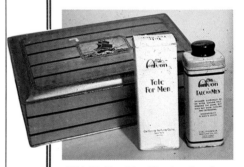

*Available from Avon at time of publication

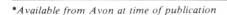

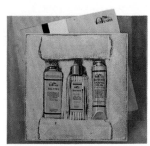

1932 *Assortment No. 7 Talc, Bay Rum 4oz, Bayberry Shaving Cream, Cannon Towel 13½x19", 2 Washcloths $2* **MP $165**

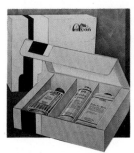

1932 *Assortment No. 2. Lilac Vegetal 2oz, Shaving Cream, Talc $1.40* **MP $120**

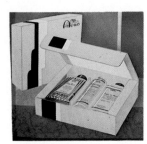

1931 *Assortment No. 1. Bay Rum 4oz, Shaving Cream, Talc $1.20* **MP $120**

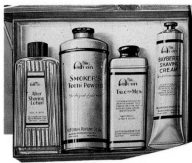

1934-35 *Men's Package. (Div. on label, rare) After Shaving Lotion 4oz, Smoker's Tooth Powder, Talc and Bayberry Shaving Cream $1.61* **MP $200 with rare labels**

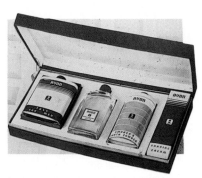

1936-37 *Avon Men's Package. Talc, After Shaving Lotion, Smoker's Tooth Powder and Shaving Cream $1.65* **MP $120**

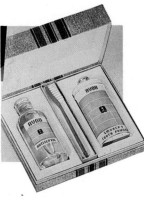

1938 *Smoker Trio. Antiseptic, Toothbrush and Smoker's Tooth Powder $1.39* **MP $90**

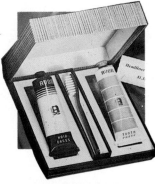

1938 *Headliner for Boys. Hair Dress, Toothbrush and Toothpaste $1.10* **MP $50**

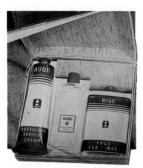

1936-38 *Assortment No. 2. Brushless Shaving Cream, After Shaving Lotion 4oz and Talc $1.10* **MP $85**

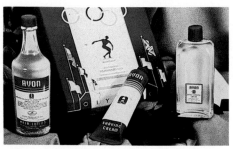

1939-46 *Olympic Set. Hair Lotion, Shaving Cream and After Shave Lotion $1.29* **MP $110**

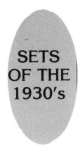

SETS OF THE 1930's

1939 *Esquire Set. Shaving Cream, Bay Rum 4oz, Talc $1.15* **MP $90** *(1936-38 Same set called Assortment No. 1* **MP $95)**

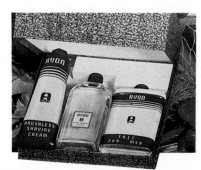

1939 *Brushless Shave Set. Brushless Shaving Cream, After Shaving Lotion and Talc $1.10* **MP $90**

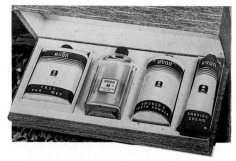

1938-39 *The Valet. Talc, After Shaving Lotion, Smoker's Tooth Powder and Shaving Cream $1.65* **MP $105**

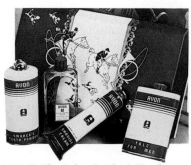

1940-42 *The Valet. Smoker's Tooth Powder, After Shaving Lotion, Shaving Cream and Talc $1.69* **MP $105**

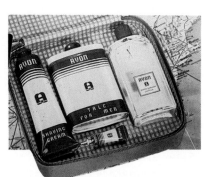

1938 *Men's Traveling Kit. Shaving Cream, Talc, After Shaving Lotion and Styptic Cream $2.16* **MP $120**

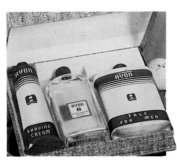

1940 *Country Club. Shaving Cream, After Shaving Lotion 4oz and Talc $1* **MP $90**

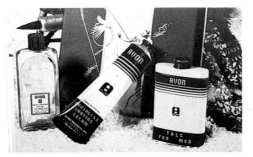

1940 *Brushless Shave Set. After Shaving Lotion. Brushless Shaving Cream and Talc $1.10* **MP $90**

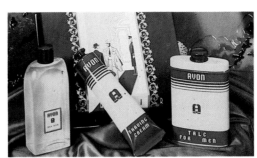

1940 *Esquire. Bay Rum 4oz, Shaving Cream and Talc $1.15* **MP $90**

SETS OF THE 1940's

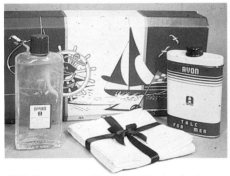

1940 *Commodore Set. After Shaving Lotion, Talc and 2 cotton Handkerchiefs $1.39* **MP $90**

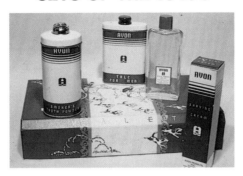

1940-42 only *Valet Set. Smoker's Tooth Powder, Talc, After Shaving Lotion and Shaving Cream $1.69* **MP $115**

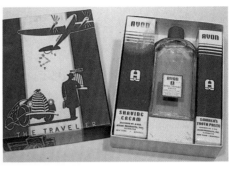

1942-45 *The Traveler. Shaving Cream, After Shaving Lotion and Smoker's Toothpaste $1.10* **MP $85**

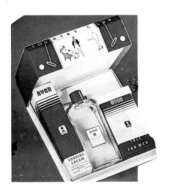

1943 *Country Club. Shaving Cream 3¹/₈oz, After Shaving Lotion 4oz and Talc 2⁵/₈oz $1.15* **MP $105**

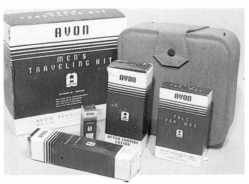

1944 *Men's Traveling Set. Styptic Cream, After Shaving Lotion, Talc and Shaving Cream $2.57, with Brushless Shaving Cream $2.65* **MP $140, $170 boxed**

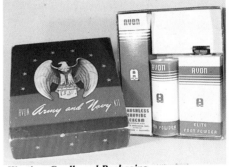

Wartime Cardboard Packaging —
1944-45 *Army & Navy Set. Brushless Shaving Cream, Tooth Powder and Elite Foot Powder $1.46* **MP $105**
(1940-42 Set, as above, held After Shaving Lotion, Shaving Cream and Elite Powder $1.35 **MP $110)**

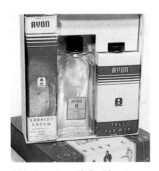

1945 *Country Club. Shaving Cream, After Shaving Lotion, Talc $1.13* **MP $100**

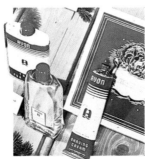

1946 *Country Club. Talc, After Shaving Lotion and choice of Shaving Cream $1.35* **MP $75**

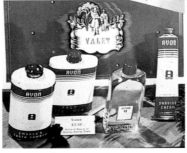

1946 *Valet Set. Smoker's Tooth Powder, Talc, After Shaving Lotion and Brushless or Lather Shaving Cream $2* **MP $90**

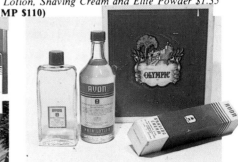

1946-49 *Olympic Set. After Shaving Lotion, Hair Lotion and Shaving Cream $1.65* **MP $100**

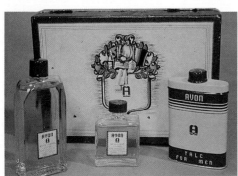

1947 *Modern Knight Set. After Shave Lotion 4oz, Deodorant 2oz and Talc $1.75* **MP $80**

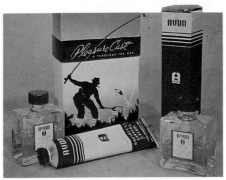

1948 *Pleasure Cast. Cologne, Deodorant for Men 2oz each and Lather or Brushless Shaving Cream 3oz $1.69* **MP $75**

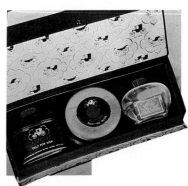

1949-51 *Pleasure Shave. Talc, Shaving Bowl and After Shave Lotion 4oz $2.25* **MP $90, $50 Shaving Bowl only**

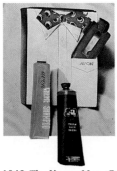

1949 *The Young Man. Creme Shampoo, Cream Hair Dress, Comb and Nail File in pocket case $1.50* **MP $50**

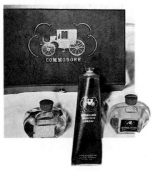

1949-51 *Commodore. Cologne, Deodorant 2oz each and choice of Brushless or Lather Shaving Cream $1.90* **MP $50**

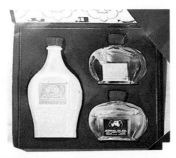

1949-51 *Deluxe Trio. Cologne, Deodorant 2oz each and choice of Liquid or Creme Hair Lotion 4oz $2* **MP $50** (1952 *Deluxe Trio, not shown. Same as above, but box had removable lid* **MP $45**)

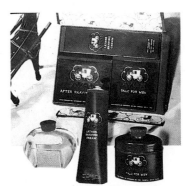

1949-51 *Country Club. After Shave Lotion 4oz, choice of Brushless or Lather Shaving Cream and Talc $1.75* **MP $45**

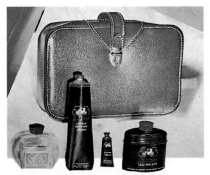

1949 *Men's Traveling Kit. After Shave Lotion 4oz, choice of Shaving Cream, Styptic Cream and Talc $4.66* **MP $80**

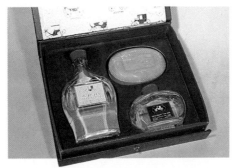

1950-51 *Classic Set. Cream or Liquid Hair Lotion 4oz, Deodorant 2oz and Men's Toilet Soap $1.75* **MP $60**

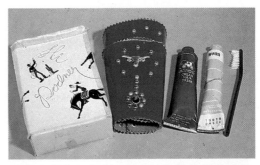

1950 *Hi Podner. Red leatherette Cuffs hold choice of Cream Hair Dress or Creme Shampoo, Toothbrush and Ammoniated or Dental Cream Toothpaste $2.39* **MP $65**

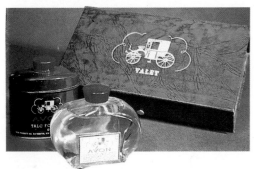

1949 *Valet Set. Cologne 4oz with choice of Talc (shown) or Shaving Soap $1.65* **MP $40, $50 with Shaving Soap**

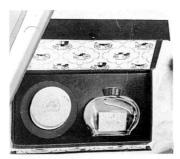

1950 *Valet Set. Cologne 4oz with choice of Shaving Soap (shown) or Talc $1.65* **MP $55, $40 with Talc**

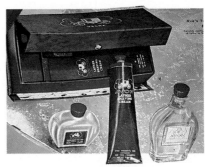

1951 *Valet Set. Deodorant 2oz, choice of Brushless or Lather Shaving Cream and Liquid or Cream Hair Lotion 4oz $2* **MP $48**

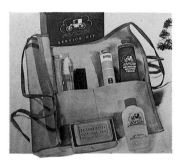

1951 *Avon Service Kit. Military Waist Pocket Apron holds Brushless Shaving Cream, Toothpaste, Comb, Toothbrush, Dr. Zabriskie's Soap and unbreakable bottle of After Shave Lotion $3.90* **MP $125**

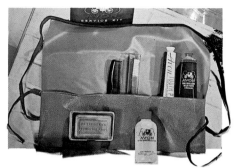

1953 *Avon Service Kit. Leatherette Military Waist Pocket Apron holds Comb, Toothbrush, Brushless Shaving Cream, Dr. Zabriskie's Soap, Toothpaste and unbreakable bottle of After Shave Lotion $3.95* **MP $125**

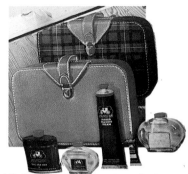

1953-55 *Men's Traveling Kit, Plaid or pigskin Leatherette holds Talc, Deodorant 2oz, Shaving Cream, Styptic Cream and After Shaving Lotion 4oz $7.50* **MP $90**
(1950-52 *Traveling Kit in Leatherette only, contents as above $6.50* **MP $90)**

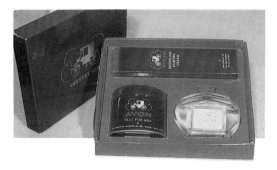

1953 *Country Club. Choice of Brushless or Lather Shaving Cream, Talc and After Shave Lotion $1.85* **MP $50**

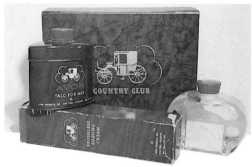

1952 *Country Club. After Shave Lotion 4oz, choice of Brushless or Lather Shaving Cream and Talc $1.85* **MP $50** *(Box has flip-open lid)*

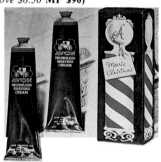

1952 *Pleasure Shave. 2 tubes of Brushless or Lather Shaving Cream 98¢* **MP $30**

SETS OF THE 1950's

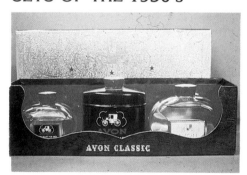

1952 *Avon Classic Cologne 4oz, Deodorant 2oz and Talc $2.25* **MP $50**

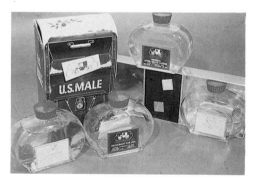

1952 *U.S. Male. Choice of 2 bottles After Shave, Cologne or Deodorant 4oz each $1.22* **MP $35**
1957 *Cuff Links Set. Cologne and Deodorant 4oz each and 2 gold-plated Cuff Links $3.50* **MP $55**

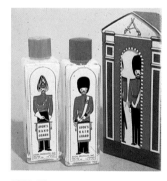

1952 *Changing of The Guard. Hand Guard and Hair Guard 2oz each $1* **MP $65, $25 each bottle**

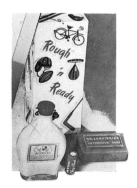

1953 *Rough 'n' Ready. Cream Hair Lotion, Chap Check and Dr. Zabriskie's Soap $1.25* **MP $60**

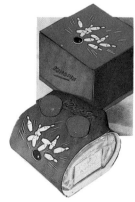

1953 *King Pin. Two bottles After Shave Lotion 4oz each $1.18* **MP $55**

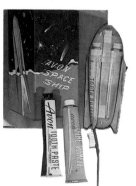

1953 *Space Ship. Plastic ship holds Chlorophyll Toothpaste, Toothbrush, and Creme Shampoo $2.10* **MP $55**

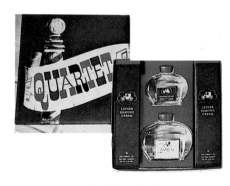

1953 *Quartet. After Shave Lotion 4oz, Deodorant 2oz and choice of 2 Brushless or Lather Shaving Cream $2.20* **MP $65**

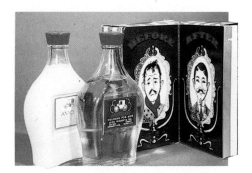

1953 *Before and After. Cologne 4oz and choice of Cream or Liquid Hair Lotion 4oz $1.69* **MP $50**

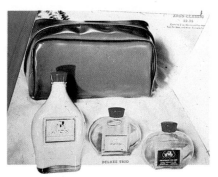

1953 *Deluxe Trio. Toilet Kit contains choice of Liquid or Cream Hair Lotion 4oz, Cologne and Deodorant 2oz each $2.25* **MP $60**

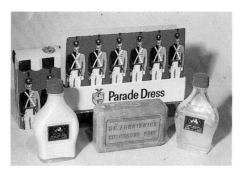

1953 *Parade Dress. Cream Hair Lotion and Liquid Shampoo 1oz each and Dr. Zabriskie's Soap $1.19* **MP $80, $25 each bottle**

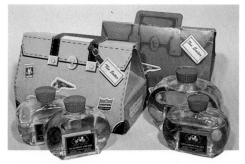

1953 & 1954 *Two Suiter Sets. Holds choice of two 2oz Deodorant or one Deodorant and After Shave 4oz or Deodorant and Cologne 2oz $1.26* **MP $55 set**

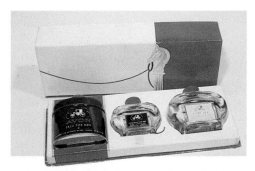

1954 *Classic Set. Talc, Deodorant 2oz and Cologne 4oz $2.25 (rare)* **MP $90**

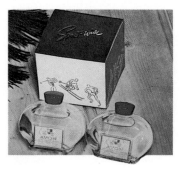

1954 *Sport-wise. Two bottles After Shaving Lotion 4oz each $1.18* **MP $55**

. . . . SETS OF THE 1950's

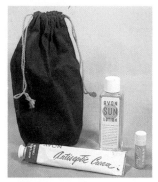

1954 only *Camping Kit for Boys or Girls. 2oz Sun Lotion, Anticeptic Cream, Chap Check and Cream Hair Dress or Creme Shampoo $1.95* **MP $80, $25 Sun Lotion only**

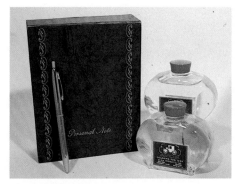

1954-56 *Personal Note. After-use box that looks like memo pad holds 4oz Cologne, 4oz Deodorant and gold Ball Point Pen $2.95* **MP $55**

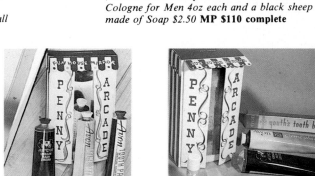

1954-56 *Black Sheep Set. Deodorant and Cologne for Men 4oz each and a black sheep made of Soap $2.50* **MP $110 complete**

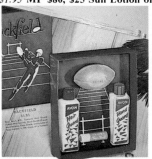

1954 *Backfield Set. Two 2oz bottles of Hair Guard and Hand Guard and Football shaped Soap $1.95* **MP $75, $20 each bottle**

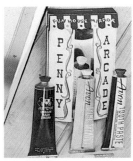

1955 *Pigskin Parade. Creme Shampoo, Hair Guard, Toothbrush and Chap Check $1.95* **MP $60**

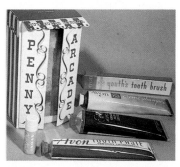

1954 *Penny Arcade. Cream Hair Dress, Creme Shampoo, Toothpaste, Youth's Toothbrush and Chap Check $2.25* **MP $70**

1955 *Penny Arcade. Toothpaste, Cream Hair Dress, Creme Shampoo, Toothbrush and Chap Check $2.25* **MP $70**

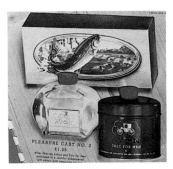

1954 *Pleasure Cast No. 2 After Shaving Lotion 4oz and Talc $1.25* **MP $45**

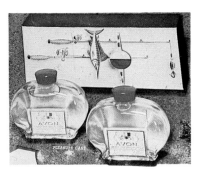

1955 *Pleasure Cast. Two 4oz bottles After Shaving Lotion $1.25* **MP $55**

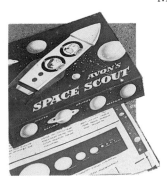

1955 *Space Scout. Toothbrush, White Toothpaste, Hair Guard, Antiseptic Cream and Chap Check $2.25* **MP $65**

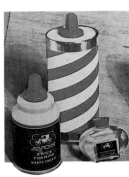

1955 *'Round the Corner. Kwick Foaming Shaving Cream and 2oz Deodorant $1.59* **MP $45**

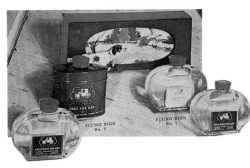

1955 *Flying High Set No. 2. (left) Deodorant and Talc 4oz each $1.49* **MP $40**
No. 1 (right) After Shaving Lotion and Deodorant 4oz each $1.49 **MP $50**
1956 *Happy Hours. Above box held same items as No. 1 Set (above right) $1.59* **MP $50**

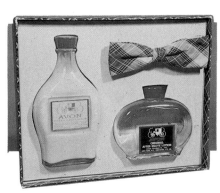

1955 *Saturday Knight. Choice of Cream or Liquid Lotion and 4oz Deodorant and Bow Tie $2.69* **MP $60**
(1956 *Same set re-named Varsity $2.19* **MP $60)**

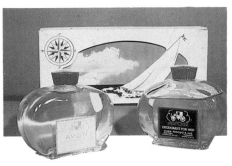

1955 & 1956 *Father's Day Set. Holds two 4oz After Shaving Lotion or 1 After Shaving Lotion and choice of Deodorant 4oz or Talc $1.29* **MP $55**

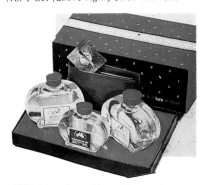

1956 *More Love Than Money. 4oz Cologne and After Shave Lotion, 2oz Deodorant, Wallet and* **1956** *penny $5.95* **MP $85**

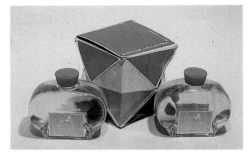

1956 *Before and After. Electric Pre-Shave Lotion and After Shaving Lotion 4oz each $1.59* **MP $55**

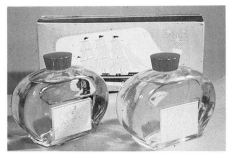

1956 *Sailing, Sailing. Two 4oz After Shaving Lotion $1.29* **MP $55**

. . . . SETS OF THE 1950's . . . .

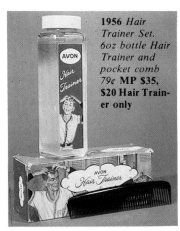

1956 *Hair Trainer Set. 6oz bottle Hair Trainer and pocket comb 79¢* **MP $35, $20 Hair Trainer only**

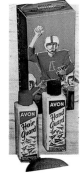

1956-57 *Touchdown Set. Soap in football shape. Hair Guard and Hand Guard $1.29* **MP $60**

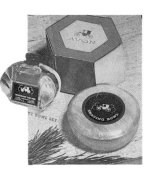

1956 *Shave Bowl Set. Shaving Bowl and choice of 4oz Deodorant or After Shave Lotion $2.50* **MP $65, $45 Shaving Bowl only**

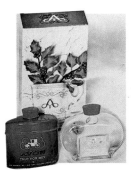

1956 *Holiday Holly. Talc and 4oz After Shave Lotion $1.29* **MP $40**

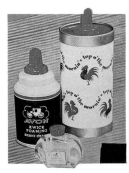

1956 *Top O'The Mornin' set. Kwick Foaming Shave Cream and 2oz After Shaving Lotion $1.59* **MP $45, $18 Shave Cream only**

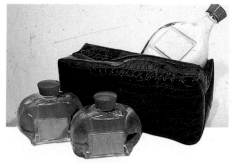

1956 *Overniter. Zippered case holds choice of 4oz Hair Lotions, 2oz Deodorant and 2oz Cologne $2.50* **MP $57**

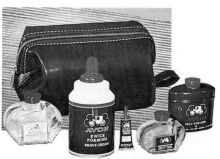

1956-57 *The Traveler. Travel Kit holds choice of Shaving Cream (Kwick, Lather, Brushless) 4oz, After Shave Lotion, 2oz Deodorant, Talc and Styptic Cream $7.95* **MP $85**

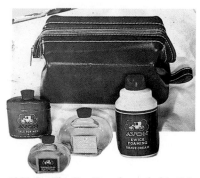

1957 *On The Go. Travel case holds Talc, 2oz Deodorant, 4oz After Shave Lotion and choice of Shaving Creams $8.95* **MP $70**

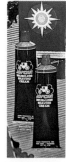
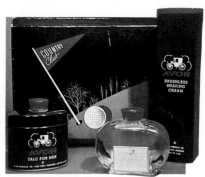

1956 *Smooth Shaving. Two tubes Brushless or Lather Shaving Cream $1.29* **MP $35**

1956-57 *Country Club Set. Talc, 4oz After Shave Lotion and choice of Brushless or Lather Shaving Cream $2.19* **MP $50**

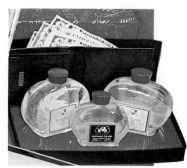

1957 *Money Isn't Everything. 4oz bottles of Cologne and After Shave, 2oz Deodorant and Cowhide Wallet $5.95* **MP $80**

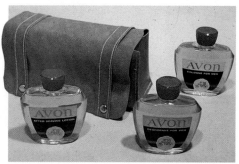

1958 *Happy Hours. Substitute set (see pg. 249) Italian-Luggage design case holds After Shave Lotion, Cologne and Deodorant 2oz each $1.98* **MP $70**

SETS OF THE 1950's

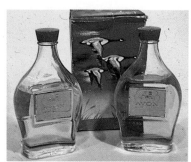

1956 *Good Morning. Two 4oz Hair Lotions, choice of Liquid or Cream $1.29* **MP $40**

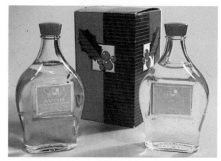

1957 *Attention Set. After Shave and choice of Liquid or Cream Hair Lotion $1.49* **MP $40**

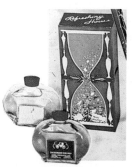

1957 *Refreshing Hours. 4oz After Shave Lotion and 4oz Deodorant $1.69* **MP $40**

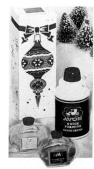

1957 *Merrily. Kwick Foaming Shave Cream and 2oz bottles of A/S & Deodorant $1.98* **MP $45, $15 Shave Cream only**

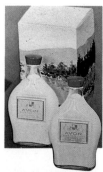

1957 *Man's World. Two 4oz Cream or Liquid Hair Lotions $1.49* **MP $40**

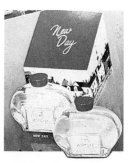

1957 *New Day. 4oz bottles of After Shave and Pre-Electric Shave Lotion $1.59* **MP $45, $20 Pre-Electric Shave only**

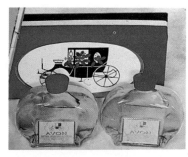

1957 *Send Off. Two 4oz bottles of After Shave Lotion $1.49* **MP $55**

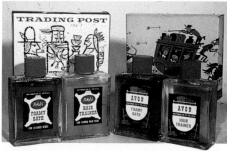

1957 *Trading Post. Hair Trainer and Foamy Bath 2oz each 98¢* **MP $65, $23 each bottle**
1958 *Stage Coach. Hair Trainer and Foamy Bath 2oz each 98¢* **MP $65, $23 each bottle**

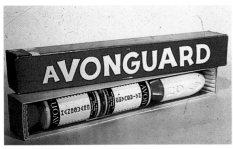

1958 *AvonGuard Set. 2oz Hairguard and Handguard and rocket shaped Soap $1.39* **MP $70, $15 each bottle, $25 Soap**

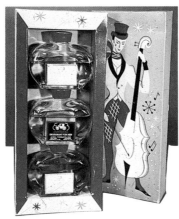

1957 *Good Cheer. After Shaving Lotion, Deodorant & Cologne 2oz each $1.98* **MP $55**

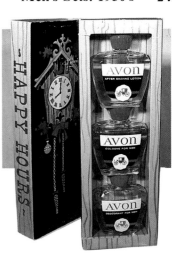

1958 *Happy Hours. After Shave Lotion Cologne & Deodorant 2oz each $1.98* **MP $50** *(See substitute set page 248)*

. . . . SETS OF THE 1950's

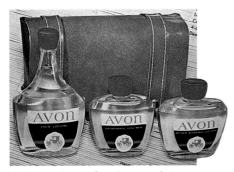

1958 *Overniter. Italian-Luggage design case holds a choice of Cream or Liquid Hair Lotion and 2oz Deodorant and After Shave Lotion $2.98* **MP $55**

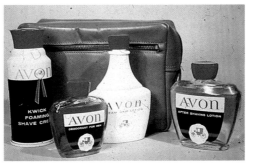

1958 *Neat Traveler. Glove leather case, moisture proof lining, holds 2oz Deodorant, 4oz After Shave Lotion, choice of Shaving Cream or Pre-Electric Shave and choice of Hair Lotion $8.95* **MP $60**

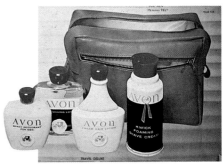

1959 *Travel Deluxe. Spray Deodorant. After Shaving Lotion 4oz, Hair Dress (Cream, Liquid or Attention) and choice of Shaving Cream (Kwick, Lather, Brushless or Electric Pre-Shave Lotion) $8.95* **MP $60**
1960 *Travel Deluxe, as above, but with Roll-On Deodorant (see Deodorant pg. 250) $9.95* **MP $55**

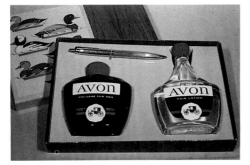

1958 *Modern Decoy. 4oz Cologne and Hair Lotion for Men and gold Papermate Pen $4.50* **MP $50**

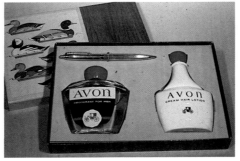

1958 *Modern Decoy with 4oz Deodorant and Cream Hair Lotion and gold Papermate Pen $4.50* **MP $40**

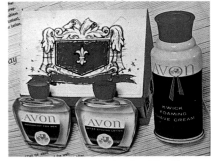

1958 *Coat of Arms. 2oz bottles After Shave Lotion and Deodorant and 6oz Kwick Foaming Shave Cream $1.98* **MP $45**

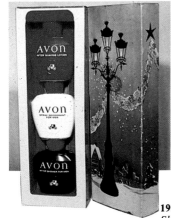

1959 *Lamplighter. 2oz After Shaving and After Shower Lotions and 1½oz Deodorant $2.98* **MP $55**

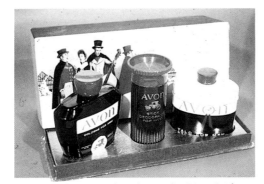

1959 *Carollers Set. After Shower for Men, Stick Deodorant and Talc $3.10* **MP $55**

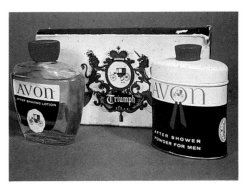

1959 *Triumph Set. Choice of 2 products in combination of After Shave Lotion, Electric Pre-Shave or After Shower Powder 4oz each $1.79* **MP $35**

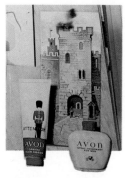

1959 Captain of The Guard. Tube of Cream Hair Dress and Spray Deodorant $1.98 **MP $40**

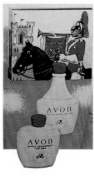

1959 Out in Front. 2³/₄oz Spray Deodorant and choice of Cream or Liquid Hair Lotion $1.98 **MP $40**

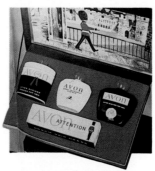

1959 Grooming Guards. Attention Cream Hair Dress, After Shower Powder, Spray Deodorant and choice of After Shower or After Shave Lotion 4oz $4.95 **MP $55**

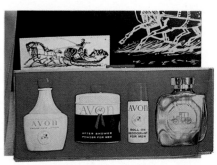

1960 Dashing Sleighs. Cream Hair Lotion, After Shower Powder, Roll-On Deodorant and choice of 'Vigorate or After Shower for Men 8oz $4.98 **MP $65**

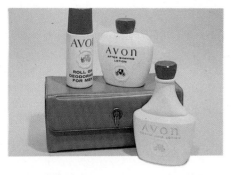

1960 Overniter. Travel Case holds Roll-On Deodorant, After Shaving Lotion 3.5oz and Cream Hair Lotion $3.98 **MP $35**

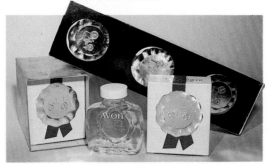

1960 First Prize. Combination of any three 2oz bottles from a choice of 8. After Shave for Dry or Sensitive Skin and Cream Hair Lotion are plastic, all other glass. $2.50 **MP $12 glass bottle, $20 boxed; $10 plastic bottle, $18 boxed; $6 sleeve only**

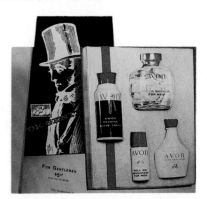

1961 For Gentlemen. 4oz Cream Hair Lotion, Roll-On Deodorant, choice of Kwick Foaming Shave Cream or Electric Pre-Shave and choice of After Shower or 'Vigorate Lotion 8oz $5.17 **MP $65**

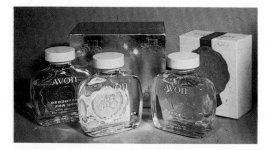

1961 Gold Medallion. Combination of any three bottles from a choice of 10. After Shave for Dry or Sensitive Skin and Cream Hair Lotion are plastic, all others glass. $2.50 **MP same as the First Prize Set, above center**

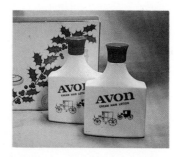

1962 Holly Time Set. 2 Cream Hair Lotions 4oz each $1.78 **MP $27**

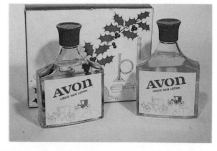

1962 Holly Time. 2 Liquid Hair Lotions 4oz each $1.78 **MP $32**

SETS OF THE 1960's . . . .

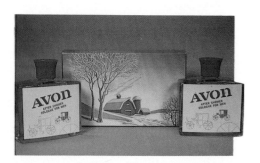

1962 Christmas Classic. Choice of 2 Spicy or 2 Original After Shave Lotions $1.78 **MP $24**, or 2 'Vigorate or 2 After Shower Colognes $2 **MP $27**

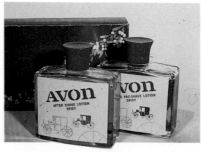

1962 Under The Mistletoe. Electric Pre-Shave and Spicy After Shave Lotions $1.78 **MP $24**

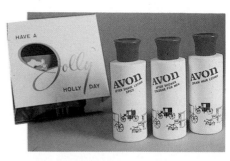

1963 Jolly Holly Day Set shows 3 lotions from a choice of 8, plastic 2oz each $1.98 **MP $20 set**

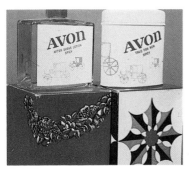

1962 *Good Cheer Set. 4oz Spicy or Original After Shave Lotion and 3oz Spicy Talc $1.78* **MP $30**
1964 *Holly Star Set. 4oz Spicy After Shave and 3oz Spicy Talc $1.78* **MP $30**

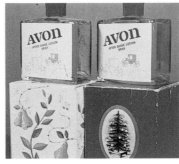

1962 *Christmas Day Set. 4oz Spicy or Original After Shave and 4oz Liquid Deodorant $1.78* **MP $23**
1964 *Christmas Morning Set. 2 bottles Spicy After Shave Lotion 4oz each $1.78* **MP $23**

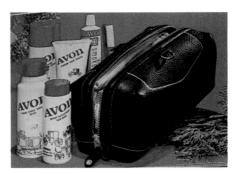

1963 *Men's Travel Kit. Vinyl kit by Amity with Foam Shave Cream (Regular or Mentholated), After Shave-After Shower Spray in Spicy, Cream Hair Dress, Smoker's Tooth Paste, Tooth Brush and Spray Deodorant (Gentle or Normal) $11.95* **MP $70**

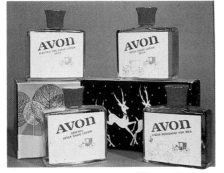

1964 *Holiday Greetings Set. Electric Pre-Shave and After Shave Lotion, both Spicy 4oz each $1.78* **MP $25**
1964 *Santa's Team Set. Spicy After Shave and Liquid Deodorant 4oz each $1.78* **MP $25**

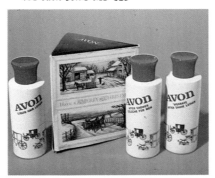

1964 *Christmas Trio. Three 2oz bottles with a choice of any 3 of 9 different products $1.98* **MP $22**

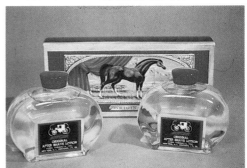

1965 *Orignial Set. (Father's Day Only) Two 4oz Original After Shave Lotions $1.96* **MP $25, $6 each bottle**

. . . . SETS OF THE 1960's . . . .

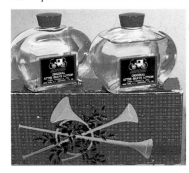

1965 *Christmas Call. Two 4oz Original After Shave Lotions $1.95* **MP $22**

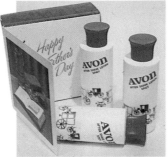

1965 *(Father's Day Only) King for A Day. Three 2oz bottles in choice of 5 assortments $1.98* **MP $28**

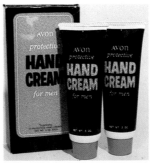

1966 *Protective Hand Cream for Men, two 2oz $2.50* **MP $12**

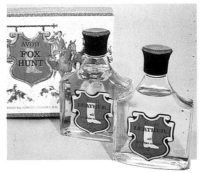

1966 *(Father's Day) Fox Hunt Set. 2 Avon Leather All-Purpose Lotion for Men $4* **MP $40, $15 each bottle**

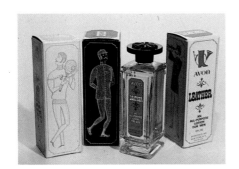

1965 *Fragrance Wardrobe. Three 2oz bottles in choice of 4 assortments fit into sleeve (not shown) $3.50 each set* **MP $45 with sleeve**

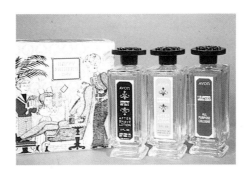

1966 *After Shave Selection in Father's Day Gift Box. Three 2oz bottles in a choice of 3 combinations $2.98* **MP $40, $9 each bottle**

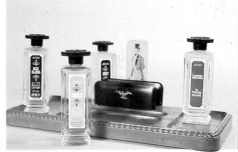

1966 *Bureau Organizer. 2oz Tribute, Spicy, Blue Blazer After Shave and Leather All Purpose Cologne $11.95* **MP $60, $20 tray**

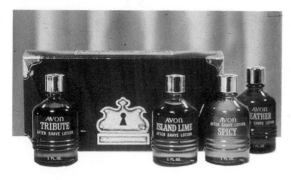

1966 *Fragrance Chest. After Shave Lotion in 4 frag. 1oz each $4* **MP $48, $9 each bottle**

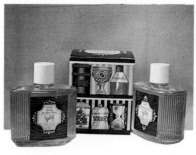

1966 *Fore 'N' After Set. Spicy Pre-Shave and After Shave Lotion 4oz each $1.96* **MP $25, $10 each bottle**

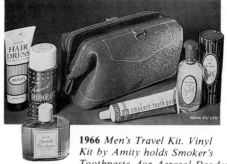

1966 *Men's Travel Kit. Vinyl Kit by Amity holds Smoker's Toothpaste, 4oz Aerosol Deodorant 4oz Clear Hair Dress, 3½oz Spicy Talc, 4oz Spicy After Shave Lotion, plus choice of Electric Pre-Shave Lotion or 6oz Foam Shave Cream $12.95* **MP $65**

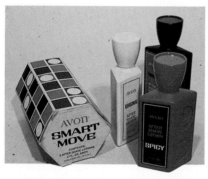

1967 *Smart Move. Spicy, Tribute and Original After Shave Lotion 2oz $4* **MP $55, $13 each bottle**

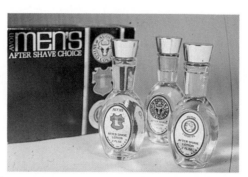

1967 *Men's After Shave Choice. Tribute, Leather and Wild Country Lotion 2oz each $5* **MP $25, $6 each bottle**

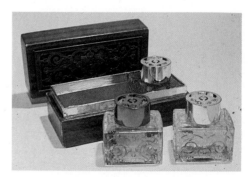

1968 *Gentleman's Collection. 1 each of Leather, Wild Country and Windjammer Cologne 2oz each $8* **MP $30, $13 box only**

SETS OF THE 1960's and 1970's

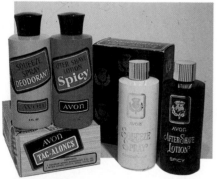

1967 *Tag-Alongs. 3oz Spicy After Shave Lotion & 3oz Squeeze Spray Deodorant $2.50* **MP $18**
1968 *Overnighter. Squeeze-Spray Deodorant 3oz & Spicy After Shave Lotion $2.50* **MP $15**

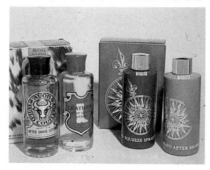

1968 *Boots and Saddle (glass) Leather and Wild Country After Shave Lotion 3oz each $3* **MP $22**
1969 *Traveler Set. Bravo or Spicy After Shave 3½oz and 3oz Squeeze-Spray Deodorant $2.50* **MP $13**

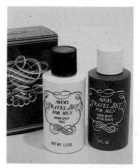

1974 *Travel Set for Men. Talc 1.5oz and After Shave 3oz in Wild Country, Deep Woods, Oland or Spicy $4* **MP $7**

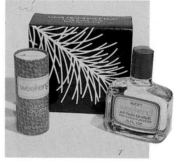

1980 *Fragrance Duo. Talc 1.5oz and After Shave 5oz in Wild Country, Trazarra, Weekend or Clint $8.50* **MP $7**

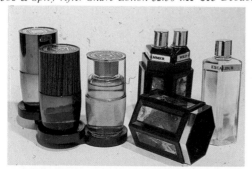

1969 *Structured for Man: Glass, Wood and Steel Cologne 3oz each $8.50* **MP $25**
1969 *Colgone Trilogy. Windjammer, Wild Country and Excalibur Cologne 1½oz each $8* **MP $25, $6 each bottle**

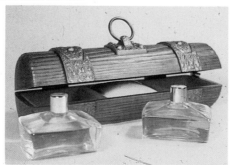

1970 *Master Organizer. Oland or Excalibur Cologne and After Shave 3½oz each and 6oz Soap. Set $25* **MP $50**

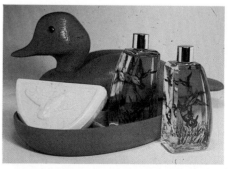

1971 *Collector's Organizer in Tai Winds or Wild Country After Shave and Cologne 3oz each with Soap, 5oz $25* **MP $55**

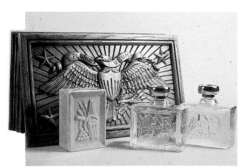

1972 American Eagle Bureau Organizer in Deep Woods or Tai Winds Cologne and After Shave 3oz each with 5oz Soap $25 **MP $45**

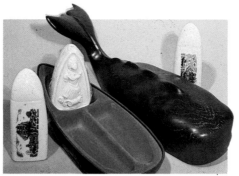

1973 Whale Bureau Organizer. Blend 7 or Deep Woods Cologne and After Shave 3oz each and 5oz Soap $30 **MP $45**

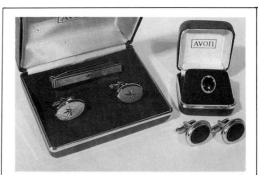

1971 Starburst Cuff Links and Tie Bar $10 **MP $20**
1971 Classic Accent Tie Tac $4 **MP $10**
1971 Classic Black Cuff Links $8 **MP $15**

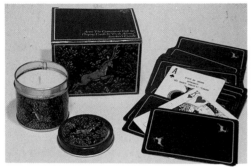

1981 Gamesman Gift Set. Playing cards 2½"x3½" and covered tin container with Fresh Aroma Smoker's Candle $12 **MP $12**

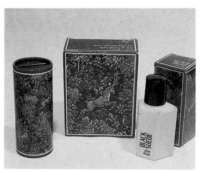

1981 Traveler Gift Set. Talc 1½oz and After Shave 2oz in Weekend, Wild Country or Black Suede $7.50 **MP $2**

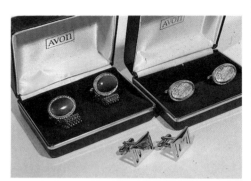

1971 Convertible Cuff Links $12 **MP $20**
1971 Brushed Oval Cuff Links $7 **MP $14**
1971 Geometric Cuff Links $8 **MP $14, $16 boxed**

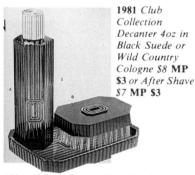

1981 Club Collection Decanter 4oz in Black Suede or Wild Country Cologne $8 **MP $3** or After Shave $7 **MP $3**

1981 Club Collection Hair Brush $8.50 **MP $6***
1981 Club Collection Caddy, 4x6" glass tray $9.50 **MP $6***

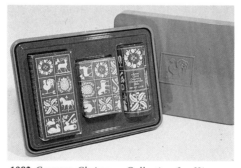

1982 Country Christmas Collection for Him. Plastic box holds 2oz Cologne, 3oz Soap and 1.5oz Talc in Wild Country, Black Suede, Weekend or Clint $14.50 **MP $6**

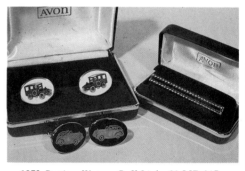

1972 Station Wagon Cuff Links $9 **MP $17**
1971 Rope Twist Tie Bar $5 **MP $11**
1972 Rolls Royce Cuff Links $9 **MP $17**

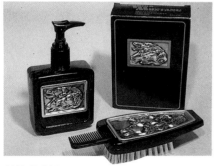

1982 Wild Mustang After Shave Soother Dispenser in Wild Country or Black Suede 5oz $12.50 **MP $8, $8.50 boxed**

1982 Wild Mustang Brush and Comb Valet $12.50 **MP $8, $8.50 boxed**

EARLY MEN'S JEWELRY

In 1971 and 1972 the men's jewelry line consisted of cuff links, tie bars and button covers. In 1976 the first piece of men's body jewelry was introduced — the Clint Wrist Chain. In 1977 men wore their first Avon neckchain, the Ankh Pendant. All handsome designs, each piece is crafted in a masculine style.

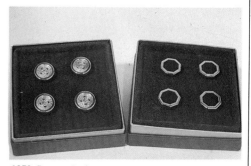

1972 Button Style Button Covers $5 **MP $12**
1972 Blue Enamel Button Covers $5.50 **MP $13**

(See also Men's Fragrance Lines pgs. 228-235)

*Available from Avon at time of publication

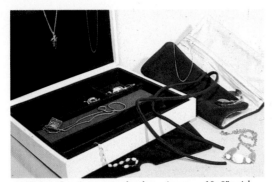

1977 Jewelry Case, sim. leather. Approx, 10x8" with removable velvety pad. $5 with a $10 purchase, one Campaign only **MP $12**
1977 Jewelry Wrap, sim. suede. $3.50 with purchase of 2 jewelry items in C-14 only **MP $7**

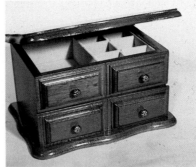

1978 Decorator's Jewelry Chest, wood, dated for collectors. $6 with $10 order in C-15 only (because Avon rejected the entire shipment, only those sold to Reps as demos were issued) **MP $40**

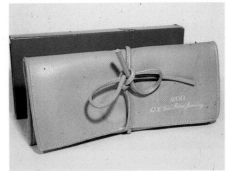

1977 Jewelry Wrap demo to hold 14k Gold Jewelry $2.50 **MP $7**

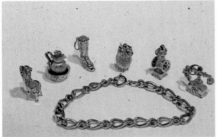

Classic Charms created by Avon's own designers, 14k gold-electroplated.
1973 Sweet Shoppe $4 **MP $10**
1973 Victoriana Pitcher and Bowl $4 **MP $9**
1973 Fashion Boot $4 **MP $9**
1973 Precious Owl $4 **MP $9**
1973 Country Store Coffee Mill $4 **MP $9**
1973 French Telephone $4 **MP $9**

1973 Classic Charm Bracelet, 7" long, 14k gold-electroplated $5 **MP $11**

EARLY WOMEN'S JEWELRY

Featured here are only the early collectibles in Avon's large collection of jewelry. The charms shown are miniature reproductions of classic Avon decanters of the past . . . so popular with collectors.

FRAGRANCE JEWELS BY AVON

The precious look of jewelry with a secret cache of Perfume or Perfume Glace —

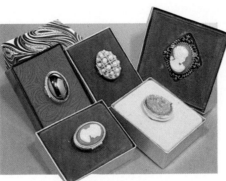

(rear)
1969 Patterns Perfume Glace Ring $6 **MP $12**
1969 Ring of Pearls. Charisma, Brocade or Regence Perfume Glace $7.50 **MP $12**
1970 Cameo Pin Perfume Glace in Bird of Paradise, Elusive, Charisma, Brocade or Regence $10 **MP $16**

(front)
1970 Cameo Ring Perfume Glace in Elusive, Charisma, Brocade or Regence $10 **MP $16**
1970 Bird of Paradise Ring, Perfume Glace Bird of Paradise only $10 **MP $12**

(See Table Top Glace Jewelry pg. 180)

1969 Golden Leaf Pin. Perfume Glace in 11 frag. $6.50 to $7 **MP $11**

(below left)
1968 Golden Charmer Necklace/Bracelet in 9 frag. $9.25 $9.50 & $10 **MP $15**

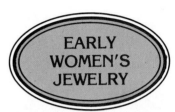

1968 Jeweled Owl Pin Perfume Glace in 10 frag. $5.75, $6 & $6.50 **MP $11**

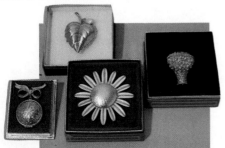

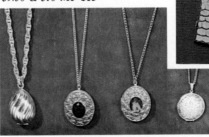

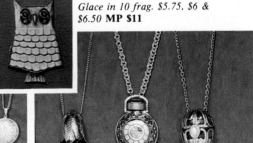

1965 Solid Perfume Jewel Locket. Choice of 9 frag. $5.25, $5.50 and $6 **MP $19**
1969 Daisy Pin. Perfume Glace in 9 frag. $5.75, $6 and $6.50 **MP $10**
1970 Flower Basket Pin. Perfume Glace in 5 frag. $7 **MP $9**

1966 Solid Perfume Locket/Pin. 1½gr in 9 frag. $8, $8.25 and $8.50 **MP $19**
1966 Solid Perfume Locket/Pin. 1½gr $8, $8.25 and $8.50 **MP $19**
1965 Jewel Locket/Chain. Solid Perfume in 9 frag. $5.25, $5.50 and $6 **MP $19**

1970 Perfume Pendant in Elusive, Charisma, Brocade or Regence ⅛oz $14 **MP $17**
1971 Golden Moments Pendant Perfume in 5 frag. ⅛oz $14 and $15 **MP $17**
1972 Perfume Pendant in Moonwind or Sonnet ⅛oz $12.50 **MP $17**

PIN PALS

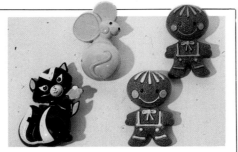

— little girls' jewelry that looks all grown-up. A little girls' fragrance glace hides in a decorative container she will delight in wearing.

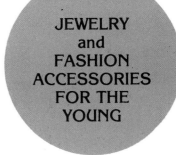

Small World —
1970 *Polynesian Pin Pal Perfume Glace $2.50* **MP $7**
1971 *Scandinavian Miss Pin Pal Perfume Glace $2.50* **MP $7**

Pin Pals *— Fragrance Glace each .02oz*
1972 *Sniffy $2.50* **MP $5**
1971 *Blouse Mouse $2.50* **MP $6** *(pink trim),* **MP $7** *(white trim)*
1972 *Gingerbread Man (white trim) $2.50* **MP $6**
1976 *Gingerbread Man (pink trim) $3.50* **MP $4**

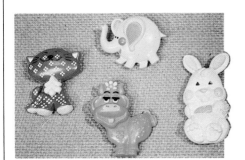

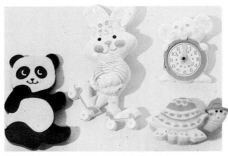

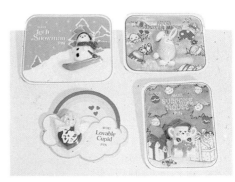

Pin Pals *— Fragrance Glace each .02oz*
1973 *Calico Cat $2.50* **MP $5,** *Blue* **MP $5**
1973 *Elphie $2.50* **MP $5**
1973 *Blue Moo $2.50* **MP $5**
1973 *Funny Bunny $2.50* **MP $5**

1973 *Pandy Bear Pin $2.25* **MP $5**
1974 *Rapid Rabbit Pin Pal Glace .02oz $3* **MP $4**
1974 *Minute Mouse Pin $2.50* **MP $4**
1974 *Myrtle Turtle Pin Pal Glace .02oz $2.50* **MP $4**

1982 *Let It Snowman Pin $5* **MP $3**
1982 *Easter Bunny Pin on gift card $5* **MP $3.50**
1983 *Lovable Cupid Pin on gift card $5* **MP $3.50**
1981 *Surprise Mouse Pin on card $5* **MP $3.50**

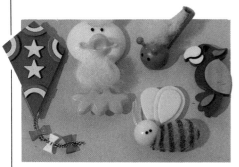

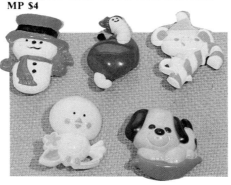

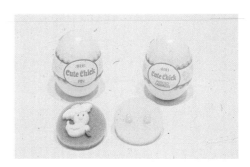

Pins —
1973 *Fly-A-Kite $2.25* **MP $5**
1973 *Luv-A-Ducky $2.50* **MP $5**
1973 *Fuzzy Bug $2.25* **MP $5**
1973 *Perky Parrot $2.25* **MP $5**
1973 *Bumbly Bee $2.25* **MP $5**

1974 *Wee Willy Winter $3* **MP $5**
1974 *Willy the Worm $3* **MP $5**
1974 *Lickety Stick Mouse Pin (not a Pin Pal Glace) $1.75* **MP $4**
1975 *Chicken Little $3.50* **MP $5**
1975 *Puppy Love $4* **MP $5**

1983 *Cute Chick Pin in plastic egg $5* **MP $4***
1983 *Cute Chick Pierced Earrings in plastic egg $5* **MP $3.50**

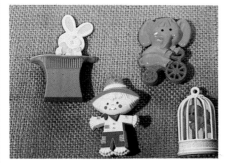

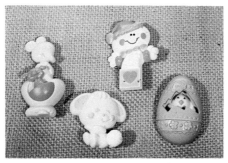

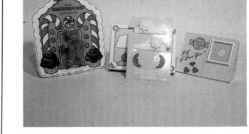

1975 *Magic Rabbit Pin $2.50* **MP $4**
1975 *Pedal Pusher Pin $2.25* **MP $4**
1975 *Peter Patches Pin Pal Fragrance Glace .02oz $3.50* **MP $5**
1975 *Bobbin' Robin Pin $2.50* **MP $4**

Pin Pals *— Fragrance Glace each .02oz*
1975 *Rock-A-Roo $3.50* **MP $4**
1976 *Jack-In-The-Box $3.50* **MP $3**
1976 *Cottontail $3.50* **MP $3**
1977 *Chick-A-Peep $3.50* **MP $3**

*Available from Avon at time of publication

1983 *Gingerbread Man Scented Pin on "house" card $5* **MP $3.50**
1983 *Magic Cloud Convertible Hair Clips. Two moon and two sun ornaments $4 set* **MP $3.50 set**
1984 *Love N'Frame with Earrings. Plastic frame 2⅞"x2⅛" $7 set* **MP $6***

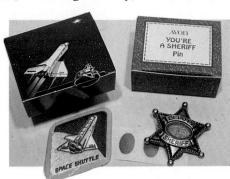

1982 *Space Shuttle Ring and Patch 2"x2½" and membership card* $6 **MP $5***
1983 *You're A Sheriff Pin with personalized stick-um labels* $5 **MP $3.50 complete**

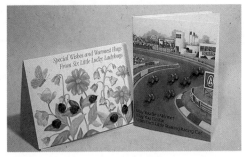

1984 *Lucky Ladybug Buttons. Six plastic buttons on 4⅜"x6" greeting card* $5 **MP $4***
1984 *Roaring Racing Car Buttons. Six plastic buttons on 4⅜"x6" greeting card* $5 **MP $4***

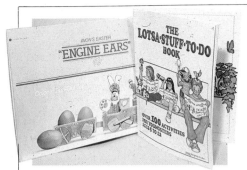

1982 *"Engine Ears" Color 'n Pop-Out Toy to hold Easter Eggs. Free with purchase* **MP $1**
1982 *The Lotsa-Stuff-To-Do Book 7½"x10", 80 pgs. (1 Campaign only)* $2.99 with $7 purchase **MP $6 value**

JEWELRY and FASHION ACCESSORIES FOR THE YOUNG

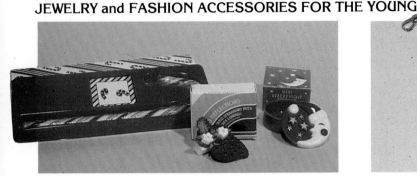

1983 *Candy Cane Treat Earrings with real 6" candy cane* $6 **MP $3** **earrings only**
1983 *Strawberry Patch and Flower Pierced Earrings. Fabric patch 2¼"x1½" and plastic earrings* $7 set **MP $5 set**
1983 *Starry Night Trinket Box with pierced Star earrings. Lid serves as pin. Box 1½" diam.x½ high. All plastic* $7 **MP $6 complete**

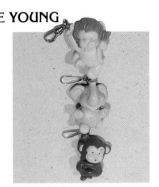

1983 *Zip-A-Zoo. Lion, elephant or monkey plastic zipper pull* $6 **MP $5 each**

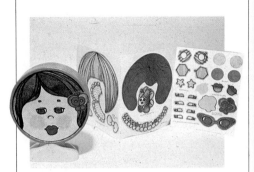

1982 *Maria Makeover. Comes with sheet of reusable decals. Decanter holds Non-Tear Shampoo or Children's Liquid Cleanser 6oz* $7 **MP $4 with decals**

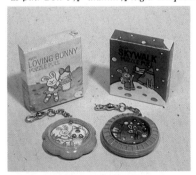

1984 *Loving Bunny Puzzle Pull 1⅝" diam.* $6 **MP $5***
1984 *Skywalk Puzzle Pull 1⅝" diam.* $6 **MP $5***

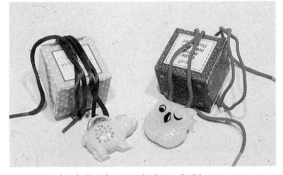

1982 *Piggybank Pendant, with slot to hold penny, on rayon cord 28"* $5 **MP $3**
1982 *Glow-in-the-Dark Owl Pin/Pendant with rayon cord 30"* $6 **MP $3**

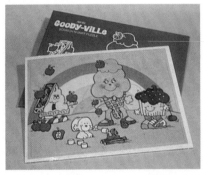

1983 *Goody-ville Scratch 'n Sniff Puzzle. Heavy cardboard 12"x9½"* $6 **MP $3**

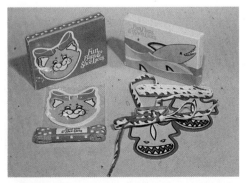

1983 *Fun Flaps and Shoelaces. Two kitty's head shoe flaps and shoelaces with cat's paw pattern or two shark's head flaps and shoelaces with shark's fins pattern. Laces 30"* $5 each set **MP $4 each set**

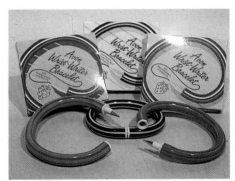

1983 *Wrist-Writer Bracelet. Flexible bracelet with ball-point pen on one end. Scented, colored ink. Grape-scented with purple ink, chocolate chip mint with brown ink or strawberry with red ink* $4 **MP $2 each**

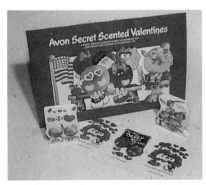

1984 *Scratch 'n Sniff Valentines. 14"x9" book holds 12 punch-out cards in 6 designs and 3 fruit fragrances (2 Campaigns only)* $4.50 **MP $3**

*Available from Avon at time of publication

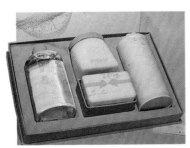

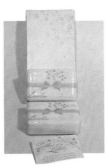

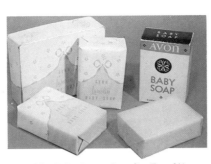

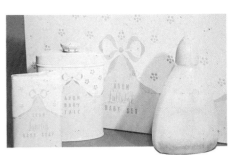

1946 Lullabye Baby Set. Baby Soap, Cream, Oil and Talc and Baby Gift Card $3.55 **MP $160**
(Sold individually: Boxed Soap 69¢ **MP $25**; *Baby Oil $1* **MP $50**; *Baby Cream 89¢* **MP $25**; *Talc 65¢* **MP $20**)

1946 Lanolin Baby Soap 86¢ for box of two cakes **MP $55, $20** **one cake**

1951 Baby Soap, Lanolin Two 3¼oz cakes 69¢ **MP $35**
1955 Baby Soap, Castile with Lanolin 29¢ **MP $15**

1952 Lullabye Baby Set. Baby Soap 3¼oz, Baby Talc and 4oz Baby Lotion $2.35 **MP $100**

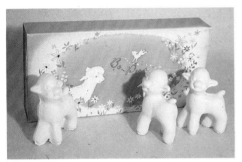

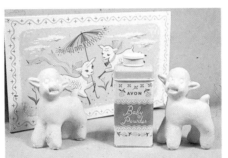

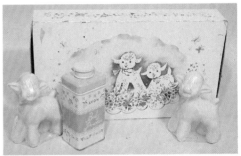

1953 Bo Peep Soap Set. Three molded lamb Soaps $1 **MP $120**

1956 Little Lambs Set. 2 molded Soaps and 2oz Baby Powder $1.39 **MP $100**, *Baby Powder Container only* **MP $20**

1954-55 Little Lambs Set. 2 molded Soaps and 2oz Baby Powder $1.25 **MP $100**

FOR BABY

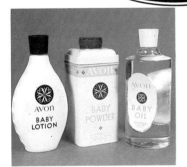

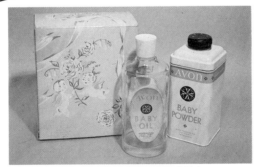

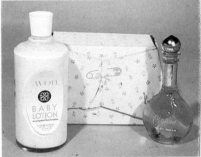

1958 Baby Lotion 6oz 98¢ **MP $10**
1955 Baby Powder 9oz 59¢ **MP $15**
1955 Baby Oil 8oz 79¢ **MP $25**

1955 Lullabye Set. Baby Oil 8oz and Baby Powder 9oz $1.39 **MP $60**

1957 Baby and Me. Baby Lotion 8oz and Cotillion Toilet Water 2oz $1.98 **MP $60**

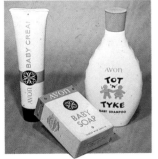

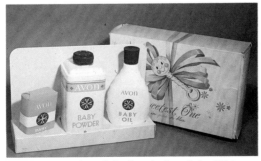

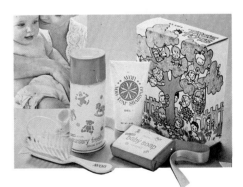

1962 Baby Cream 2oz 89¢ **MP $7**
1955 Baby Soap, Castile with Lanolin 29¢ **MP $15**
1960 only Tot 'n' Tyke Baby Shampoo 6oz 89¢ **MP $15** **with light blue cap**

1962 Sweetest One. Baby Powder 9oz, Baby Oil 6oz and Soap $2.07 **MP $40** *(1961 Set with same items, but Soap wrapper is white with blue center band* **MP $42**)

1966 Tree Tots. Hair Brush, Nursery Fresh Room Spray, Non-Tear Shampoo and Soap $3.98 **MP $30**

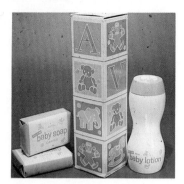

1964 *Lullabye Set. Baby Lotion 6oz, 2 Baby Soaps 3oz each $1.76* **MP $27,** *Soaps* **$8 ea.**

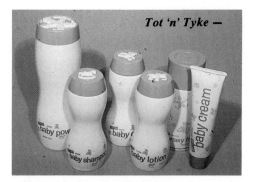

Tot 'n' Tyke —

1964 *Baby Powder 9oz 98¢* **MP $6**
1964 *Baby Shampoo 6oz 98¢* **MP $6**
1964 *Baby Oil 6oz 98¢* **MP $7**
1964 *Baby Lotion 6oz 98¢* **MP $6**
1965 *Nursery Fresh Spray 6oz $1.35* **MP $4**
1964 *Baby Cream 2oz 98¢* **MP $4**

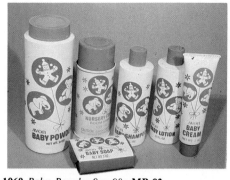

1969 *Baby Powder 9oz 98¢* **MP $2**
1969 *Nursery Fresh Room Spray 6oz $1.50* **MP $2**
1969 *Baby Shampoo 6oz 98¢* **MP $2**
1969 *Baby Lotion 6oz 98¢* **MP $2**
1969 *Baby Cream 2oz 98¢* **MP $2**
1969-74 *Baby Soap 3oz 59¢* **MP $4**

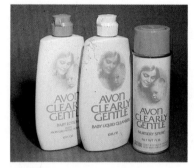

Clearly Gentle —
1975 *Baby Lotion 10oz $2.50* **MP $1**
1975 *Liquid Cleanser 10oz $2.50* **MP $1**
1975 *Nursery Spray 7oz $1.98* **MP $2**

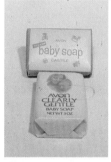

1964-69 *Tot 'n' Tyke Baby Soap 3oz 49¢* **MP $8**
1975 *Clearly Gentle Baby Soap 3oz 69¢* **MP $1**

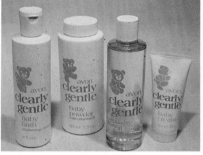

1983 *Clearly Gentle —*
Baby Bath 8oz $1.99 **MP $2***
Baby Cream 2oz $1.99 **MP $2***
Baby Oil 8oz $2.99 **MP $3***
Baby Powder 7.5oz $2.49 **MP $2.50***

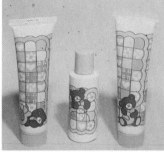

1983-84 *Mother's Little Helpers —*
Baby Bath 1oz $2 **MP 25¢**
Baby Oil 1oz $2 **MP 25¢**
Baby Cream 1oz $2 **MP 25¢**

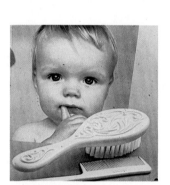

1974 *Baby Brush and Comb Set. Brush 6" long, comb 5" long $3.50* **MP $4**

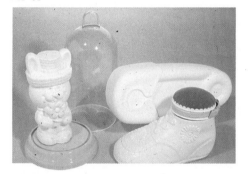

1973 *Sunny Bunny Baby Pomander 5oz $6* **MP $7**
1973 *Safety Pin Decanter Baby Lotion 8oz $4* **MP $5**
1973 *Baby Shoe Pin Cushion Baby Lotion 7oz $5* **MP $6**

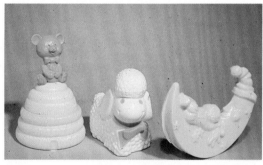

1974 *Honey Bear Baby Cream Decanter 4oz $5* **MP $6**
1974 *Precious Lamb Baby Lotion 6oz $5* **MP $6**
1980 *Rock-A-Bye-Baby hanging pomander Nursery Fresh fragrance $8.50* **MP $7**

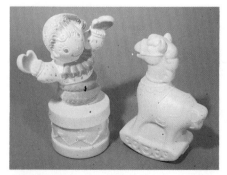

1974 *Jack-in-the-Box Baby Cream 4oz $5* **MP $6**
1975 *Rock-A-Bye Pony 6oz Clearly Gentle Baby Lotion $5* **MP $5**

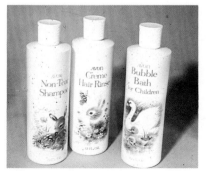

1975 *Non-Tear Shampoo 12oz (deer) $2.49* **MP $2.49***
1975 *Creme Hair Rinse 12oz (rabbit) $1.69* **MP $1**
1975 *Bubble Bath 12oz (swan) $2.19* **MP $1**

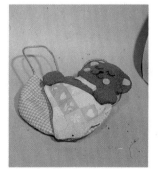

1984 only *Shh . . . Baby's Scented Door Message. Nursery Fresh scent 6" high $10* **MP $4**

**Available from Avon at time of publication*

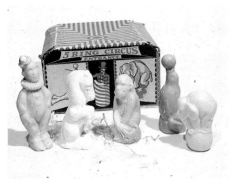

1939 *Five Ring Soap Circus, 5 molded Soaps $1.19* **MP $200**

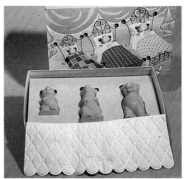

1954 *Three Little Bears, 3 molded castile Soaps $1.19* **MP $135**

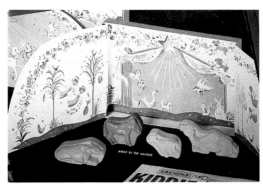

1955 *Away in a Manger. 4 molded Soaps $1.49* **MP $135**

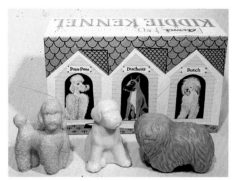

1955 *Kiddie Kennel, 3 molded Soaps $1.49* **MP $135**

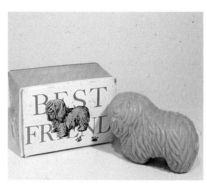

1956 *Best Friend molded Soap 59¢* **MP $45**

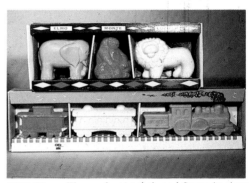

1957 *Circus Wagon, 3 animal shaped Soaps in circus wagon box $1.25* **MP $95**
1956 *Casey Jones, Jr., 3 Soaps boxed $1.19* **MP $95**

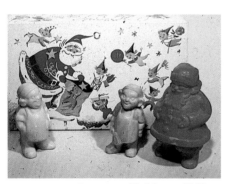

1955 *Santa's helpers, 3 molded Soaps $1.19* **MP $125**

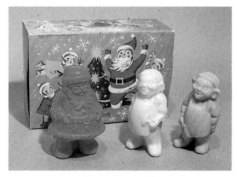

1956 *Santa's Helpers, 3 molded Soaps $1.19* **MP $135**

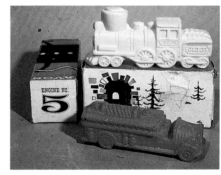

1958 *"Old 99" Train engine Soap 69¢* **MP $40**
1957 *Fire Engine No. 5 Soap 59¢* **MP $45**

CHILDREN'S SOAPS and SOAP SETS

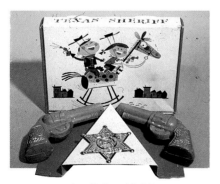

1958 *Texas Sheriff, 2 molded Soap guns and metal badge $1.19* **MP $60**

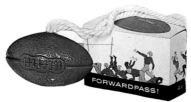

1958 *Forward Pass. Football Soap-On-a-Rope 7½oz $1* **MP $40**

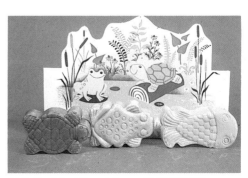

1959 *Pool Paddlers, 3 Soaps $1.39* **MP $40**

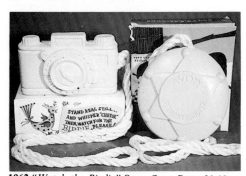

1962 *"Watch the Birdie" Soap-On-a-Rope $1.19* **MP $25**
1962 *Sheriff's Badge Soap-On-a-Rope $1.19* **MP $25**

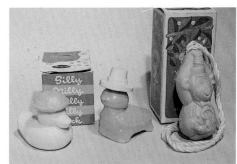

1960 *Frilly Duck Soap 5¾oz 89¢* **MP $25**
1962 *L'il Tom Turtle Soap 5½oz 98¢* **MP $25**
1965 *Mr. Monkey Soap 5½oz $1.35* **MP $17**

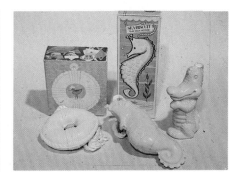

1963 *Life Preserver Soap-On-a-Rope 6oz $1.19* **MP $20**
1964 *Sea Biscuit Soap-On-a-Rope $1.25* **MP $20**
1971 *Al E Gator Soap-On-a-Rope 5oz $2* **MP $9**

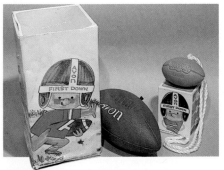

1965 *First Down Set. Junior size rubber Football and Football Soap-On-a-Rope 6oz $3.95* **MP $50, $17 Soap, $20 Football**

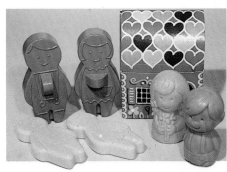

1965 *Gingerbread Soap Twins. Two 2½oz bars and 2 plastic cookie cutters $1.50* **MP $30**
1965 *Hansel and Gretel Soaps in box 3oz each. Set $1.35* **MP $27**

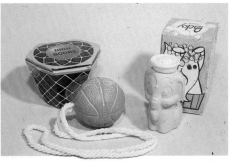

1959 *High Score Soap-On-a-Rope $1.19* **MP $40**
1964 *Packy the Elephant Soap 5½oz 98¢* **MP $20** *(See also pg. 269)*

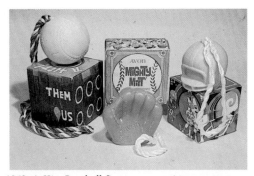

1962 *A Hit. Baseball Soap on a cord $1.19* **MP $25**
1969 *Might Mitt French milled Soap 4oz $2* **MP $9**
1973 *Football Helmet Soap-On-a-Rope 5oz $2.50* **MP $7**

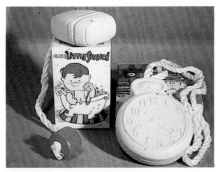

1966 *Little Shaver Soap-On-a-Rope 4oz $1.35* **MP $22**
1961 *Li'l Folks Time Alarm Clock Soap-On-a-Rope 5½oz $1.19* **MP $25**

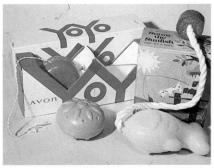

1966 *Yo Yo Set. Yo Yo and Soap 3oz $1.50* **MP $32, $13 each Yo Yo and Soap**
1966 *Sunny the Sunfish Soap-On-A-Rope $1.35* **MP $16**

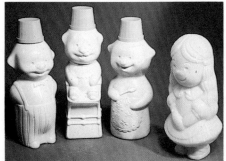

1966 *Papa Bear Baby Oil 3oz $1.25* **MP $11**
1966 *Baby Bear Tot 'n' Tyke Shampoo 3oz $1.25* **MP $10**
1966 *Mama Bear Baby Lotion 3oz* **MP $10**
1966 *Goldilocks molded Baby Soap 5oz* **MP $15**

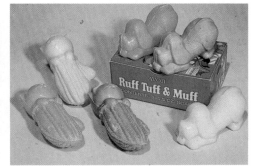

1969 *Mitten Kittens, 3 bars Soap 1⅞oz each $1.50* **MP $10**
1968 *Ruff, Tuff and Muff Soaps in box 1½oz each. Set $1.35* **MP $12**

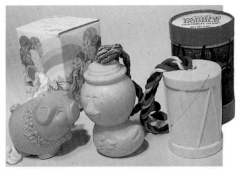

1973 *Petunia Piglet Soap-On-a-Rope 5oz $2.50* **MP $7**
1968 *Easter Quacker Soap-On-a-Rope 5oz $1.35* **MP $10**
1969 *Yankee Doodle Soap 6oz $2* **MP $11**

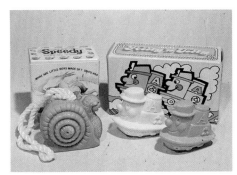

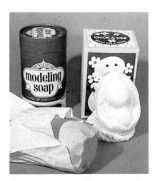

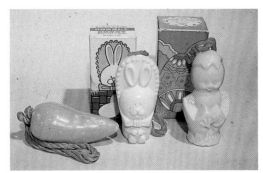

1966 *Speedy the Snail Soap-On-a-Rope 4oz $1.35* **MP $20**
1973 *Hooty & Tooty Tugboat Soap 2oz each $1.75* **MP $7**

1969 *Modeling Soap 6oz $2* **MP $8**
1966 *Chick-A-Dee Soap-On-a-Rope $1.35* **MP $15**

1967 *Bunny Dream Soap-On-a-Rope $1.25* **MP $20**
1969 *Easter Bonnet Bunny Soap 5oz $1.35* **MP $9**
1970 *Peep-A-Boo Soap 5oz $1.35* **MP $8**

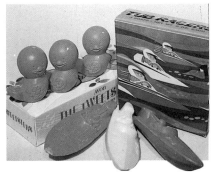

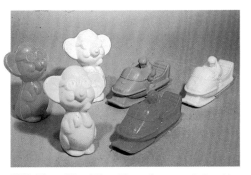

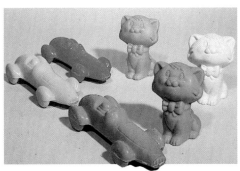

1971 *Tweetster's Soaps. Three 1½oz Soaps $2* **MP $8**
1970 *Tub Racers, Three 3oz Soaps $2* **MP $9**

1971 *Three Nice Mice. Three Soaps each 2oz $2* **MP $8**
1973 *Sure Winner. Three Snow Buggy Soaps each 2oz $2.25* **MP $7**

1969 *Tub Racers. Three 3oz Soaps $1.75* **MP $10**
1971 *Aristocrat Kittens Soap Trio. Each 1½oz $2* **MP $8**

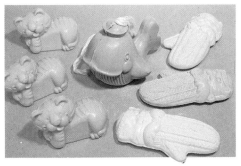

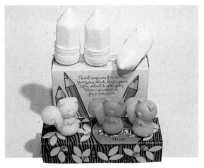

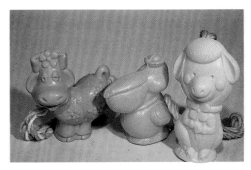

1974 *Tubby Tigers Soap Set. 2oz each $3.50* **MP $6**
1974 *Wilbur the Whale Soap-On-a-Rope 5oz $2.50* **MP $5**
1978 *Furry, Purry, Scurry. Three 2oz Soaps $5* **MP $6**

1980 *Scribble Dee-Doo, three 2.5oz pencil-shaped Soaps $6* **MP $6**
1970 *Tree Tots, three 1.5oz squirrel-shaped Soaps $1.75* **MP $9**

1972 *Blue Moo Soap-On-a-Rope 5oz $1.75* **MP $7**
1972 *Percy Pelican Soap-On-a-Rope 5oz $2* **MP $7**
1971 *Honey Lamb Soap-On-a-Rope 5oz 99¢* **MP $8**

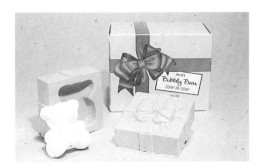

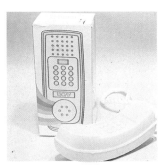

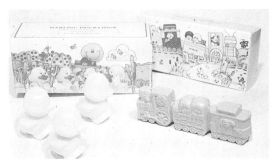

1980 *Bubbly Bear Soap-In-Soap, three 2oz Soaps $7.50* **MP $7.50**

(see also pages 268, 272 & 273)

1982 *Party Line Soap-On-a-Rope 5oz $5.50* **MP $5.50**

1983 *Darling Duckling. Three 1.5oz soaps in "egg carton" Fresh Fun fragrance $5* **MP $5**
1982 *Avon R.R. Three 1oz snap-apart soaps. Fresh Fun fragrance $4.50* **MP $4.50**

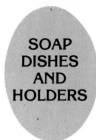

SOAP
DISHES
AND
HOLDERS

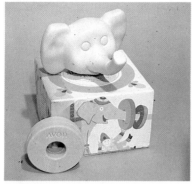

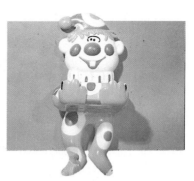

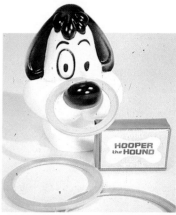

*1966 Ring-Around-Rosie.
Elephant's trunk holds 3oz Soap
$2.25* **MP $25**

*1973 Clancey the Clown Soap Holder
and Soap 3oz $4.50* **MP $9**

*1974 Hooper the Hound Soap
Holder and Soap 3oz $5* **MP $8**

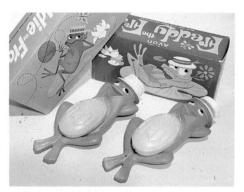

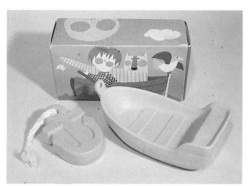

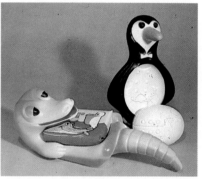

*1965 Freddie the Frog Floating Soap Dish and 3oz
soap $1.75* **MP $20**
*1969 Freddy the Frog Soap Dish and 3oz soap
(right) $2.50* **MP $10**

*1966 Wash Aweigh floating Soap Dish and 3oz
anchor-shaped Soap-On-a-Rope $1.98* **MP $20**

*1967 Gaylord Gator. 9½" long, holds 3oz
Soap $2.25* **MP $12**
*1966 Perry the Penguin Floating Soap
Dish and Soap $1.98* **MP $20, $8 Penguin,
$12 Soap**

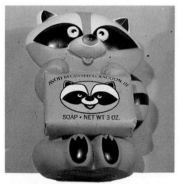

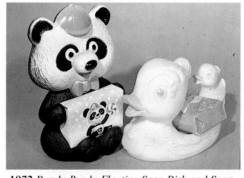

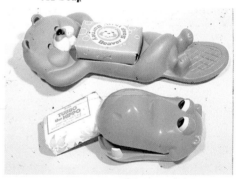

*1970 Reginald G. Racoon III Soap 3oz
and Floating Soap Dish 7" long $2.50*
MP $10

*1972 Randy Pandy Floating Soap Dish and Soap
3oz $3.50* **MP $8**
*1974 Quack and Doodle Floating Soap Dish and
Soap 3oz $4.50* **MP $7**

*1971 Barney Beaver Soap Dish and 3oz Soap
$3.50* **MP $8**
*1979 Tubbo the Hippo Soap Dish and 3oz Soap
$6.50* **MP $6**

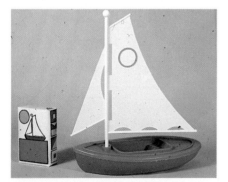

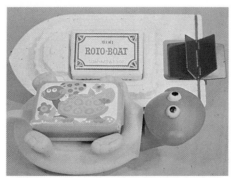

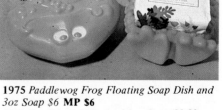

*1972 Soap Boat Floating Soap Dish &
Soap 3oz $3* **MP $10**

1973 Roto-Boat Soap Dish and Soap 3oz $3.75
MP $6
*1973 Topsy Turtle Floating Soap Dish and Soap
3oz $3.75* **MP $6**

*1975 Paddlewog Frog Floating Soap Dish and
3oz Soap $6* **MP $6**
1977 Terrible Tubbles and 3oz Soap $5.50
MP $5

(see also page 267)

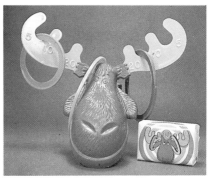

1972 *Loop-A-Moose with Soap 3oz $3.50* **MP $9**

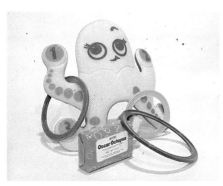

1980 *Oscar Octopus Ring Toss Game with 3 plastic rings and 3oz Soap $7* **MP $7**

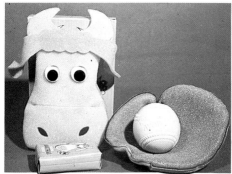

1965 *Minnie the Moo Sponge Puppet and Soap 3oz $1.75* **MP $17**
1966 *Little Pro Soap 'n' Sponge. Mitt Sponge and Soap 6oz $2.25* **MP $16**

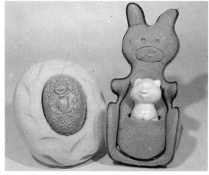

1967 *Nest Egg Soap 'n' Sponge 3oz $2.25* **MP $13**
1966 *Spongaroo. Kangaroo foam Sponge and Baby Ru Soap 3oz $2.25* **MP $16**

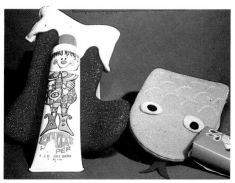

1967 *Santa's Helper Xmas stocking Sponge and tube of Gel Bubble Bath 6oz $2.50* **MP $15**
1968 *Clarence the Sea Serpent Puppet Sponge and 3oz Soap $2.25* **MP $12**

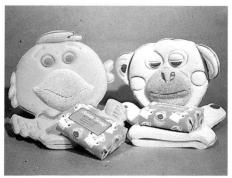

1969 *Parrot Puppet Sponge and Soap 3oz $3* **MP $10**
1969 *Monkey Shines Puppet Sponge and 3oz $3* **MP $10**

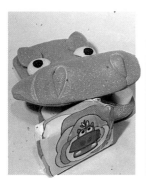

1970 *Hubie the Hippo Sponge and 3oz Soap $4* **MP $9**

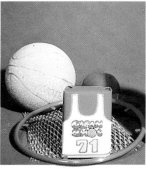

1971 *Clean Shot Basketball shaped Sponge and 3oz Soap $4.50* **MP $10**

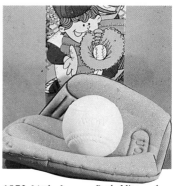

1973 *Little League Bath Mitt and Soap 3oz $3* **MP $11**

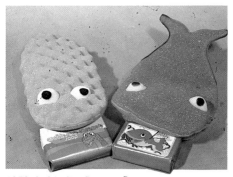

1973 *Cedric Sea Serpent Puppet Sponge and Soap 3oz $3* **MP $9**
1973 *Soapy the Whale Bath Mitt and Soap 3oz $3* **MP $9**

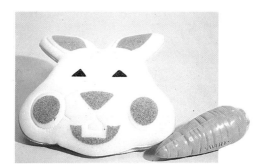

1974 *Good Habit Rabbit Bath Mitt and Soap 3oz $3.50* **MP $7**

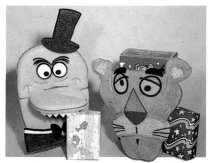

1978 *Misterjaw Bath Mitt and 3oz Soap $6.50* **MP $6.50**
1977 *Pink Panther Sponge and Soap 3oz $6* **MP $7**

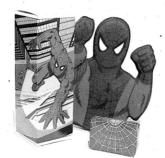

1980 *Spider-Man Sponge Mitt and 3oz Soap $6.50* **MP $6.50**

(see also pages 267 & 268)

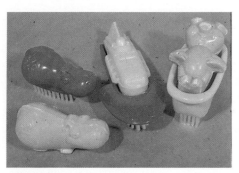

1972 *Happy Hippos Nail Brush and Soap 2oz $3* **MP $6**
1972 *Hydrojet Scrub Brush and Soap 2oz $2.50* **MP $6**
1973 *Pig-In-a-Tub Nail Brush and Soap 2oz $2.75* **MP $6**

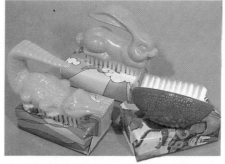

1974 *Gaylord Gator Scrub Brush and Soap 3oz $3.50* **MP $5**
1974 *Good Habit Rabbit Nail Brush and Soap 3oz $3.50* **MP $5**
1975 *Gridiron Scrub Brush and 3oz Soap $4* **MP $5**

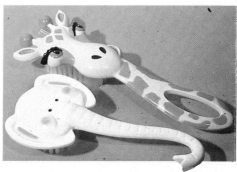

1976 *Giraffabath Bath Brush $6* **MP $6**
1974 *Scrubbo the Elephant Bath Brush $5* **MP $7**

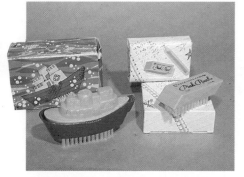

1971 *Scrub Tub Nail Brush and Soap 2oz $2.50* **MP $7**
1977 *Scrub Away Nail Brush and Soap 3oz $4* **MP $5**

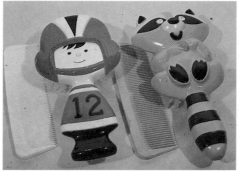

1972 *Grid Kid Comb and Brush $3.50* **MP $6**
1972 *Reggie Raccoon Brush and Comb $3.50* **MP $6**

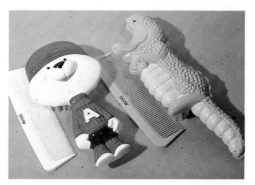

1974 *Arch E. Bear Brush and Comb $4* **MP $5**
1974 *Al E. Gator Brush and Comb $4* **MP $5**

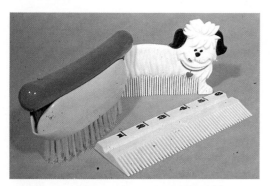

1975 *Hot Dog! Brush and Comb $5* **MP $5.50**
1976 *Shaggy Dog Comb $2.50* **MP $3**
1976 *School Days Ruler Comb $3* **MP $3.50**

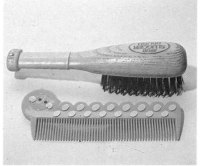

1974 *Slugger Hairbrush 7" long $4* **MP $5**
1975 *Curly Caterpillar Comb 6" long $2* **MP $3**

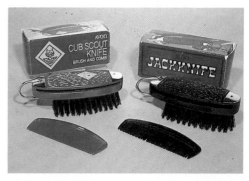

1977 *Cub Scout Knife Brush and Comb $6* **MP $6**
1973 *Jackknife Brush and Comb $4.50* **MP $6**

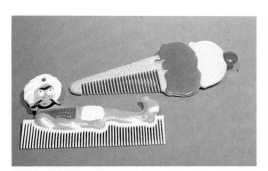

1977 *Ice Cream Comb $3* **MP $3**
1978 *Bed of Nails Comb $3.50* **MP $3**

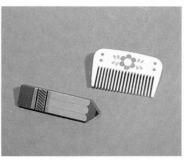

1973 *School Days Barrette $1.50* **MP $2**
1973 *Comb Barrette $2* **MP $2**

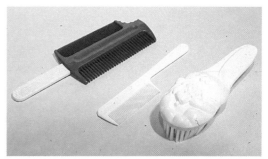

1979 *Combsicle Comb $3* **MP $3**
1981 *Good Habit Rabbit Brush and Comb. Both, 5½" long $6.50* **MP $6**

(see also pages 267 & 268)

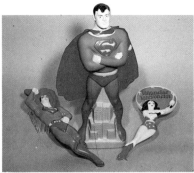
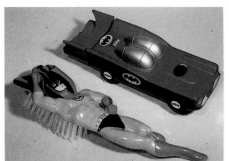
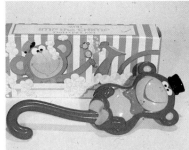
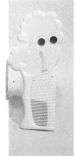

1976 *Superman Styling Brush 8½" long $6* **MP $6**
1978 *Superman Bubble Bath 6oz $8* **MP $7**
1978 *Wonder Woman Mirror 7½" $7.50* **MP $6**

1977 *Batman Styling Brush $6* **MP $6**
1978 *Batmobile Bubble Bath 6oz with decals $6.50* **MP $5.50**

1979 *Imp the Chimp Bath Brush $8.50* **MP $7**

1984 *Pocket Peepers Comb, Yellow, Green or Purple 6" long $5.50 ea.* **MP $4***

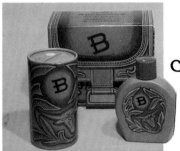

FOR YOUNG COWBOYS

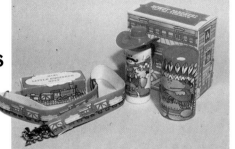

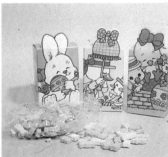

1981 *Buckaroo Gift Set for Boys. Buckaroo fragranced Cologne and Talc 2oz each $7* **MP $3**

1983 *Little Engineer Belt with metal train buckle 1" wide $7* **MP $7**
1983 *Howdy Pardners Set. Buckaroo fragranced Cologne and Talc 2oz each $6.50* **MP $2.50**

1984 *Easter Sweetkins. Lemon, Fruit Punch, Orange and Grape Candies in choice of three punch-out designed cartons 2oz each (2 Campaigns only) $1.69 each* **MP $1.69, carton only MP 50¢**

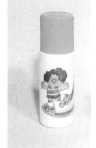

COLORING SOAPS for KIDS

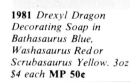
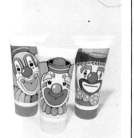
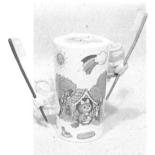

1984 *Roll-A-Soap in Green, Red or Blue $3 ea.* **MP $2***

1981 *Drexyl Dragon Decorating Soap in Bathasaurus Blue, Washasaurus Red or Scrubasaurus Yellow. 3oz $4 each* **MP 50¢**

1982 *Clowning Around Decorating Body Soap in Blue, Yellow or Red 1.5oz $2 each* **MP 50¢**

1982 *Tweethouse Paper Cup Toothbrush holder. Cup dispenser comes with two toothbrushes and vinyl decals 5¼" high $10* **MP $10 complete**

BEDROOM BUDDIES

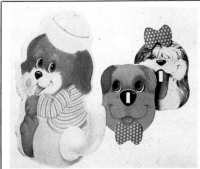
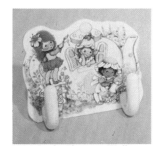
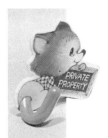
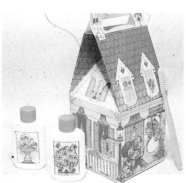

Playful Pups —
1981 *Wall Hook 3x5" with adhesive backing $4* **MP $4**
1981 *Light Switch Cover with Fragranced Bow 3½x5½", plastic loveable puppy or sheepdog design $5.50* **MP $4.50***

1984 *Little Blossom Wall Hook 5" wide with adhesive backing $7* **MP $7**

1982 *Felix Fox Wall Hook 4"x4½" with adhesive backing $5* **MP $5**

1982 *Going to Grandma's House. Cardboard house 8" high holds toothbrush, 1.25oz Bubble Bath and 1.25oz Buckaroo Cologne for boys or Little Blossom Cologne for girls $6.50* **MP $4 complete**

**Available from Avon at time of publication*

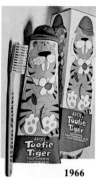

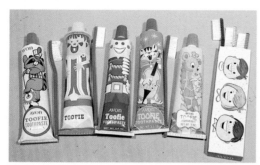

TOOFIE

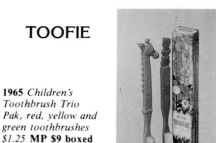

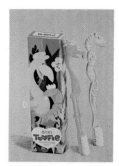

1965 *Children's Toothbrush Trio Pak, red, yellow and green toothbrushes* $1.25 **MP $9 boxed**

1966
Toofie Tiger Twosome Toothpaste 3.5oz and Brush $1.35 **MP $15**

Toothpaste/Toothbrush Sets *3½oz —*
1967 *Toofie (Raccoon design) magenta toothbrush* $1.25 **MP $12**
1964 *Toofie Twosome (Clown design) red, blue or green toothbrush* $1.25 **MP $16**
1968 *Toofie on Guard, green toothbrush* $1.25 **MP $11**
1969 *Toofie (Hi Diddle Diddle design) red toothbrush* $1.35 **MP $10**
1970 *Toofie Toothpaste (Giraffe and Bunny design) 3.5oz* 89¢ **MP $8**

1970 *Toofie Toothbrush Duo, Bunny and Giraffe* $1.75 **MP $4 boxed**

1972 *Toofie Toothbrush Duo, Bird and Worm* $2 **MP $5 boxed**

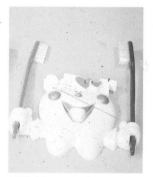

1973 *I Love Toofie Toothbrush Holder and 2 Brushes* $2.75 **MP $6**

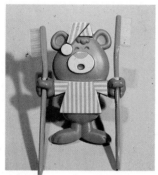

1974 *Ted. E. Bear Toothbrush Holder and 2 Brushes* $2.75 **MP $6**

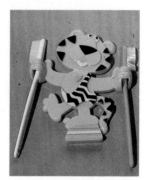

1976 *Toofie Tiger Toothbrush Holder and 2 Brushes* $3.50 **MP $5**

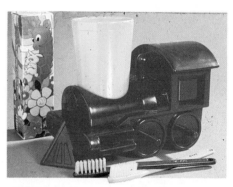

1974 *Toofie Train. Tube of Toofie Toothpaste, 2 Toothbrushes and a plastic Cup* $6 **MP $8**

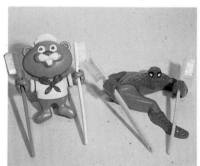

1973 *Barney Beaver Toothbrush Holder and 2 Brushes* $2.75 **MP $6**
1979 *Spider-Man Toothbrush Holder and 2 Brushes* $6 **MP $6**

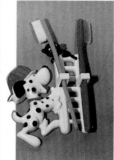

1976 *Spotty to the Rescue Toothbrush Holder and 2 Brushes* $3.75 **MP $5**

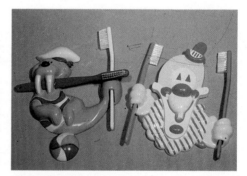

1977 *Wally Walrus Toothbrush Holder and 2 Brushes* $4 **MP $5**
1978 *Toofie the Clown Toothbrush Holder and 2 Brushes* $4.50 **MP $5**

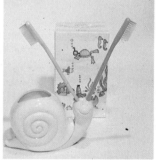

1980 *Smiley Snail Toothbrush Holder and 2 Brushes* $7.50 **MP $6**

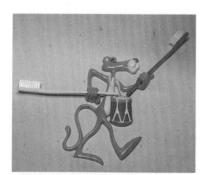

1979 *Pink Panther Toothbrush Holder and 2 Toothbrushes 6" high with adhesive backing* $6 **MP $6**

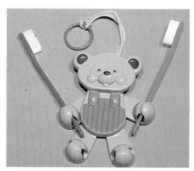

1980 *Tuggable Teddy moveable Toothbrush Holder and 2 Brushes* $6.50 **MP $6**

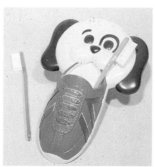

1981 *Playful Pups Toothbrush Holder and 2 Toothbrushes 4"x6" with adhesive backing* $8 **MP $6**

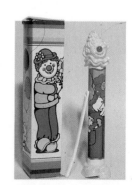

1983 *Toofy the Tooth Clown with toothbrush 8¼" high* $6.50 **MP $5**

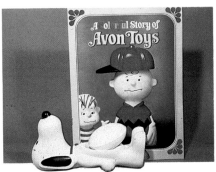

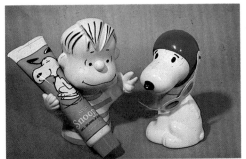

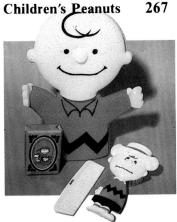

1968 *Snoopy Soap Dish and Soap 3oz*
$3 **MP $7**
1968 *A Colorful Story of Charlie Brown.*
Coloring Books sold to Representatives
only **MP $3**

1968 *Linus Bubble Bath Holder with Gel*
Bubble Bath, tube 4oz $3.50 **MP $8**
1969 *Snoopy the Flying Ace Bubble Bath*
4oz $3 **MP $6 with goggles**

1969 *Charlie Brown Bath Mitt &*
Soap 3oz $3 **MP $8**
1971 *Charlie Brown Brush & Comb*
$3.50 **MP $7**

PEANUTS

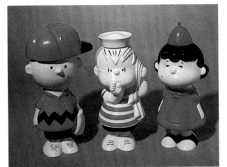

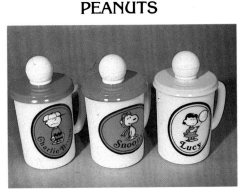

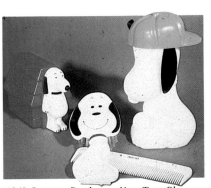

1968 *Charlie Brown Non-Tear Shampoo*
4oz $2.50 **MP $6**
1970 *Linus Non-Tear Shampoo 4oz $3*
MP $6
1969 *Lucy Bubble Bath 4oz $2.50* **MP $6**

1969 *Charlie Brown Mug Bubble Bath 5oz $3.50*
MP $11 with lid
1969 *Snoopy Mug Liquid Soap 5oz $3.50*
MP $11 with lid
1969 *Lucy Mug Non-Tear Shampoo 5oz $3.50*
MP $11 with lid

1969 *Snoopy Doghouse Non-Tear Shampoo*
8oz $3 **MP $7**
1970 *Snoopy Brush and Comb $3.50* **MP $7**
1969 *Snoopy Surprise Package. Excalibur or*
Wild Country After Shave or Sports Rally
Lotion (glass) 5oz $4 **MP $7**

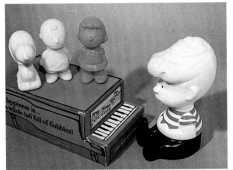

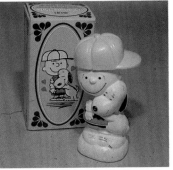

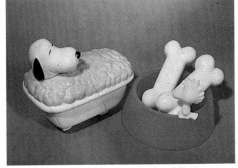

1970 *Peanuts Gang Soaps, three 1¾oz cakes*
$2 **MP $12**
1970 *Schroeder Bubble Bath 6oz $3.50*
MP $8, $11 with piano box

1971 *Peanuts Pals. Charlie Brown &*
Snoopy Non-Tear Shampoo 6oz
$3.50 **MP $7**

1971 *Snoopy's Bubble Bath Tub $4* **MP $6**
1973 *Snoopy's Pal Soap Dish and 2 Soaps 2oz*
each $3.75 **MP $9**

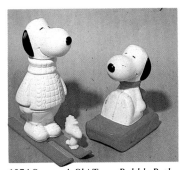

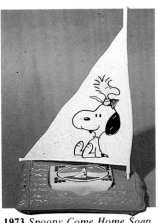

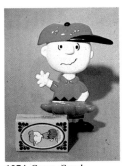

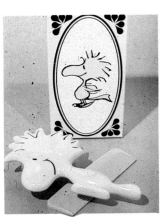

1974 *Snoopy's Ski Team Bubble Bath*
8oz $6 **MP $6**
1972 *Snoopy Snow Flyer Bubble*
Bath 10oz $5 **MP $6**

1973 *Snoopy Come Home Soap*
Dish and Soap 3oz $4.50 **MP $9**

1974 *Great Catch.*
Charlie Brown Soap
Holder and Soap 3oz
$5 **MP $8**

©*PEANUTS Characters:*
1950, 1951, 1952, 1958, 1965
United Features Syndicate, Inc.

1975 *Woodstock Brush and*
Comb $6 **MP $6**

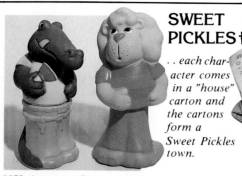

SWEET PICKLES†

. . each character comes in a "house" carton and the cartons form a Sweet Pickles town.

1978 *Accusing Alligator Bubble Bath 6oz $8* **MP $8**
1978 *Loving Lion Non-Tear Shampoo 6oz $8* **MP $8**

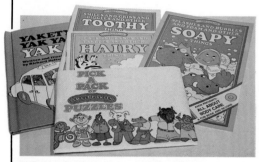

1978 *Fun Books and Records. Each "All About. book 11x7" with a built-in sing-along record $2.50 each* **MP $3.50**
Yakety Yak Yak hard cover book **MP $4**
1978 *Pick a Pack Puzzles. Three Sweet Pickles puzzles 25¢ with any Sweet Pickles purchase during C-20-78 only* **MP $2 in sealed package** *(front)*

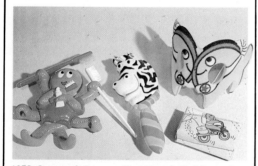

1978 *Outraged Octopus Toothbrush Holder and 2 Brushes, red and white $5.50* **MP $6**
1978 *Zany Zebra Hair Brush 7½" $6.50* **MP $6**
1979 *Fearless Fish Sponge Mask and Soap 3oz $6.50* **MP $7**

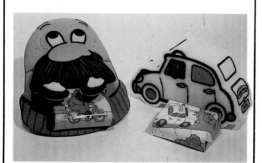

1979 *Worried Walrus Sponge Mitt and Soap 3oz $6.50* **MP $6.50**
1978 *Yakety Yak Taxi Sponge and Soap 3oz $6.50* **MP $6.50**

†*Characters © Perle/Reinach/Hefter 1979*

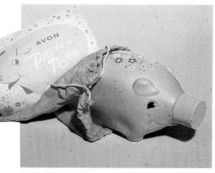

1960 *Pig in a Poke Bubble Bath 8oz $1.79* **MP $20**

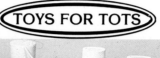

TOYS FOR TOTS

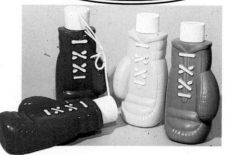

1960 *A Winner Set. Hair Guard and Hand Guard 4oz each $1.98* **MP $25**
1967 *Little Champion Set. (blue glove) Non-tear Shampoo, (yellow glove) Hair Trainer 4oz each $2* **MP $17**

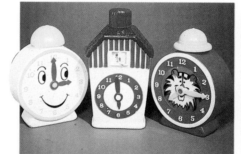

1961 *Li'l Folks Time Bubble Bath 8oz $1.79* **MP $16**
1965 *Cuckoo Clock Bubble Bath 10oz $2.50* **MP $14**
1967 *Tic Toc Tiger Bubble Bath 8oz $1.75* **MP $11** *(Moveable hands on all clocks)*

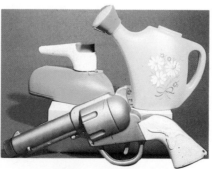

1962 *Little Helper plastic iron Bubble Bath 8oz $1.98* **MP $16**
1962 *Watering Can, plastic Bubble Bath 8oz $1.98* **MP $16**
1962 *Six Shooter, plastic No-tears Shampoo 6oz $1.98* **MP $21**

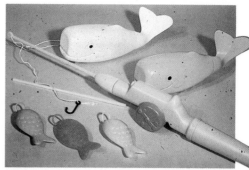

1959 *Whitey the Whale Bubble Bath 8oz $1.69* **MP $18**
1967 *Smiley the Whale Bubble Bath 9oz $1.98* **MP $9**
1968 *Tub Catch Fishing Rod and 3 plastic fish. Rod holds Bubble Bath 6oz $3.50* **MP $14 complete**

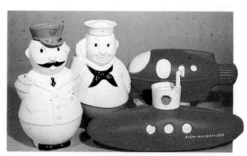

1963 *Captain Bubble Bath 8oz $1.79* **MP $15**
1963 *First Mate's Shampoo 8oz $1.98* **MP $15**
1964 *Aqua Car Bubble Bath 8oz $1.98* **MP $18**
1961 *Naughty-Less plastic sub with Bubble Bath 8oz $1.79* **MP $22**

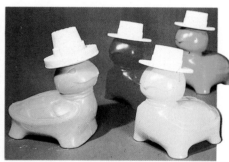

1962 *L'il Tom Turtle. Green molded Soap 98¢* **MP $25**. *Yellow Shampoo, blue Baby Oil, red Baby Lotion 3oz each $1.10* **MP $16 each**

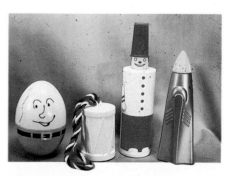

1963 *Humpty Dumpty Bubble Bath 8oz $1.98* **MP $15**
1969 *Yankee Doodle Soap 6oz $2* **MP $11**
1960 *Clean As a Whistle Bubble Bath 8oz $1.79* **MP $20**
1968 *Space Ace Hair Trainer 4oz $1.50* **MP $11**

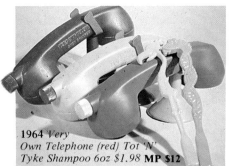

1964 *Very Own Telephone (red) Tot 'N' Tyke Shampoo 6oz $1.98* **MP $12**
1967 *Tub Talk (yellow) Non-tear Shampoo 6oz $1.75* **MP $10**
1969 *Tub Talk (blue) Non-tear Shampoo $2.25* **MP $8**
1972 *Toofie Toothbrush Duo, Bird & Worm $2* **MP $5**

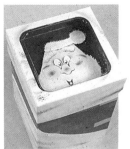

1964 *Santa's Chimney. Powdered Bubble Bath 5oz. Top of box is game $1.98* **MP $20**

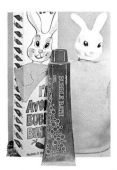

1964 *Bubble Bunny Gel Bubble Bath 6oz $1.98* **MP $22 complete**

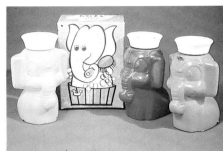

1964 *Packy Elephant. Blue Baby Oil, yellow Baby Shampoo, red Baby Lotion 3oz each $1.10* **MP $17 each**
(See Soap pg. 260)

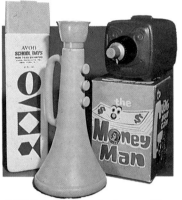

1966 *School Days plastic pencil box. Non-tear Shampoo 8oz $1.98* **MP $10**
1965 *Avon Bugle Non-tear Shampoo 6oz $1.98* **MP $14**
1965 *Safe Sam Bubble Bath 8oz $1.98* **MP $15**

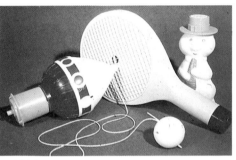

1966 *Spinning Top Bubble Bath 4oz $1.75* **MP $11**
1966 *Paddle Ball Set. Shampoo 6oz $1.98* **MP $15**
1967 *Good Habit Rabbit Tot 'N' Tyke Shampoo 3oz $1.50* **MP $10**

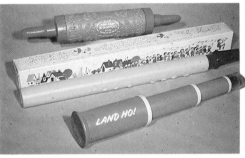

1966 *Little Missy Rolling Pin Shampoo 8oz $2.25* **MP $12**
1965 *Avon Fife Hand Lotion or Hair Trainer 6oz $1.75* **MP $14**
1961 *Land Ho! plastic telescope with Hair Trainer 8oz $1.49* **MP $22**

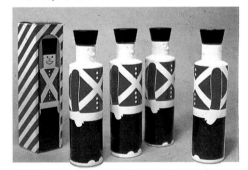

1964 *Toy Soldiers: Hair Trainer, Shampoo, Hand Lotion and Bubble Bath each 4oz $1.25 each* **MP $13 each**

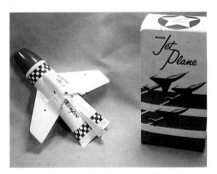

1965 *Jet Plane Gel Bubble Bath, Gel Shampoo or Hair Trainer 3oz each $1.50* **MP $17**

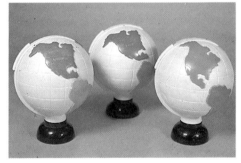

1966 *Globe Bank Bubble Bath, plastic 10oz $2.50 each* **MP $18 complete**
(3 different colors of snap-on countries)

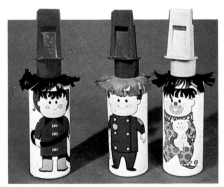

1966 *Whistle Tots: Fireman Tot 'n' Tyke Shampoo, Policeman Hair Trainer, Clown Bubble Bath 4oz each $1.50* **MP $11 each**

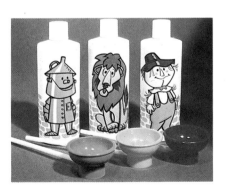

1967 *Tin Man blue Pipe and Non-tear Shampoo 4oz $1.50* **MP $10**
1967 *Mr. Lion red bubble Pipe and Bubble Bath 4oz $1.50* **MP $10**
1967 *Straw Man yellow bubble Pipe and Hand Lotion 4oz $1.50* **MP $10**

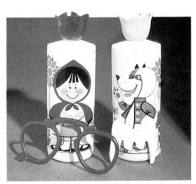

1968 *Little Red Riding Hood Bubble Bath 4oz and "Granny" Glasses $1.50* **MP $10**
1968 *The Wolf Non-tear Shampoo 4oz and "Funny Fangs" $1.50* **MP $10**

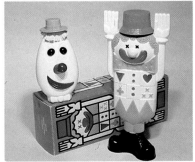

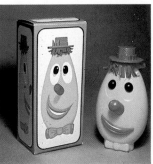

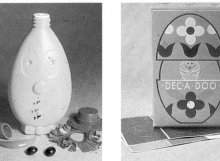

1965 *Mr. Many Moods with moveable eyes, nose and mouth. Non-tear Shampoo 6oz $1.98* **MP $16**
1965 *Topsy Turvy Clown Bubble Bath 10oz $2.50* **MP $20**

1968 *Mr. Presto-Chango Non-tear Shampoo 6oz $2.25* **MP $12 complete**

1968 *Easter Dec-A-Doo Bubble Bath 8oz $2.50* **MP $7 with decals**

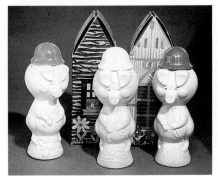

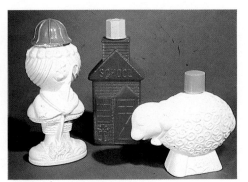

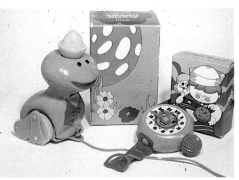

1967 *Little Piggy (yellow) Baby Shampoo 3oz $1.35* **MP $10**
1967 *Little Piggy (blue) Bubble Bath 3oz $1.35* **MP $10**
1967 *Little Piggy (pink) Baby Lotion 3oz $1.35* **MP $10**

1968 *Mary Non-tear Shampoo 3oz $1.35* **MP $10**
1968 *Schoolhouse Bubble Bath 3oz $1.35* **MP $10**
1968 *Little Lamb Baby Lotion 3oz $1.35* **MP $10**

1969 *Jumpin' Jimminy Bubble Bath 8oz $3.50* **MP $7**
1969 *Wrist Wash Bubble Bath 2oz $3* **MP $8**

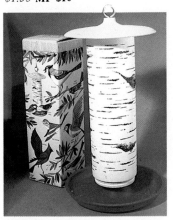

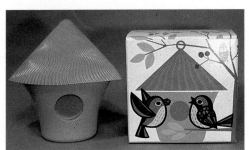

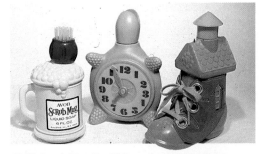

1967 *Birdfeeder Powdered Bubble Bath 7½oz $3.50* **MP $12**

1969 *Birdhouse Powdered Bubble Bath 8oz $3.75* **MP $11**

1968 *Scrub Mug liquid Soap 6oz $2.50* **MP $6**
1968 *Tic Toc Turtle Bubble Bath 8oz $2.50* **MP $7**
1968 *One, Two. . . Lace My Shoe Bubble Bath 8oz $2.98* **MP $9**

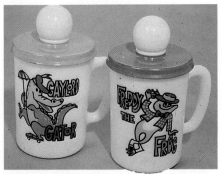

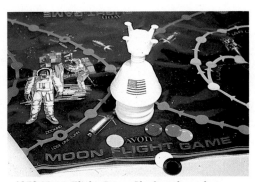

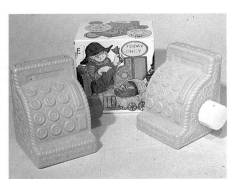

1970 *Gaylord Gator Mug Non-tear Shampoo 5oz $3.50* **MP $9**
1970 *Freddy the Frog Mug Bubble Bath 5oz $3.50* **MP $9**

1970 *Moon Flight Game. Playboard, markers, Lem, Space Capsule Non-tear Shampoo 6oz $4* **MP $12 complete.**

1970 *Ring 'Em Up Clean Non-tear Shampoo 8oz $2.50* **MP $6**
1970 *As above (with white lid) $2.50* **MP $9**

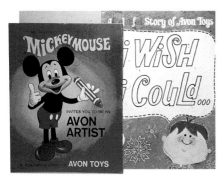
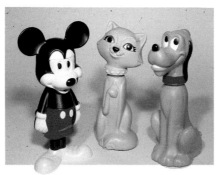
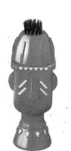
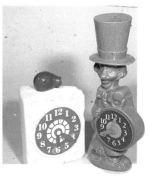

1969 *Mickey Mouse© Coloring Book of Avon Toys* **MP $4**
1967 *A Colorful Story of Avon Toys. Coloring Book not for sale, except to Representatives* **MP $5**

1969 *Mickey Mouse© Bubble Bath 4¹/₂oz $3.50* **MP $9**
1971 *Aristocat Non-Tear Shampoo 4oz $3* **MP $7**
1970 *Pluto© Non-tear Shampoo 4oz $4* **MP $8**

1969 *Chief Scrubbem Liquid Soap 4oz $2.50* **MP $8**

1971 *Hickory Dickory Clock Non-Tear Shampoo 8oz* **MP $8**
1970 *Mad Hatter Bubble Bath 6oz $3* **MP $10**

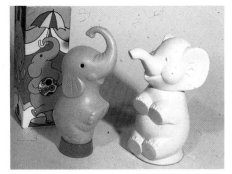
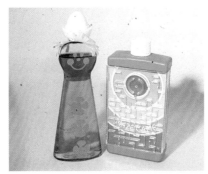
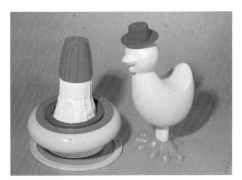

1970 *Bo-Bo the Elephant Non-Tear Shampoo 5oz $2.50* **MP $7**
1973 *Bo-Bo the Elephant Baby Shampoo 6oz $4* **MP $5.50**

1970 *Topsy Turvy Bubble Bath 4oz $2* **MP $7**
1971 *Maze Game Non-Tear Shampoo 6oz $2.50* **MP $9**

1970 *Splash Down Bubble Bath 8oz $4* **MP $7 complete**
1971 *Cluck-A-Doo Bubble Bath 8oz $3* **MP $7**

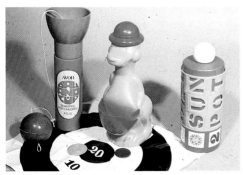
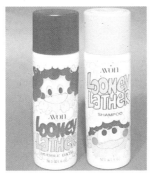
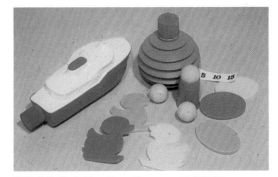

1972 *Ball and Cup Shampoo for Children 4oz $3.50* **MP $10**
1971 *Kanga Winks. Tiddley-Wink Game and Bubble Bath 8oz $4* **MP $9**
1972 *Turn-A-Word Bubble Bath 8oz $3.50* **MP $6**

1971 *Looney Lather Bubble Bath 6oz $2* **MP $8**
1971 *Looney Lather Shampoo 6oz $2* **MP $8**

1970 *S.S. Suds Non-Tear Shampoo $3* **MP $7**
1971 *Pop-A-Duck Bubble Bath Game 6oz $3.50* **MP $9**

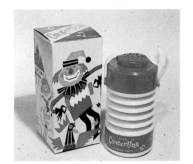
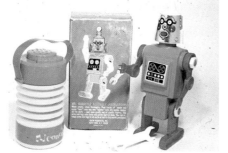
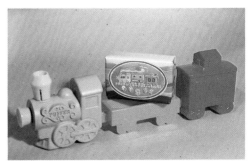

1962 *Concertina Bubble Bath 8oz $1.98* **MP $17**

1970 *Concertina Bubble Bath 8oz $2.50* **MP $9**
1971 *Mr. Robottle Bubble Bath 5oz $3.50* **MP $7**

1971 *Puffer Chugger Bubble Bath 4oz, Soap Coach 3oz and Caboose Non-Tear Shampoo 4oz each $2.25* **MP $6 each**

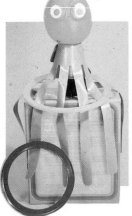

1973 *Little Wiggley Game Bubble Bath 8oz $4.50* **MP $7**

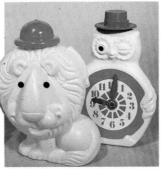

1974 *Loveable Leo Children's Shampoo 10oz $4* **MP $4**
1975 *Winkie Blink Clock Bubble Bath 8oz $5* **MP $5.50**

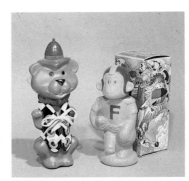

1971 *Huggy Bear Bubble Bath 8oz $3.50* **MP $7**
1979 *Most Valuable Gorilla Bubble Bath 4oz $7.50* **MP $5**

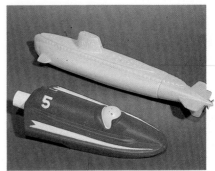

1972 *Red Streak Bubble Bath 5oz $2.50* **MP $8**
1978 *Tub Sub Bubble Bath for Children 6oz $6* **MP $4**

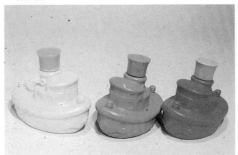

1980 *Tub Tug Non-Tear Shampoo (Yellow), Liquid Cleanser (Blue), Bubble Bath (Red) 5oz each $5* **MP $4 each**

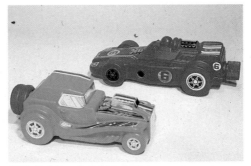

1979 *Red Streak Bubble Bath 7oz and Decals $5.50* **MP $4**
1976 *Custom Car Bubble Bath 7oz and Decals $5* **MP $5**

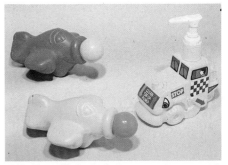

1982 *Clean Flight Bath Decanter. Orange, with Children's Liquid Cleanser or Yellow with Non-Tear Shampoo 6oz $5.50* **MP $3**
1981 *Clean-'Em-Up-Pump with Children's Liquid Cleanser and set of decals 8oz $8.50* **MP $5**

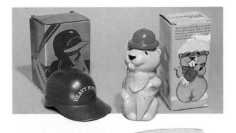

1978 *Heavy Hitter Non-Tear Shampoo 4oz $7* **MP $4**
1979 *Willie Weatherman Non-Tear Shampoo 6oz $7.50* **MP $4**
1961 *Avonville Slugger (bat) Non-Tear Shampoo 6oz $1.49* **MP $18**

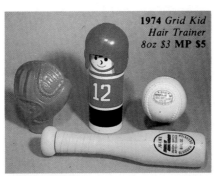

1974 *Grid Kid Hair Trainer 8oz $3* **MP $5**
1974 *Sure Winner Catcher's Mitt Hair Trainer 6oz $3* **MP $5**
1973 *Sure Winner Slugger Decanter. Hair Trainer, Bracing Lotion or Spicy After Shave 6oz $3* **MP $7**
1973 *Sure Winner Baseball Hair Trainer 4oz $2.50* **MP $6**

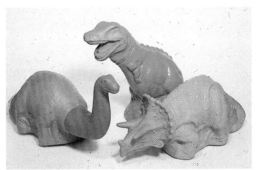

1975 *Brontosaurus Bubble Bath 10oz $5* **MP $5**
1976 *Tyrannosaurus Rex Bubble Bath 9oz $5.50* **MP $5**
1977 *Triceratops Bubble Bath 8.5oz $5.50* **MP $5**

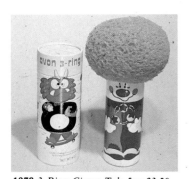

1978 *3-Ring Circus Talc 5oz $3.50* **MP $1**
1981 *Spongie The Clown Liquid Cleanser 6oz $6* **MP $4**

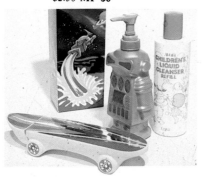

1978 *Hang Ten Skateboard Bubble Bath 5½oz $6.50* **MP $5**
1980 *I.M. Clean II Pump Dispenser Liquid Cleanser 8oz and decals $8* **MP $8**
1980 *Children's Liquid Cleanser Refill 8oz $4* **MP $1**

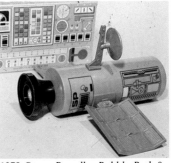

1979 *Space Patroller Bubble Bath 8oz and decals $7* **MP $5**

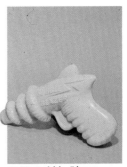

1982 *Bubble Blazer Space Gun Soap 4oz $5* **MP $5**

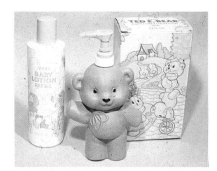

1981 *Baby Lotion Dispenser Refill 9.5oz $4* **MP $1**
1981 *Ted E. Bear Baby Lotion Dispenser in pink or blue 10oz $8.50* **MP $7**

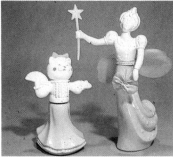

1976 *Felina Fluffles Pink & Pretty Cologne 2oz $6* **MP $6**
1978 *Good Fairy Cologne in Delicate Daisies 3oz $8* **MP $6**

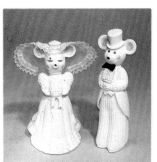

1977 *Church Mouse Bride. Delicate Daisies Cologne 2oz $6* **MP $6**
1979 *Church Mouse Groom. Delicate Daisies Cologne .75oz $7* **MP $6**

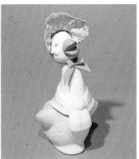

1979 *Mrs. Quackles with fabric bonnet, Delicate Daisies Cologne 2oz $8* **MP $7**

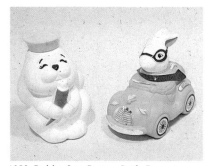

1982 *Bubba Lee Bunny Bath Decanter with Non-Tear Shampoo or Children's Bubble Bath 6oz $7.50* **MP $5.99***
1983 *The Wabbit with Non-Tear Shampoo or Children's Bubble Bath 5oz $7.50* **MP $4**

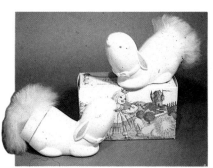

1969 *Bunny Puff. Her Prettiness Perfumed Talc 3½oz $3.75* **MP $8**
1979 *Bunny Fluff Puff with children's Talc 3½oz $8* **MP $6**

...FOR CHILDREN and TEENS

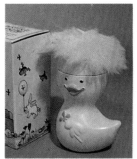

1978 *Duster D. Duckling Fluff Puff. Delicate Daisies Talc 3½oz $6.50* **MP $4**

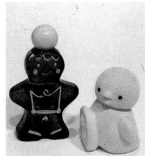

1979 *Cute Cookie. Hello Sunshine Cologne 1oz $5.50* **MP $4**
1980 *Fluffy Chick. Hello Sunshine Cologne 1oz $7* **MP $3**

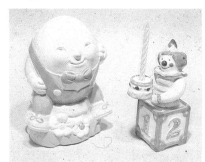

1982 *Humpty Dumpty Keepsake Bank. Earthenware, dated "1982" 5" high $14* **MP $12**
1983 *Year-to-Year Birthday Candle with candle $13.50* **MP $11**

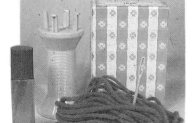

1972 *Spool-A-Doo Rollette .33oz $3* **MP $7 complete**

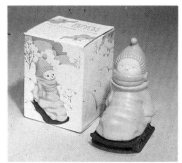

1980 *Bundle of Fun in Hello Sunshine Cologne or Sure Winner Lotion .75oz $6.50* **MP $4**

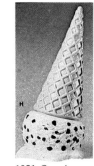

1981 *Oops! Cologne in Country Breeze or Sweet Honesty 1.5oz $7.50* **MP $4**

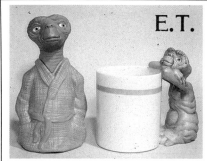

E.T.

1983 *E.T. Bath Decanter Children's Bubble Bath 7oz $11* **MP $9**
1983 *E.T. Everything Caddy. Porcelain figurine and holder 4½" high $25* **MP $25**

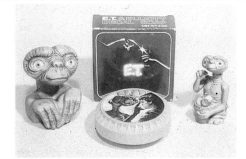

1983 *E.T. Porcelain Pot Pal $12.50* **MP $12.50**
1983 *E.T. and Elliott Decal Soap, Fresh Fun fragrance 3" diam $4* **MP $4**
1984 *E.T. "Flowers" Porcelain Figurine 2½" high $12.50* **MP $10***

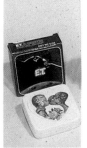

1984 *E.T. and Gertie Decal Soap, Strawberry fragrance 3oz $5.50* **MP $4***

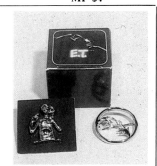

1983 *E.T. Tac Pin 1" high $12* **MP $12**
1983 *E.T. Touch of Love Pin 1" diam. $12* **MP $10***

Available from Avon at time of publication

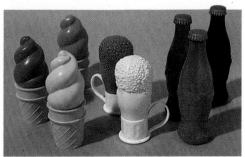
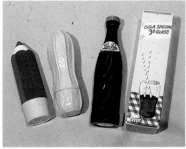
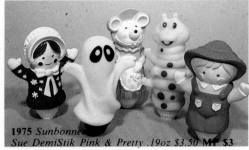

Flavored Lip Pomades —
1974 *Ice Cream Cone in Cherry, Strawberry, Tutti-Frutti $2.50* **MP $3**
1974 *Ice Cream Soda in Cherry, Strawberry, Tutti-Frutti $3* **MP $3**
1973 *Lip Pops in Cola, Cherry or Strawberry $1.75* **MP $3** *Solid red issue in Strawberry* **MP $7**

1975 *School Days Lip Pomade in Cherry, Strawberry or Tutti-Frutti Pomade .13oz $3.50* **MP $3**
1974 *In a Nutshell Color Magic Lipstick 2 shades .13oz $3* **MP $3**
1978 *Lip-Pop Pomade Cola-colored and flavored lip balm .13oz $3.75* **MP $3**

1975 *Sunbonnet Sue DemiStik Pink & Pretty .19oz $3.50* **MP $3**
1976 *Gilroy the Ghost Finger Puppet. Care Deeply Lip Balm .19oz $3.50* **MP $3**
1977 *Millicent Mouse Finger Puppet DemiStik. Pink & Pretty .19oz $3.75* **MP $3**
1977 *Glow Worm Finger Puppet. Care Deeply Lip Balm .19oz $3.50* **MP $2**
1977 *Huck L. Berry Finger Puppet Lip Balm .20oz $3.75* **MP $2**

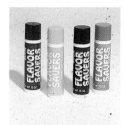
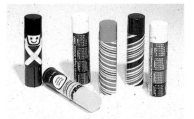
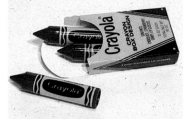
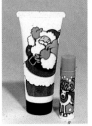
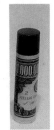

1979 *Flavor Savers, flavored Lip Gloss in Grape, Cherry, Chocolate, Strawberry, Lime and Orange .15oz $2* **MP $1** *ea.*

Care Deeply Lip Balm *.15oz each —*
1979 *Toy Soldier $1.29* **MP $1**
1979 *Wilson Championship $1.29* **MP $1**
1979 *Smooth Days Ahead $1.29* **MP $1**
1980 *Candy Cane, Wintergreen or Peppermint (red) $1.49* **MP 50¢**
1980 *Smooth Days Ahead $1.49* **MP 50¢**

1980 *Crayola Lip Glosses in Grape, Strawberry and Chocolate, each .15oz $6.50* **MP $5**

1980 *Santa's Helpers Care Deeply Hand Cream 1.5oz and Lip Balm $2.79* **MP $1.50**

1981 *Cool Million Lip Balm .15oz $2* **MP 50¢**

LIP POMADES, GLOSSES and CREAMS

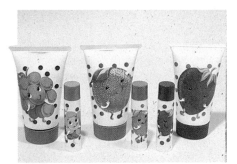
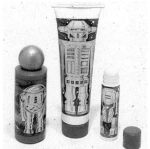
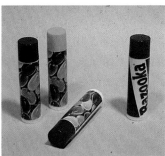
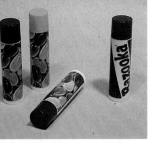
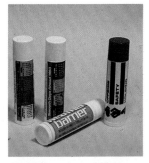

1981 *Fruit-For-All Sets. Lip Balm .15oz and Hand Cream 1.5oz in Grape, Orange and Strawberry fragrance $3.50 each set* **MP $2 ea.**

1981 *Avon-In-Space 1oz Non-Tear Shampoo, 1oz Liquid Cleanser and .15oz Lip Balm $2 each* **MP 50¢ each**

1982 *Jelly Bean Lip Balm in Cherry, Grape and lime, each .15oz (2 Campaigns only) $2 each* **MP $1**

1982 *Bazooka Lip Balm .15oz $2* **MP 50¢**

Lip Balms *.15oz ea* **MP 50¢ ea.**
1981 *Smooth Days Ahead $1.49*
1982 *Smooth Days Ahead $1.50*
1982 *Referee $2*
1982 *Weather Barrier $1.29*

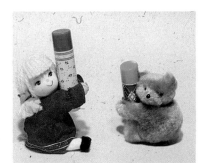
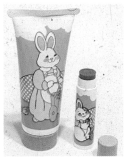

1982 *Little Rag Doll and DemiStik in Sweet Honesty .15oz $7.50* **MP $5**
1981 *Bearing Gifts. Miniature stuffed bear and Lip Balm .15oz $7* **MP $5**

1983 *Strawberry Hand Cream 1.5oz and Strawberry Lip Balm .15oz $3.50 set* **MP $1 set**

1982 *Halloween Make-A-Face Kit. White Base 2.25oz and Make-up Sticks in black, rust and blue .15oz each $7.50 set* **MP $3.50 set in carton**

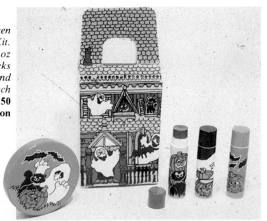

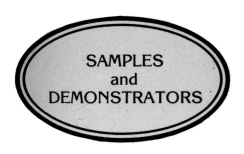

AVON

. . . *Demonstration and sample products are usually offered during the introduction of a particular product. Representatives have found that use of these demonstration and sample products help increase sales. Because demonstrators eventually become outdated, and samples are quickly distributed to customers, these items are extremely scarce. Many issues have become prized and valuable collector items.*

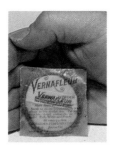

1923 *Vernafluer Adherent Face Powder Sample* **MP $50**

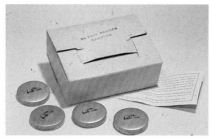

1930 *Purse size Face Powder Samples. Box of 30* **MP $130**

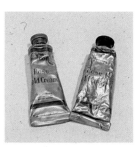

1931 *Rose Cold Cream samples* **MP $12 each**

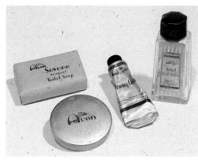

1928-36 Samples —
Savona Bouquet Toilet Soap **MP $20**
Ariel Face Powder **MP $4**
Cleansing Cream Tube **MP $12**
Ariel Bath Salts **MP $60**

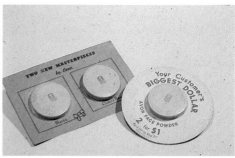

1937 *Face Powder Demo. introducing 2 new shades* **MP $25**
1937 *Your Customers Biggest Dollar Demo.* **MP $25**

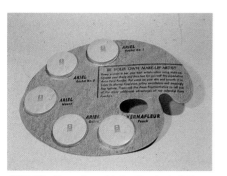

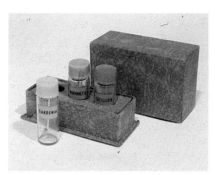

1937 *"Be Your Own Make-Up Artist" Face Powder Palette* **MP $45**

1938 *Fragrance Demonstrator. Cotillion, Marionette, Gardenia* **MP $100**

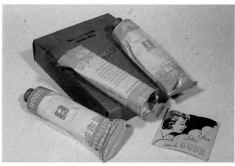

1937-41 *Cleansing Cream Demonstrator. Three 2½oz tubes for normal, oily and dry skin* **MP $60 with folder**

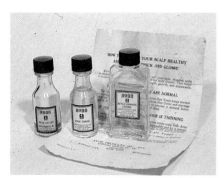

1940 *Hair Lotion* **MP $50**
1939 *Hair Tonic* **MP $50**
1942 *After Shave Lotion* **MP $36**

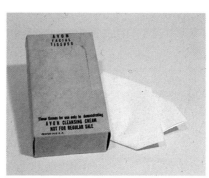

1940 *Avon Facial Tissues* **MP $15**

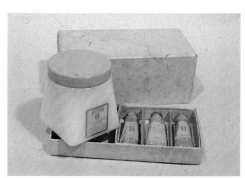

1942 *Cleansing Cream Demonstrator* **MP $50**

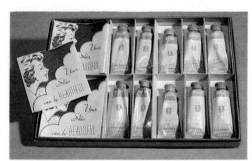

1937 *Cleansing Cream Sampler Box for new Representatives. Ten ¼oz tubes and "Your Skin Can Be Beautiful" folders* **MP $60 complete**

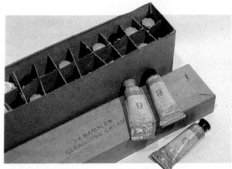

1937-41 *Cleansing Cream Samples, box of 24, ¼oz 50¢* **MP $95 complete, $3 each**

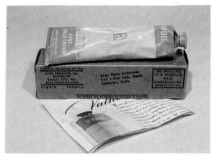

1937 *Rose Cold Cream Demonstrator. Tube reads "Not for Sale"* **MP $35 boxed**

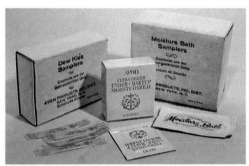

1960 *Dew Kiss Samplers, box of 45* **MP $40, 75¢ each**
1969 *Ultra Sheer Under-Makeup Moisturizer, box of 10* **MP $3, 25¢ each**
1961 *Moisture Bath, box of 40* **MP $40, 75¢ each**

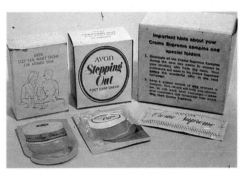

1966 *Stay Fair Night Cream, box of 10, 20¢* **MP $12, $1 each**
1969 *Stepping Out Foot Cream, box of 10, 25¢* **MP $3, 25¢ each**
1961 *Creme Supreme, box of 30* **MP $25, 75¢ each**

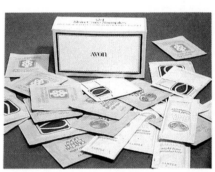

1976 *Skin Care Samples, box of 24 given only to those attending C-11 Sales Meetings. 8 each of Perfect Balance, Delicate Beauty & Moisture Secret* **MP $5 complete**

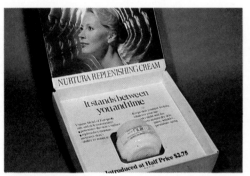

1979 *Nurtura Replenishing Cream Demo* **MP $6 jar, $7 as shown**

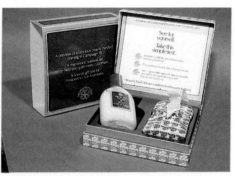

1980 *Beauty Fluid 3oz and package of Tissue, gift to President's Club Members* **MP $4*** **Beauty Fluid, $7 complete**

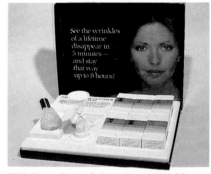

1980 *Time Control Temporary Wrinkle Smoother Kit holds 7 bottles Time Control .75oz each and a 5-minute timer. Only to Representatives pre-ordering 6 bottles Time Control at C-14 Sales Meeting* **MP $4**

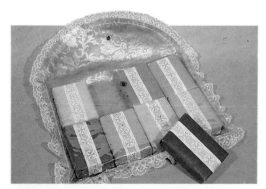

1961 *Perfumed Soap Demonstrator 8½ x 11", plastic, holds eight 3oz cakes soap in new wrap. Somewhere, Here's My Heart, Rose Geranium, Lemonol, Topaze, To A Wild Rose, Cotillion and Royal Jasmine* **MP $80 complete, $5 each soap**

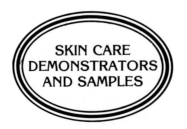

SKIN CARE
DEMONSTRATORS
AND SAMPLES

Little sample treats that make a lasting impression on both Avon customers and Avon collectors . . .

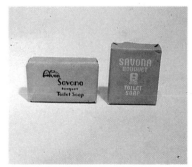

1931 *Savona Bouquet Toilet Soap sample* **MP $20**
1937 *Savona Bouquet Toilet Soap sample* **MP $15**

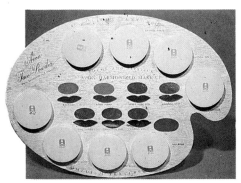

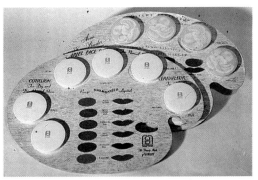

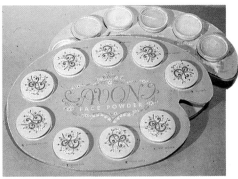

1941 *Palette, 8 Face Powder shades 20¢*
MP $40

1942 *Palette (top) 8 shades, metal 20¢* **MP $42**
1940 *Palette, 6 shades in Cotillion, Ariel &*
Vernafleur frag. 20¢ **MP $45**

1946 *Palette (top) 9 shades have Heavenlight*
printed on lid 20¢ **MP $35**
1943 *Palette, 8 shades in cardboard*
containers 20¢ **MP $40**

FACE POWDER DEMONSTRATORS AND SAMPLES

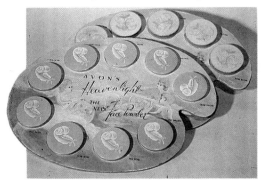

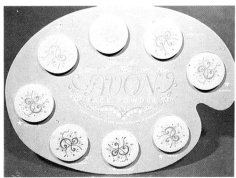

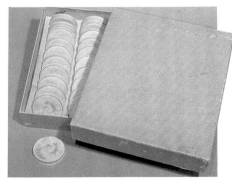

1944 *(top) Heavenlight Face Powder, 9 shades*
cardboard 20¢ **MP $38**
1948 *Heavenlight Face Powder, 9 shades, metal*
30¢ **MP $33**

1949 *Face Powder Palette, 8 shades 30¢*
MP $33

1957 *Face Powder Selector (top) 10 shades*
50¢ **MP $28**
1951 *Face Powder Palette, 9 shades 30¢*
MP $30

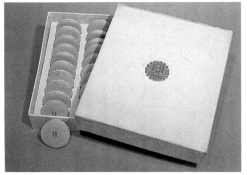

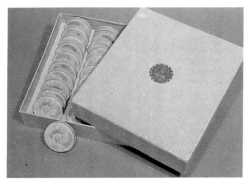

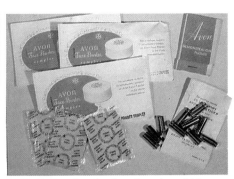

1940 *Face Powder, box of 30 Samples 50¢*
MP $115 *complete, $3 each sample*

1943-44 *Face Powder Samples, box of 30*
cardboard containers 50¢ **MP $140** *complete,*
$4 each sample

1944-45 *Face Powder Samples, box of 30*
cardboard containers 50¢ **MP $140**
complete, $4 each sample

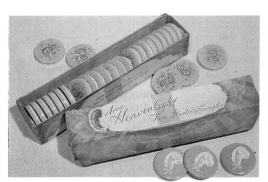

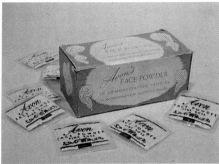

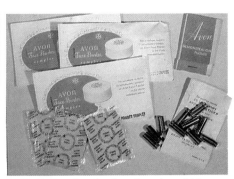

1949-52 *Face Powder, box of 30 samples 50¢*
$90 complete, $2.25 each sample
1948 *Heavenlight Face Powder, box of 30*
samples 50¢ **MP $120,** *$3 each*

1948-49 *Face Powder, box of 30 samples 50¢*
MP $40 *complete, $1 each*

1953-57 *Face Powder Samples, pkg. of 10*
MP $12, *$1 each*
1948-49 *Demonstration Tissues by Kleenex,*
pkg. of 10 **MP $16**
1950's *Lipstick Samples, pkg. of 10* **MP $8**

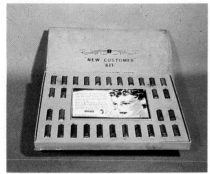

1937-39 *New Customer Kit of 30 Lipstick samples* **MP $55**

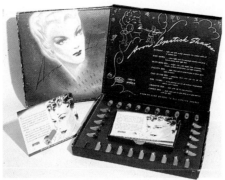

1940-42 *Lipstick Demonstrator Case of 30 samples* **MP $45**

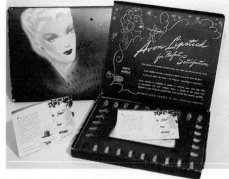

1945-47 *Lipstick Demonstrator Case of 30 samples* **MP $40**

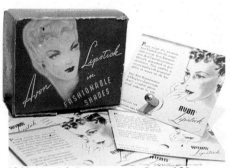

1948 *Lipstick Demonstrator Case of 30 samples 4 x 3½"* **MP $35**

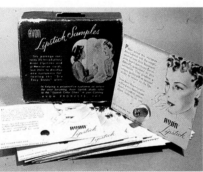

1949 *Box of 30 Lipstick Samples and Cards 50¢* **MP $30**

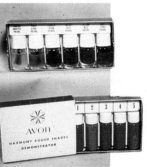

1950 *Nail Polish Demonstrator, six ½ dram bottles* **MP $22**
1956 *Harmony Rouge Demonstrator, 5 bottles* **MP $18**

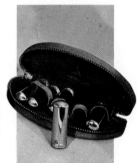

1952 *Fashion Lipstick Demonstrator Case of 5 colors* **MP $32**

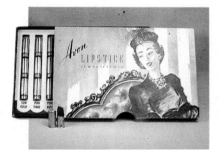

1950 *Lipstick Sample Case, 10 shades* **MP $30**

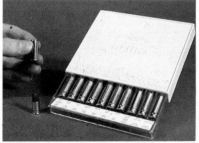

1951 *Jewel-Etched Lipstick Demonstrator* **MP $25**

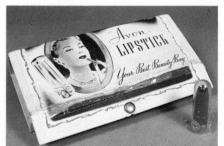

1952 *Lipstick Demonstrator with 4 regular lipsticks and 1 refill (shown)* **MP $45 complete**

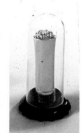

1961 *Introductory Demo of Deluxe Lipstick on black plastic pedestal, topped with lucite dome* **MP $20**

MAKEUP DEMONSTRATORS AND SAMPLES

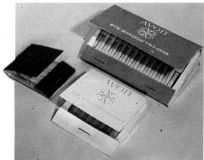

1950 *Matchstick Eye Shadow Try-Ons* **MP $20**
1960 *Matchsticks Eye Shadow Try-Ons* **MP $15 for 50 sticks**
1961 *Matchstick Eye Shadow Try-Ons* **MP $15 in Violet Mist, 15 sticks**

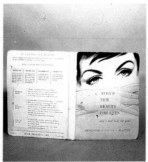

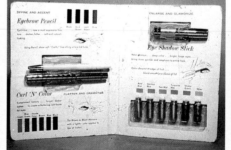

1960 *New Beauty for Eyes Demonstrator holds Curl 'N' Color Mascara, Eyebrow Pencil, Eye Shadow Stick and Try-On Demos of Eye Shadow* **MP $60**

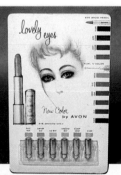

1963 *Eye Shadow Stick Demonstrator with new shade Eye Shadow Try-Ons* **MP $22**

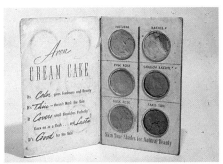

1948 *Cream Cake Demonstrator, 6 shades*
MP $25

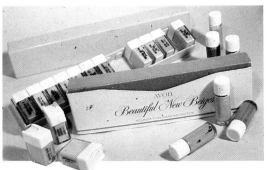

1961 *Face Powder Demonstrator, 13 shades* **MP $15**
1965 *Beautiful New Beiges Demonstrator* **MP $12**

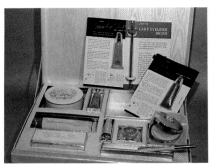

1965 *Manager's Product Case holds Face Powder, Natural Radiance, Tone 'N' Tint, Cream & Luminous Eye Shadows, Cake Eyeliner, Eyeliner Brush, Eyeliner Pencil, Eyebrow Brush-A-Line, Deluxe Lipstick and Deluxe Compact* **MP $90**

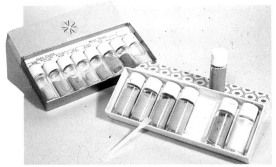

1957 *Makeup Demonstrator holds 8 shades* **MP $18**
1973 *Makeup Demonstrator holds 7 shades $1.75*
MP $6

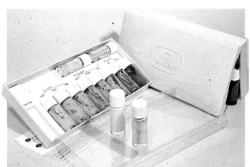

1966 *Makeup Demonstrator holds 3 shades Face Powder, 8 Foundations and 1 Dew Kiss* **MP $9**
1967 *Makeup Demonstrator holds 3 shades Face Powder, 8 shades Foundation and Dew Kiss in covered plastic case* **MP $10**

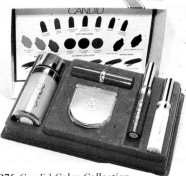

1976 *Candid Color Collection Demonstrator holds Makeup 1.5oz, Lip Color, Cheek Color, Eye Color and Mascara* **MP $16 with Color Chart in lid**

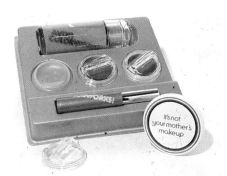

1977 *Colorworks Demo Kit holds 5 products $4.50* **MP $5 boxed**
1977 *"It's Not Your Mother's Makeup" Pin given to Reps at Sales Meetings* **MP $2**

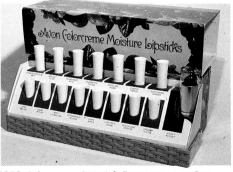

1978 *Colorcreme Lipstick Demonstrator. One Richly Russet full size lipstick and 15 samples given only to Reps attending C-16 Sales Meeting* **MP $5**

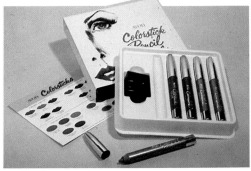

1977 *Colorstick Pencil Sampler holds 2 Colorsticks for Eyes, 2 for Lips and a Twin Sharpener, Color Chart $3.99* **MP $6 boxed**

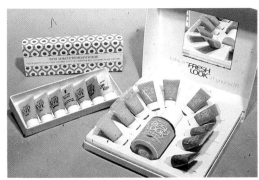

1979 *Makeup Demonstrator Kit with tube of Dew Kiss and all 6 shades of Even Tone Makeup $2*
MP $4 complete, 25¢ each tube
1979 *Fresh Look Makeup Demonstrator with one full size bottle and 10 demo tubes of makeup. Given only to those attending C-2 Sales Meeting* **MP $5, 50¢ bottle only**

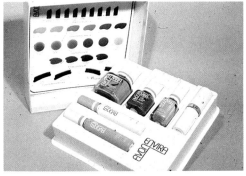

1979 *Envira Makeup Demonstrator holds Conditioning Makeup, Color Blush, Eye Color, Lipstick, Eye Definer, Mascara* **MP $17** *contents, $18 boxed*

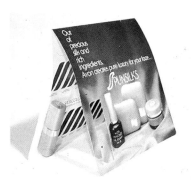

1980 *Spunsilks Color Chart Demonstrator with Spuncolor Lipstick* **MP $3** *Lipstick, $3.50 with chart*

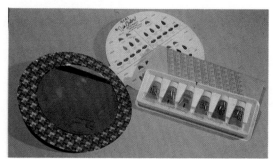

1981 *Colorcreme Color Chart and Mirror* **MP $3**
1981 *Even Tone Demonstrator* **MP $3**

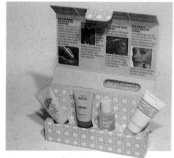

1983 *97th Anniversary Celebration Sampler. Contains 4 Trial Size Products* **MP $4**

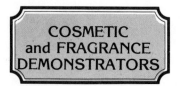

COSMETIC and FRAGRANCE DEMONSTRATORS

AVON

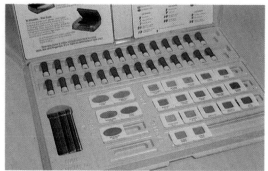

1983 *Coordinates Make-Up Demonstrator* **MP $22**

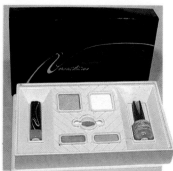

1983 *Versatilites Make-up Demonstrator* **MP $10**

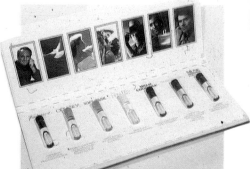

1983 *Fragrance Portfolio Demonstrator* **MP $3**

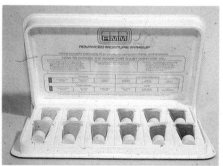

1984 *Advanced Moisture Makeup Demonstrator* **MP $5***

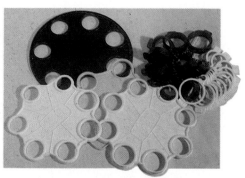

1970's & 80's *Ring Sizers* **MP $1 each**

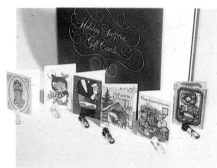

1983 *Holiday Suprise Gift Cards Demonstrator* **MP $5**

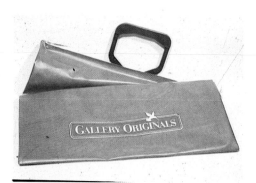

**Available from Avon at time of publication*

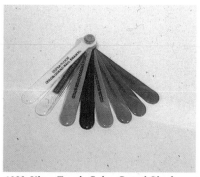

1983 *Ultra Touch Color Guard Shade Selector* **MP $1.95***

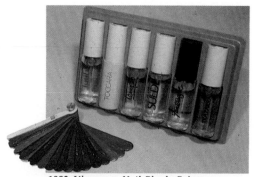

1982 *Ultrawear Nail Shade Selector* **MP $3.95***
1982 *Fragrance Demonstrator, 6 Spray Colognes* **MP $1 each, $8 set**

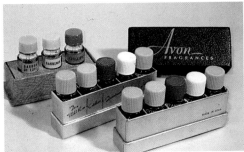

1939 *Fragrance Demonstrator. Cotillion, Garden of Love, Gardenia* **MP $100**
1951 *Fragrance Demonstrator. To A Wild Rose, Cotillion, Quaintance, Golden Promise, Forever Spring* **MP $28**
1952 *Fragrance Demonstrator. Same fragrance as above* **MP $26**

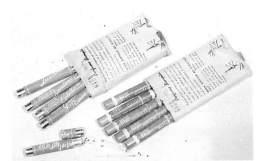

1946-50 *Perfume Samples. Each blue or pink cardboard tube holds 8 glass ampules of perfume (10 frag. available). Bottled for Avon by Nips, Inc. Each tube with 8 ampules* **MP $42,** *each ampule* **$4** *Set of 5 tubes in envelope* **MP $225**

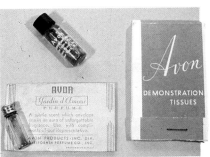

1937 *Jardin d'Amour Perfume sample and envelope* **MP $26, $20** *Perfume only*
1964 *Somewhere Perfume Oil Demonstrator Bottle* **MP $10**
1949 *Demonstration Tissues by Kleenex, pkg. of 10* **MP $15**

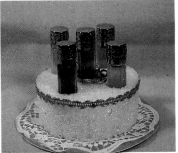

1951 *65th Anniversary Demo. Styrofoam birthday cake holds five 1 dram Perfumes in To A Wild Rose, Flowertime, Quaintance, Golden Promise and Cotillion* **MP $150 complete**

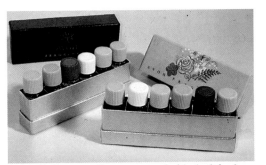

1954-58 *Fragrance Demonstrator holds 6 of the 9 fragrances offered between 1954-58* **MP $22**
1959-60 *Fragrance Demonstrator holds Topaze, Here's My Heart, Persian Wood, Cotillion, To A Wild Rose, Bright Night* **MP $20**

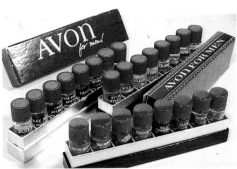

1965-66 *Avon for Men Demonstrator, 8 bottles of fragrance* **MP $15**
1970 *Avon for Men Demonstrator, 8 bottles of fragrance* **MP $15**
1972 *Avon for Men Demonstrator, 8 bottles of fragrance* **MP $10**

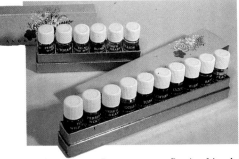

1961 *Fragrance Demonstrator. Persian Wood, Topaze, To A Wild Rose, Somewhere, Here's My Heart, Cotillion* **MP $18**
1964-65 *Fragrance Demonstrator, 10 bottles* **MP $18**

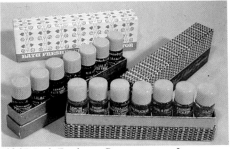

1967 *Bath Freshener Demonstrator. Lemon Friction Lotion, Lilac, Hawaiian White Ginger, Blue Lotus, Lily of the Valley, Jasmine and Honeysuckle* **MP $13**
1974 *Fragrance Demonstrator No. 2 holds Lemon Velvet, Sweet Honesty, Hawaiian White Ginger, Honeysuckle, Pink & Pretty, Raining Violets and Lilac* **MP $8**

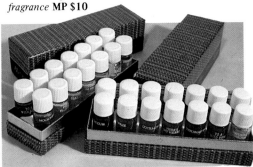

1972 *Fragrance Demonstrator, 14 bottles* **MP $10**
1973 *Fragrance Demonstrator, 14 bottles* **MP $10** (smooth lids)

FRAGRANCES DEMONSTRATORS AND SAMPLES

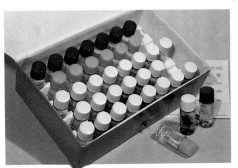

1975 *Fragrance Demonstrator, 38 bottles of Women's, Men's, Girl's and floral fragrances* **MP $15**

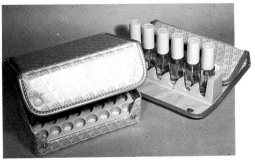

1978 *Sales Mates Sample Kit holds a variety of samples $2 (empty)* **MP $2.25**
1978 *Sales Mates Fragrance Demonstrator with a choice of 6 miniature Sprays $4.50, empty $1.75* **MP $8, $2 empty**

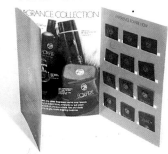

1980 *Foxfire Fragrance Folio holds 12 samples* **MP $2**

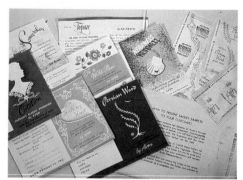

1950's & 1960's *Assortment of Powder Sachet Samples, envelope of 10 with matching Folder* **MP $12,** $1 each sachet and folder

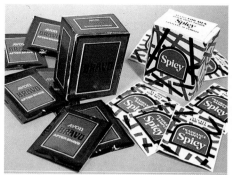

1969 *Bravo Samples, box of 10* **MP $5**
1967 *Spicy Samples, box of 10* **MP $5**

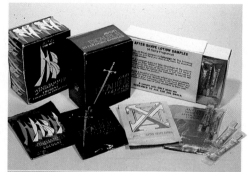

1968 *Windjammer Cologne Samples, box of 10* **MP $6**
1969 *Excalibur Cologne, box of 10* **MP $5**
1964 *"4-A" After Shave, box of 10* **MP $8**
1964 *Tribute After Shave, box of 10* **MP $8**
1961 *Spicy After Shave, box of 30* **MP $20,** 50¢ each

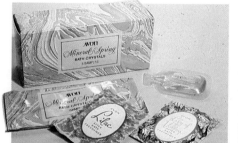

1972 *Mineral Springs Bath Crystals, box of 5* **MP $3,** 50¢ each
1963 *After Bath Freshener in Lilac, Lily of the Valley, box of 10* **MP $15,** $1.25 each
1972 *Skin-So-Soft Bath Oil, box of 10, 40¢* **MP $3,** 25¢ each

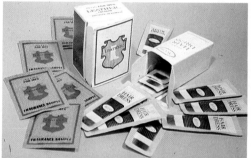

1965 *Leather Samples, box of 10* **MP $5**
1966 *Clear Hair Dress Samples, box of 10* **MP $7**

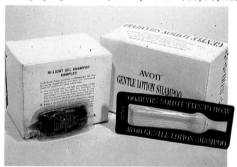

1962 *Hi-Light Gel Shampoo, box of 15* **MP $23,** $1.25 each
1969 *Gentle Lotion Shampoo, box of 10, 60¢* **MP $7,** 50¢ each

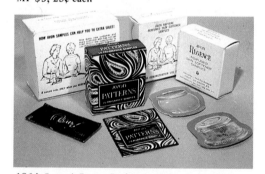

1964 *Occur! Cream Sachet Samples, box of 30 $1* **MP $18,** 50¢ each
1968 *Patterns Fragrance Samples, box of 10* **MP $2**
1965 *Rapture Skin Softener, box of 10* **MP $12,** $1 each
1967 *Regence Skin Softener, box of 10* **MP $9,** 75¢ each

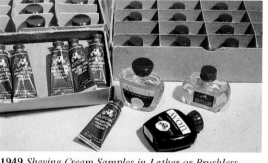

1949 *Shaving Cream Samples in Lather or Brushless ¼oz. Box of 20, 50¢* **MP $120,** $5 each
1958 *After Shave Sample ½oz. Box of 20, 50¢* **MP $250,** $12 each
1959 *After Shower Sample (black) ½oz. Box of 20, 50¢* **MP $310,** $15 each
1949 *After Shave, ½oz. Box of 20, 50¢* **MP $210,** $10 each

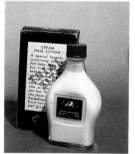

1949 *Cream Hair Lotion, 1oz trial size* **MP $25,** $35 boxed

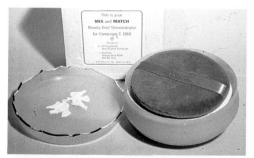

1968 *Mix and Match Beauty Dust Demonstrator* **MP $40** boxed

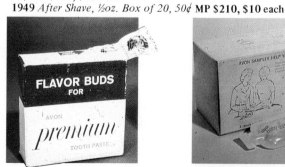

1964 *Premium Toothpaste Samples, foil-wrapped, 50 in a box* **MP $15**

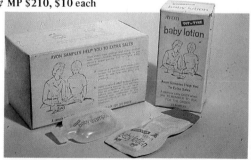

1964 *Baby Shampoo, 20 in a box* **MP $18,** 75¢ each
1964 *Baby Lotion, 10 in a box, 30¢* **MP $9,** 75¢ each

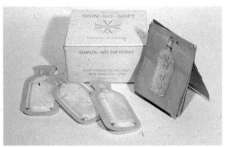

1967-72 *Box of 10 Skin-So-Soft Samples. (Left 10020 zip code)* **MP $12, $1 each**
1973 *Box of 10 Skin-So-Soft Samples. (Right 10019 zip code)* **MP $12, $1 each**

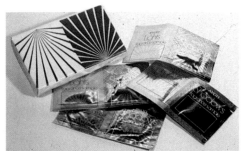

1969 *Box of 10 Lights and Shadows Samples* **MP $12, $1 each**

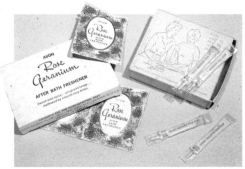

1964 *Box of 10 Rose Geranium After Bath Freshener Samples* **MP $18, $1.50 each**
1950's *Box of 10 Rich Moisture Cream Samples* **MP $20, $1.25 each**

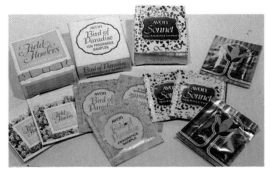

Field Flowers Samples **MP 50¢ each**
Bird of Paradise Samples **MP 50¢ each**
Sonnet Samples **MP 50¢ each**
Queen's Gold **MP 50¢ each**

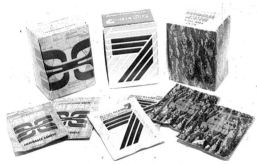

1972 *Tai Winds Samples* **MP 50¢ each**
1973 *Blend 7 Samples* **MP 50¢ each**
1973 *Deep Woods Samples* **MP 50¢ each**

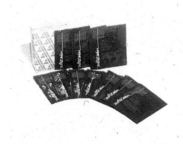

Ultrawear Box of 10 Samples **MP $3, 25¢ each**

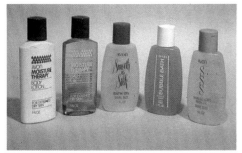

Trial Sizes —
Moisture Therapy Body Lotion 39¢ **MP 25¢**
Moisture Therapy Bath Oil 39¢ **MP 25¢**
Smooth As Silk Bath Oil 39¢ **MP 25¢**
Bubble Bath 39¢ **MP 25¢**
Skin-So-Soft Bath Oil 39¢ **MP 25¢**

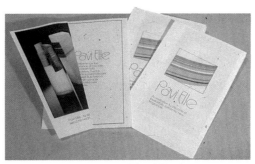

1983 *Pavi Elle Sample Folders* **MP 50¢ ea.**

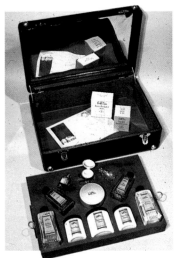

1935 *Demonstration Case. Gardenia and Cotillion Perfumes 1/4oz each. Skin Freshener and Astringent 2oz each, Rose Water, Glycerin and Benzoin Lotion 4oz, Lotus Cream 4oz, One jar each of Tissue, Cleansing and Vanishing Cream, Face Powder, Rouge Compact and Lipstick* **MP $1100**

REPRESENTATIVE'S DEMONSTRATION CASES

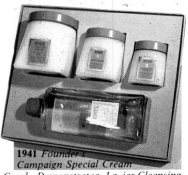

1941 *Founder's Campaign Special Cream Comb. Demonstrator. Lg. jar Cleansing Cream, med. jar Night Cream, sm. jar Foundation Cream & 4oz Skin Freshener* **MP $110**

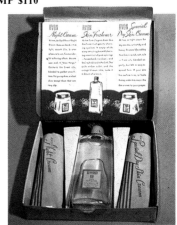

1946 *Skin Care Demonstration Kit. One tube each of Night Cream and Special Dry Skin Cream. Skin Freshener 4oz* **MP $80 complete**

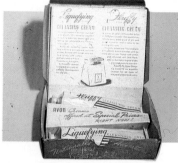

1947 Skin Care Demonstration Kit. One tube each of Liquefying Cleansing Cream and Fluffy Cleansing Cream **MP $80 complete**

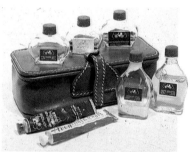

1953 Leatherette Kit holds ½oz Brushless Shaving Cream, ¾oz Toothpaste, ½oz each After Shave Lotion, Cologne and Deodorant, 1oz each Liquid Shampoo and Cream Hair Lotion **MP $200**

Highly prized collectibles, cherished by both collectors and Representatives.

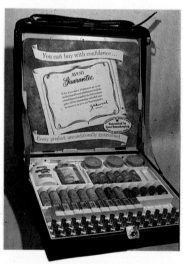

1959 Beauty Counselor Demonstration Kit. Plastic bottle of Moisture Bath, Skin Freshener 1oz. One plastic jar each of Rich Moisture and Vita Moist Cream and Strawberry Cooler. Demonstrator bottles of Perfumes, Foundations, Rouge, Face Powder and Lipstick Samples **MP $350 complete**

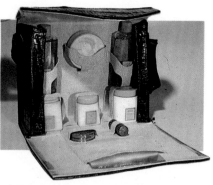

1948 Demonstration Case holds Bamboo Lipstick and Rouge Compact, Skin Freshener and Astringent, Night Cream, Foundation Cream and Super Rich Cream **MP $100**

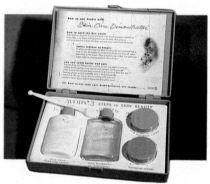

1956 Skin Care Demonstrator holds Deep Clean Cleansing Cream, Skin Freshener, Rich Moisture Cream, Hormone Cream and Spatula **MP $100**

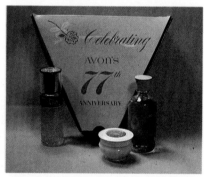

1963 77th Anniversary Gift Demonstrator. Compact, 2oz Topaze Cologne Mist, Skin-So-Soft and 1oz Cream Foundation **MP $40 complete**

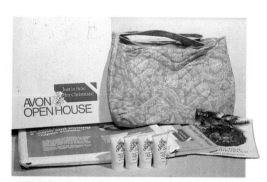

1983 Open House Kit offered only at Christmas **MP $8 complete**

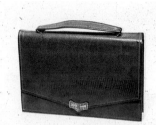

1929 Representative's Beauty Case **MP $55**

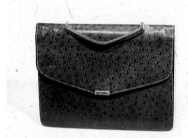

1942 Representative's Beauty Case **MP $32**

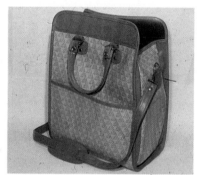

1981 Sales Notes Beauty Showcase **MP $11.50***

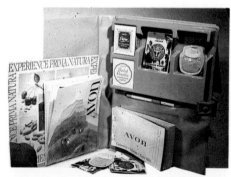

1971 Representative's Organizer Showcase holds Order Book, Samples, Color Chart, Pen and Catalog **MP $20**

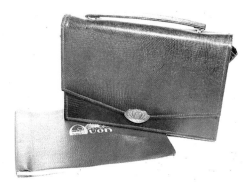

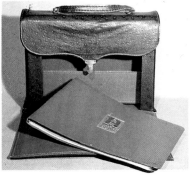

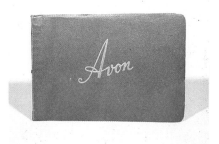

1929-36 *Sales Catalog* **MP $50**
1929 *Representative's Beauty Case* **MP $55**

1948-52 *Representative's Beauty Case*
MP $28
1937 *Sales Catalog $2.50* **MP $40**

1948-52 *Sales Catalog* **MP $30**

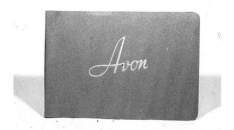

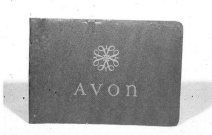

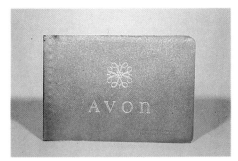

1953 *Sales Catalog* **MP $40**

1954-57 *Sales Catalog* **MP $20**

1954 only *Sales Catalog imprinted with
"Honor Representative President's Award" on
cover* **MP $35**

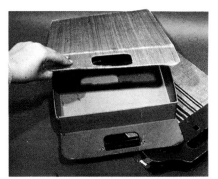

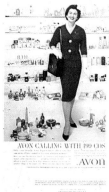

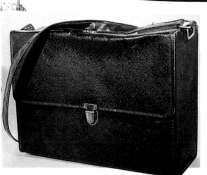

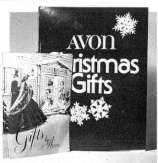

REPRESENTATIVE'S SALES AIDS

1943-44 *Gift Display Ensemble Boxes
(cardboard) to carry Xmas Gift Demos
and Sets* **MP $25 each**

1960 *Avon Ad,
Engraver's Proof:
"199 Cosmetics"*
MP $17

1952 *Representative's Beauty Case, green
plastic lining* **MP $25**

1953 *Xmas Gifts by Avon Book*
MP $25
1975 *Xmas Gift Book Cover*
MP $4

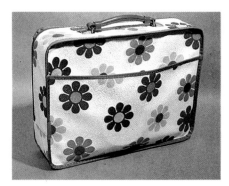

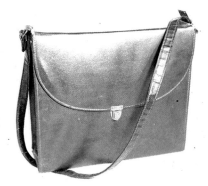

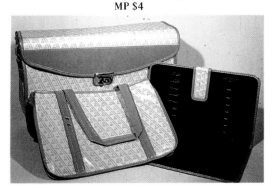

1969 *Representative's Summer Beauty
Showcase, a "Spring Fever"
Recommendation prize* **MP $22**

1950's *Representative's Beauty Case* **MP $22**

Sales Mates —
1978 *Beauty Showcase, empty $11.50* **MP $11.50**
1978 *Tote Bag, empty $4* **MP $4**
1978 *Jewelry Demonstrator, empty $5* **MP $5**

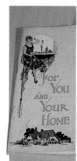
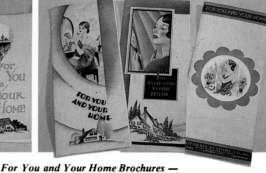
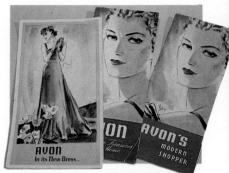

1924 *CPC Bulletin* **MP $50**

(See also CPC pages 8 & 9)

For You and Your Home Brochures —
1927 MP $50   **1934 MP $40**
1929 MP $45   **1936 MP $35**

1937 *Avon In Its New Dress* **MP $30**
1938 *Avon Brings Treasures* **MP $28**
1940-41 *Modern Shopper* **MP $25**

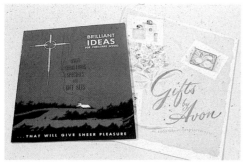
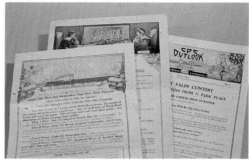
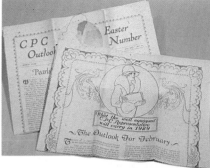

1941 *Christmas Gift Catalog* **MP $35**
1954 *Gifts by Avon* **MP $25**

1924 *California Perfume Company Outlooks*
MP $25 each

1929 *Feb. & March CPC Outlooks* **MP $**

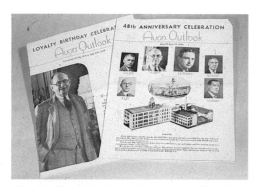
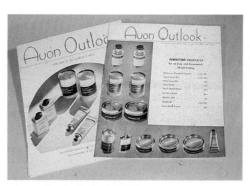
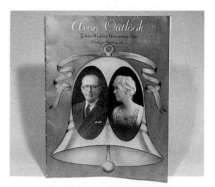

1934 *Loyalty Outlook for Mr. McConnell's 76th*
Birthday **MP $20**
1934 *Outlook for Avon's 48th Anniversary* **MP $20**

1934 *Avon Outlooks* **MP $15**

1935 *Avon Outlook for Mr. & Mrs.*
McConnell's Golden Wedding
Anniversary **MP $40**

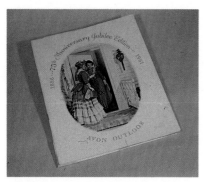
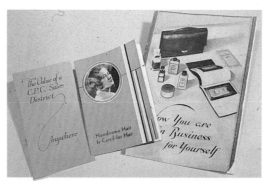
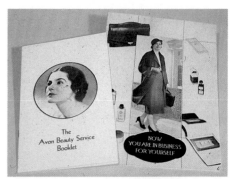

1961 *Avon Outlook Celebrating Avon's*
75th Anniversary **MP $10**

1931 *The Value of a CPC Sales District* **MP $15**
1931 *Hair Care Booklet* **MP $10**
1931 *Now You Are in Business For Yourself Booklet*
MP $15

1935 *Beauty Service Booklet* **MP $12**
1935 *Now You Are in Business for Yourself*
MP $12

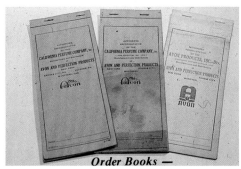

Order Books —
1930 - MP $20
1934 - MP $20
1936 - MP $17

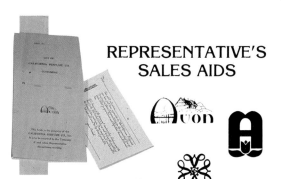

REPRESENTATIVE'S SALES AIDS

1934 *Customer List Booklet*
MP $12
1934 *Calling Card* **MP $3**

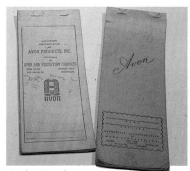

Order Books —
1939 - MP $17
1953 - MP $12

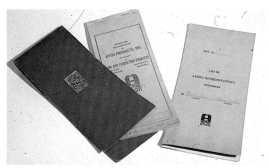

1937 *Order Book and Cover* **MP $17 each**
1940's *Customer Name Book* **MP $10**

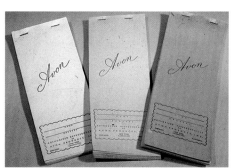

1948 - MP $15
1949 - MP $15
1950 - MP $15

Order Books —

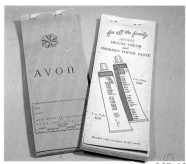

1956 - MP $8
1957 - MP $8

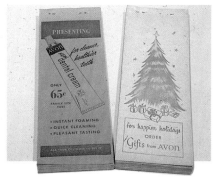

1959 *Order Books* **MP $8 ea.**

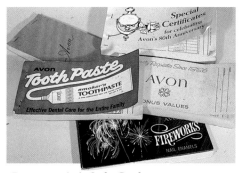

Representative's Order Books —
1940's *Script Avon on cover* **MP $15**
1966 *80th Anniversary cover* **MP $10**
1967 *Toothpaste Promotion cover* **MP $8**
1965 *Contains Bonus Value Coupons* **MP $10**
1967 *Fireworks Nail Enamels cover* **MP $8**

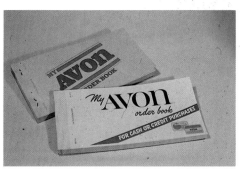

1981 *Order Books* **MP $2**

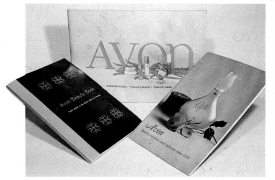

1961 *Beauty Book* **MP $5**
1964 *Catalog* **MP $5**
1965 *Catalog* **MP $5**

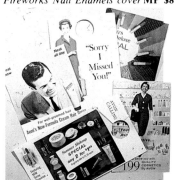

Assortment of "Make
Yourself Known"
Folders and Door-
hanger "Call-Back"
Reminders of the 60's:

4 page special "New
Products" Folder
MP $4

2 page Price Folders
MP $3

Door Hanger
Reminders **MP $1 ea.**

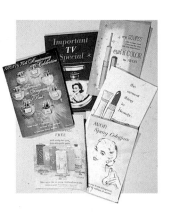

. . . REPRESENTATIVE'S SALES AIDS

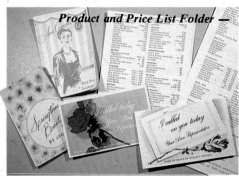

Product and Price List Folder —

top —1950 *Spring (8 pages)* **MP $5**
       1962 *C-8 (4 pgs. shown open)* **MP $4**
       1962 *C-2 (6 pgs. shown open)* **MP $4**
bottom —1955 *Spring (8 pages)* **MP $5**
       1962 *C-8 (4 pages)* **MP $4**
       1963 *C-2 (4 pages)* **MP $4**

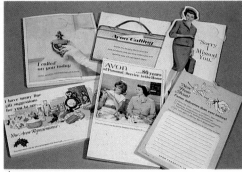

Across top —
1964-65 *Make Yourself Known Cards* **MP $1 ea.**
Across bottom —
1966-68 *Make Yourself Known Cards* **MP $1 ea.**

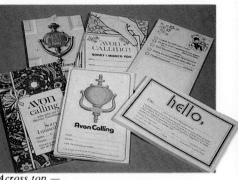

Across top —
1969-70 *Make Yourself Known Cards* **MP $1 each**
Across bottom —
1971-72-74 *Customer Service Reminders*
MP 75¢ each

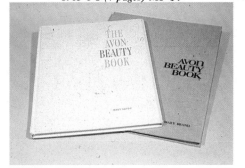

1967 *Beauty Book, hardcover, Manager's* **MP $7**
1975 *Beauty Book, hardcover* **MP $5**

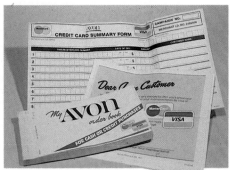

1980 *Order Book* **MP $2**
1980 *VISA, MasterCard Summary* **MP $1**

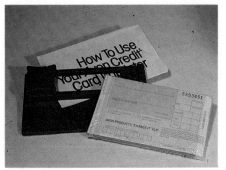

1976 *Credit Card Imprinter. Test Market
Kansas City* **MP $25**
1976 *Cards for Imprinter* **MP $5**

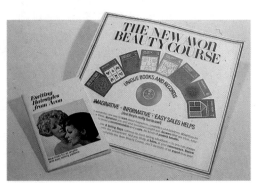

1969 *Hair Styles Book* **MP $5**
1971 *The New Avon Beauty Course* **MP $4**

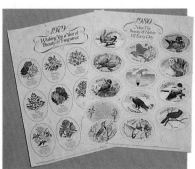

1978 *Floral Calendar (1979) sold only to
Representatives to distribute as customer
Christmas gifts 25¢* **MP $2**
1979 *Nature Calendar (1980) sold only to
Representatives to distribute as Christmas
gifts 30¢ each* **MP $2**

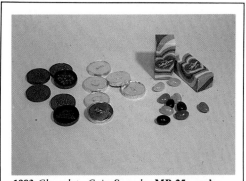

1983 *Chocolate Coin Samples* **MP 25¢ each**
1984 *Chocolate Coin Samples* **MP 25¢ each**
1983-84 *Jelly Bean Samples* **MP 50¢ each box**

CANDY SAMPLES

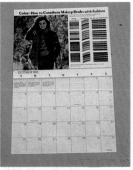

1980 *How-To Beauty
Calendar (1981) sold only
to Representatives to
distribute as customer
Xmas gifts 20¢* **MP $1**

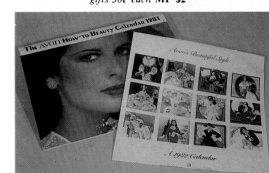

1980 *Avon Calendar. How-To Beauty Calendar (1981)
Sold only to Representatives to distribute as Christmas
gifts* **MP $1**
1981 *Avon Calendar. Avon's Beautiful Style (1982) sold
only to Representatives to distribute as Christmas gifts*
MP $1

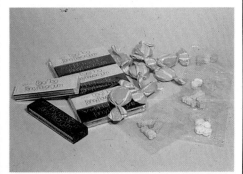

1983 *Fancy Flavor Gum Samples* **MP $1 pkg.**
1984 *Easter Sweetkins Samples* **MP $1 pkg.**
1984 *Mother's Day Bouquet Samples* **MP 25¢ ea**

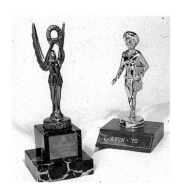

1950's *"Woman of the Year" Award given thru 1959 to the top Representative in each District*
MP $125
1970 *Avon Trophy* **MP $50**

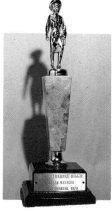

1970 *Stellar Manager Award, 2nd Quarter*
MP $100

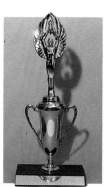

1978 *Customer Service Trophy (Pasadena Branch) to Rep in each District who served most customers during the year*
MP $25

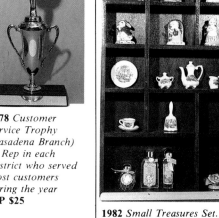

1982 *Small Treasures Set. Awarded in 5 Sales Achievement Steps. Complete with display case*
MP $150

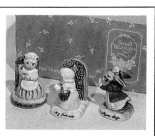

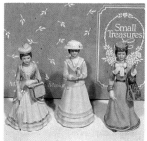

1982 *Small Treasures Cherished Moments Mini Award, Step 4*
MP $35
1982 *Small Treasures Albee Miniatures Award. Step 5*
MP $40

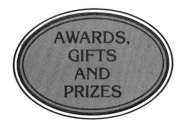

AWARDS, GIFTS AND PRIZES

O ver the years the world's largest cosmetic company has presented these trophies of success to those who have helped make it great.

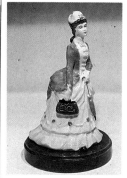

1961 *Woman of Achievement Award, one in each District "Western Germany"*
MP $300

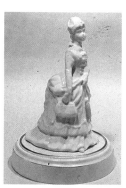

1969 *"Better Way" Award, one in each Division "Western Germany Dresdner Art"*
MP $325

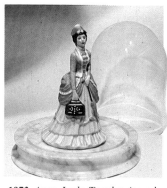

1973 *Avon Lady Trophy Award given to approximately 6,000 Representatives of 5 winning Districts in each Branch* **MP $250**

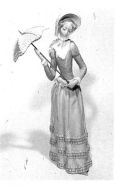

1975-76 *Division Managers Albee. Made by Lladro in Spain. Does not say Avon.* **MP $70**

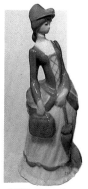

1976 *First Avon Lady Porcelain Figurine made in Spain. Anniversary Sales Award to President's Club Members* **MP $55**

O ver ninety years ago, Mrs. Albee, the California Perfume Company's first Representative, knocked on a door, launching Avon's tradition of door-to-door selling and personal service. The legacy of Mrs. Albee lives on with charming statuettes in her image. The Avon "First Ladies" are awarded to Representatives for outstanding achievement — Avon's very best!

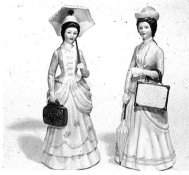

1978 *Albee Trophy Award, 10 in each District* **MP $140**
1979 *Albee Trophy Award, 10 in each District* **MP $130**

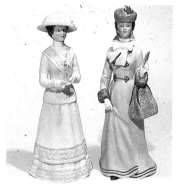

1980 *Albee Trophy Award, 10 in each District* **MP $125**
1981 *Albee Trophy Award, to all Representatives attaining President's Club Membership* **MP $60**

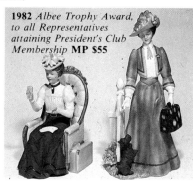

1982 *Albee Trophy Award, to all Representatives attaining President's Club Membership* **MP $55**

1983 *Albee Trophy Award to all Representatives attaining President's Club Membership* **MP $50**

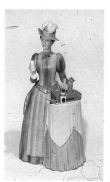

1984 *Albee Trophy Award to Presidents Club Member*
MP $50

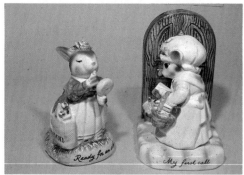

1980 *"Ready for an Avon Day" awarded for sales of $175 each in Campaigns 4, 5 and 6* **MP $25**
1980 *"My First Call" for sales of $250 each in each of three campaigns* **MP $35**

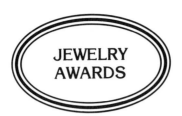

JEWELRY AWARDS

In 1928 Avon introduced the Award Pin Program. The designs of the pins and the requirements to earn them have changed many times, but the Program has continued since 1928.

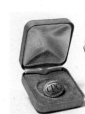

1910 *CPC Identification Pin* **MP $160**

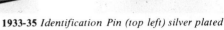

1933-35 *Identification Pin (top left) silver plated* **MP $55**
1935-38 *Identification Pin (top right) silver plated* **MP $50**
1930-33 *Identification Pin (bottom left) silver plated (left leg of "A" and "N" intersect lower rim of oval)* **MP $65**
1935-38 *Honor Award Pin, Gold Filled* **MP $60**

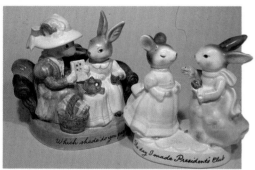

1980 *"Which Shade Do You Prefer?" for sales of $350 in each of three campaigns* **MP $50**
1980 *"The Day I Made President's Club" awarded for membership in President's Club* **MP $40**

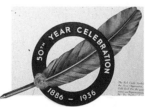

1936 *50th Anniversary Gift to Representatives. Quill Pen and Certificate* **MP $55**
Certificate only **MP $35**

1936 *50th Anniversary Award 24k gold-plated pin.* **MP $55, $65 boxed**

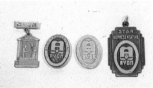

1938 *Service-Counsel-Satisfaction Medallion* **MP $58**
1938-45 *Identification Pin* **MP $40**
1938-43 *Honor Award Pin* **MP $45**
1938-45 *Star Representative Medallion 1/20-10k Gold Filled* **MP $55**

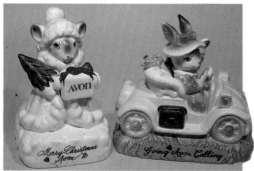

1980 *"Merry Christmas Avon '80" awarded for two successful Recommendations, only in C-22, 23 and 24. Limit of 1 per Representative* **MP $60**
1982 *Going Avon Calling awarded for successful recommendations* **MP $70**

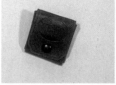

1945 *Jeweled Pearl Pin, highest honor case* **MP $20**

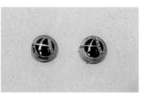

1945 *Identification Pin, leaf patterned* **MP $25**
1945-61 *Jeweled Pin Award with 5 seed Pearls, 10k Gold* **MP $35**

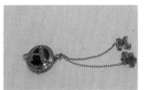

1945 *Manager's Identification Pin with plain M for Field Managers* **MP $75**, *with 11 seed Pearls for City Managers* **MP $100**

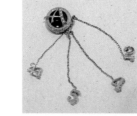

1945-56 *Jeweled Pin with Numeral Guards, given for each consecutive $1,000 in sales. Numeral 2 through 5* **MP $15**, *6 through 10* **MP $20**, *11-15* **MP $30**, *16-20* **MP $40**, *21-30* **MP $50**, *31-40* **MP $60**, *41-50* **MP $70**, *51 and up* **MP $85**, *Pin serves as Numeral 1* **MP $30**

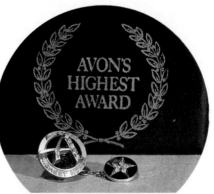

1956-61 *Representative's Highest Award, 5 diamonds on "A" of pin and 5 diamond Star Guard for sales of $26,000 within a year* **MP $300**

1956-61 *Diamond Star Guards replace Numeral Guards #5 and higher. Star Guard with 1 diamond for sales of $6,000 in a year or less* **MP $20** *Guard only, with 2 diamonds for sales of $11,000 in a year or less* **MP $30**, *with 3 diamonds for sales of $16,000 in a year or less* **MP $50**, *with 4 diamonds for sales of $21,000 in a year or less* **MP $100**

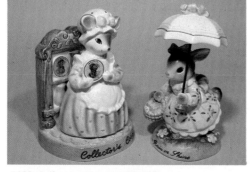

1982 *Collectors Corner* **MP $35**
1983 *Come Rain or Shine* **MP $25**

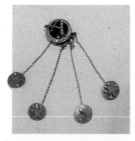

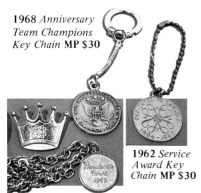

1968 Anniversary Team Champions Key Chain **MP $30**

1962 Service Award Key Chain **MP $30**

1964 Crown Pin Award for top sales **MP $20**
1969 President's 22k Court Charm & Bracelet **MP $30, $20 charm only**

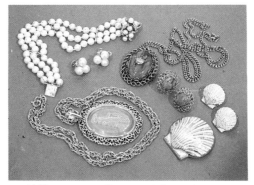

1962 Manager's Christmas Gift. Pearl & Diamond Bracelet & Earrings **MP $300**
1966 Regence Crown Performance Pendant/Pin Combo & Earrings to winning team in General Manager's Branch contest **MP $100, $125 boxed**
1967 Pin/Pendant incentive Award to Managers **MP $50, $65 boxed**
1975 Avon Lady Pendant to top 15 Reps in each district **MP $40**
1968 Shell Pin and Earrings recommendation prizes **MP $7 each**

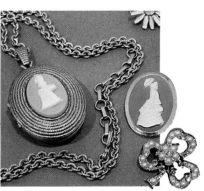

1966 Cameo Glace Brooch Locket, Honor Award **MP $30**
1965 Avon Lady Award Pin **MP $20**
1951 Three-Leaf Clover Pin by Coro, Award for Customer Service **MP $40**

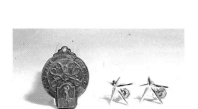

1960 Golf League Tournament Charm to Pasadena Branch employees **MP $50**
1961 Star Award Earrings Representative incentive Award **MP $15**

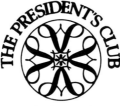

The President's Club — an elite group of special Representatives who share the pride of being Avon's very best . . .

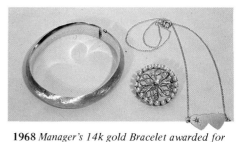

1968 Manager's 14k gold Bracelet awarded for high achievement in the General Manager's Contest **MP $100 with certificate**
1969 Manager's diamond and pearls Circle of Excellence Pin **MP $300**
1976 Diamond Sterling Silver/Necklace, engraved "1976 #1" on back **MP $75**

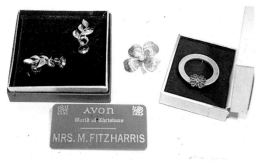

1964 Christmas Bells Earrings to winning team in each Division, General Manager's Contest **MP $35**
1964 Four Leaf Clover Pin, simulated pearl, by Coro. To Reps in "Lucky 7" contest **MP $20**
1970 Five year Avon Employees Service Pin **MP $25, $35 boxed**
1976 Manager's Xmas Conference Name Badge **MP $7**

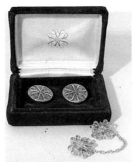

1966 Cuff Links worn by Avon Executives in 10k gold **MP $450** *(in other metals awarded to employees* **MP $50)**
1973 Branch Tour Guide's Jacket Guard **MP $35**

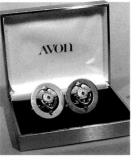

1974 Sterling Silver Doorknocker Cuff Links with Sapphire, incentive Award to Manager's, only 200 to 300 made **MP $250**

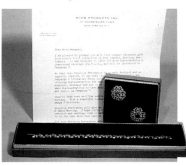

1971 Manager's Valentine Gift of Precious Pretenders Bracelet & Earrings **MP $45 boxed with letter, $15 letter only**

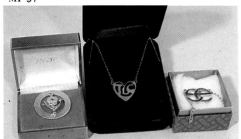

1976 Sterling Silver Doorknocker Circle Pin (left) with Sapphire. **MP $80 boxed with letter, $50 without letter**
1976 Team Leader Christmas Gift **MP $25**
1976 Double "e" Necklace, gift to Team Leaders for Emprise Survey **MP $25**

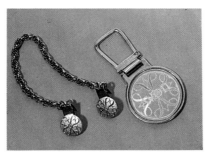

1968 Sweater Guard, General Manager's Honor Award, given to winning teams in each Branch **MP $25**
1973 Key Ring, Representative's Prize, "What's In It For You" Program **MP $10**

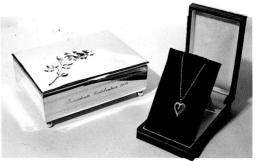

1974 Curio Box. Red lined with embossed Rose and engraved "President's Celebration '74". To Reps in winning districts **MP $65**
1974 Diamond Necklace. Given to top ten Reps of each winning District during President's Campaign. 14k pendant with 3pt diamond **MP $85**

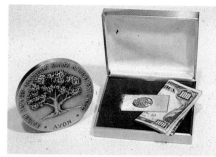

1980 Manager's Sales Achievement, President's Celebration Award **MP $200**
1979 Male Manager's 10k gold and diamond Money Clip engraved DM **MP $175**
1979 Male Team Leader Xmas Gift (not shown) as above **MP $130**

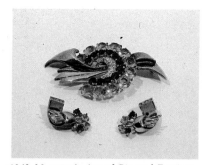

1943 Manager's Award Pin and Earrings. Given in Loyalty Campaign March 2-22, 1943. **MP Pin only $125, MP set $175**

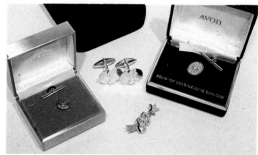

1969 Male Executive Tie Tac with blue Sapphire **MP $200**
1976 Male Manager #1 Cuff Links **MP $125**
1978 Male Team Leader Christmas Gift, 10k gold and diamond Tie Tac **MP $150**
1980 Manager's Shooting Star Pin. Box sleeve reads "We're Going To Be Stronger and Better Than Ever" **MP $40**

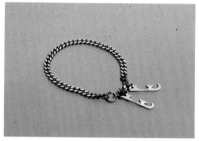

1951 Figure 8 Charm Bracelet Awarded for interviewing 120 customers in C-3 **MP $55**

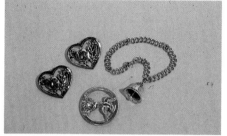

1955 Sterling Silver Robin Pins, given in pairs to Representatives for reaching customer goals in "Red Robin" Campaign 7 **MP $28 pair**
1967 Representative's Sterling Silver Bracelet by Tiffany with Bell and clapper **MP $40**
1964 Rapture Dove Pin, antique silver finish awarded in General Manager's Contest **MP $35**

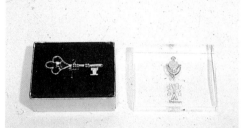

1962 Key Pin awarded for activity **MP $20**
1970's Lucite Paper Weight Doorknocker. Given to Shawnee Div. **MP $30**

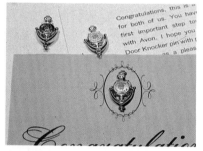

1964 Manager's Sterling Silver Door-knocker Pin **MP $40**
1964 Representative's Gold-plated Door-knocker Pin on green card **MP $12, $10 on white card**

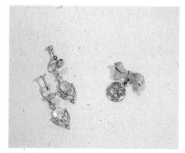

1967 Representative's Doorknocker Earrings awarded to Championship Teams from each Branch **MP $25**
1967 Ten year Service Pin awarded to Representatives on retirement, engraved on back and rare **MP $100**

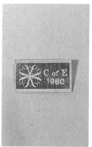

1980 Circle of Excellence Pin **MP $25**

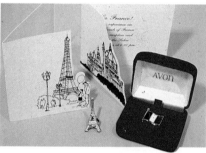

Circle of Excellence Manager Gifts, Paris —
1979 Eiffel Tower Pin **MP $25**
1979 French Flag Pin **MP $20**

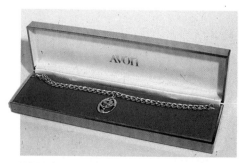

1974 Silver Doorknocker Bracelet awarded to only 40 Managers in each Branch **MP $150**

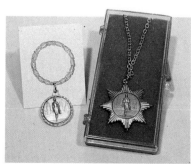

1975 Springdale Branch Medallions left **MP $10**, *right* **MP $25**

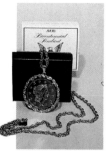

1976 Bicentennial Coin Pendant. Anniversary Sales Award **MP $30**

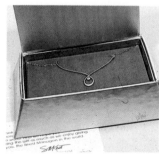

1977 Manager's Diamond Loop Necklace in gold presentation box **MP $40**

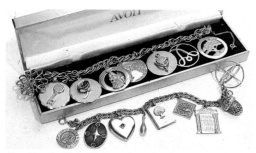

President's Club Highest Award, Charm Bracelet and Charms (in box) complete **MP $320**
1971 *Bracelet and "4-A" Charm* **MP $35**
1972 *Avon Rose* **MP $25**
1972 *First Lady Charm with topaze* **MP $35**
1973 *World of Avon with aquamarine* **MP $40**
1973 *Doorknocker with amethyst* **MP $40**
1974 *Jeweled A with sapphire* **MP $45**
1974 *Key with garnet* **MP $45**
1975 *Great Oak* **MP $55**

1963-65 *Manager's Circle of Leadership Bracelet with 10k gold filled Charms and genuine jewels. (Listed in Achievement sequence)*
1. *Circle of Leadership, 4 diamonds & Bracelet* **MP $65**
2. *Heart Locket, ruby* **MP $40**
3. *Cotillion Cologne* **MP $45**
4. *Great Oak Book* **MP $50**
5. *Women of Achievement* **MP $55**
6. *Emerald Charm (square)* **MP $60**
7. *Acorn* **MP $65**
8. *Door Charm Locket* **MP $70**
9. *Oval with star and 4 sapphires* **MP $75**
10. *11 & 12 not shown, are same shape as Charm 9, but set with rubies, emeralds and diamonds, consecutively* **MP $85, $100 and $150**

Avon's Exclusive Symbols —
The "4-A" design is the world-wide Avon corporate symbol.
Avon Rose *symbolizes beauty made possible by Avon products.*
First Avon Lady *represents Mrs. P.F.E. Albee, mother of the California Perfume Company.*
The **"World of Avon"** *is the symbol of the 31 countries Avon served in 1981.*
Doorknocker *is the symbol of personal and loyal service.*
The **"Jeweled A"** *honors Representative's Achievement.*
Avon Key *is the symbol of "key" to success.*
The Great Oak *signifies the growing success and solid foundation on which Avon is based.*

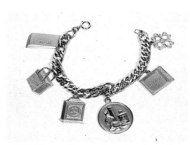

1959 *Silver Charm Bracelet Award. Awarded to two Districts in each Branch only. Very few awarded for Sales Achievement, rare* **MP $190**

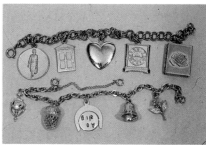

1965 *Representative's Golden Circle of Service Charm Bracelet (top) 22k gold finish and 5 charms* **MP $75 complete, $10 each charm**
Charms awarded in following sequence —
Avon Lady
The Door, *inscribed "Avon Calling . . . Guaranteed to Please"*
Heart, *inscribed "Quality and Service Are the Heart of Avon"*
Clock, *inscribed "Avon Hours . . . Time for Opportunity"*
Rose Locket, *inscribed "Avon . . . a History of Beauty since 1886"*

1969 *Representative's Charm Bracelet, with Doorknocker, Bell, Avon Rose, Spinner and Acorn charms* **MP $50 complete, $8 each charm**

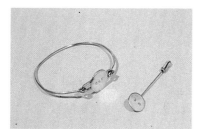

1979 *Circle of Excellence Sterling Silver Bracelet and Stick Pin. Bracelet* **MP $90,** *Pin* **MP $30**

1979 *Circle of Excellence Winners Pin* **MP $20**

Avon, the world's largest cosmetic company, presents these symbols of success to those who helped the company to greatness.

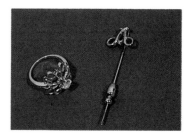

1968 *Manager's ¼ carat Diamond Ring* **MP $425**
1978 *President's Celebration Award. Sterling Silver Stickpin to top ten Reps in each District* **MP $25**

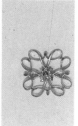

1961 *Manager's 4-A Pin with 11 diamond "M"* **MP $130**

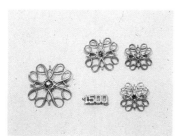

1961 *Representative's Diamond 4-A Pin Award* **MP $55**
1963 *Sapphire 4-A Pin Award* **MP $35**
1963-70 *Pearl 4-A Pin Award* **MP $28**
1973 *Ruby 4-A President's Club Membership Pin* **MP $18**

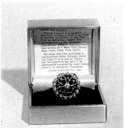

1971 *Manager's diamond and pearls Circle of Excellence Ring* **MP $300**

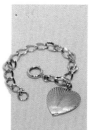

1953 *Valentine's Gift to Representatives. Sterling Silver Bracelet and Heart charm inscribed "1953"* **MP $65**

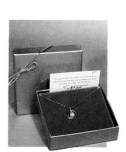

1978 *Manager's specially boxed Cultured Pearl Necklace* **MP $75 boxed with card**

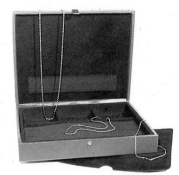

January – Carnation
February – Violet
March – Daffodil
April – Daisy
May – Lily of the Valley
June – Rose
July – Lily
August – Gladiolus
September – Aster
October – Calendula
November – Chrysanthemum
December – Jonquil

1967 *81st Anniversary Sterling Silver Pins. Winning Reps could choose 1 of 12 exclusive flower-of-the-month designs* **MP $25, $35 boxed**

The grace and fragrance of a Year of Flowers, each one a favorite in someone's collection. . .

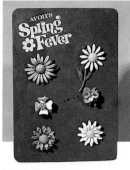

1968 *Spring Fever Pins. Representative's recommendation prizes* **MP $6 each pin, $50 with card**

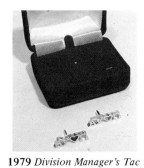

1979 *Division Manager's Tac Pin with red enamel heart* **MP $35**
1979 *Manager's Tac Pin, "Thanks America" promotion, engraved DM on back* **MP $25**
1979 *Representative's Pin, as above, not engraved* **MP $15**

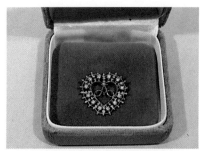

1977 *Gold and 12-diamond Pin, Sales Achievement Award to Representative with highest yearly sales in each Division* **MP $1000**

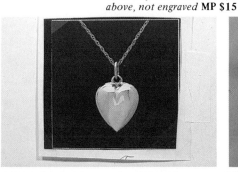

1978 *Valentine Sweepstakes 14k gold Pendant and chain. A winning Rep in each District, 2500 total. Retail value $50* **MP $70 boxed**

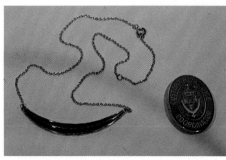

1978 *Smile Necklace, engraved "Team Leader March 1978"* **MP $15**, *Manager's engraved "D.M."* **MP $20**
1977 *Division Manager's Award, Pasadena Branch* **MP $15**

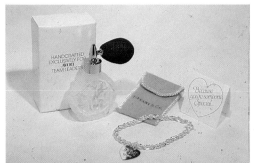

1975 *Representative's Jewelry Display Case for reaching sales goal* **MP $7**

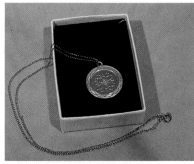

1977 *Representative's Sales Achievement Award Pendant to top 10% in each Division* **MP $25**

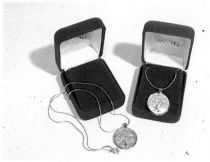

1980 *President's Celebration goldtone Oak Tree Pendant awarded to 20 Representative's in each District* **MP $20**
1980 *Silvertone Oak Tree Pendant Representatives of Number One District in each Division* **MP $50**

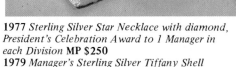

1980 *Team Leader Cologne Atomizer, embossed "TL" on bottom* **MP $10, Manager's emb. DM MP $20**
1980 *Manager's Sterling Silver Bracelet by Tiffany with heart Charm engraved "DM"* **MP $110**

1977 *Sterling Silver Star Necklace with diamond, President's Celebration Award to 1 Manager in each Division* **MP $250**
1979 *Manager's Sterling Silver Tiffany Shell Award inscribed "1979 Sales Leader"* **MP $150**

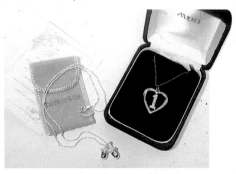

1981 *Manager Silver Acorn Necklace by Tiffany* **MP $125**
1976 *Manager's Necklace Award* **MP $100**

1977 *Silvery Pendant Necklaces* hold "Inch of Ariane" fragrance —

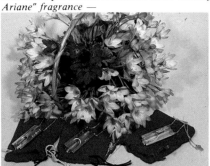

Manager's Bouquet with Silvery Pendant engraved "August Conference 1977" in bag with red drawstrings **MP $50**
Representative's Pendant in bag with black drawstrings **MP $15**
President's Club Members Pendant engraved "P.C." in bag with silver drawstrings **MP $25**

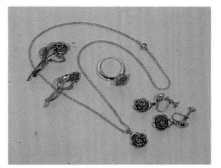

1971 *85th Anniversary Awards of 22k gold-plated sterling silver in shape of roses with diamond, large Pin (President's Club Members)* **MP $35.**, *small Pin* **MP $25**, *Pendant* **MP $40**, *Ring (2 awarded per District)* **MP $85**, **Earrings MP $35**

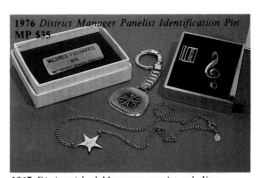

1976 *District Manager Panelist Identification Pin* **MP $35**

1967 *Distinguished Management Award, Key Chain and Fob* **MP $35**
1968 *Manager's Award, "G" Clef Pin 14k for "Making Beautiful Music with Avon"* **MP $50, $60 boxed**
1975 *Manager's Sunny Star Necklace, engraved on back "August 1975"* **MP $15 boxed**

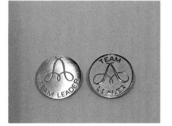

1974 *Team Leader Pin* **MP $12**
1975 *Team Leader Pin* **MP $12**

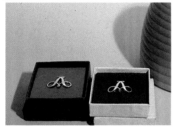

1976 *Step Up to Stardom "A" Pin Award for Sales Achievements* **MP $7**
1976 *As above, first issued in white box* **MP $9**

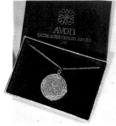

1977 *Representative's Sales Achievement Award Pendant to top 10% in each Division* **MP $25**

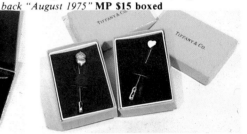

1978 *Manager's Appreciation Gifts. Sterling Silver Acorn and Heart Stickpins by Tiffany.* **MP $50 each, boxed with card.**

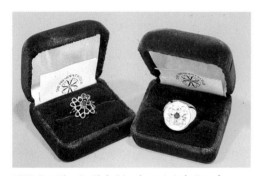

1978 *President's Club Members 4-A designed ruby Ring* **MP $50**
1978 *Men's President's Club Members ruby Ring* **MP $200**

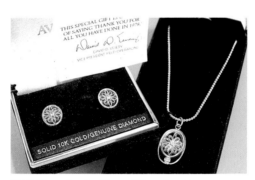

1978 *Team Leader Xmas Gift, 10k gold and diamond Earrings* **MP $55**
1979 *Manager's Xmas Gift, 10k gold with 2 diamonds. Engraved "District Manager 1979 Avon 10k" on back of Pendant* **MP $150**
1979 *Team Leaders Xmas Gift (not shown) as above* **MP $90**

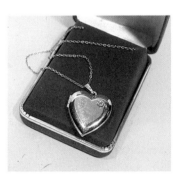

1979 *President's Celebration diamond Heart Locket Award* **MP $30.** *Same Locket inscribed DM on back* **MP $40**

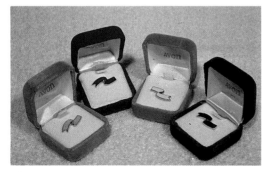

1980 *Manager's Royal Ribbons Award Pins. Yellow* **MP $20**, *Red* **MP $25**, *White* **MP $30**, *Blue* **MP $35**

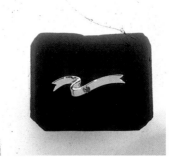

1983 *President's Club Pin. Awarded with one, two, three and four rubies. Pin with one ruby* **MP $20, add $15 ea. additional ruby**

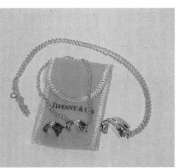

1983 *President's Celebration. Pin to Reps in Top Team* **MP $20**
Bracelet to 10 Reps each District **MP $30**
Necklace to 2 Reps each District **MP $50**

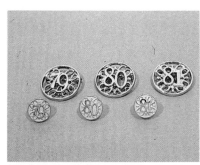

Women's President's Club Membership Pin (top row) **1979 MP $20, 1980 MP $15, 1981 MP $15** *Men's President's Club Membership Tie Tac* **1979 MP $30, 1980 MP $25, 1981 MP $25**

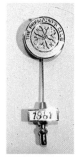

1981 *Presidents Club Pin* **MP $15**

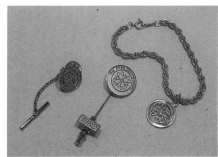

1982 *Men's President's Club Tac Pin* **MP $20** **1982** *Women's President's Club Pin* **MP $10** **1982** *Top 10 District Award Bracelet* **MP $30**

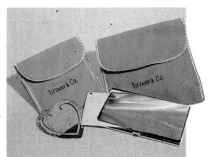

Heart Bookmark Award, sterling silver by Tiffany **MP $35** *Business Card Holder for Pres. Club Members Award, sterling silver by Tiffany* **MP $45**

The *"Jeweled A"* honors Representatives' Achievement

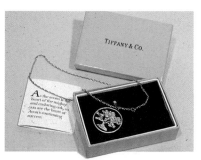

1980 *President's Celebration Oak Tree Necklace awarded to Managers* **MP $110**

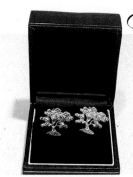

1980 *Great Oak Cuff Links. Division Manager Award* **MP $250**

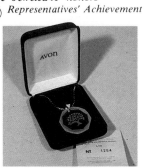

1981 *Tree of Life Pendant awarded to Managers with numbered card* **MP $45** **Add $5 with card**

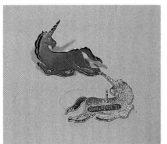

1981 *Unicorn Pin Awards Team Leader Pin* **MP $15** *Manager Pin* **MP $25**

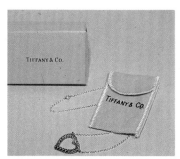

1981 *Heart Necklace. Sterling silver by Tiffany. Awarded to Test Market Managers, Opportunities Unlimited* **MP $160**

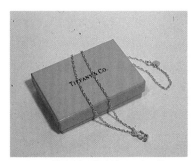

1982 *Teddy Bear Necklace. Sterling silver by Tiffany. Awarded to Team Leaders* **MP $35**

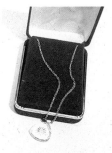

District Manager 15 year Service Award. Pendant with ruby **MP $60**

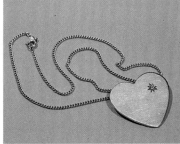

1976 *Presidents Celebration Champion. Awarded one per Division for top sales to District Manager* **MP $40**

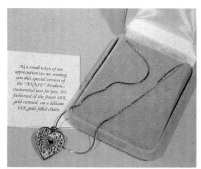

1982 *Annie Pendant awarded to District Managers. 18k gold Vermiel on 14k gold filled chain* **MP $100**

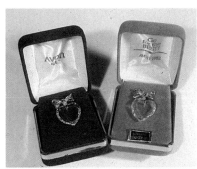

1982 *Lead Crystal Heart Sales Challenge Awards. Representative* **MP $20** *Manager* **MP $30**

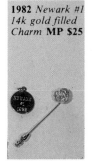

1982 *Newark #1 14k gold filled Charm* **MP $25**

Silver Rose Stick Pin, 25th Anniv. Morton Grove **MP $25**

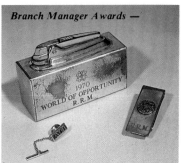

Branch Manager Awards —

1970 *"World of Opportunity" Cigarette Lighter* **MP $125** *Avon Tie Tac Pin* **MP $40** **1963** *Pathways of Achievement Money Clip* **MP $150**

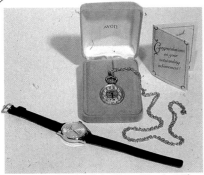
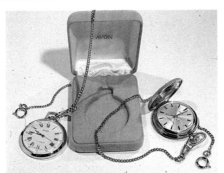
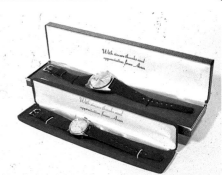

1974 *President's Club Wrist Watch. "The President's Club" and 4—A symbol on face.* **MP $55**
1980 *President's Club 17-jewel Pendant Watch with "Albee" engraved on back* **MP $55**

1980 *Men's President's Club Pocket Watches, both engraved "President's Club 1981"* **MP $150 each**

1977 *Male Manager's Wrist Watch* **MP $200**
1977 *Manager's Wrist Watch* **MP $125**

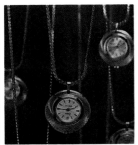
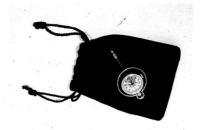
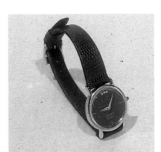
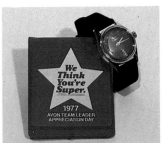

1970 *Sheffield Pendant Watch awarded to 6 Representatives from each District for superior sales achievement* **MP $50**

1979 *Manager's Stick Pin Watch* **MP $75**

Managers Three Diamond **Feraud** *Watch Award* **MP $150**

1977 *Team Leader Mirror, Appreciation Day gift* **MP $8**
1977 *Team Leader Christmas Gift, Jeweled Wrist Watch with floating "Avon" second hand* **MP $70**

WATCHES

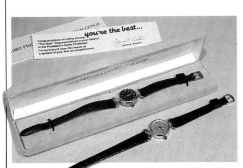
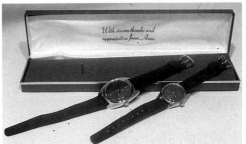
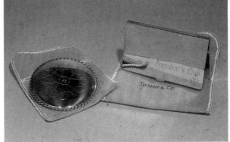

1982 *President's Sales Challenge Watches. Black face, one per District* **MP $110,** *Gold face, 20 per District* **MP $55**

1977 *Team Leader Christmas Gift, jeweled wrist watch with floating "Avon" second hand. Male Team Leader* **MP $150,** *Female Team Leader* **MP $70**

1980 *10 Year Service Award, 3" Purse Mirror by Tiffany* **MP $45**
Sterling Business Card Holder by Tiffany, Pres. Club **MP $45**

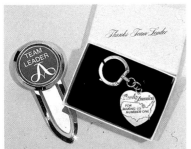
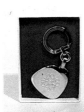
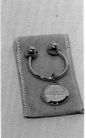
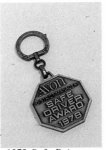
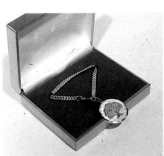

1974 *Team Leader Bookmark* **MP $18**
1979 *Team Leader Key Ring & Heart Medallion inscribed "Thanks for Making Us No. 1"* **MP $15**

1975 *Manager's Boca or Bust Key Ring with 4-A design* **MP $20**

1971 *Key Ring, gift to employees. Medallion reads "Avon" on one side and "You're In Demand" on reverse* **MP $30**

1978 *Safe Driver Award Key Chain to Managers* **MP $20**

1980 *Men's President's Celebration Award Key Chain* **MP $100**

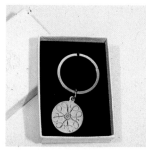

1982 *Key Chain Award for 12 new recruits* **MP $15**

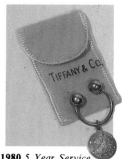

5 Year Service Award Key Chain **MP $20**

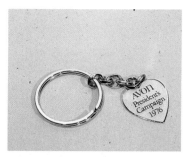

1980 *5 Year Service Award Key Ring* **MP $25**

1976 President's Celebration Key Chain **MP $15**

EMPLOYEE SERVICE AWARDS

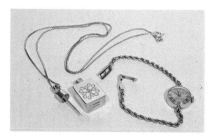

1980 *Perfume Vial 10 Year Service Award Sterling Silver by Tiffany* **MP $65** *25 Year Service Award Watch* **MP $100**

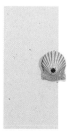

1954 15 Year Service Award Pin **MP $25**

Perfect Attendance Pin Award **MP $20**

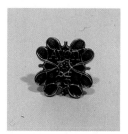

1970 *25 Year Employee Service Award, rare* **MP $150**

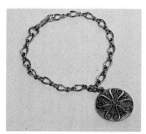

15 Year Service Award 10k gold Charm and Chain Bracelet Awarded to Employees **MP $150**

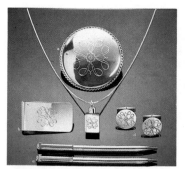

1980 *10 Year Service Awards. Sterling by Tiffany. Purse Mirror* **MP $45**, *Money Clip* **MP $45**, *Perfume Vial Pendant* **MP $65**, *Cufflinks* **MP $50**, *Pen and Pencil* **MP $55**

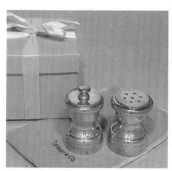

15 Year Service Award. Salt and Pepper. Sterling by Tiffany **MP $75**

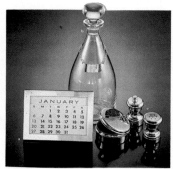

1980 *15 Year Service Awards by Tiffany. Choice of Perpetual Calendar, Crystal Decanter, Salt & Pepper, Pin and Stud Box* **MP $75 each**

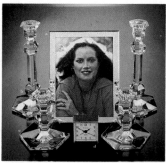

1980 *20 Year Service Awards by Tiffany. Choice of Sterling Picture Frame, Quartz Brass Clock* **MP $100 ea.** *9¼" Crystal Candlesticks, 4½" Crystal Candlesticks* **MP $75 each**

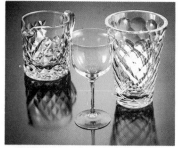

1980 *20 Year Service Awards by Tiffany. Choice of Crystal Pitcher, Crystal Vase* **MP $60 ea.** *or 6 Crystal Tulip Wine Glasses* **MP $75 set**

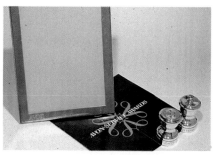

1980 *20 Year Service Award. Sterling Silver by Tiffany 9x7" Picture Frame* **MP $100**

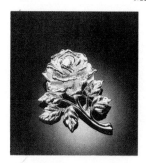

Representative 30 Year Service Award Pin 14k gold with diamond **MP $150**

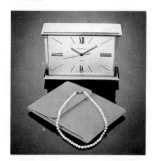

1980 *30 Year Service Awards. Choice of Polished Brass Quartz Clock or Cultured Pearl Necklace with 14k gold clasp* **MP $150 each**

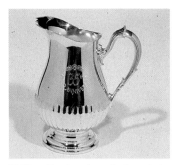

35 Year Service Award. Awarded to Representatives for 35 years service. Silver plated by Tiffany **MP $180**

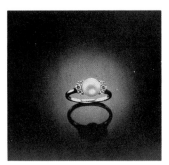

1983 Representatives 35 Year Service Award. 14k gold Ring with pearl and diamonds **MP $180**

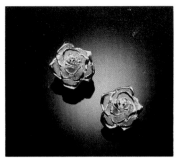

1983 Representatives 35 Year Service Award. 14k gold Rose Bud Earrings with diamonds **MP $180**

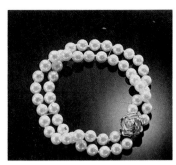

1983 Representatives 40 Year Service Award. Pearl Bracelet, 14k Rose Bud Clasp with diamond **MP $180**

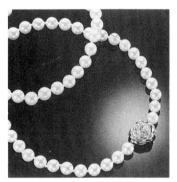

1983 Representatives 45 Year Service Award. 20" Strand of Pearls with 14k clasp and a diamond **MP $210**

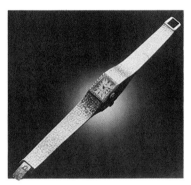

1983 Representatives 50 Year Service Award. 14k gold Tiffany Watch with diamonds **MP $300**

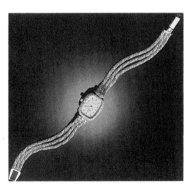

1983 Representatives 50 Year Service Award. 14k gold Tiffany Watch with diamonds **MP $300**

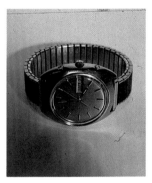

Employees 25 Year Service Award. Omega Watch **MP $150**

COMPREHENSIVE MODELS

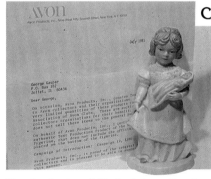

Little Miss Muffet **MP $250**

Test Production of Mother's Love Figurine with Avon Certification Letter. Approx. 24 issued **MP $150**

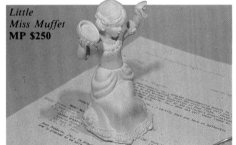

*O*ne-of-a-kind comprehensive mock-ups used for photography in Avon Brochures. Each is shown with a letter of certification from Avon Products, Inc.

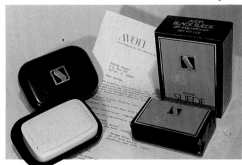

1980 Black Suede Soap Dish and Soap **MP $175**

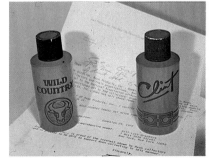

1977 Lotions from Men's Travel Sets, Wild Country and Clint **MP $50 each**

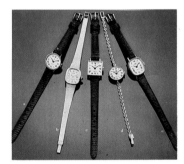

Women Employee 25 Year Service Award. Choice of 14k gold Watches, different straps **MP $130**

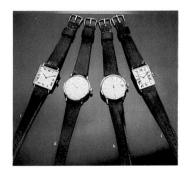

Male Employee 25 Year Service Award. Choice of 14k gold Watches, different straps **MP $150**

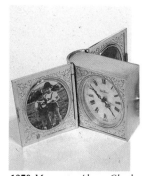
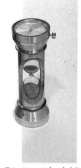
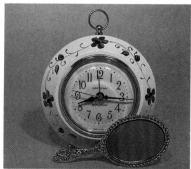
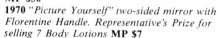
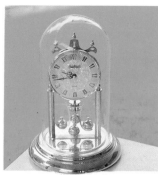

1970 *Memento Alarm Clock by Seth Thomas. Recommendation Gift. (No engraving on back)* **MP $35**

1968 *Distinguished Management Award. Brushed gold paperweight/clock in one end, engraved on other end and a 3-minute timer in center* **MP $175**

1971 *"Tole-Alarm" Solid Wood, Hand Painted Clock by Seth Thomas. Recommendation Prize* **MP $30**
1970 *"Picture Yourself" two-sided mirror with Florentine Handle. Representative's Prize for selling 7 Body Lotions* **MP $7**

40 Year Service Award Clock **MP $250**

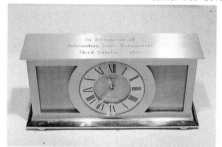
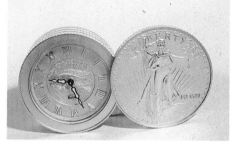
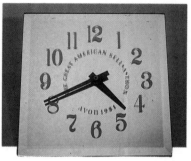

1977 *Manager's 15-jewel Clock Award engraved "Outstanding Sales Management Third Quarter 1977"* **MP $125**

1977 *Million Dollar Baby Clock by Bulova awarded only to 40 Managers for outstanding sales increase* **MP $150**

1981 *Great American Sell-A-Thon Clock Prize* **MP $50**

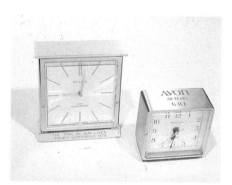
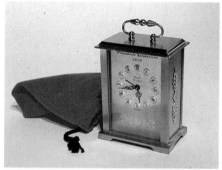
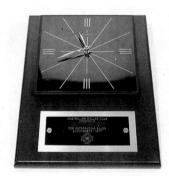

District Manager 20 year Service Award Clock by Tiffany **MP $75**
1978 *"The Time of Our Lives" District Manager's August Conference Gift.* **MP $75**

1974 *President's Celebration Award Clock by Relide. Awarded to top Representatives in three Divisions. Approx. 250 awarded.* **MP $200**

1977 *Division Manager's Million Dollar Club Clock* **MP $200**

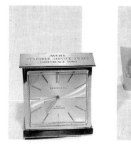
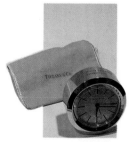
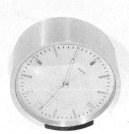
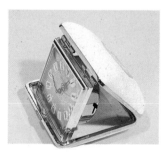

1980 *Conference, Customer Service Clock Award* **MP $140**
Circle of Excellence Award Clock **MP $60**

1981 *Division Manager's Clock by Tiffany. Opportunities Unlimited Christmas Gift* **MP $100**

1982 *Manager's Recruiting Award Clock by Tiffany* **MP $100**

1977 *Hours for Excellence Travel Clock awarded to C of E Managers* **MP $40**

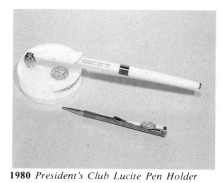
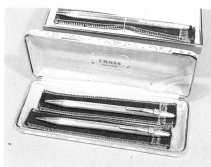
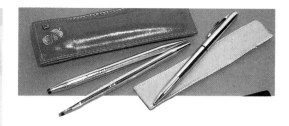

1980 *President's Club Lucite Pen Holder and Pen* **MP $25**
1950 *Gold Lead Pencil* **MP $50**

1969 *Cross Sterling Pen and Pencil Set. 4-A insignia on clips* **MP $45**

1970 *Avon employees 15 year Award, 14k gold Cross Pen and Pencil set, engraved "Avon 15 years" and initials. Case has ruby in 4-A* **MP $65**
1969 *14k gold Cross Pen with 4-A symbol on clip* **MP $40**

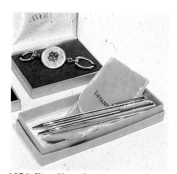
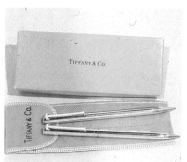
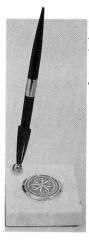
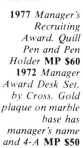
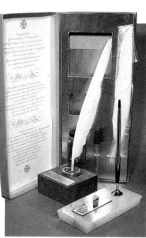

1974 *Five Year Service Award to employees, come-apart Key Ring with 4-A design* **MP $35 boxed**
1979 *Ten Year Service Award to employees, gold Pen and Pencil Set by Tiffany. Personalized with initials* **MP $50 boxed**

Manager's Sterling Silver Pen and Pencil Set by Tiffany, letter "T" serves as pocket clip **MP $125**

1974 *88th Anniversary Award. Marble Pen Stand and Pen for $125 order* **MP $25**

1977 *Manager's Recruiting Award. Quill Pen and Pen Holder* **MP $60**
1972 *Manager Award Desk Set, by Cross. Gold plaque on marble base has manager's name and 4-A* **MP $50**

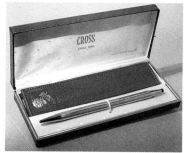
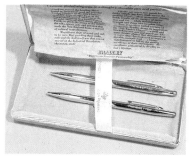
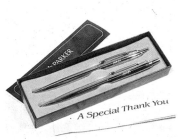
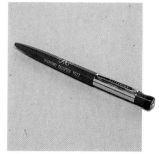

1976 *Cross 14k gold filled Pen engraved "Avon Calling" with Rose embossed case. Recommendation gift* **MP $25**

Chrome plated Pen and Pencil Set Award, engraved "Trendsetter" **MP $25**

Parker Pen and Pencil Set Award, engraved "Avon 3rd Quarter Achievement" **MP $30**

1977 *Diamond Quarter Pen. Simulated diamond on lid, Springdale Branch Award* **MP $25**

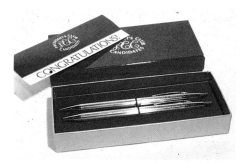
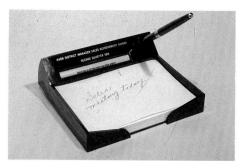
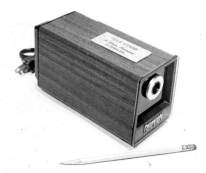

1980 *Representative's Gold Pen and Pencil Set engraved "President's Club Candidate" awarded to new Representatives for sales of $250 in 4 consecutive campaigns* **MP $27 with pen refill**

1979 *Manager's Sales Achievement Award 2nd Quarter* **MP $25**

1979 *Manager's Panasonic Pencil Sharpener with engraved nameplate. Christmas Conference gift* **MP $40**

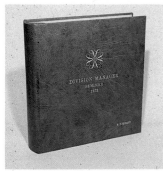

1973 *Division Manager's Seminar loose-leaf Binder* **MP $50**

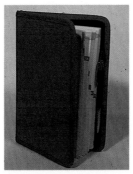

1977 *Team Leader gift, Address Book with note pad and pen has a suede-like cover* **MP $7**

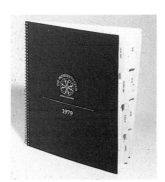

1979 *Date Book, only to President's Club Members attending annual luncheon* **MP $15**

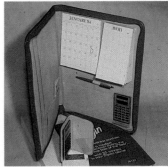

Sales Award. Zippered Portfolio with Calendar, Calculator, Pen and Note Pad **MP $125**
Sales Award. Solar Calculator with case **MP $15**

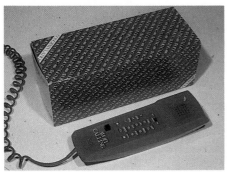

1983 *Zip Telephone. President's Club Award* **MP $37**

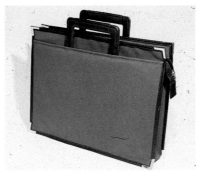

1981 *Manager's Attache Case* **MP $35**

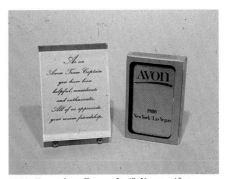

1970 *Frameless Frame 3x4" Xmas gift to Team Captains (later called Team Leaders)* **MP $20**
1979 *Boxed deck of Playing Cards. N.Y. to Las Vegas promotional gift to all Division Managers* **MP $30**

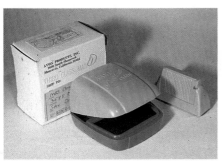

1972 *Name Stamp, President's Club members Award* **MP $8**

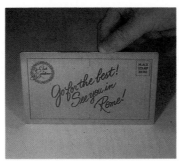

Circle of Excellence Brass Postcard Award **MP $75**

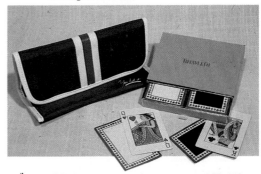

"You Did It!" Wallet Award to Managers **MP $12**
Tiffany Playing Cards. Manager Award **MP $17**

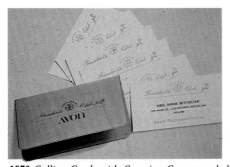

1970 *Calling Cards with Carrying Case awarded to President's Club Members* **MP $10**

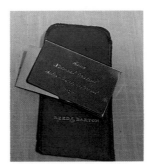

1982 *National District Sales Manager Panel. Business Card Holder* **MP $50**

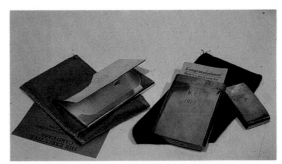

1979 *District Manager Quarterly Sales Increase, engraved Card Case Award, silver* **MP $50**, *brass* **MP $40**

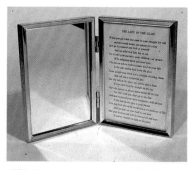

1979 *Manager Conference Gift Framed Mirror and "The Lady in The Glass" Poem* **MP $20**

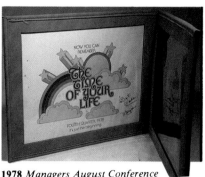

1978 *Managers August Conference Picture Frame. Suede like cover* **MP $20**

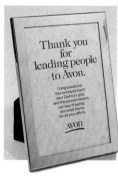

1978 *Picture Frame to Team Leaders for soliciting recommendations* **MP $12**

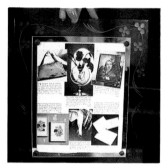

1943 *Etched Glass Frame shown holding page from Dec. 1943 Outlook that offered frame as prize to Representatives with $75 to $99.99 in customer sales* **MP $200**

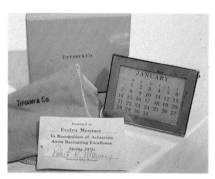

1979 *District Managers Calendar Award by Tiffany for recruiting* **MP $40**

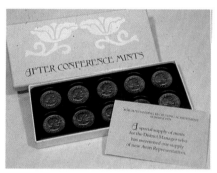

1979 *After Conference Mints Manager Recruiting Award. Holds 50 Susan B. Anthony Dollars* **MP $100**

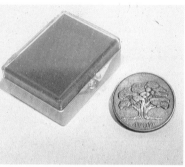

1980 *Coin Award, Pasadena Branch, pictures Oak tree. Opposite side, with Avon crest reads "Pasadena #1 1980"* **MP $50 boxed**

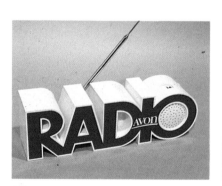

1980 *Avon Transistor Radio* **MP $75**

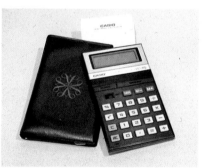

1980 *Customized Casio Calculator in wallet cover with Avon crest. Recommendation prize* **MP $22**

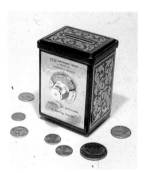

1980 *Bank Award to Managers in Springdale Branch* **MP $45**

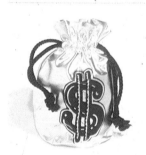

1980 *Money Bag Award. Bag only* **MP $20**

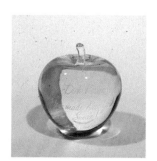

1978 *"Big Apple" Glass Paperweight etched "Dick Kovac You Made New York Smile" Sales Achievement Award* **MP $110**

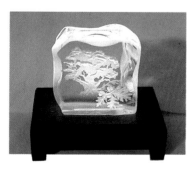

1980 *Great Oak Lamp. Awarded to Managers at Conference* **MP $110**

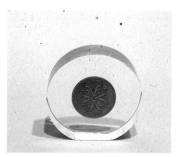

1980 *Pasadena Branch Paper Weight Award with Avon crest, inscribed "Pasadena #1" Reverse pictures Oak Tree* **MP $100**

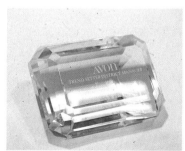

1981 *Trendsetter District Manager Award. Lucite Paper Weight by Tiffany* **MP $90**

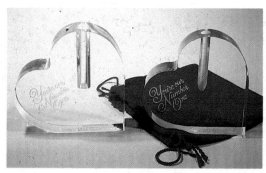

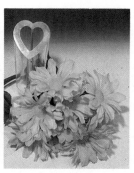

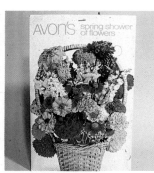

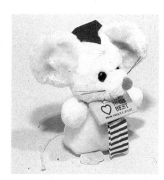

1979 *President's Celebration Commemorative Lucite Heart Bud Vase to Representatives in winning Districts* **MP $25 boxed**
1979 *Manager's Lucite Heart Bud Vase in suede-like drawstring bag* **MP $35**

1981 *Subtle Reflections Lucite Vase & Silk Flowers awarded to Pres. Club Members* **MP $15**

Avon's Spring Shower of Flowers. Packet of Flower Seeds **MP $10**

1982 *Valentine's Day Gift to Managers "To the Best from your N.Y. Buddy"* **MP $30**

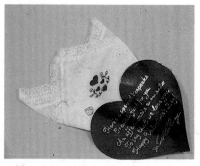

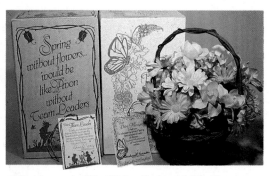

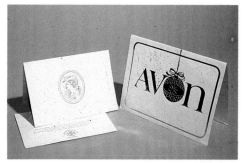

1982 *Valentine's Day Gift to President's Club Members* **MP $8**

1980 *Manager's Gift. Wicker Basket of Silk Flowers* **MP $35**
1980 *Team Leader Gift. Wicker Basket of Silk Flowers.* **MP $25**

1980 *President's Club Members token gift, Box of 25 Note Cards and matching Envelopes* **MP $8**
1980 *Avon Christmas Card given to Managers to send to Representatives* **MP $2 each**

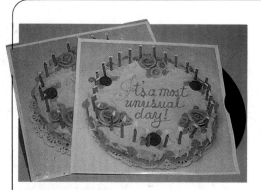

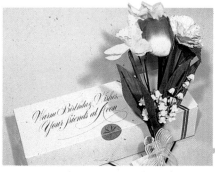

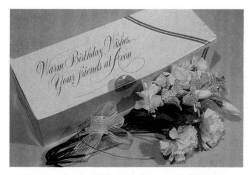

1981 *Happy Birthday Record. "It's A Most Unusual Day" given to President's Club Members* **MP $8**

1980 *President's Club Members Birthday Gift. Bouquet of fabric Flowers, boxed* **MP $17**

1980 *President's Club Members Birthday Gift. Bouquet of fabric Flowers, boxed* **MP $17**

REPRESENTATIVE BIRTHDAY GIFTS

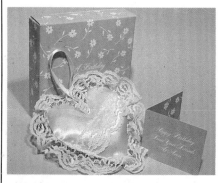

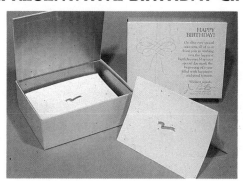

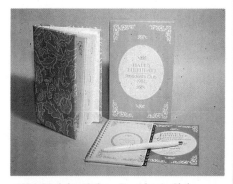

1982 *Birthday Gift to Representatives. Lace-trimmed Pillowette* **MP $8**

1983 *Birthday Gift to Representatives* **MP $7**

1984 *Birthday Gift to President's Club Members* **MP $7**

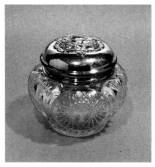

1912 CPC Powder Puff Jar, crystal with silverplate lid. For sales of $50 in December, Canadian orders of $66.65 **MP $250**

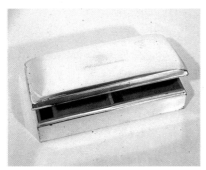

1961 Christmas gift. Cigarette Case, lid engraved with 4-A design and Christmas 1961 **MP $55**

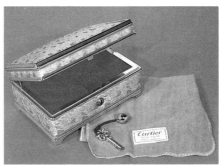

1966 "Sound of the Seasons" Music Box by Cartier, with Key and jingle bell, plays Sound of Music. To managers for reaching 4th quarter sales projections. (No pin included) **MP $90 with felt bag, $70 box only**

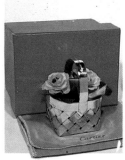

1978 Sterling Silver Basket of Roses by Cartier. Increased Sales Award to one Manager in each Division **MP $110**

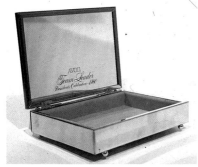

1980 Jewelry Box engraved "Avon Team Leader President's Celebration 1980" **MP $22**

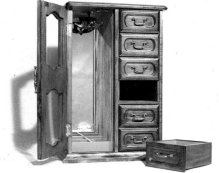

1981 Christmas Gift to Managers and Team Leaders. Musical, plays "You Light Up My Life", engraved Team Leader **MP $75**, *engraved Manager* **MP $125**

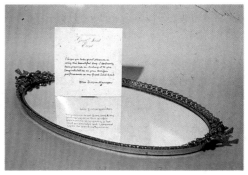

1980 Scent Event Vanity Tray to 15 Representatives per District for top sales of Cologne Sprays in C-9 **MP $25 with letter**

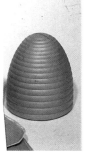

1968 Beehive Bank, Manager's Gift introducing Silk & Honey **MP $18**

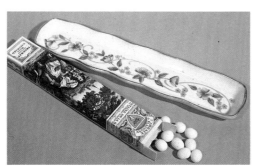

1977 Port O'Call Pasadena Candy Dish and candy **MP $20**

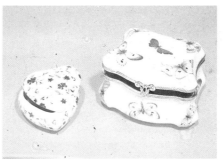

1979 Manager Award Limoges Trinket Box **MP $35**
1980 Manager Award Limoges Porcelain Hinged Trinket Box **MP $30**

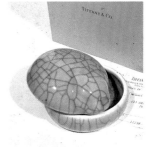

1980 Manager Award. China Trinket Box **MP $25**

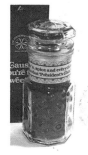

1980 Candy Jar and Candy gift to President's Club Members **MP $15 boxed**
1980 Covered Crystal Dish, Valentine's Gift to Team Leaders **MP $18 with card**

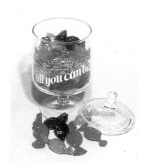

1983 "All You Can Be" Candy Jar to Managers at Conference **MP $15**

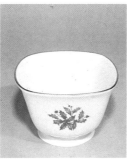

1982 Managers Lenox Candy Dish from Division Manager **MP $20**

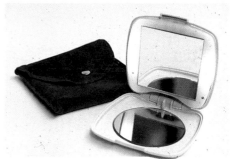

1981 Representative's Award. Look-A-Lite lighted makeup mirror by Schildkraut, made exclusively for Avon, with carrying bag **MP $32 with bag and boxed**

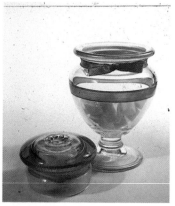

1924 *CPC American Beauty Fragrance Jar, painted. Representative's Gift* **MP $300**

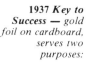

FRAGRANCE and PRODUCT INTRODUCTION AWARDS and GIFTS

Awards and gifts of jewelry, china, perfumes, cosmetics and more . . . each in specially designed packaging created exclusively for Avon Representatives.

1937 *Key to Success* — *gold foil on cardboard, serves two purposes:*

Representative's Award for writing letters on their success selling a particular Avon product. Only 2 awarded each campaign **MP $20**

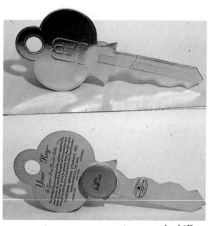

(top) With miniature container attached (Face Powder shown). Token gift for "Greater Face Powder Sales", etc. **MP $35** *(with product)*

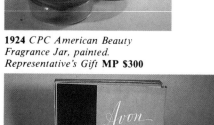

1942 *56th Anniversary Gift. The Album holds pictures and messages from Avon personnel and two sachet pillowettes. Gold imprinted on back "From Your Friends at the Avon Laboratories. . . 56th Anniversary 1942."* **MP $125 complete, $30 each pillowette**

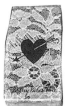
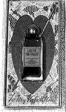

1940's *Valentine's Day Gift Perfume 1/8oz* **MP $80**

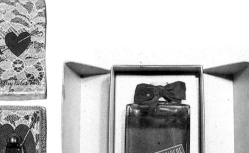

1943 *57th Anniversary Gift Avon Cologne 6oz* **MP $100, $135 boxed**

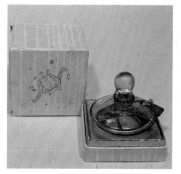

1945 *Ballad Perfume Award 3/8oz, rare* **MP $400**

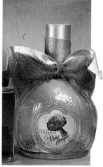

1945 *59th Anniversary Gift, Violet Bouquet Cologne 16oz* **MP $150, $180 boxed**

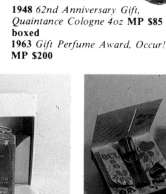

1948 *62nd Anniversary Gift, Quaintance Cologne 4oz* **MP $85 boxed**
1963 *Gift Perfume Award, Occur!* **MP $200**

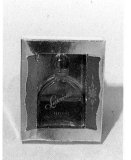

1950 *Luscious Perfume Award 3 drams* **MP $165 boxed**

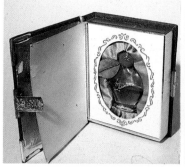

1949 *Representative's 63rd Anniversary Gift Quaintance Perfume 3 dram for selling 63 products during Anniversary campaign* **MP $75, $110 boxed**

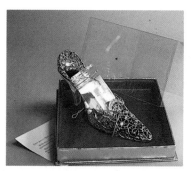

1947 *61st Anniversary Gift, Wishing Cologne* **MP $85, $110 boxed**

1951 *Oct. 8 Gift. 1 dram Forever Spring. introduced October 8th* **MP $55 boxed**

1959 *Golden Slipper Award. Topaze Perfume 1oz to one winning District of each Branch in Avon's 73rd Anniversary contest. Slipper and perfume* **MP $200, $250 boxed**

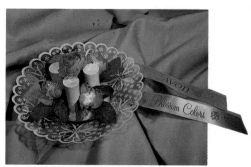

1960 *Representative's Gift, styrofoam Nosegay of Blossom Colors holds 4 new Lipsticks in Peach, Cherry, Plum and Orange Blossom Shades* **MP $75 as shown**

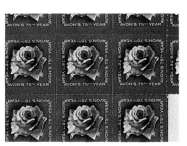

1961 *75th Anniversary Rose Stamps, sheet of 75* **MP $40 sheet, 50¢ each stamp**

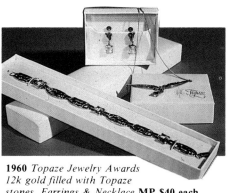

1960 *Topaze Jewelry Awards 12k gold filled with Topaze stones. Earrings & Necklace* **MP $40 each** *14k solid gold Bracelet, highest level* **MP $100**

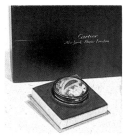

1967 *Hawaiian White Ginger Glace Compact, Representative's Honor Award in President's Campaign* **MP $22**

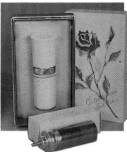

1961 *75th Anniversary Gift, Perfume Mist in Somewhere* **MP $16 as shown**

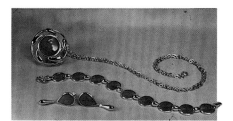

1968 *Charisma Jewelry Awards —*
Convertible Necklace/Pin **MP $15**
Bracelet **MP $15**
Earrings **MP $15**

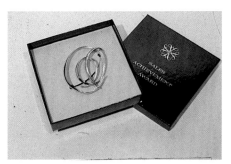

1968 *Sales Achievement Award, Charisma Pin* **MP $25**

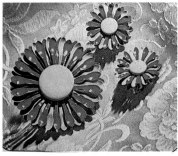

1970 *Hana Gasa Jewelry. Enameled Pin and Earrings, Recommendation Prize* **MP $30 set**

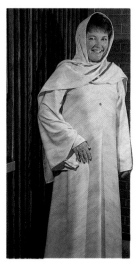

A delightful array of Fragrance Introduction awards for high sales achievement.

1974 *Timeless Caftan. Given to Managers at August Conference on introduction* **MP $50**

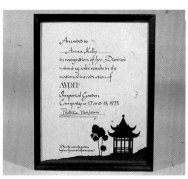

1973 *Imperial Garden framed Award Certificate. For sales in C-17 — C-18 1973* **MP $70**

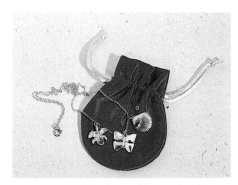

1979 *Manager's Tasha Necklace, 18k gold over Sterling Silver with flower, butterfly and seashell Charms. Satin-like drawstring bag serves as box* **MP $35 in bag**

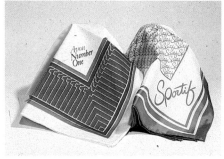

1979 *"Avon Number One" Scarf* **MP $8**
1980 *Sportif Signature Scarf for Representative's order of 10 bottles Cologne Spray in C-6* **MP $6**

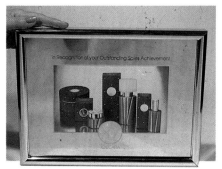

1981 *Toccara Sales Achievement Award* **MP $50**

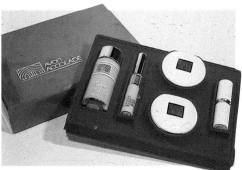

1982 *Accolade Make-Up Set to District Managers* **MP $50**

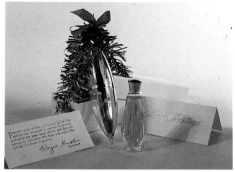

1964 *78th Anniversary Gift (not a Xmas gift) tree ornament holds .4oz Rapture Cologne, Avon's major pre-Christmas fragrance introduction* MP $65 **complete with card,** $45 **ornament and bottle**

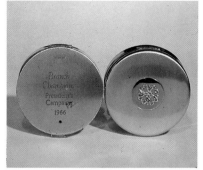

1966 *Deluxe Compact, engraved to Branch Champions, President's Campaign* MP $25

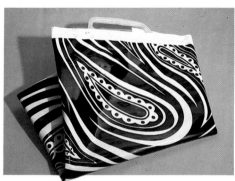

1969 *Patterns designed plastic carry-all bag. For submitting recommendation names* MP $6

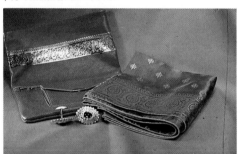

1969 *Elusive Awards: Mini Bag lettered "An S. M. Kent exclusive for Avon by Enger Kress" Scarf with S. M. Kent signature and Avon embossed Cuff Links. Cuff Links* MP $12, *Purse* $15, *Scarf* MP $10. *Blouse (not shown)* MP $20

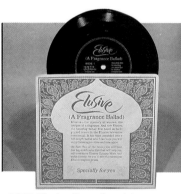

1969 *Elusive Record sent to Representatives at time of Elusive introduction* MP $10

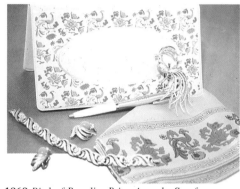

1969 *Bird of Paradise Prize Awards, Scarf* MP $10, *Order Book Cover and Pen* MP $7, *Bracelet and Earrings* MP $20 each, *Pin* MP $15, *Robe (not shown)* MP $35

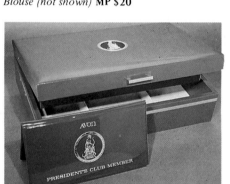

1971 *Moonwind Prizes. Order Book Cover and Pen* MP $7 *Jewelry Box* MP $25 *Robe (not shown)* MP $35

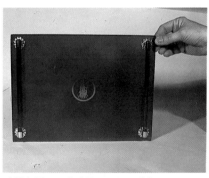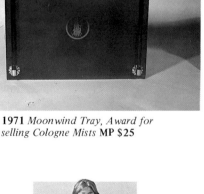

1971 *Moonwind Tray, Award for selling Cologne Mists* MP $25

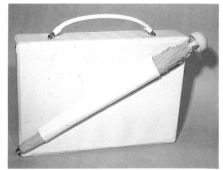

1971 *Field Flowers Awards: Tote Bag* MP $12, *Umbrella* MP $10, *Cape (not shown) with Sash* MP $20

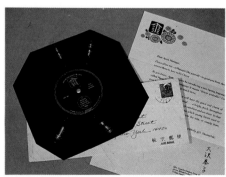

1970 *Hana Gasa 33-1/3 rpm Record with emblem. Given to all Representatives prior to fragrance introduction* MP $16
1970 *Hana Gasa Manager's Letter, from Japanese Manager, relating story of "Hana Gasa"* MP $30 **with envelope**

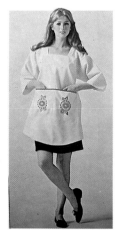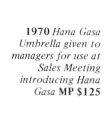

1970 *Hana Gasa Happi-Coat Recommendation gift* MP $35

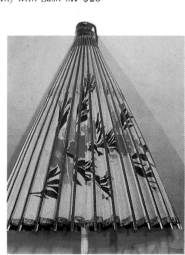

1970 *Hana Gasa Umbrella given to managers for use at Sales Meeting introducing Hana Gasa* MP $125

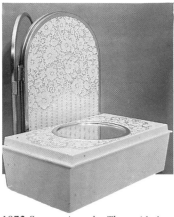

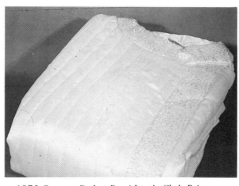

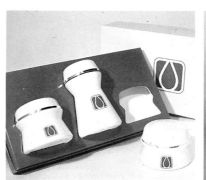

1972 *Sonnet Awards: Three sided mirror* **MP $28** *Vanity Box* **MP $18**

1972 *Sonnet Robe, President's Club Prize* **MP $38**
1972 *Vanity Tray (not shown)* **MP $12**

1975 *Moisture Secret Gift Set to Managers. 4oz Cremegel Cleanser, 5oz Freshener, 3oz Night Concentrate* **MP $25**
1975 *Moisture Secret Night Cream Concentrate 3oz. President's Club Members Gift* **MP $9 boxed with sleeve**

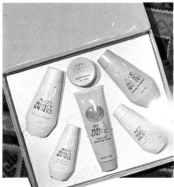

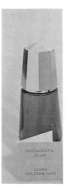

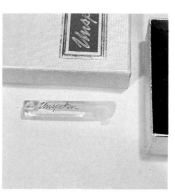

1974 *Perfect Balance Manager's Gift. Freshener and Astringent 6oz each, Cleansing Cream and Lotion 4oz each, Night Cream 2½oz, Moisturizer 3oz* **MP $40**

1974 *President's Club Members Gift. Collector's Edition of Ultra Timeless Cologne Mist 2oz. Embossed 4-A on base of bottle* **MP $15 with card**
1974 *Manager's Timeless Gift Set. 2oz Cologne Mist, .66oz Creme Perfume and Perfume Rollette* **MP $37**

1975 *Vial of Unspoken to Managers only* **MP $15 boxed**

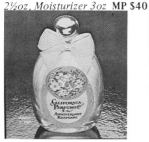

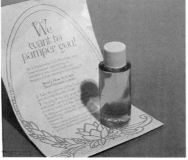

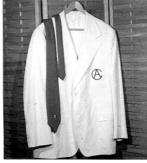

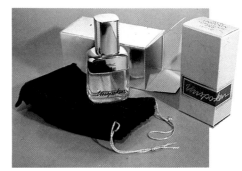

1975 *Manager's California Perfume Co. Anniversary Keepsake Bottle. Limited edition carries the 4-A design on base beneath the label* **MP $20**

1975 *Gift Sample of Queen's Gold Foaming Bath Oil given to President's Club Members, with "Pamper You. . ." Card* **MP $10**

1977 *Candid Blazer and Tie* **MP $110**

1975 *Unspoken, Manager's Gift. Blue velour drawstring bag holds 3oz Cologne Spray, silver outer box* **MP $25 with box**

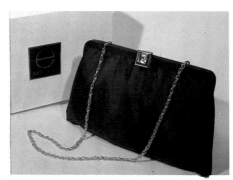

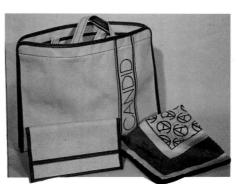

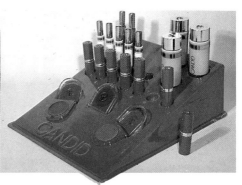

1976 *Emprise Evening Bag. Awarded for highest Emprise sales* **MP $20**

1977 *Candid Prize Awards. Tote Bag* **MP $10**, *Purse Organizer for highest Candid sales* **MP $8**, *Scarf, a gift to President's Club members* **MP $7**

1977 *Manager's Display Tray used at Sales Meetings to hold Candid makeup products* **MP $9 empty**

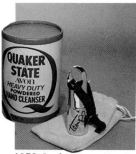

1978 *Quaker State Hand Cleanser, empty container used by Managers as demo at Sales Meeting. Note different lid* **MP $10**
1978 *Manager's Tempo Cologne Portable in drawstring bag* **MP $20**

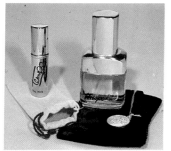

1978 *Tempo Cologne Spray in drawstring bag, designed for Reps only at C-20 Meeting* **MP $12**
1975 *President's Club Members blue velvet drawstring Bag with silver plastic medallion (to carry Unspoken Cologne Spray demo not included)* **MP $5 Bag only**

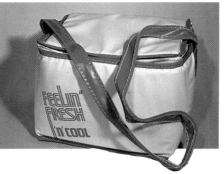

1978 *Feelin' Fresh Insulated Bag, free to Reps with purchase of C-14 demonstration product assortment* **MP $12**

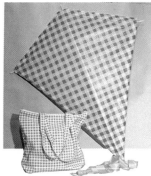

1980 *Country Breeze Kite* **MP $6**
1980 *Country Breeze Tote to Representatives selling 10 bottles Cologne Spray in C-12* **MP $8**

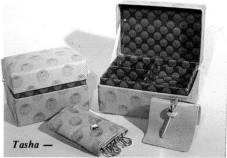

Tasha —
1979 *Wishing Box to Representatives for Cologne Spray pre-order of 10 bottles* **MP $8**
1979 *Dream Box and Fantasy Pin to President's Club Members, 20 bottle order* **MP $25**, **$7 pin only**
1979 *Key Case Award to Representatives with a 40-customer list in Name Book* **MP $6**

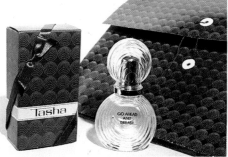

Tasha —
1979 *Manager's Gift Cologne Spray in ribboned box* **MP $15**
1979 *Manager's Tasha-designed Conference Folder* **MP $4**

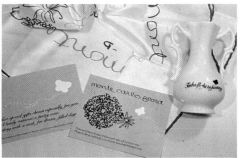

Tasha — Gifts to "Flight to Fantasy" Monte Carlo winners:
1979 *Gift Scarf from Princess Grace Boutique* **MP $35 with card**
1979 *Tasha Flight to Fantasy Vase* **MP $40 with card**

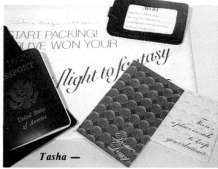

Tasha —
1979 *Flight to Fantasy Passport in suede case* **MP $15 with folder**
1979 *Flight to Fantasy suede Luggage Tag* **MP $10**
1979 *Dream Diary to Representatives at Sales Meeting* **MP $1**

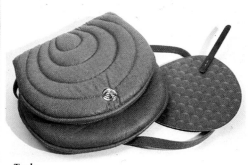

Tasha —
1979 *Stowaway Bag won in Fantasy Sweepstakes by 7 finalists from each District* **MP $30**
1979 *Fantasy Fan to Representatives at C-22 Sales Meeting* **MP $2**

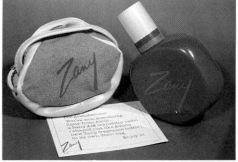

1979 *Zany Sweepstakes AM Transistor Radio and Disco Bag to 25,000 customer Sweepstakes winners* **MP $45, $35 radio only**

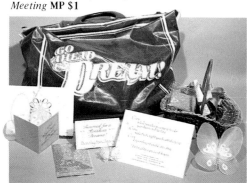

Tasha —
1979 *Manager's Conference Gifts: Tote Bag* **MP $4**, *Basket with Nail Polish and packet of sand from Hawaii* **MP $6**, *Butterflies and Gift Cards* **MP $1 each**

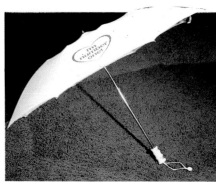
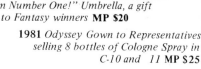

1979 *"I'm Number One!" Umbrella, a gift to Flight to Fantasy winners* **MP $20**

1981 *Odyssey Gown to Representatives selling 8 bottles of Cologne Spray in C-10 and 11* **MP $25**

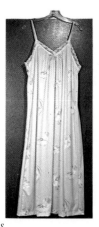
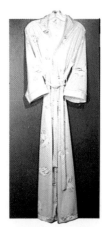

1981 *Robe for selling 15 bottles of Cologne Spray in C-10 and 11* **MP $35**

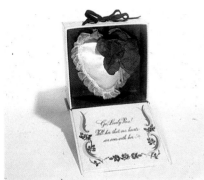

1944 *58th Anniversary Gift to Representatives. Heart shaped Sachet* **MP \$110**

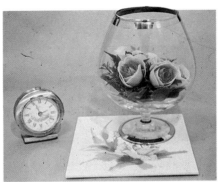

1972 *Roses, Roses Prizes: Clock* **MP \$22,** *Corningware Trivet* **MP \$12,** *Bowl of Roses* **MP \$15**

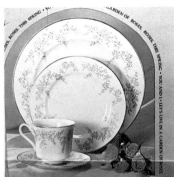

1972 *Mikasa "April Roses" Dinnerware, 65 piece set. One winner in each District in Roses, Roses Spring Sweepstakes, total 1900* **MP \$200 complete set**

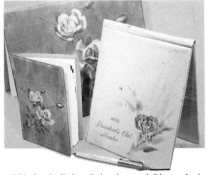

1971 *Desk Folio Calendar and Phone Index Gifts for sending in C-1 & 2 orders* **MP \$13 set**
1972 *Roses, Roses Order Book Cover & Pen* **MP \$7**

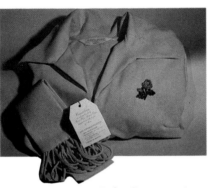

1972 *Roses, Roses Robe. Representative Prize Award* **MP \$35**

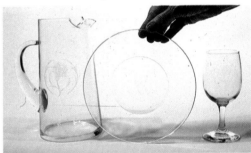

1980 *Avon Rose 94th Anniversary Collection —*
3rd Level: Pitcher, 64oz capacity **MP \$25**
2nd Level: Four 8" diam. Luncheon Plates with rose motif **MP \$8 each**
1st Level: Four 8½oz Goblets with rose motif **MP \$6 each**

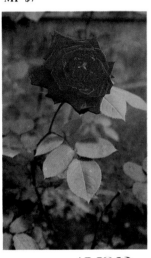

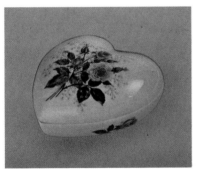

1976 *Porcelain Treasure Box, awarded to each Representative in 252 winning Districts. Bottom inscription "Avon President's Club 1976. Made in Spain"* **MP \$45**

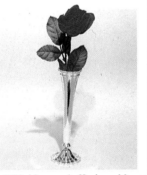

1978 *Manager's Hudson Manor silverplated Bud Vase. Bottom inscription "Avon August Conference"* **MP \$30**

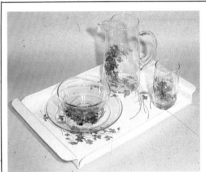

1984 *Wild Violets Collection. 4 different levels. Representative's Sales Award. Entire 20 pc. collection* **MP \$60**

(The Avon Rose is presently grown by Kimbrew-Walter, rose growers of Wills Point, Texas.)

The AVON ROSE

—symbol of beauty and fragrance

Throughout the years, the rose had special significance for Avon. The Queen of Flowers symbolizes 95 years of bringing beauty and fragrance to the American woman.

The loveliness of the Rose is captured in these exclusive Avon creations, designed especially for Representatives as a reward for superior sales achievement.

The living "Avon Rose", developed by Jackson & Perkins, world's largest rose growers, has one of the most intense and persistent fragrances to be found in any rose variety. It was introduced in 1961 in honor of Avon's 75th Anniversary and made its debut at the Annual International Flower Show in New York.

The Avon Rose has a family history that can be traced back 136 years! Its earliest recorded ancestor was a rose called Gloire des Rosomanes that flourished in 1825. Its nearest "kin" are the famous roses Nocturne and Chrysler Imperial. It is also a very close relative of the popular Crimson Glory, another gorgeous rose.

The Avon Rose is a brilliant, scarlet-red hybrid tea rose, particularly noted for its amazing fragrance. It is tall and elegant and keeps its color and perfume as long as it lives.

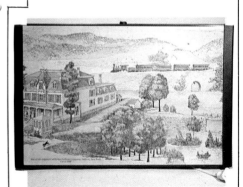

1981 *Electric Warm-O-Tray personalized with a California Perfume Company picture* **MP \$30**

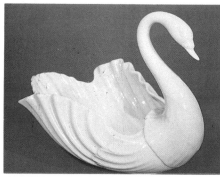

1964 *78th Anniversary Prize. Lenox China Swan* **MP $75**

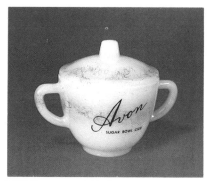

1942 *Representative's Sugar Bowl Award* **MP $60**

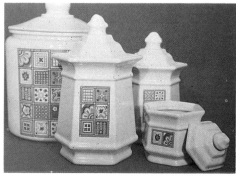

1972 *Patchwork Prize Awards. Patchwork Cookie Jar* **MP $20**, *Canister Set, 3 pieces* **MP $22**

CHINA and CERAMICS

Imperial Garden Prizes

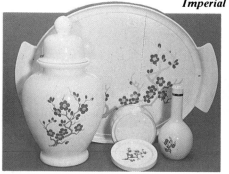

1973 *Melamine Serving Tray* **MP $12**
1973 *Ginger Jar, hand-blown Italian glass 10¾" high* **MP $25**
1973 *Mikasa Garden Bud Vase* **MP $12**
1973 *Coasters, gifts at meeting* **MP $7 each**
1973 *Robe (not shown)* **MP $35**

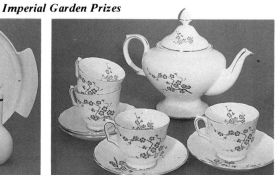

1973 *English Bone China Tea Set with Imperial Garden Motif by Crown Staffordshire, Ltd. of England. Teapot, 4 cups and saucers won by 1 Representative in each District, 2067* **MP $150** *(Rare, limited edition)*

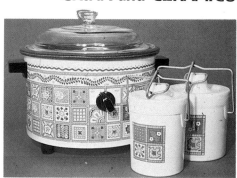

1971 *Patchwork Prize Awards. Crock-Pot Cooker* **MP $35** *Two refrigerator containers* **MP $6 each**

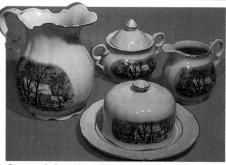

Currier & Ives Porcelain, trimmed in 22k gold. Each piece is marked "Awarded Exclusively to Avon Representatives"
1978 *Pitcher, 1 qt.* **MP $20**
1977 *Sugar & Creamer* **MP $20**
1978 *Butter Dish* **MP $15**

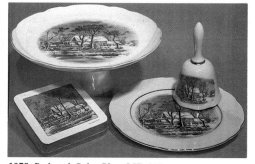

1978 *Pedestal Cake Plate* **MP $50**
1977 *Sweets Plate 8"* **MP $6**
1978 *Dinner Bell* **MP $12**
1978 *Set of 6 Coasters for submitting two Recommendation names* **MP $8 set**

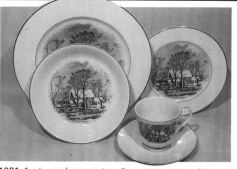

1981 *5 piece place setting Recruiting Award. Plate, Salad Plate, Soup Bowl, Cup and Saucer* **MP $30 set**

Currier & Ives

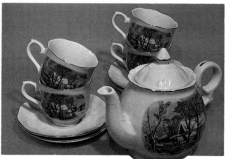

1977 *Four Teacups & Saucers* **MP $35**
1977 *Teapot, 5 cup* **MP $15**

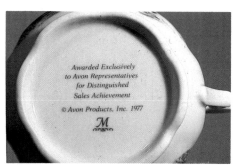

1977 *Manager's Currier & Ives Porcelain marked with "M" on base. Add* **MP $10** *to each piece with "M"*

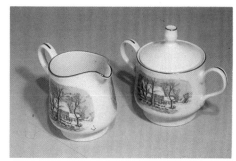

1981 *Creamer & Sugar Recruiting Award* **MP $17**

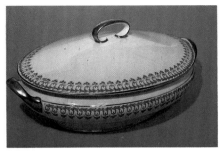

1930's *Covered Vegetable Dish with CPC-Avon printed on bottom of bowl. One of several prizes offered for submitting an order of $35 to $49.99* **MP $110**

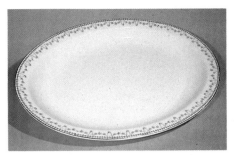

1930's *12"x16" Platter with CPC-Avon printed on bottom. One of several prizes offered for submitting an order of $35 to $49.99* **MP $70**

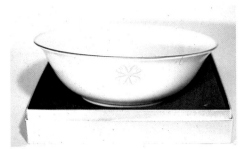

1980 *Lenox Bowl awarded to each member of the 1980 President's Club* **MP $40**

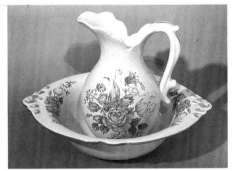

1975 *Pitcher and Bowl, an exclusive Avon Recommendation Prize* **MP $55**

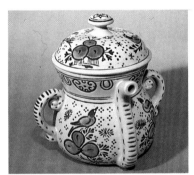

1975 *Posset Pot made in Brazil exclusively for Avon as a Recommendation Prize* **MP $40**

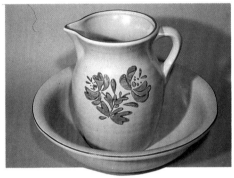

1978 *Stoneware Pitcher and Bowl by Pfaltzgraff, Recommendation Prize* **MP $40**

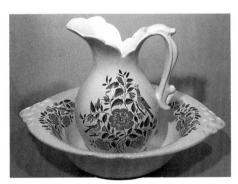

1977 *Pitcher and Bowl, an exclusive Avon Recommendation Prize* **MP $50**

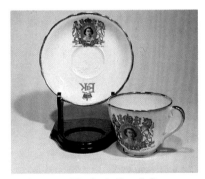

1953 *Queen Elizabeth Cup & Saucer awarded at Avon's 67th Anniversary Celebration* **MP $80**

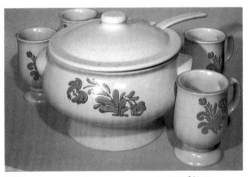

1977 *Yorktowne stoneware soup tureen 3½qt with ladle and 10" serving plate (not shown) Recommendation Prize* **MP $35 boxed**
1978 *Set of four handcrafted Coffee Mugs, Recommendation Prize* **MP $20 boxed**

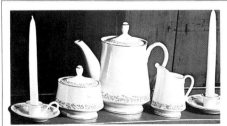

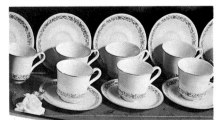

1972 *Mikasa Montclair China. Representatives Sales Achievement Prizes. Candleholders* **MP $8 each,** *Sugar & Creamer* **MP $9 each,** *Beverage Server* **MP $18**

1972 *Mikasa Montclair China. Eight cups and saucers, President's Club Members only* **MP $10 per Cup/Saucer**

Mikasa Montclair China

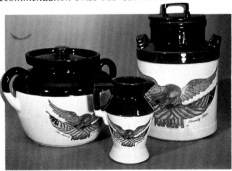

1973 *Nelson McCoy's Pottery Prizes (in Avon boxes only) Bean Pot* **MP $15,** *Pitcher* **MP $7,** *Cookie Jar* **MP $20**

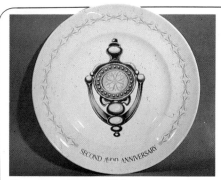

Second Anniversary, "The Avon Doorknocker" **MP $15**

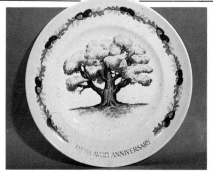

Fifth Anniversary, "The Great Oak" **MP $20**

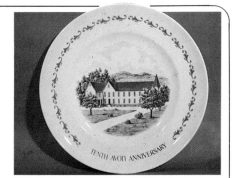

Tenth Anniversary "The California Perfume Co." **MP $30**

1973 *Anniversary Commemorative Award Plates — created to honor Representatives on their Avon Anniversaries.*

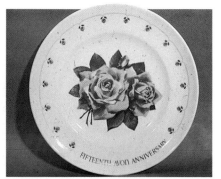

Fifteenth Anniversary, "Avon Roses" **MP $40**

Produced by Enoch Wedgwood (Tunstall) Ltd., England

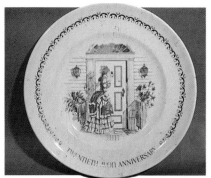

Twentieth Anniversary, "The First Avon Lady" **MP $60**

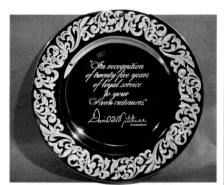

Twenty-Fifth Anniversary "A Message from Avon's President" Sterling Silver Plate accompanied by a letter suitable for framing **MP $140**

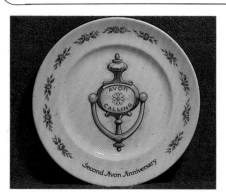

Second Anniversary "The Avon Door-knocker" **MP $7**

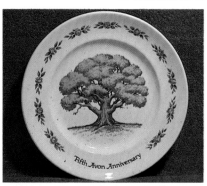

Fifth Anniversary "The Great Oak" **MP $15**

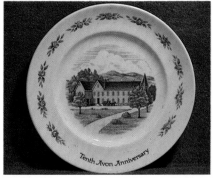

Tenth Anniversary "The California Perfume Co." **MP $22**

1981 *Anniversary Commemorative Award Plates*

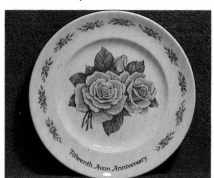

Fifteenth Anniversary "Avon Roses" **MP $30**

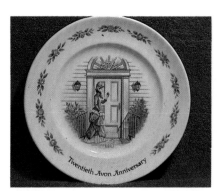

Twentieth Anniversary "The First Avon Lady" **MP $45**

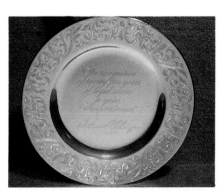

Twenty-Fifth Anniversary "A Message From Avon's President" **MP $65**

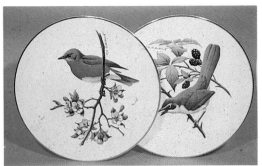

1975 *Representative's Sales Achievement Award Plates. Bluebird* **MP $22**, *Yellow Breasted Chat* **MP $30**

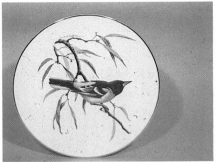

1975 *Representative's Sales Achievement Award Plate. Baltimore Oriole* **MP $37**

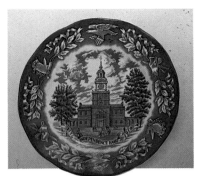

1976 *Independence Hall Plate. Representative's Sales Achievement Prize* **MP $30**

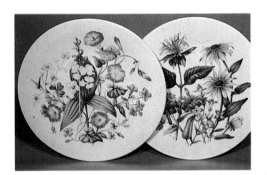

1976 *American Wildflower Plates* — *Exclusive Avon Sales Awards by Wedgwood*

Southern Wildflower Plate **MP $22**
Eastern Plate **MP $22**

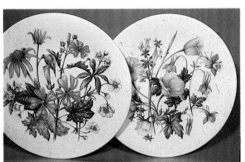

Northern Plate **MP $28**
Western Plate **MP $28**

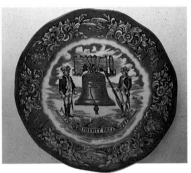

1976 *Liberty Bell Plate, Representative's Sales Achievement Prize* **MP $40**

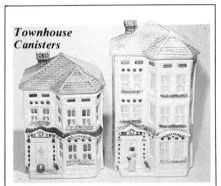

Townhouse Canisters

1983 *Townhouse Canister 3rd Level Award* **MP $35**
1983 *Townhouse Cookie Jar 4th Level Award* **MP $55**

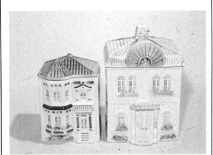

1983 *Townhouse Canister 1st Level Award* **MP $15**
1983 *Townhouse Canister 2nd Level Award* **MP $25**

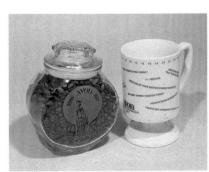

1977 *Managers Prospecting Coffee Mug & Jar of Coffee Beans* **MP $40 set**

Mugs . . .

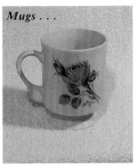

1977 *Sales Achievement Award Mug. 4th Quarter* **MP $15**

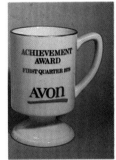

1978 *Team Achievement Award, First Quarter. Coffee Mug* **MP $15**

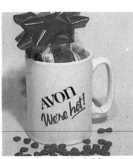

Avon "We're Hot" Mug Award. Came with Heart shaped Hot Cinammon Candies **MP $12**

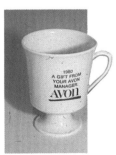

1980 *Plastic Mug Award "A Gift from your Avon Manager"* **MP $6**

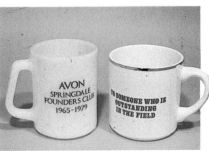

1979 *Springdale Founders Club Award Mug. Given to all employees who had worked from 1965* **MP $20**
1981 *District Managers Award Mug* **MP $17**

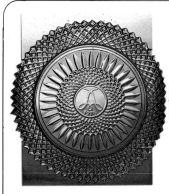

Jewelled "A" Plate **MP $15**

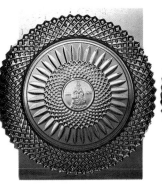

First Representative Plate **MP $15**

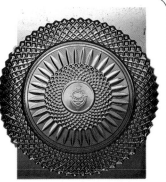

Doorknocker Plate **MP $15**

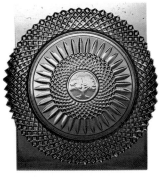

Great Oak Plate **MP $15**

ℱostoria

1978 *92nd Anniversary Fostoria Lead Crystal Plates. A different Avon symbol in the center of each plate. First 4 plates awarded for sales of $250 in C-12, 13 and 14. Last 4 to President's Club Members only for sales of $300 in each of 3 campaigns.*

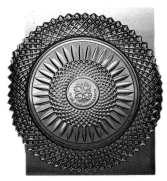

The "4-A" Plate **MP $20**

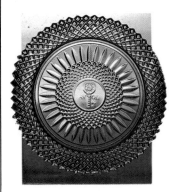

Avon Key Plate **MP $20**

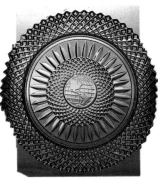

World of Avon Plate **MP $20**

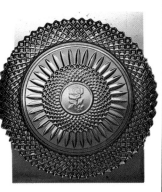

Avon Rose Plate **MP $20**

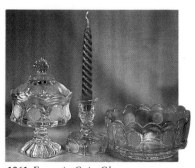

1961 *Fostoria Coin Glass Representative's Prize Award dated 1886: Wedding Bowl and Cover, 7" bowl* **MP $35 with Avon box** *Pair Candleholders* **MP $30 with Avon box** *Oval Bowl* **MP $25 with Avon box**

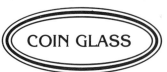

COIN GLASS

Except for the 91st Anniversary Awards, all Fostoria Coin Glass Awards have at least one coin motif inscribed "1886", Avon's founding date. Although these were exclusive Representative Awards, many pieces with the "1886" date have been seen in retail stores. The glassware must be in its original Avon gift box to be considered an Avon collectible.

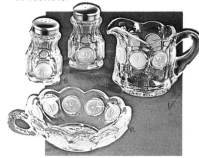

1971 *President's Campaign Fostoria Coin Glass Awards Salt & Pepper Shakers* **MP $15** *Creamer* **MP $15** *Nappy Serving Dish* **MP $15 boxed**

AVON GLASS AWARDS

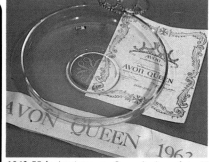

1963 *77th Anniversary Queen's Award, to 10 Reps in each District. Fostoria Serving Dish* **MP $60.** *Rhinestone Tiara, Certificate and Ribbon* **MP $60**

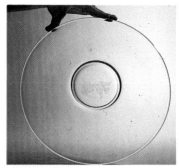

1965 *79th Anniversary Award to winning team of Representatives. Fostoria Bowl with Rapture dove motif. 12"* **MP $40**

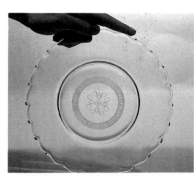

1967 *Manager's Distinguished Management Award* **MP $50**

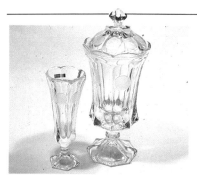

Fostoria Coin Glass Vase **MP $25**
1960's Compote Fostoria Coin Glass Award **MP $70 in Avon box**

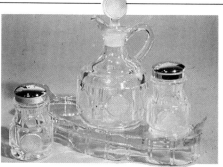

1964 *78th Anniversary Representative's Prize. Fostoria Condiment Set.*
MP $50 with Avon box

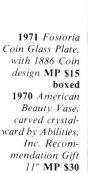
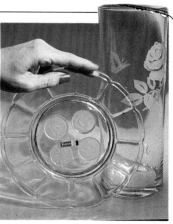

1971 *Fostoria Coin Glass Plate, with 1886 Coin design* **MP $15 boxed**
1970 *American Beauty Vase, carved crystal- ward by Abilities, Inc. Recom- mendation Gift 11"* **MP $30**

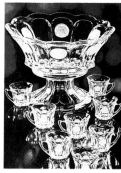

1969 *Fostoria Coin Glass Punch Set. Eight Cups and 1½ gallon capacity Bowl. Coin Motif inscribed with "1886" date (see left). A selection from "Avon in Wonderland" prize program* **MP $70 boxed**

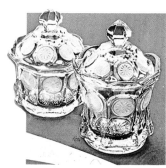

1971 *Fostoria Coin Glass Sugar Bowl with 1886 Coin design* **MP $15 boxed**
1971 *Fostoria Coin Glass Covered Candy Jar with 1886 Coin design* **MP $18 boxed**

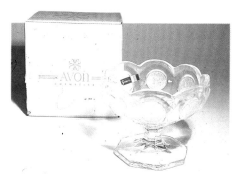

1971 *Fostoria Coin Glass Jelly Dish with 1886 Coin design* **MP $15 boxed**

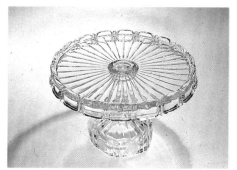

1975 *Fostoria Coin Glass Cake Salver, 1 in a choice of 3 Xmas gifts to Team Leaders* **MP $100 with card**

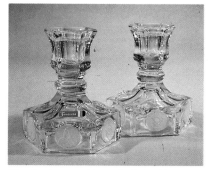

91st Anniversary Fostoria Coin Glass Awards *(Avon Symbol Motifs in coins)*
1977 *President's Club only, set of Candleholders* **MP $40**

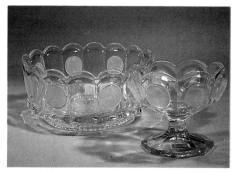

1977 *Centerpiece Bowl* **MP $30**
1977 *Footed Compote* **MP $20**

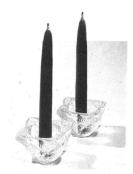

1980 *Candlestick Holders and Candles engraved "The President's Celebration 1980"* **MP $40 pair**

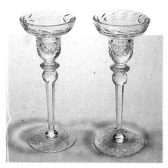

1980 *Crystal Candleholders. Representative 30 year Service Award, inscribed "30th Avon Anniversary"* **MP $125 pr**

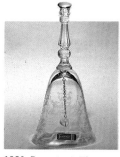

1980 *Recruit-A-Thon, Fostoria Glass Bell awarded to Team Leaders* **MP $40**

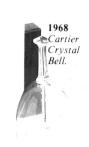

1968 *Cartier Crystal Bell.*
Awarded to 1 Rep in each District for most Recommendation appointments **MP $50, $65 boxed**

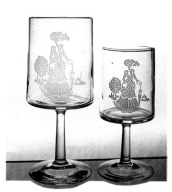

1975 *Avon Lady Stemware, set of six 6oz and six 10oz glasses awarded to winning District in each Branch* **MP $60**

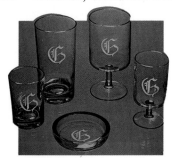

1970 *84th Anniversary Monogrammed Awards. President's Club Members won 6 5½oz and 6 11oz goblets* **MP $5 each.** *Non-PC Members won 6 6oz and 6 12oz glasses* **MP $4 each.** *Representatives who won both sets received six coaster-ash trays* **MP $3**

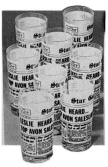

1971 *Eight 14oz Front Page Tumblers headlined with Representative's name and "Top Avon Sales Lady", Recommendation gift* **MP $25 set**

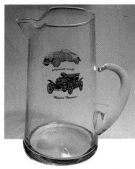

1971 *Antique Car Pitcher, with silver Duesenberg & Stanley Steamer, rare* **MP $45**

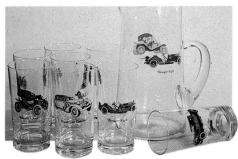

1971 *Antique Car Glasses, set of 8 for selling Avon Car Decanters* **MP $7 each**
1971 *Antique Car Pitcher, prize program and gift of recommendation* **MP $30**

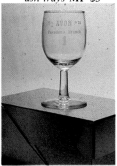

1974 *Manager's Wine Glass, etched "Avon 1974 Pasadena Branch 1"* **MP $25**

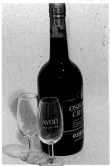

Circle of Excellence Managers —
1975 *Madrid, Spain, Gift of Osborne Cream Sherry and 2 engraved wine glasses* **MP $130 set**

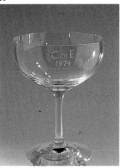

1974 *Circle of Excellence etched Champagne Glass* **MP $60**

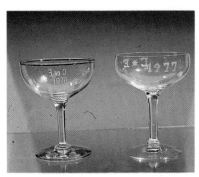

1976 *Circle of Excellence Champagne Glass* **MP $60**
1977 *Circle of Excellence Champagne Glass* **MP $60**

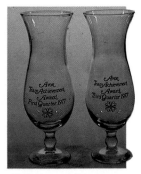

1977 *Team Achievement Awards, First and Third Quarters* **MP $22 each**

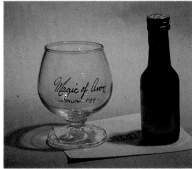

1977 August *Christmas Conference, Rye Branch Managers only — Miniature of Christian Brothers Brandy* **MP $2,** *Brandy Snifter* **MP $25,** *and Card* **MP $3** *(Card reads "The Magic of Avon has just begun, Sleep well.")*

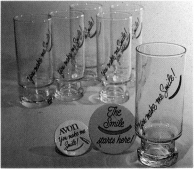

1978 *Smile Glasses, six 15oz by Anchor Hocking. Bonus Recommendation prize* **MP $20 boxed set, $3 each**
1978 *Smile Buttons* **MP $1 each**

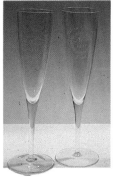

1981 *Ultra Crystal Event Award by Tiffany. Awarded by drawing at Sales Meeting for those meeting goal.* **MP $50**

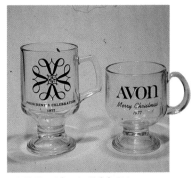

1977 *President's Celebration Award Mug* **MP $15**
1979 *Merry Christmas Award Mug* **MP $15**

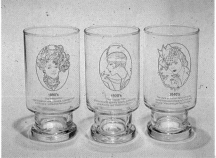

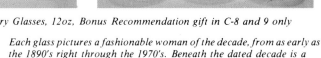

1980 *Six Avon Fashion History Glasses, 12oz, Bonus Recommendation gift in C-8 and 9 only* **MP $45 boxed set, $7 each**

Each glass pictures a fashionable woman of the decade, from as early as the 1890's right through the 1970's. Beneath the dated decade is a description of the particular era and how Avon was involved.

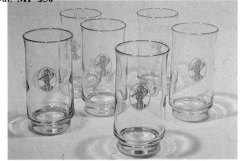

1983 *6 Avon Albee Award Glasses. Awarded to President's Club Members* **MP $32 boxed set, $5 each**

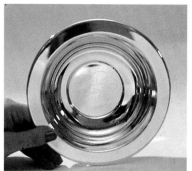

1977 Silver-plated Bowl engraved "President's Celebration 1977" awarded to Representatives in the two winning Districts from each Division **MP $29**

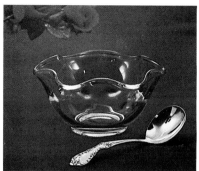

1971 Representative's Sweepstakes Prize. Glass Sauce Dish and silver-plated spoon **MP $15**

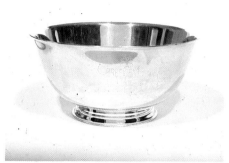

1962 Silver-plated bowl awarded to Representatives from winning Districts in President's Campaign **MP $45**

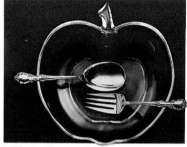

1973 Tic-Tac-Toe Prize Program Award. 10" apple shaped, clear glass bowl and silver-plated fork and spoon, Grand Elegance pattern by Wm. Rogers **MP $20**

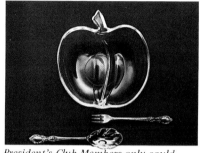

President's Club Members only could win 6" divided Apple Relish Dish with silver-plated fork and spoon by William Rogers **MP $25**

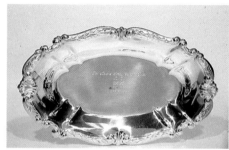

1977 Pasadena Branch silver-plated Tray engraved "Top Ariane Spray Cologne Sales 1977 Award" **MP $25**

1972 "People Who Like People" *Prize Program Awards*

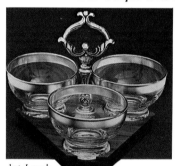

1st Level:
6oz crystal and silver bowls in walnut base **MP $15**

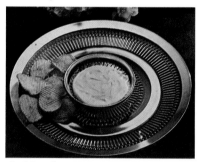

2nd Level:
Chip 'n Dip Serving Set, crystal and silver tray and bowl **MP $20**

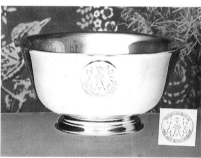

1974 88th Anniversary Award. Silver-plated Paul Revere Bowl by Oneida. Ten per District **MP $22 with plain insignia, $25 with President's Club insignia**

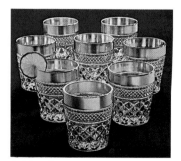

3rd Level:
Eight 10oz crystal and sterling silver faceted glasses **MP $5 each**

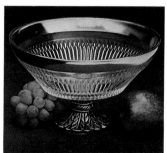

4th Level:
Footed crystal and sterling silver Fruit Bowl **MP $25**

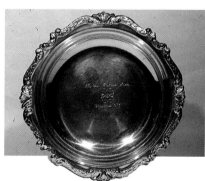

1976 Pasadena Branch Sales Award **MP $30**

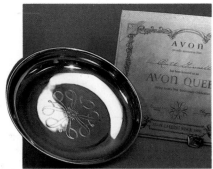

1964 *78th Anniversary Queen's Award to 10 Reps in each District. Wm. A. Rogers gold lined, silver plated bowl with Queen's Certificate, Crown Award Pin and colorful cardboard Tiara (not shown)* **MP $45 Bowl, $30 Certificate, Pin and Tiara**

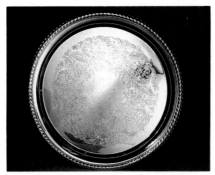

1978 *Commemorative Silver plated Tray 12" diam. engraved "President's Celebration 1978" awarded to Representatives in the two winning Districts from each Branch (3000)* **MP $40**

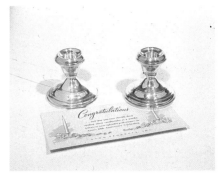

1952 *Candlestick Awards. Sterling Silver, awarded to Representatives for calling on 120 customers in the 66th Anniversary Campaign* **MP $65**

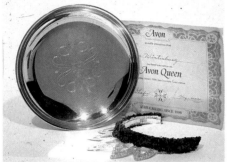

1965 *79th Anniversary Queen's Award to 10 Reps in each District. Silver plated bowl with Queen's Certificate, cardboard Tiara* **MP $40 Bowl, $30 Certificate, Pin and Tiara**

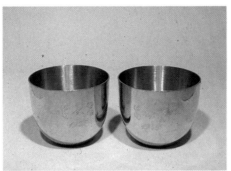

1976 *Circle of Excellence Award. Two polished Pewter Cups engraved "C of E 1976"* **MP $65**

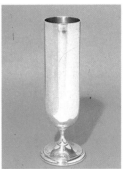

1974 *Silver Vase awarded to 250-300 Canadian and U.S. Circle of Excellence Managers* **MP $75**

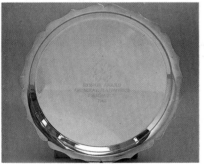

1965 *Honor Award General Manager's Campaign. Silver plated tray 9¾" diam. to Representatives in 1 winning District from each Branch* **MP $60**

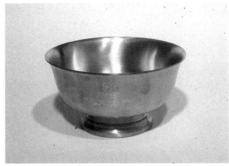

1977 *Sales Excellence Award C-23-76, C9-77. Jostens Pewter, awarded to top sales Representative* **MP $30**

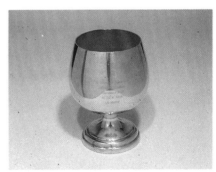

1978 *Million Dollar Increase Goblet. Managers Award for 1 million dollar sales increase* **MP $75**

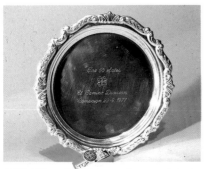

1977 *Silver plated Tray, sales award C-23-76 to C-9-77 to Top 50 in El Camino Division, Pasadena Branch* **MP $20**

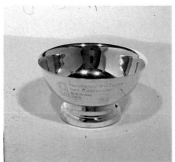

1979 *President's Day Trophy. Golf Championship Silverplate Bowl* **MP $50**

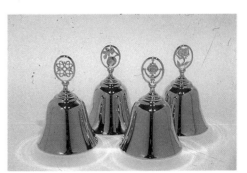

1983 *Golden Bell Award Collection. Brass Bells awarded for meeting sales goals. 1st Bell "4A"* **MP $10,** *2nd Bell "Acorn"* **MP $10,** *3rd Bell "Doorknocker"* **MP $15,** *4th Bell "Rose"* **MP $20**

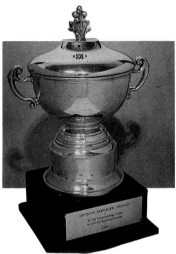

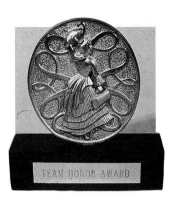

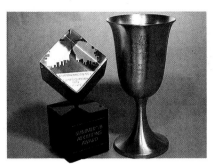

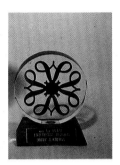

1972 *Team Honor Award to winning team in each District* **MP $35**

1978 *Additions Award for recruiting Representatives* **MP $20**
1977 *Sales Excellence Award to Representatives in the top 2% of each Division* **MP $50**

1977 *Award Trophy to top 10 Representatives in each Division for highest yearly sales* **MP $75**

1966 *Divisional Manager's Loving Cup, Pewter* **MP $160**

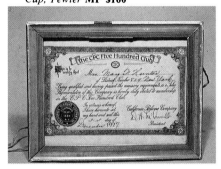

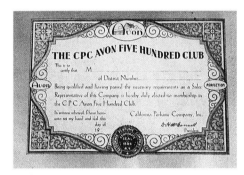

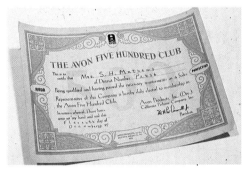

1927 *California Perfume Co. 500 Club Certificate* **MP $40**

1935 *California Perfume Co. 500 Club Certificate* **MP $30**

1937 *Avon 500 Club Certificate* **MP $20**

500 **Club Certificates** *were Awarded for $500 worth of net business*

TROPHIES and PLAQUES

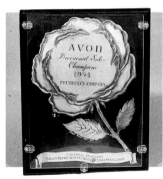

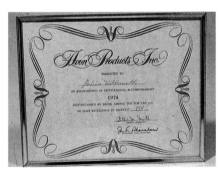

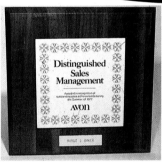

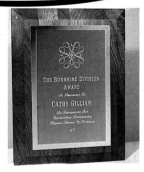

1954-56 *Divisional Sales Campaign Award to top 20 Managers* **MP $250**

1974 *Sales Achievement Certificate. Awarded to top 10 Representatives in each District* **MP $10**

1977 *Distinguished Sales Management Award Plaque* **MP $35**

1977 *Pasadena Branch Division Award for highest percent of increased sales in 1977* **MP $30**

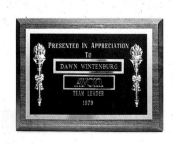

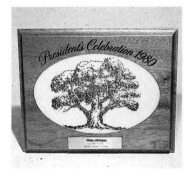

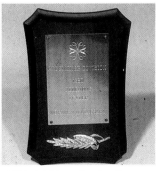

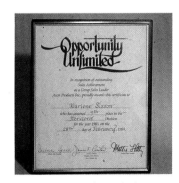

1979 *Team Leader Award Plaque* **MP $30**

1980 *President's Celebration wood and ivory plaque* **MP $25**

1980 *Additions Leader Plaque* **MP $20**

Opportunity Unlimited Plaque. Group Sales Leader Award **MP $20**

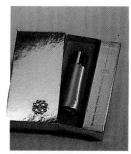

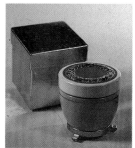

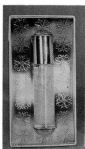

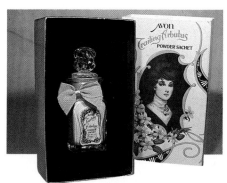

1960 *Representative's Xmas Gift, Deluxe Lipstick* **MP $15 boxed**

1961 *Christmas Gift. Specially designed Cream Sachet Decanter for Representatives. Somewhere 1½oz* **MP $15, $20 boxed**

1962 *Perfume Creme Rollette, Xmas Gift to Representatives* **MP $15 boxed as shown**

1975 *Representative's Christmas Gift. 1oz Trailing Arbutus Powder Sachet* **MP $15 boxed**

REPRESENTATIVE CHRISTMAS GIFTS

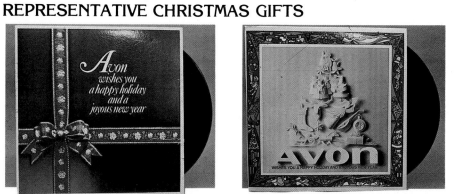

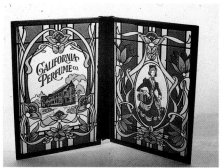

1970 *Christmas Gift. Nelson Riddle Xmas music recorded for Avon* **MP $15**

1969 *Christmas Gift. Longine's Xmas music recorded for Avon* **MP $15**

1976 *Representative's Christmas Gift* **MP $20**

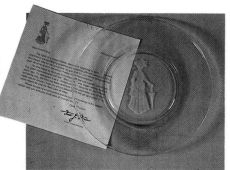

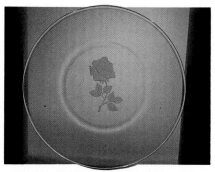

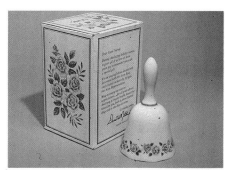

1971 *Representative's Christmas gift. Fostoria Plate 8" diam. "limited edition".* **MP $30 boxed with letter**

1972 *Representative's Christmas gift. Fostoria Plate 8" diam. "limited edition".* **MP $25 boxed with letter**

1973 *Christmas Gift. Mikasa China Bell (only to Representatives with Avon for less than two years)* **MP $20**

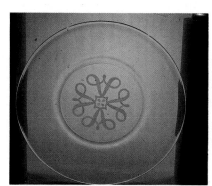

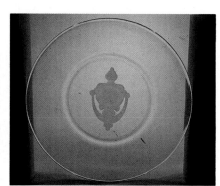

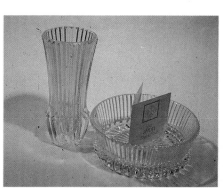

1973 *Representative's Christmas gift. Fostoria Plate 8" diam. "limited edition".* **MP $20 boxed with letter**

1974 *Representative's Christmas gift. Fostoria Plate 8" diam. "limited edition".* **MP $20 boxed with letter**

Representative's Xmas Gifts by Fostoria, inscribed with date and "4-A" symbol
1977 *Cut-crystal Bud Vase* **MP $18, $25 boxed**
1978 *Lead Crystal Candy Dish* **MP $18, $25 boxed**

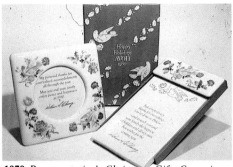

1979 *Representative's Christmas Gift. Ceramic Picture Frame 5" square with message from William Chaney* **MP $15**
1980 *Representative's Christmas Gift. Matching Note Paper Holder with note from Mr. Chaney* **MP $12**

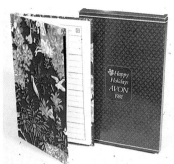

1981 *Representatives Christmas Gift. Tapestry Book* **MP $10**

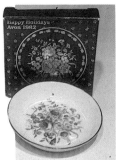

1982 *Representative Christmas Gift* **MP $10**

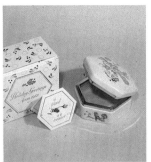

1983 *Presidents Club Christmas Gift. Porcelain, hinged Trinket Box* **MP $20**

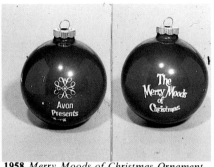

1958 *Merry Moods of Christmas Ornament, given to Managers at Christmas Conference* **MP $50 each**

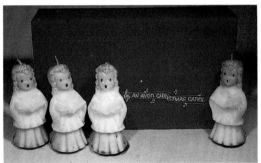

1959 *"An Avon Christmas Carol" awarded to Managers at Christmas* **MP $130**

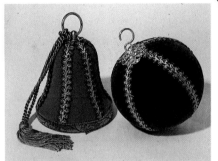

1974 *Christmas Ornament Music Boxes. Representative Recommendation Prizes* **MP $35 each, $75 set**

CHRISTMAS GIFT ORNAMENTS

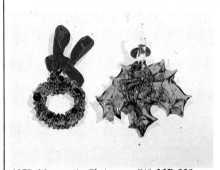

1979 *Manager's Christmas Gift* **MP $30**

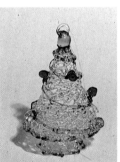

1977 *Manager's Christmas Ornament, first in a series* **MP $30**

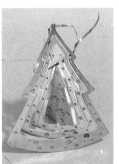

1978 *Manager's Christmas Ornament, hand-crafted by renowned metal sculptor, Bijan* **MP $30**

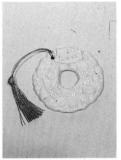

1980 *Manager's Ceramic Wreath Xmas Ornament. Personalized with gold initials* **MP $30**

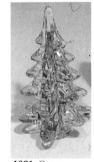

1981 *Great American Sell-A-Thon Christmas Tree Award* **MP $40**

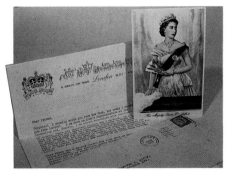

1953 *67th Anniversary Celebration letter from Irene Nunemaker, Editor of the Avon Outlook, to Representatives. Envelope postmarked 5/22/53, London, England* **MP $65**

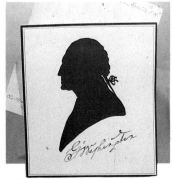

1976 *Recommendation Gift. George Washington's acceptance letter of Office of President, April 14, 1789. Reproduced especially for Avon Representatives by permission of the Lilly Library, Indiana University* **MP $8**

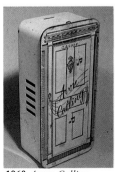

1960 *Avon Calling "Ding Dong" Doorbell used by Managers at Sales Meetings* **MP $100**

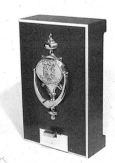

1979 *Manager's Doorknocker/Doorbell Award for reaching appointment goal during 3rd quarter. Full-size brass doorknocker and "Ding-Dong" door chime* **MP $100**

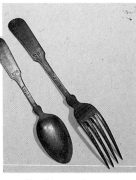

. . . Whether received as an Anniversary gift, a Recommendation prize or an Achievement Award, Silver Flatware has been a long-time favorite with both Representatives and Avon collectors.

1920-30 *CPC Silverware. Used in employee eating areas at CPC factories* **MP $10 each**

TABLEWARE and CUTLERY

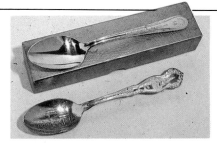

1936 *CPC Souvenir Spoon, stamped "50th Anniversary of Mr. and Mrs. D.H. McConnell". Gold wash Argyle silver plate* **MP $75, in Hammer tone box MP $110**
1915 *CPC Panama Pacific Exposition Spoon awarded to Representatives selling 12 cans of Bath Powder during May and June. Not sold or given away at the Exposition. (Reference: April 1915 Outlook)* **MP $125**

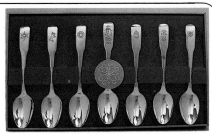

1969 *83rd Anniversary silver-plated demitasse spoons, fragrance symbol on handles. Center spoon only to reps in winning District each Branch* **MP $75 boxed set, $7 each, $20 center spoon**

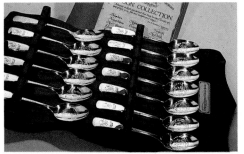

1976 *Recommendation Gift Award for 2 appointments. Bicentennial original 13 Colonies Commemorative Spoons* **MP $35 set**

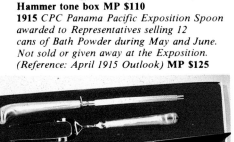

1972 *Six Steak Knives in Avon Award Box* **MP $20** *President's Club also received Oneida Carving Set in Award box* **MP $20**

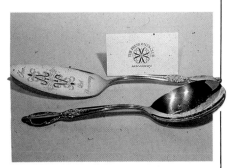

1978 *92nd Anniversary Cake Server. Silver, awarded to all President Club members* **MP $20, $25 boxed with card**
1979 *93rd Anniversary Serving Spoon, silver, awarded to all President Club members* **MP $15, $20 boxed with card**

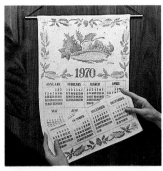

1970 *Representative's Gift for sending in a C-1-70 order. 15½x 28½" linen wall calendar* **MP $8**

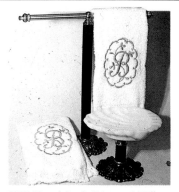

1972 *Towel Rack Prize and Milk Glass Soap Dish, an exclusive Avon prize. Rack* **MP $10,** *Soap Dish* **MP $15,** *Towels* **MP $7**

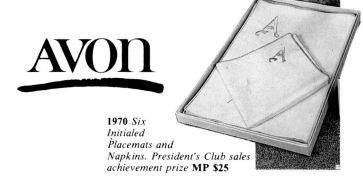

1970 *Six Initialed Placemats and Napkins. President's Club sales achievement prize* **MP $25**

1980 *Grandma Wheaton's Blue Ribbon Gift Sets with Gift Card from National Sales Manager of each Avon Branch. District Manager prizes for reaching appointment goals in "Beat the Clock Program".*

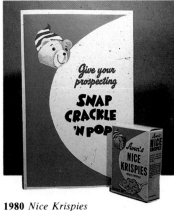

1980 *Nice Krispies Box, served as gift box for Team Leader cash award* **MP $6**

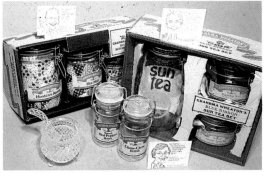

Kitchen Canister Set, *3 glass canisters hold Apron, Hot Mitt & Towel* **MP $25 with card**
Relish Set, *2 jars relish, glass Kettle and Spoon* **MP $15 with card**
Sun Tea Set, *2 glass canisters hold loose Tea and Tea Bags* **MP $20**

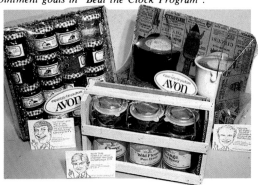

Jams and Jellies, *set of 12 small jars* **MP $15**
Cheese Kettle Set, *2 handled kettles of cheese & cheese spreader* **MP $15**
Honey Set, *3 jars Clover, Wild Flower and Orange flavored honey* **MP $20 with card**

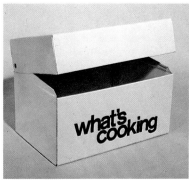

1974 *What's Cooking Recipe Box,* metal **MP $8**

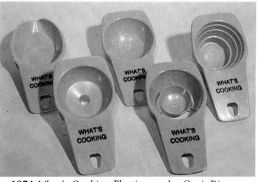

1974 *What's Cooking Plasticware by Geni, Div. of Avon. Scoop, strainer, measurer, funnel and egg separator, gifts to Representatives for Sales Meeting Attendance* **MP $3 each**

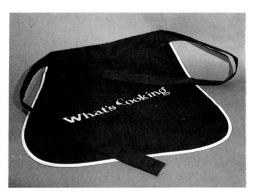

1974 *"What's Cooking Apron, Recommendation Prize* **MP $15**

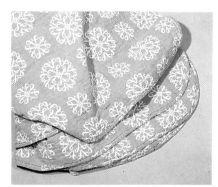

1969 *"4-A" Quilt by Barclay, tape-bound edges, in gold, avocado or pink, Recommendation prize* **MP $50**

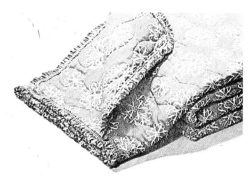

1971 *"4-A" Quilt by Barclay, reversible, ruffle-edged comforter 76 x 86" in gold, avocado or blue. Recommendation prize* **MP $50**

(back) *(front)*

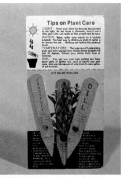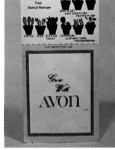

1974-75 *Grow with Avon Plant Spikes with herb, flower or vegetable seed, ready to plant. To Representatives attending Sales Meetings* **MP $5**

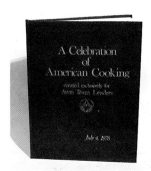

1978 *Cookbook, created exclusively for Team Leaders, dated July 4, 1978* **MP $20**

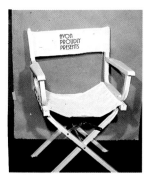

1981 *Director's Chair, "Avon Proudly Presents" used at Conference and then sent to Managers* **MP $35**

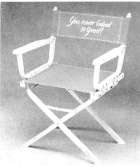

1980 *Director's Chair, "You Never Looked So Good" by Domestic Industries with 2 slip-on backs, one plain* **MP $35**

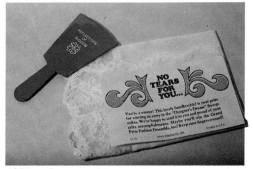

1975 *Reflections of Success. Purse Mirror awarded to Representatives of Enterprise Division, Pasadena Branch, approx. 3500* **MP $13**
1971 *No More Tears for You, Representatives Sweepstakes Gift Handkerchief* **MP $8 with card**

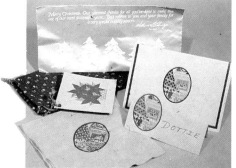

1980 *Manager's Xmas Card and Calico drawstring bag held Xmas bonus check, Xmas Conference Invitation, Place Card and Napkin* **MP $7**

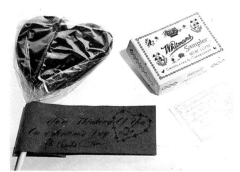

1981 *Manager's Valentine Heart-shaped Sucker* **MP $10 with card**
1976 *Representative's Valentine gift, Whitman's Sampler Candy* **MP $12**

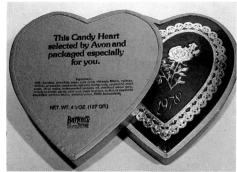

1978 *President's Club Members luncheon gift. Heart-shaped box of Barton's Candy 4½oz* **MP $5 box only** *(candy can be replaced)*

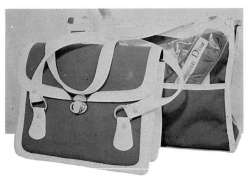

1974 *Representative's Prizes: President's Club Kadin Handbag* **MP $20**
Exclusive Christian Dior Scarf **MP $10**
Tote Bag **MP $15**

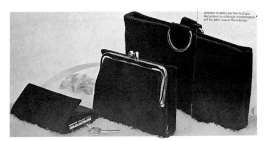

1973 *Representative's Prizes of suede by St. Thomas.*
1st level: Key Case **MP $10**
2nd level: French Purse **MP $15**
3rd level: Clutch Bag **MP $20**

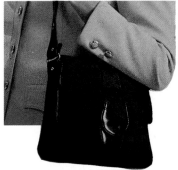

1973 *President's Club Members 4th level prize. Suede Shoulder Handbag by Kadin* **MP $30**

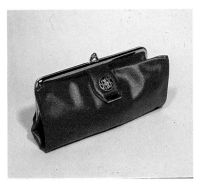

1967 *Representative's Pursette Award for sales achievement* **MP $20**

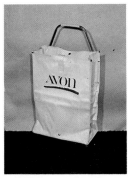

1980 *Sales-Aid-on-Wheels to carry orders and demos. C-16 Sales Meeting prize* **MP $25**

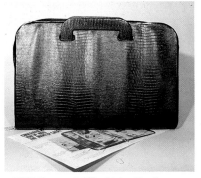

1976 *Sunny Griffin Make-Up Case. Representative's Sales Prize* **MP $15 with certificate**

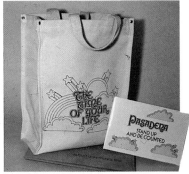

1978 ***Pasadena Manager's Conference Gifts —***
Tote Bag **MP $20**, *Portfolio* **MP $18**, *Invitation* **MP $3**

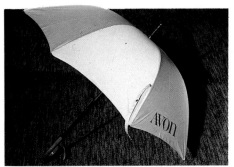

1976 *Avon Umbrella. Recommendation Prize* **MP $30**

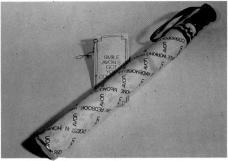

1977 *Manager's Advertising Media Umbrella. Imprinted with names of TV shows and magazines that carry the Avon commercials and ads* **MP $30**

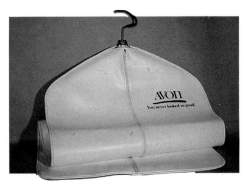

1977 *Circle of Excellence Manager gift. Leather-like Garment Bag to use on New York-Bermuda trip* **MP $60**

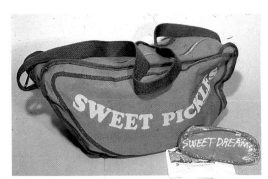

1978 ***Manager's Conference Gifts —***
Sweet Pickles Tote Bag **MP $15**
Sweet Pickles Cooky **MP $5**
Sweet Pickles Napkin (not shown) **MP $1**

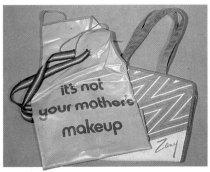

1978 *Manager's "It's Not Your Mother's Makeup" Apron* **MP $8**
1979 *Zany Tote Bag. With pre-order of 10 Zany Cologne Sprays at Sales Meetings* **MP $6**
"I've Gone Zany" buttons (not shown) **MP 75¢ each**

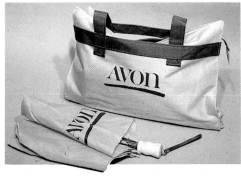

1980 *Avon Bag 'n Brella, President's Club Members incentive prize* **MP $40**

— CIRCLE OF EXCELLENCE —

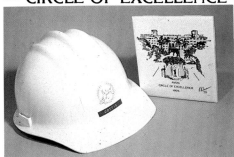

1979 *Manager's Circle of Excellence* contender gift, Pasadena Branch. Hard Hat, plastic **MP $10**
1975 *Manager's Circle of Excellence Trivet* **MP $25**

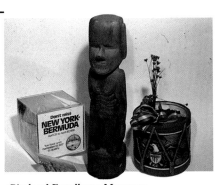

Circle of Excellence Managers —
1977 *New York-Bermuda, Plastic Photo Cube* **MP $10**
1976 *Hawaii, Wood Tiki God* **MP $35**
1975 *Florida, Ceramic Planter* **MP $40**

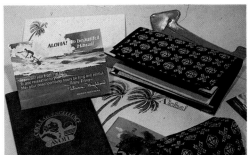

Circle of Excellence Manager's Awards, Hawaii—
1976 *Stationery and Imprinted Notebook* **MP $15**
1976 *Pocket Organizer and Matching Key Case* **MP $40** set with card signed by Pat Neighbors

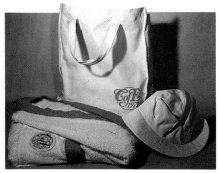

Manager's Circle of Excellence Awards —
with C of E monogram
1977 *New York-Bermuda. Robe* **MP $45,**
Tote Bag **MP $15,** *Hat* **MP $15**

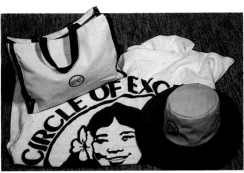

Circle of Excellence Manager Awards, Hawaii —
1976 *Beach Towel* **MP $20**
1976 *Tote Bag* **MP $15**
1976 *Hat* **MP $15**

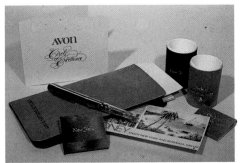

1977 *Manager's Circle of Excellence Memorabilia, Honor Banquet in New York City. Invitation and Matchbooks* **MP $3** each, *Match Holders* **MP $4** each, *Notebook and Pen with penlight* **MP $13** set

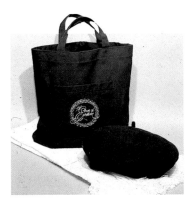

Circle of Excellence Manager Gifts, Paris —
1979 *Tote Bag* **MP $15**
1979 *French Cap* **MP $10**
1979 *Shawl* **MP $15**

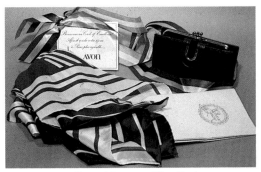

Circle of Excellence Manager Gifts, Paris —
1979 *Banner* **MP $8**
1979 *Scarf* **MP $12**
1979 *French Purse* **MP $20**
1979 *Menu* **MP $3**

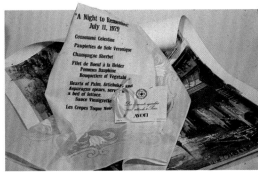

Circle of Excellence Manager Gifts, Paris —
1979 *Napkin Menu* **MP $20**
1979 *French Print Poster* **MP $12** with card

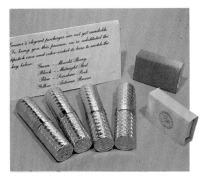

Circle of Excellence contender gifts, Paris —
1979 *Envira Lipstick, 4 shades* **MP $6 each**
1979 *Matchbox* **MP $3 each**

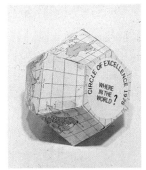

1978 *Circle of Excellence* Cardboard, "Where in the World?" **MP $5**

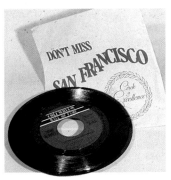

Circle of Excellence —
Don't Miss San Francisco Record **MP $7**

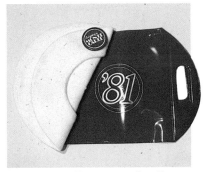

Circle of Excellence contender gifts, Monte Carlo —
1981 *French Beret with Monte Carlo button* **MP $15**
1981 *Handled vinyl organizer* **MP $5**

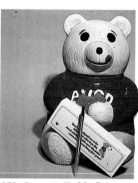

1978 *Team Leader's Teddy Bear Mascot, Xmas gift* **MP $30**
1978 *Team Leader's Shopping Bag* **MP $2**

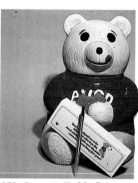

1979 *Ceramic Teddy Bear Cookie Jar, Team Leader Gift* **MP $35**
1980 *Chrome Pen by Cross with "Teddy Bear" clip, Team Leader gift* **MP $25**

TEDDY BEAR

In 1978 the lovable Teddy Bear was chosen as mascot for Avon's Team Leaders. The Teddy Bear proved to be a gift delight for Representatives and pure joy for collectors.

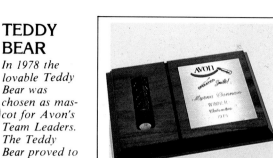

1978 *Operation Smile Plaque with Lipstick* **MP $15**

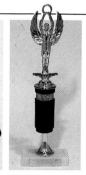

1978 *Operation Smile Trophy. Awarded to Managers* **MP $20**

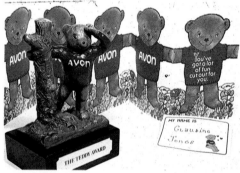

1979 *Teddy Bear Cut-Out Table Decoration. Team Leader Appreciation Day* **MP $2**
1980 *Teddy Award to 1 Team Leader per District for recommendation support* **MP $75**

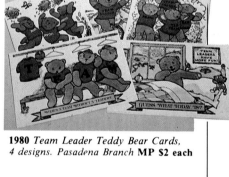

1980 *Team Leader Teddy Bear Cards, 4 designs. Pasadena Branch* **MP $2 each**

OPERATION SMILE

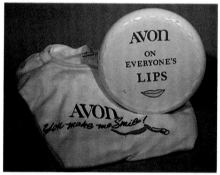

1978 *Smile T-Shirt* **MP $10** *and Frisbee (Not all Branches)* **MP $4**

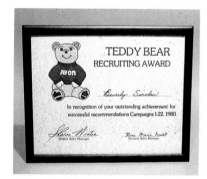

1980 *Teddy Bear Recruiting Award Plaque* **MP $15**

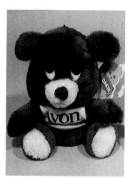

1980 *Bean Bag Teddy Bear. Awarded at President's Club Luncheon* **MP $25**

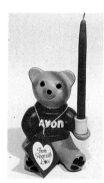

1980 *Team Leader Award. Teddy Bear Candle Holder* **MP $30**

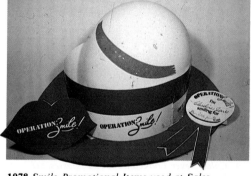

1978 *Smile Promotional Items used at Sales Meetings. Cardboard Hat* **MP $1**, *Lips* **MP 50¢**, *Balloon* **MP 50¢**, *Name Badge* **MP 50¢**

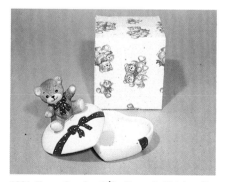

1981 *Team Leader Gift. Ceramic Trinket Box* **MP $20**

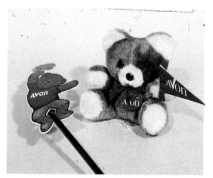

1981 *Team Leader Decoration* **MP $4**
1982 *Stuffed Teddy Bear Award for Brand Switch Sales* **MP $15**

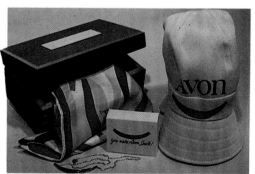

1978 *Smile Music Box awarded to team winners of the Lipstick competition* **MP $40**
1978 *Smile Scarf, only to Representatives attending C-11 Sales Meeting* **MP $7**
1978 *Team Leader Smile Necklace* **MP $15**
1978 *Manager's white duck hat* **MP $15**

GREAT AMERICAN SELL-A-THON

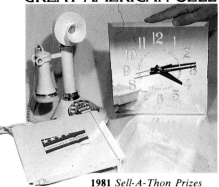

1981 *Sell-A-Thon Prizes*
Telephone **MP $100**
Warming Tray **MP $25**
Clock **MP $50**

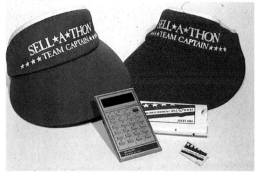

1981 *Team Leader Caps* **MP $3 ea.**
1981 *Calculator* **MP $20**
1981 *Pin Awarded to Representatives on Winning Team* **MP $2**

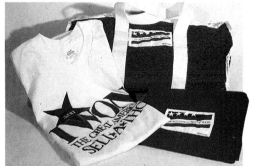

1981 *T-Shirt* **MP $5**
1981 *Tote Bag* **MP $15**
1981 *Poncho* **MP $10**

S.M. KENT designed Awards

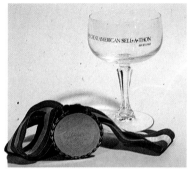

1981 *President's Celebration Outstanding Sales Achievement Medallion* **MP $150**
1981 *Sell-A-Thon Champagne Glass* **MP $20**

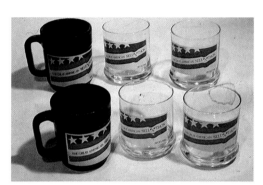

1981 *Coffee Mugs* **MP $15 set of 2**
1981 *Glasses, set of 4* **MP $15**

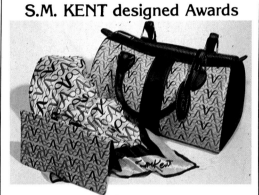

Order Book Cover **MP $5**
Scarf **MP $8**
Cosmetics Case **MP $15**

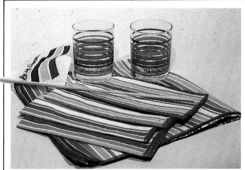

1979 *"Color Never Looked So Good" glasses, set of 6. Prize at C-11 Sales Meeting* **MP $24 set**
1979 *Tablecloth used in Manager's kick-off "Color Up America" Luncheon* **MP $20**
1979 *Luncheon Napkin, Manager's* **MP $5 each**
1979 *Banner* **MP $4**

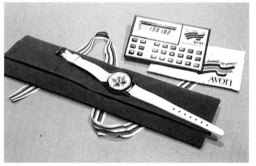

1979 *Calculator, auction prize at C-11 Sales Meeting* **MP $30**
1979 *Watch, 15 per District for customer service* **MP $50**

COLOR-UP

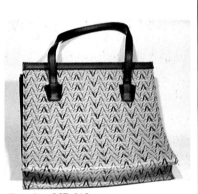

Tote Bag **MP $15**

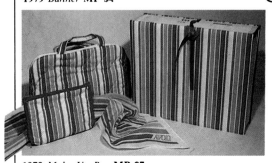

1979 *Make-Up Bag* **MP $7**
Clutch Purse **MP $4**
Scarf **MP $3**
Manager's File Organizer **MP $6**

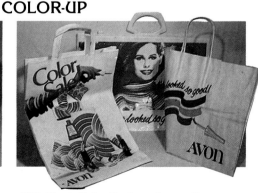

1979 *Plastic Color Up Bags given to Reps attending sales meeting* **MP $2**
1979 *Delivery Bags* **MP $1**

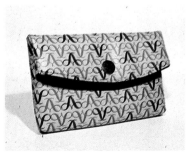

Clutch Purse **MP $15**

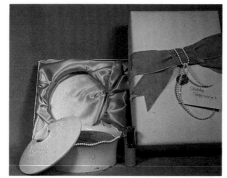

1958 *Here's My Heart Beauty Dust, Lotion Sachet and Top Style Lipstick* **MP $75** *(Spray Perfume shown, not in set)*

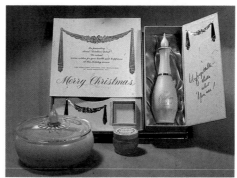

1961 *Cotillion Beauty Dust 6oz, Cream Sachet .66oz and Cologne Mist 3oz* **MP $65**

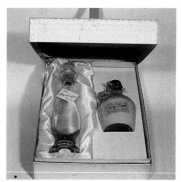

1962 *Skin-So-Soft Bud Vase and Bay Rum Jug* **MP $65**

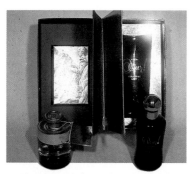

1963 *Occur! Cologne Mist 3oz and Tribute Cologne 4oz. One bottle each side* **MP $60**

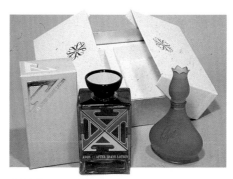

1964 *Rapture Cologne 2oz and 4-A After Shave Lotion 6oz* **MP $60**

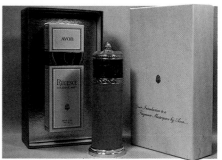

1966 *Regence Cologne Mist 3oz* **MP $50**

STOCKHOLDER'S GIFTS

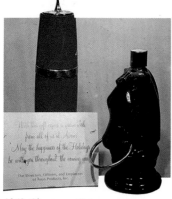

1968 *Charisma Cologne Mist 3oz and Pony Post Decanter 4oz Windjammer* **MP $45**

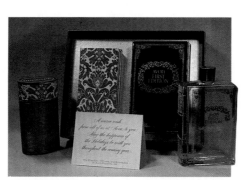

1967 *First Edition Wild Country Cologne 6oz and Brocade Cologne 4oz* **MP $50**

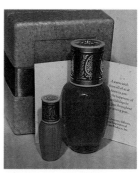

1969 *Elusive Cologne Mist 3oz and Rollette .33oz* **MP $40 with card**

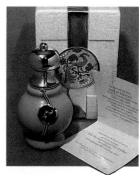

1970 *Bird of Paradise Cologne Mist 3oz with card* **MP $40**

STOCKHOLDER'S GIFTS

Stockholders Gifts not shown—
1957 *Persian Wood Perfume Mist and Persian Wood Beauty Dust* **MP $80**
1959 *Topaze Spray Perfume, Topaze Cologne Mist and After Shower Lotion for Men* **MP $75**
1960 *Topaze Treasure Set. Beauty Dust, 3oz Cologne Mist, Cream Sachet and 8oz Spice After Shave Lotion* **MP $80**
1965 *Just Two Set. 3oz Rapture Cologne and 3oz Tribute After Shave Lotion* **MP $100**

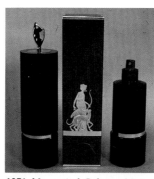

1971 *Moonwind Cologne Mist 3oz* **MP $35**

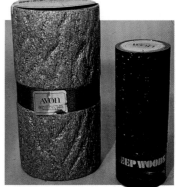

1972 *Deep Woods Cologne 5oz* **MP $35**

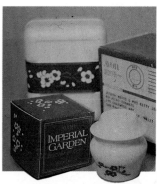

1973 *Imperial Garden Cream Sachet .66oz* **MP $30**

Specially designed Stockholder's Gifts were sent as Christmas Gifts from 1957 through 1973.

I N D E X

All Avon items of a *particular fragrance or product line*, with the same in-line design packaging, are found under the proper name unique to the line. For example, each Cotillion item or set is not individually listed, but can be found under the name *COTILLION* in the Index. Use the same method for the other specific fragrance or product lines, such as *TEMPO, BRONZE GLORY, HI-LIGHT, DELICATE BEAUTY, FASHION MAKEUP* and others.

Sub-group listings are found under *AWARDS, JEWELRY* and *PERFECTION*.

Where *many fragrances share* the same bottle and packaging design, they may be found under a common title, such as *PERFUMES, TALCUM, COLOGNE MINIATURES* and other categories.